Oxford American Handbook of
Pediatrics

Published and forthcoming Oxford American Handbooks

Oxford American Handbook of Clinical Medicine
Oxford American Handbook of Anesthesiology
Oxford American Handbook of Clinical Dentistry
Oxford American Handbook of Critical Care
Oxford American Handbook of Emergency Medicine
Oxford American Handbook of Nephrology and Hypertension
Oxford American Handbook of Obstetrics and Gynecology
Oxford American Handbook of Oncology
Oxford American Handbook of Otolaryngology
Oxford American Handbook of Pediatrics
Oxford American Handbook of Psychiatry
Oxford American Handbook of Pulmonary Medicine
Oxford American Handbook of Rheumatology
Oxford American Handbook of Surgery

Oxford American Handbook of **Pediatrics**

Edited by

F. Bruder Stapleton, MD
Professor and Chair
Ford/Morgan Endowed Chair
Department of Pediatrics
University of Washington School of Medicine

and

Chief Academic Officer
Seattle Children's Hospital

With the assistance of the
University of Washington faculty at
Seattle Children's Hospital

with

Robert C. Tasker

Robert J. McClure

Carlo L. Acerini

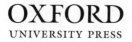

OXFORD
UNIVERSITY PRESS

Oxford University Press, Inc., publishes works that further
Oxford University's objective of excellence
in research, scholarship, and education.

Oxford New York
Auckland Cape Town Dar es Salaam Hong Kong Karachi
Kuala Lumpur Madrid Melbourne Mexico City Nairobi
New Delhi Shanghai Taipei Toronto

With offices in
Argentina Austria Brazil Chile Czech Republic France Greece
Guatemala Hungary Italy Japan Poland Portugal Singapore
South Korea Switzerland Thailand Turkey Ukraine Vietnam

Library of Congress Cataloging-in-Publication Data

Oxford American handbook of pediatrics/edited by F. Bruder Stapleton; with the
assistance of the University of Washington faculty at Seattle Children's Hospital;
with Robert C. Tasker, Robert J. McClure, Carlo L. Acerini.
p. ; cm.
Adapted from: Oxford Handbook of Paediatrics/Robert C. Tasker,
Robert J. McClure, and Carlo L. Acerini. 2008.

Includes bibliographical references and index.
ISBN 978-0-19-532904-9 (flexicover : alk. paper)
1. Pediatrics—Handbooks, manuals, etc. I. Stapleton, F. Bruder, 1946-
II. Title: Handbook of pediatrics.
[DNLM: 1. Pediatrics—Handbooks. WS 39 O98 2009]
RJ48.O94 2009
618.92—dc22   2008030814

9 8 7 6 5 4 3 2 1

Printed in China
on acid-free paper

Preface

Plunging into a career in pediatrics is both exhilarating and daunting. New medical knowledge, genetic breakthroughs, and clinical evaluation tools are growing at a dazzling pace. Our handbook is intended for residents, fellows, and students as a concise, convenient, portable pediatric reference that provides clinically useful information and professional advice for any clinical setting. It also will be an excellent tool for reviewing the most pertinent data for pediatric cognitive examinations. Our text includes some valuable Web-based references for specific tools, guidelines, and databases to allow ready access for these more detailed resources.

Possession of knowledge alone, of course, does not create a complete pediatrician. Our handbook also addresses key ethical, communication, and public health issues as a complement to the clinical science. The aphorism, "No one cares how much you know, until they know how much you care," has particular relevance for all who care for children and their families. The practice of pediatrics requires a gentle, healing heart in order to apply most effectively the information contained in our handbook.

You are now traveling on a demanding medical journey in the land of pediatrics, which will present extraordinary and unexpected rewards. We hope that our handbook becomes a valuable map to aid you in your travels.

F. Bruder Stapleton, MD

Acknowledgments

The editors gratefully acknowledge the expert editorial contributions of the following faculty members at the University of Washington:

Heath Ackley
Kym Ahrens
Maneesh Batra
Thomas J. Benedetti
Henry Berman
Julia M. Bledsoe
Cora C. Breuner
Dena Brownstein
Jane Burns
Edward Carter
Shilpi Chabra
Dennis Christie
Helen Emery
Janet A. Englund
Brianna Enriquez
Patricia Y. Fechner
Kenneth Feldman
Joseph Flynn
Debra Friedman
Ron L. Gibson
Ann Giesel
Ian Glass
Christine A. Gleason
Michael Goldberg
Sidney M. Gospe, Jr.
Sihoun Hahn
Nicole Hamblett
Douglas Hawkins
W. Alan Hodson
Robin Hornung
Simon Horslen
J. Craig Jackson
Brian D. Johnston
Sandra E. Juul
Ron L. Kaplan
Maureen Kelley
Yemiserach Kifle

Eileen Klein
Isabella Knox
Mary Len
James Lymp
Marcella Mascher Denen
Dana Matthews
Dennis E. Mayock
Suzan Mazor
Ann Melvin
John Lawrence Merritt, II
Soheil Meshinchi
Erica Michiels
Russell Migita
Yosuke Miyashita
Megan Moreno
Karen Murray
Michael D. Neufeld
Annie Nguyen Vermillion
Audrey Odom
Melissa Parisi
Julie R. Park
Janna Patterson
Catherine Pihoker
Linda Quan
Gregory Redding
Jennifer R. Reid
Stephanie Richling
Joan Roberts
Robert Sawin
Jessica Slusarski
Charles V. Smith
Thomas P. Strandjord
Amanda Striegl
David Suskind
Jordan Symons
James A. Taylor
Blythe Thomson

Troy Torgerson
Kevin Urdahl
Christopher Varley
Margaret M. Vernon
Ghassan Wahbeh
Leslie R. Walker
William O. Walker, Jr.

Theresa Walls
Benjamin Wilfond
David E. Woodrum
George A. Woodward
Paige Wright
Joan C. Zerzan
Samuel H. Zinner

We also thank Brooke A. Freed for providing invaluable editorial oversight for this project.

Contents

Detailed contents

9 Respiratory issues 291

Symbols and abbreviations

?	controversial topic
↑	increased
↓	decreased
↔	normal
→	leading to
2°	secondary
♂	male
♀	female
AAP	American Academy of Pediatrics
ABC	airway, breathing, circulation
ABCD	airway, breathing, circulation, disability
ABPA	allergic bronchopulmonary aspergillosis
ABR	auditory brainstem response
ACE	angiotensin-converting enzyme
ACh	acetylcholine
ACL	anterior cruciate ligament
ACR	American College of Rheumatology
ACTH	adrenocorticotrophin
AD	autosomal dominant
ADH	antidiuretic hormone
ADHD	attention deficit hyperactivity disorder
ADP	adenosine 5-diphosphate
ADPKD	autosomal dominant polycystic kidney disease
ADR	adverse drug reaction
AFP	α-fetoprotein
AG	anion gap
AHA	American Heart Association
AIS	androgen insensitivity syndrome
ALD	adrenoleukodystrophy
ALL	acute lymphoblastic leukemia
ALP	alkaline phosphatase
ALS	advanced life support
ALT	alanine transferase

AML	acute myeloid leukemia
AN	anorexia nervosa
ANA	anti-nuclear antigen
ANCA	anti-neutrophil cytoplasmic antibodies
ANLL	acute non-lymphoblastic leukemia
AOM	acute otitis media
AP	anteroposterior
APC	activated protein C
APD	automated peritoneal dialysis
APH	antepartum hemorrhage
APTT	activated partial thromboplastin time
AR	autosomal recessive
ARA	American Rheumatism Association
ARDS	acute respiratory distress syndrome
ARF	acute renal failure
ARM	artificial rupture of membranes
ARR	absolute risk reduction
AS	Angelman syndrome
ASA	5-aminosalicylic acid
ASD	atrial septal defect
ASIS	anterior superior iliac spine
ASO	anti-streptolysin
AT	ataxia–telangiectasia
ATN	acute tubular necrosis
ATP	adenosine triphosphate
AV	arteriovenous or atrioventricular
AVP	arginine vasopressin
AZA	azathioprine
BA	bone age
BAL	bronchoalveolar lavage
BCG	bacille Calmette–Guérin
bid	twice a day
BIH	benign intracranial hypertension
BLS	basic life support
BMD	Becker muscular dystrophy
BMI	body mass index
BMT	bone marrow transplantation
BO	bronchiolitis obliterans

BP	blood pressure
BPD	bronchopulmonary dysplasia
BSA	body surface area
BSS	Bernard–Soulier syndrome
BUN	blood urea nitrogen
BVM	bag-valve mask
BWS	Beckwith–Wiedemann syndrome
BXO	balanitis xerotica obliterans
CACT	carnitine–acylcarnitine translocase
CAD	coronary artery disease
CAH	congenital adrenal hyperplasia
CBC	complete blood count
CBT	cognitive–behavioral therapy
CCAM	congenital cystic adenomatoid malformation
CCNU	Lomustine
CD	Crohn's disease
CDG	congenital disorder of glycosylation
CDGP	constitutional delay in growth and puberty
CDH	congenital diaphragmatic hernia
CER	control event rate
CF	cystic fibrosis
CFRD	cystic fibrosis–related diabetes
CFS	chronic fatigue syndrome
CFTR	cystic fibrosis transmembrane receptor
CGD	chronic granulomatous disease
CGH	comparative genomic hybridization
CGMS	continuous glucose monitoring system
CH	cystic hygroma
CHARGE	coloboma, heart defects, choanal atresia, retarded growth, genital anomalies, ear abnormalities
CHC	choriocarcinoma
CHD	congenital heart disease
CHO	carbohydrate
CI	confidence interval
CK	creatine kinase
CKD	chronic kidney disease
CLD	chronic lung disease
CLE	congenital lobar emphysema
CML	chronic myeloid leukemia

CMV	cytomegalovirus
CNS	central nervous system
CO	carbon monoxide
CoA	coarctation of aorta
CONS	coagulase-negative staphylococci
CP	cerebral palsy
CPAP	continuous positive airway pressure
CPK	creatine phosphokinase
CPP	central precocious puberty
CPR	cardiopulmonary resuscitation
Cr	creatinine
CRF	chronic renal failure; corticotrophin-releasing factor
CRH	corticotrophin-releasing hormone
CRP	C-reactive protein
CRRT	continuous renal replacement therapy
CRT	capillary refill time
CS	Caesarean section
CSF	cerebrospinal fluid
CSII	continuous subcutaneous insulin infusion
CT	computerized tomography
CVP	central venous pressure
CVS	cardiovascular system
DALY	disability-adjusted life-year
DAT	direct antiglobulin test
DBP	diastolic blood pressure
DCD	developmental coordination disorder
DCT	direct Coombs' test
DDAVP	deamino-8-d-arginine vasopressin (desmopressin)
DDH	developmental dysplasia of the hip
DEXA	dual-energy X-ray absorptiometry
DHEAS	dehydroepiandrosterone sulfate
DHR	dihydrorhodamine
DI	diabetes insipidus
DIC	disseminated intravascular coagulation
DIOS	distal intestinal obstruction syndrome
DIP	distal interphalangeal (joint)
DJF	duodenojejunal flexure
DKA	diabetic ketoacidosis

DM	diabetes mellitus
DMARD	disease-modifying antirheumatic drug
DMD	Duchenne muscular dystrophy
DMSA	dimercaptosuccinic acid
DPG	diphosphoglycerate
DPI	dry powder inhaler
DQ	Developmental Quotient
DSD	disorders of sexual development
DSM	*Diagnostic and Statistical Manual of Mental Disorders*
DTaP	diptheria, tetanus, acellular pertussis
DTPA	diethylenetriamine pentaacetic acid
EA	esophageal atresia
EAR	estimated average (nutritional) requirement
EBM	expressed breast milk
EBV	Epstein–Barr virus
EC	embryonal carcinoma
ECG	electrocardiogram
ECMO	extracorporeal membrane oxygenation
ED	emergency department
EEG	electroencephalogram
EER	experimental event rate
EFM	electronic fetal (heart rate) monitoring
EGD	esophagogastroduodenoscopy
EHEC	enterohemorrhagic *E. coli*
EIA	exercise-induced asthma; enzyme immunoassay
ELISA	enzyme-linked immunosorbent assay
ELBW	extremely low birth weight
EM	electron microscopy
EMDR	eye movement desensitization and reprocessing
EMG	electromyogram
EMU	early-morning urine
ENT	ear, nose, throat
ERCP	endoscopic retrograde cholangiopancreatography
ERT	enzyme replacement therapy
ES	Ewing sarcoma
ESR	erythrocyte sedimentation rate
ESRD	end-stage renal disease
$ETCO_2$	end-tidal carbon dioxide

ETT	endotracheal tube
FA	fluorescent antibody; Friedreich's ataxia
FB	foreign body
FBAO	foreign-body airway obstruction
FBC	full blood count
FDA	(U.S.) Food and Drug Administration
FDP	fibrin/fibrinogen degradation products
FENA	fractional excretion of sodium
FEV_1	forced expiratory volume in 1 second
FFP	fresh frozen plasma
FH	familial hypercholesterolemia
FiO_2	fractional inspired oxygen
FISH	fluorescence in situ hybridization
FLAG	fludarabine, ara-C, and G-CSF (regime)
FMR	fetal mortality rate
FRAXA	fragile X syndrome
FRC	functional residual capacity
FSGS	focal segmental glomerulosclerosis
FSH	follicle-stimulating hormone
fT4	free thyroxine
FTT	failure to thrive
FVC	forced vital capacity
FVL	factor V Leiden
GA	general anesthesia; glutaric aciduria
GAD	glutamic acid decarboxylase; generalized anxiety disorder
GBS	group B streptococcus; Guillain–Barré syndrome
GCS	Glasgow coma scale
G-CSF	granulocyte colony-stimulating factor
GCT	germ cell tumor
GERD	gastroesophageal reflux disease
GFR	glomerular filtration rate
GH	growth hormone
GHIS	growth hormone insensitivity syndrome
GHRH	growth hormone-releasing hormone
GI	gastrointestinal
GIR	glucose infusion rate
GMFCS	gross motor function classification system
GN	glomerular nephritis

GnRH	gonadotropin-releasing hormone
G6PD	glucose-6-phosphate dehydrogenase
GSD	glycogen storage disease
GU	genitourinary
GVHD	graft versus host disease
Hb	hemoglobin
HBeAg	hepatitis B virus e antigen
HBL	hepatoblastoma
HBsAg	hepatitis B surface antigen
HCC	hepatocellular carcinoma
hCG	human chorionic gonadotropin
HCM	hypertrophic cardiomyopathy
Hct	hematocrit
HD	hemodialysis; Hirschsprung's disease
HE	hereditary elliptocytosis
HELLP	hemolytic anemia–elevated liver enzymes–low platelet count
HFOV	high-frequency oscillatory ventilation
hGH	human growth hormone
HH	hypogonadotropic hypogonadism; hiatus hernia
HHNK	hyperosmolar hyperglycemic nonketotic coma
HHV	human herpes virus
HiB	*Haemophilus influenzae* type B
HIDA	hepatoiminodiacetic acid
HIE	hypoxic–ischemic encephalopathy
HIPAA	Health Insurance Portability & Accountability Act
HIV	human immunodeficiency virus
HL	Hodgkin's lymphoma
HLH	hemophagocytic lymphohistiocytosis
HLHS	hypoplastic left heart syndrome
HMD	hyaline membrane disease
HOCM	hypertrophic obstructive cardiomopathy
HPA	human platelet antigen
HPI	history of past illness
HPS	hypertrophic pyloric stenosis
HPV	human papillomavirus
HRCT	high-resolution computerized tomography
HS	hereditary spherocytosis
HSCT	hematopoietic stem cell transplantation

HSP	Henoch–Schönlein purpura
HSV	herpes simplex virus
HTN	hypertension
HUS	hemolytic–uremic syndrome
HVA	homovanillic acid
IAA	insulin auto-antibody
IBD	inflammatory bowel disease
ICA	islet cell antibody
ICD	International Classification of Diseases
ICF	International Classification of Functioning, Disability, & Health
ICP	intracranial pressure
ICS	inhaled corticosteroid(s)
IDDM	insulin-dependent diabetes mellitus
I:E	ratio of inspiratory time to expiratory time
IEM	inborn errors of metabolism
IEP	individualized education program
IGF	insulin-like growth factor
Ig	immunoglobulin
IGT	impaired glucose tolerance
IHPS	idiopathic hypertrophic pyloric stenosis
ILAR	International League of Associations for Rheumatology
IM	intramuscular
IMD	inherited metabolic disease
IMR	infant mortality rate
INR	international normalized ratio
IO	intraosseous
IOM	Institute of Medicine
IPPV	intermittent positive pressure ventilation
IPV	inactivated polio virus
IRT	immunoreactive trypsinogen
IT	intrathecal
ITP	idiopathic thrombocytopenic purpura
ITT	insulin tolerance test
IU	international units
IUGR	intrauterine growth restriction
IUT	intrauterine blood transfusion
IV	intravenous
IVA	isovaleric academia

IVC	inferior vena cava
IVH	intraventricular hemorrhage
IVI	intravenous infusion
IVIG	intravenous immunoglobulin
IWL	insensible water loss
JDM	juvenile dermatomyositis
JIA	juvenile idiopathic arthritis
JMML	juvenile myelomonocytic leukemia
JVD	jugular venous distension
JVP	jugular venous pressure
KS	Kallmann syndrome
LBW	low birth weight
LCH	Langerhan's cell histiocytosis
LD	learning disability
LDH	lactate dehydrogenase
LDL	low-density lipoprotein
LES	lower esophageal sphincter
LFT	liver function test
LGA	large for gestational age
LH	luteinizing hormone
LIP	lymphoid interstitial pneumonitis
LKM	liver/kidney microsomal (antibodies)
LOC	level of consciousness
LP	lumbar puncture
LR	likelihood ratio
LRD	living related donor
LRTI	lower respiratory tract infection
LSCS	lower-segment Cesarean section
LV	left ventricular
MA	microalbuminuria; mesenteric adenitis
MAG-3	mercaptoacetyltriglycine
MAHA	microangiopathic hemolytic anemia
MAP	mean airway pressure
MAS	meconium aspiration syndrome; McCune–Albright syndrome; macrophage activation syndrome
MCD	minimal-change disease
MCDK	multicystic dysplastic kidneys
MCH	mean cell hemoglobin
MCHC	mean corpuscular hemoglobin concentration

MCP	metacarpal phalangeal (joint)
M, C & S	microscopy, culture, and sensitivity
MCTD	mixed connective tissue disease
MCUG	micturating cystourethrography
MCV	mean cell volume
MDI	metered dose inhaler
MDS	myelodysplastic syndrome
MELAS	mitochondrial encephalopathy–lactic acidosis and stroke-like episodes (syndrome)
MEN	multiple endocrine neoplasia
MEP	maximal exhibitory pressure
MFS	Marfan syndrome
MGN	membranous glomerulonephritis
MIBG	meta-iodo-benzylguanidine
MIP	maximal inhibitory pressure
MLD	metachromatic leukodystrophy
MMA	methylmalonic academia
MMF	mycophenolate mofetil
MMR	measles, mumps, rubella (vaccination)
MODY	maturity onset diabetes of young
MPA	microscopic polyangiitis
MPGN	membranoproliferative glomerulonephritis
MPS	mucopolysaccharidosis
MRCP	magnetic resonance cholangiopancreatography
MRD	minimal residual disease
MRI	magnetic resonance imaging
MRSA	methicillin-resistant *Staphylococcus aureus*
MSbP	Munchausen syndrome by proxy
MSH	melanocyte-stimulating hormone
MSU	midstream urine
MTHFR	methyltetrahydrofolate reductase
MTP	metatarsal phalangeal (joint)
MTX	methotrexate
NAI	nonaccidental injury
NAIT	neonatal alloimmune thrombocytopenia
NAS	neonatal abstinence syndrome
NAT	nonaccidental trauma
NC	nasal cannula; nonconvulsive
NEC	necrotizing enterocolitis

NF	neurofibromatosis (NF1, NF2)
NFCS	Neonatal Facial Coding System
NG	nasogastric
NHL	non-Hodgkin's lymphoma
NHLBI	National Heart, Lung, & Blood Institute
NICU	neonatal intensive care unit
NIH	National Institutes of Health
NK	natural killer (cells)
NNU	neonatal unit
NMJ	neuromuscular junction
NNT	number (of patients) needed to treat
NPO	nothing by mouth (nil per os)
NS	Noonan syndrome
NSAID	nonsteroidal anti-inflammatory drug
NSE	neuron-specific enolase
NTD	neural tube defect
OAE	otoacoustic emissions
OCD	obsessive–compulsive disorder
OD	observed difference
OE	otitis externae
OFC	occipitofrontal circumference
OG	orogastric
OGTT	oral glucose tolerance test
OI	osteogenesis imperfecta; oxygenation index
OME	otitis media with effusion
OMIN	Online Mendelian Inheritance in Man (database)
O&P	ova & parasite exam
ORS	oral rehydration solution
OSA	obstructive sleep apnea
OSAS	obstructive sleep apnea syndrome
OTC	over-the-counter
PA	posteroanterior; propionic acidemia
$PaCO_2$	arterial carbon dioxide tension
PAN	polyarteritis nodosa
p-ANCA	perinuclear antineutrophil cytoplasmic antibody
PaO_2	arterial oxygen tension
PAP-A	pregnancy-associated protein A
PBSC	peripheral blood stem cell(s)
PCA	patient-controlled analgesia

PCKD	polycystic kidney disease
PCP	*Pneumocystis carinii* pneumonia
PCR	polymerase chain reaction
PCV	packed cell volume; pneumococcal conjugate vaccine
PD	peritoneal dialysis
PDA	patent ductus arteriosus
PDD	pervasive developmental disorder
PDPE	psychologically determined paroxysmal events
PEEP	positive end-expiratory pressure
PEFR	peak expiratory flow rate
PEG	polyethylene glycol
PET	positron emission tomography; pressure-equalization tube
PFT	pulmonary function test
PGE1	prostaglandin E1
PHP	pseudohypoparathyroidism
PHVD	post-hemorrhagic ventricular dilatation
PICC	peripherally inserted central catheter
PICU	pediatric intensive care unit
PIE	pulmonary interstitial emphysema
PIP	peak inspiratory pressure; proximal interphalangeal (joint)
PIPP	Premature Infant Pain Profile
PK	pyruvate kinase
PKU	phenylketonuria
PMDI	propellant metered dose inhaler
PML	promyelocytic leukemia
PMN	polymorphonuclear leukocytes
PMR	perinatal mortality rate
PN	parenteral nutrition
PNDM	permanent neonatal diabetes mellitus
PNET	primitive neuroectodermal tumor
PNH	paroxysmal nocturnal hemoglobinuria
PNMR	postneonatal mortality rate
PO	orally, by mouth (per os)
PP	precocious puberty
PPHN	persistent pulmonary hypertension of the newborn
PPI	proton pump inhibitor
PPROM	preterm prolonged rupture of membranes
PPS	peripheral pulmonary stenosis

PROM	prolonged rupture of membranes
PR	rectally, per rectum
PSC	primary sclerosing cholangitis
PSS	progressive systemic sclerosis
PT	prothrombin time
PTH	parathyroid hormone
PTSD	post-traumatic stress disorder
PTT	partial thromboplastin time
PTV	patient-triggered ventilation
PUBS	percutaneous umbilical blood sampling
PUJ	pelviureteric junction
PUV	posterior urethral valve
PV	vaginally, per vagina
PVH	periventricular hemorrhage
PVL	periventricular leukomalacia
PWS	Prader–Willi syndrome
qid	four times a day
RA	rheumatoid arthritis
RAS	reflex anoxic syndrome
RAST	radioallergosorbent test
RBC	red blood cell
RCC	red cell count
RCM	red blood cell mass
RCT	randomized, controlled trial
RDS	respiratory distress syndrome
RDW	red cell distribution width
RF	rheumatoid factor
rhGH	recombinant human growth hormone
RIF	right iliac fossa
RMS	rhabdomyosarcoma
ROM	range of movement
ROP	retinopathy of prematurity
RP	retinitis pigmentosa
RPGN	rapidly progressive glomerulonephritis
RRR	relative risk reduction
RSV	respiratory syncytial virus
RTA	renal tubular acidosis; road traffic accident
RV	residual volume; right ventricular
RVH	right ventricular hypertrophy

SAD	separation anxiety disorder
SaO_2	arterial oxygen saturation
SBFT	small bowel follow-through
SBP	systolic blood pressure
SBR	serum bilirubin
SC	subcutaneous
SCHIP	State Children's Health Insurance Program
SCID	severe combined immunodeficiency
SCL	subcortical leukomalacia
SCM	sternocleidomastoid muscle
SD	standard deviation
SE	standard error; status epilepticus
SEER	Surveillance Epidemiology & End Results (U.S.)
SGA	small for gestational age
SIADH	syndrome of inappropriate antidiuretic hormone
SIDS	sudden infant death syndrome
SIMV	synchronized intermittent mandatory ventilation
SIPPV	synchronized intermittent positive pressure ventilation
SLE	systemic lupus erythematosus
SMA	spinal muscular atrophy; superior mesenteric artery; smooth muscle antibody
SN	sensorineural
SOB	shortness of breath
SPA	suprapubic aspiration
SpO_2	pulse oximetry measurement of oxyhemoglobin saturation
SR	steroid-resistant
SS	steroid-sensitive
SSc	systemic sclerosis
SSPE	subacute sclerosing panencephalitis
STI	sexually transmitted infection
SUDI	sudden unexpected death in an infant
SUFE	slipped upper femoral epiphysis
SVC	superior vena cava
SVT	supraventricular tachycardia
SWL	sensible water loss
T3	triiodothyronine
T4	thyroxine

TA	tricuspid atresia; Takayasu arteritis
TaGVHD	transfusion-associated graft versus host disease
TAPVD	total anomalous pulmonary venous drainage
TAR	thrombocytopenia–absent radius (syndrome)
TAT	trans-anastomotic tube
TB	tuberculosis
TBI	total body irradiation
TBM	tuberculous meningitis
TBW	total body weight
TcCO$_2$	transcutaneous carbon dioxide pressure
TcO$_2$	transcutaneous oxygen pressure
TDC	thyroglossal duct cyst(s)
TDD	total digitalizing dose (for digoxin)
T1DM	type 1 diabetes mellitus
T2DM	type 2 diabetes mellitus
TdT	terminal deoxynucleotidyl transferase
tid	three times a day
TE	expiratory time
TEF	tracheoesophageal fistula
TFT	thyroid function test
TGA	transposition of great arteries
T$_i$	inspiratory time
TIBC	total iron binding capacity
TLC	total lung capacity
TNDM	transient neonatal diabetes mellitus
TNF	tumor necrosis factor
TORCH	toxoplasmosis, others, rubella, cytomegalovirus, herpes virus II
t-PA	tissue plasminogen activator
TPN	total parenteral nutrition
TPPS	Toddler–Preschooler Postoperative Pain Scale
TRALI	transfusion-related acute lung injury
TSC	tuberous sclerosis complex
TSH	thyroid stimulating hormone
TST	tuberculin skin test
TT	thrombin time
TTN	transient tachypnea of newborn
UA	urinalysis

UAC	umbilical arterial catheter
UC	ulcerative colitis
UCD	urea cycle disorder
U&E	urea and electrolytes
UGI	upper gastrointestinal
UNC	urine net charge
UPJ	ureteropelvic junction
UP:UCr	urinary protein to urinary creatinine (ratio)
URI	upper respiratory infection
UTI	urinary tract infection
UVC	umbilical venous catheter
UVJ	ureterovesicular junction
VACTERL	vertebral anomalies, anal atresia, cardiac malformations, tracheoesophageal fistula, renal and limb anomalies
VATS	video-assisted thoracoscopic surgery
VCA	viral capsid antigen
VCFS	velocardiofacial syndrome
VCUG	voiding cystourethrogram
VDDR	vitamin D–dependent rickets
VDRL	Venereal Disease Research Laboratory (test)
VF	ventricular fibrillation
VHL	von Hippel–Lindau (disease)
VIP	vasoactive intestinal polypeptide
VLBW	very low birth weight
VLDL	very low density lipoprotein
VMA	vanillylmandelic acid
V/Q	ventilation–perfusion ratio
VSD	ventricular septal defect
VT	ventricular tachycardia
VUJ	vesicoureteric junction
VUR	vesicoureteric reflux
vWD	von Willebrand's disease
vWF	von Willebrand's factor
VZV	varicella zoster virus
WAGR	Wilms, aniridia, gonadal dysplasia, retardation (complex)
WAS	Wiscott–Aldrich syndrome
WBC	white blood cell
WCC	white cell count

WG	Wegener's granulomatosis
WHO	World Health Organization
WS	Williams syndrome
XLP	X-linked lymphoproliferative disease
YST	yolk sac tumor
ZIG	zoster immunoglobulin

Practicing pediatrics

Reading and learning about pediatrics

Welcome to pediatrics and child health! You will find this area of medicine challenging, rewarding, and, above all, fun. We have written this handbook to help you develop your clinical skills—whether in the office, emergency department, or hospital.

Six basic goals in your learning

If you are a novice in the field you will find that every day requires new skills, and sometimes this can seem daunting. Take heart. We hope that this experience will provide an education in the aspects of general pediatrics, important for all health professionals who care for children. Your curriculum goals should include the following:

- *Acquire basic knowledge of growth and development.* Learn about physical, physiological, and psychosocial change from birth through adolescence and see how this applies to clinical practice.
- *Develop communication skills* that will help you speak to children, adolescents, and their families.
- *Become competent in physical examination* of babies, infants, toddlers, children, and adolescents.
- *Learn enough core knowledge* so that you can make a diagnosis and start treatment for common acute and chronic pediatric illnesses.
- *Improve your clinical problem-solving skills.*
- *Take a broad perspective* and understand more about raising healthy children in modern society, and recognize the differences between communities and cultures.

As you scan through the handbook you will see that all of the chapters will assist you in reaching these goals. We hope that this book will continue to be a useful tool in your practice in the future.

What's next after this foundation?

For those who are using this handbook as an aid in becoming a pediatrician, we offer a more prescriptive approach in the next sections. We have itemized certain objectives deemed essential for professional conduct, attitudes, skills, and knowledge. Use these as a checklist and monitor your progress as you work through the handbook.

Professional conduct and attitudes

- *Have you learned to adapt your clinical approach to patients of all ages?* Can you communicate with the child or adolescent and family in the clinic? What about dealing with confidentiality and privacy?
- *Can you communicate clearly and sensitively?* How do you break bad news to new parents, or to the newly diagnosed adolescent with chronic illness or disability?
- *Do you work well in a team?* Do you treat each member of the team with courtesy and recognize the contributions of each?
- *Are you aware of the foundations of professional behavior?* Do you demonstrate these values in your professional interactions?
- *Are you aware of cultural, ethnic, and socioeconomic factors in your practice?*
- *Do you have a foundation in basic ethical principles?* Do you appreciate the ethical challenges specific to pediatrics and child health?

Professional skills

Interviewing

- *Can you obtain a complete medical history?* The history of the perinatal period, immunizations, development, diet, family and social history, and systems review is unique to pediatrics. Can you collect this information in a timely manner—40 minutes in a complex case history? You should also be able to modify the medical history according to the age of the child, with particular attention given to the following age groups: neonate, infant, toddler, school age, and adolescence.
- *Can you obtain a focused medical history?* In an emergency or acute-care encounter, you will need to know the important questions to ask in order to gain the essential information needed to guide therapy.

Physical examination

- *Can you complete a full physical examination of an infant, child, and adolescent, including the observation and documentation of normal physical findings?* You should be able to do this "long-case" examination in less than 10 minutes.
- *Can you carry out a problem-oriented examination?* For example, in the child with a limp, what are the important positive and negative clinical findings?
- *Are you a good observer?* Do you take time to look first?
- *Can you assess behavior, neurodevelopment, and pubertal staging?*

Communication

- *Can you establish rapport with the patient and family?* Are you able to identify the main concerns of the patient and family? Can you communicate information to both the patient and parent, making sure both understand the diagnosis and treatment plan, and do you give them the opportunity to ask questions?
- *Can you write a discharge letter for a referring physician?*
- *Can you write a well-constructed daily progress note, transfer note, and discharge summary?*
- *Can you present a well-organized summary of your patient to colleagues?* Can you communicate effectively with other health-care workers, including nurses and social workers, and explain the thought process that led to your diagnosis and treatment?
- *Can you communicate effectively through the use of an interpreter for families unable to communicate in English?*

Clinical problem-solving

- *Can you compile a problem list and differential diagnosis for each of the common clinical presentations?* Can you use your knowledge of key signs and symptoms and the frequency and prevalence of diseases at different ages to develop a likely differential diagnosis?
- *Can you develop a diagnostic plan?* Can you interpret the results of commonly ordered laboratory tests, such as the full blood count, urinalysis, and serum electrolytes, and recognize that the normal values of some tests may vary with the age of the patient?

- Can you use the medical pediatric literature and Web-based medical literature search resources to research the diagnosis and management of clinical problems? Can you critically appraise a topic and decide on best evidence for treatment?

Practical procedures
- Do you know when common procedures are needed (e.g., lumbar puncture, intravenous line, nasogastric tube, etc.)?
- Can you explain these procedures to parents and children?
- Pediatric residents should be able to perform the procedures listed in Box 1.1 by the completion of training.

Box 1.1 Diagnostic and therapeutic procedures

Diagnostic procedures
- Venopuncture and venous cannulation
- Blood sampling from central lines and umbilical arterial lines
- Capillary blood sampling
- Peripheral arterial blood gas sampling
- Electrocardiogram
- Lumbar puncture
- Suprapubic aspiration of urine
- Noninvasive blood pressure measurement
- Urethral catheterization
- Urine analysis using standard bedside tests
- Blood sugar measurement using standard point-of-care glucometers

Diagnostic procedures with supervision
- Needle aspiration of the knee for microbiology and cytology studies

Needle thoracentesis of pleural effusion for microbiology and cytologyTherapeutic procedures
- Bag, valve, and mask ventilation
- Placement of an oral airway
- Cardiopulmonary resuscitation
- Tracheal intubation of children at all ages
- Removal and replacement of a blocked tracheotomy tube
- Percutaneous central-line insertion
- Placement of nasogastric tube
- Repair of superficial lacerations
- Incision and drainage of superficial abscesses
- Splinting of non-displaced fractures

Therapeutic procedures with supervision
- Injections: intradermal, subcutaneous, intramuscular, intravenous
- Insertion of an intraosseous needle
- Administer surfactant
- Tracheal intubation of pre-term and older child
- Chest tube insertion for pneumothorax

Knowledge

During your reading you should consider the following questions as a starting point to the knowledge expected of a pediatrician.

Growth

- What are the intrauterine factors that affect growth of the fetus? Can you explain how growth charts are used in the longitudinal evaluation of height, weight, and head circumference?
- Can you recognize abnormalities of growth that warrant further evaluation?
- What is the significance of crossing centiles on a growth chart?
- What is the significance of discrepancies between height, weight, and head circumference?
- What are short stature, constitutional delay, failure to thrive, obesity, microcephaly, and macrocephaly?

Development

- Why is following development important in clinical pediatrics?
- What are the normal changes in reflexes, tone, and posture in the infant?
- What is the normal progression in motor milestones in the first year?
- What are the signs of cerebral palsy?
- What are the signs of autism?

Behavior

- What are the typical presentations of common behavioral problems at various developmental levels and ages?
- What are temper tantrums?
- How may somatic complaints represent psychosocial problems?
- In what types of situations does pathology in the family contribute to childhood behavior problems?

Nutrition

- What factors contribute to the development of failure to thrive during infancy?
- What factors contribute to the development of child obesity?
- What are the special dietary needs of children with chronic illness?
- What caloric intake is needed for normal growth in infants and small children?
- What are the major differences between human milk and commonly available formulas?
- What are the advantages of breast-feeding?

Newborns

- What diseases are detected by neonatal blood screening?
- What important historical information, physical-examination findings, and laboratory data are needed for the differential diagnosis of the following problems?
- Jitteriness or seizures
- Jaundice
- Lethargy or poor feeding
- Respiratory distress
- Cyanosis
- Bilious vomiting
- Nonbilious vomiting
- Hypoglycemia
- Sepsis

Genetics and congenital malformations

- What are the effects of teratogenic agents such as alcohol and phenytoin?
- What are the findings and implications of the following common chromosomal abnormalities?
- Trisomy 21
- Sex chromosome abnormalities (e.g., Turner syndrome, fragile X syndrome)
- Other genetic disorders (cystic fibrosis, sickle cell disease)

Common pediatric illnesses

For each of the common "presentations" and "conditions" in this handbook can you review the following:

- Cause
- Pathophysiology
- Natural history
- Presenting signs and symptoms
- Initial laboratory test and/or imaging needed for diagnosis
- Plan for initial management

Epidemiology, evidence, and practice

The aim of this chapter is to provide an overview of the epidemiological concepts we find useful in supporting our everyday clinical practice. You may have read a relevant article and need a quick reference. Alternatively, you may want to examine some data published in a report and apply it to your work. To translate epidemiologic research into meaningful application, one first needs an understanding of the key measures used to quantify the existence, cause, and treatment of disease. A further requirement is knowledge of the basic statistical principles needed to assess the significance of study results.

In this chapter, we focus on the epidemiologic and statistical concepts needed to understand some of the more common applications of quantitative medical research:

- Estimating the burden of disease in the population
- Identifying risk factors for disease
- Predicting disease using a diagnostic test
- Describing the impact of treatment on disease

Although we focus on disease as the outcome of interest for presentation purposes, the definitions and concepts to follow apply more broadly to any definitive clinical outcome. We begin this chapter with a description of the relevant measures used for quantification in each of the applications above, and review the study designs that can be used to derive these measures. Beyond understanding how each of these measures are estimated, we are often interested in using statistical tests to determine their significance. We therefore end the chapter with an overview of the principles of statistical inference, followed by an overview of the approaches used to characterize levels of existing clinical evidence.

Estimating the burden of disease

The epidemiologic approach toward quantifying disease in the population is based on the measures of prevalence, incidence, and mortality.

Prevalence

This is the proportion of persons in a population who have the disease at a fixed time point, defined as

$$\frac{(\text{\# of existing cases})}{(\text{\# at risk in the population})}$$

Prevalence is typically measured at a fixed time point, called *point prevalence*. Prevalence can also be measured over a period of time, which is called *period prevalence*. Period prevalence would be calculated as above by determining the number of cases and number at risk over a specified time frame. In general, prevalence measures are used to quantify a person's likelihood of having the disease.

Incidence

This is the proportion of new persons in a population who develop disease over a period of time, defined as

$$\frac{(\text{\# of new cases over a period of time})}{(\text{\# at risk in the population in the time period})}$$

Incidence measures are used to quantify a person's probability of being newly diagnosed with the disease over a specified time period.

Mortality rate

This is the proportion of persons who die from a disease, defined as

$$\frac{(\text{\# of deaths due to disease})}{(\text{\# of persons in the population})}$$

The most common mortality rates summarized in the pediatric literature include the following:
- *Perinatal mortality*, which includes both stillbirths and deaths occurring in the first week of life
- *Infant mortality*, which includes deaths occurring from birth to 1 year
- *Post-neonatal mortality*, which includes deaths occurring between 4 weeks of age to 1 year
- *Under 5-year mortality*, which includes deaths occurring from birth to age under 5 years

Identifying risk factors for disease

The objective of many epidemiologic investigations is to evaluate associations between risk factors and disease. There are three main study designs that can be used for this research objective.

- *Prospective (cohort) study*: Persons with and without the risk factor of interest are selected (and possibly matched), and followed for a specified amount of time to determine the number of persons who develop the disease in each risk-factor group. Historical prospective studies can be performed by using existing longitudinal data, for instance, with the use of medical records.
- *Retrospective (case–control) study*: Persons with and without the disease are identified, and retrospective data are   collected to determine prior exposure to the risk factor of interest. Results from retrospective studies must be carefully interpreted on the basis of this sampling scheme, as the diseased cases may not be representative of the population of all diseased persons.
- *Cross-sectional study*: A sample of persons is identified and classified into four groups defined by the joint presence or absence of the d isease and risk factor. This study design can lead to biases if some of the four groups have a lower participation rate in the study than that of the other groups.

There are two key measures of association for these epidemiologic investigations: *relative risk* and *odds ratios*, which we define below.

	Disease status	
Risk factor	**Disease +**	**Disease –**
Exposure +	A	B
Exposure –	C	D

- Relative Risk:

$$\frac{\text{Pr (disease + | exposure +)} = A/(A+B)}{\text{Pr (disease + | exposure –)} \; C/(C+D)}$$

The relative risk is the probability of disease in the exposed group divided by the probability of disease in the unexposed group. For example, a relative risk of 5 means that an exposed person is at 5 times greater risk of developing the disease than an unexposed person. The relative risk is generally the most interpretable measure of association. The relative risk can be estimated in prospective or cross-sectional studies, since the number of diseased persons is randomly determined. The relative risk cannot be estimated in retrospective case–control studies, since the number of diseased persons is fixed by design.

- Odds Ratio:

$$\frac{\text{Pr(disease+| exposure+)}/\text{Pr(disease-| exposure+)}}{\text{Pr(disease+| exposure-)}/\text{Pr(disease-| exposure-)}} = \frac{(A/(A+B))/(B/(A+B))}{(C/(C+D))/(D/C+D))}$$

The odds ratio is the odds of disease in the exposed group divided by the odds of disease in the unexposed group. For example, an odds ratio of 5 means there is a 5-fold greater odds of having disease for those with the risk factor than without the risk factor. If the overall disease rate in the population is very small, then the odds ratio is an approximation of the relative risk. Unlike relative risk, the odds ratio can be estimated in retrospective case–control studies. This is because the odds ratio is equivalent to the odds of exposure in the diseased group divided by the odds of exposure in the nondiseased group. The odds ratio is used for measuring association in retrospective studies, and has a more meaningful interpretation when it can be assumed that it is an approximation of a relative risk. This may not be the case for all retrospective studies, and this commonly leads to misinterpretations in the medical literature.

Predicting disease using a diagnostic test

A diagnostic test is a clinical or laboratory procedure used to predict disease status. The test could be as complex as a series of laboratory measurements or as simple as a short symptom questionnaire. When developing a diagnostic test, it is important to understand how well the test predicts disease status. Some of the many parameters used to assess prediction of a diagnostic test can be illustrated by starting with a 2×2 table of disease status and test result.

	Disease status	
Test result	Diseased	Nondiseased
Positive	A (true positive)	B (false positive)
Negative	C (false negative)	D (true negative)

Individuals evaluated with the test can be classified into one of four categories:
- *True positive*: a diseased person who tests positive
- *True negative*: a nondiseased person who tests negative
- *False positive*: a nondiseased person who tests positive
- *False negative*: a diseased person who tests negative

Several measures are used to evaluate the predictive ability of diagnostic tests. Two of the most commonly used measures are sensitivity and specificity.
- *Sensitivity*: percent of diseased persons who test positive = $A/(A+C) \times 100$
- *Specificity*: percent of nondiseased persons who test negative = $D/(B+D) \times 100$

An ideal diagnostic test would have sensitivity and specificity both near 100%. These measures are sometimes combined and presented as likelihood ratios:
- *Likelihood ratio positive* (LR+): Sensitivity/(1-Specificity)
- *Likelihood ratio negative* (LR–): Specificity/(1-Sensitivity)

An ideal diagnostic test would have likelihood ratios greater than 1. Greater likelihood ratios indicate more predictive ability.

Predictive values are commonly used to estimate the probability of disease for a person with a given test result.
- *Positive predictive value*: percent of positive-testing subjects who are diseased = $A/(A+B) \times 100$
- *Negative predictive value*: percent of negative-testing subjects who are nondiseased = $D/(C+D) \times 100$

An ideal diagnostic test would have predictive values near 100%. If the individuals included in a diagnostic test study are representative of the overall population, then the predictive values can be estimated as above. However, in some study designs the proportion of diseased subjects is fixed. (e.g., case–control studies), and in this setting the known prevalence of disease can instead be used in conjunction with sensitivity and specificity estimates to estimate predictive values.

Describing the impact of treatment on disease

Understanding the impact of treatment on disease can be tricky. There are many factors potentially associated with the choice of treatment in clinical practice. When such factors are also associated with disease, the results from observational studies are subject to confounding. That is, the observed relationship between treatment and disease may not be an accurate estimate of treatment impact. There are at least two ways to address this issue. One method is to carefully measure all potential confounding factors and account for them in an analysis using statistical modeling techniques such as regression or propensity scores. Another, more direct method to account for confounding is to conduct an experimental study called a *randomized controlled trial* (RCT).

RCTs are characterized by random allocation of treatment choices with prospective follow-up to measure post-treatment disease status as compared to pre-treatment disease status. When properly designed, conducted, and analyzed, RCTs are often considered the best available study design for causal inference as well as for approval of new therapies by governmental agencies such as the U.S. Food and Drug Administration (FDA). RCTs usually incorporate blinding, or hiding the actual treatment assignment, to further control potential biases such as the "placebo effect." As further discussion of RCT methodology is beyond the scope of this chapter, recommended references are provided at the end of this chapter.

Regardless of whether the study design is observational or experimental, there are several ways to characterize treatment effect depending largely on how disease outcome is measured. For continuous quantitative measures such as systolic blood pressure (BP), examples of how disease status could be measured include BP at post-treatment follow-up, change in BP over the follow-up period, percent change in BP over the follow-up period, and rate of change in BP over the follow-up period. Treatment effect for continuous measures would typically be characterized as the absolute difference between treatment groups, for example:

Treatment Effect = (Rate of change in BP for active treatment group) −
(Rate of change in BP for placebo group).

Other common outcome measures include dichotomous yes/no indicators over the course of follow-up, or the time from randomization until an event. An example of a dichotomous outcome might be an indicator for whether the subject was hospitalized during the month following randomization. The time to event counterpart of that measure would be the time from randomization until hospitalization, if hospitalization occurred. For these measures, treatment effect is typically measured as the relative risk, for example:

Treatment Effect = (Risk of hospitalization in the active treatment
group)/(Risk of hospitalization in the placebo group)

When the results from a successful treatment study are presented, the number needed to treat is an epidemiologic measure that may also be provided. The number needed to treat is the number of individuals that need to be treated in order to reduce the expected number of cases with a disease or defined end point by 1.

Overview of statistical inference

In the prior sections, we provided the relevant context behind the estimation of some of the most common measures of interest in the medical literature. However, the objective of many clinical studies is to not only estimate the measure of interest but also evaluate the value of the observed measure with respect to an a priori hypothesized value. To achieve this objective, formal statistical inference procedures must be implemented. When reading the literature, it is important to understand the statistical measures and methods presented and to evaluate the statistical significance of the presented results. We provide a brief overview of the key statistical terms encountered in the literature.

• *Statistical inference.* The use of statistical methods to reach conclusions about a population based on a study sample.
• *Confidence interval (CI).* A range of values which we are confident contains the true value. The confidence level is often set at 95%, meaning that in repeated sampling, the CI would contain the true value 95% of the time.
• *Hypothesis test.* A statistical method for decision making based on careful evaluation of the risks of the potential incorrect decisions.
• *Null hypothesis.* The hypothesis associated with the baseline or current standard. Typically the null hypothesis will be that there is no association.
• *Alternative hypothesis.* The hypothesis associated with the treatment or proposed risk factor. Typically the alternative hypothesis will be that there is an association.
• *Type I error.* This type of error results when a hypothesis test results in a decision that there is an association when there is, in fact, no association.
• *Type II error.* This type of error results when a hypothesis test results in a decision that there is no association when there is in fact an association.
• *Significance level of a statistical test* (α). The probability of a type I error: finding an association by chance alone when there really is no association. The significance level is often set at 0.05 (5%), and this value is what is used to evaluate the p value from a statistical test.
• *Power of a statistical test* ($1-\beta$). The probability of finding an association when there is one, where (β) is the probability of a type II error, or the probability of not finding an association when there is one. The power is often set at 0.80 (80%) or 0.90 (90%) during the design phase of a study.
• *Sample size.* The number of persons included in a clinical study. The sample size is ideally large enough to achieve a sufficiently high power to detect minimally clinically relevant differences.
• *P value.* The probability of observing a value as extreme or more extreme than the one observed, when there really is no true association. This value is not the same as the probability of a finding by chance alone. If the p value is less than the preset significance level α, then the finding is considered not due to chance.

Levels of evidence

Evidence-based medicine is a method used for guiding clinical decision making based on critically analyzed information. There are now standard texts for this discipline. These approaches, however, are now commonplace and the clinician should be aware of the information available (see Table 2.1).

Systematic reviews

A *systematic review* is a summary of the medical literature that uses a standardized methodology for searching databases, appraising the content of individual studies, and synthesizing all the data in a coherent and statistically rigorous manner. When this process involves quantitative data it could be called a "meta-analysis."

Guidelines

A *clinical guideline* is a series of systematically developed statements that are used to assist clinical decisions. Guidelines should provide a summary of the evidence (quality and level) on which the statements are based, and an instruction on applying the evidence in practice.

Expert opinions

When there is little in the way of systematic or high-quality data, one may have to resort to the advice of a panel of experts. The approach can be systematized with a technique called the "Delphi" approach. In this iterative process one brings together a panel of experts who each assign a score (0 to 9) to statements about practice, management, or care. The process continues with changes to statements until consensus is achieved. Each step, for acceptance or rejection, has strict criteria.

Table 2.1 Recommended levels of evidence

Recommendation	Level of evidence
A (Best)	1. Systematic reviews, randomized controlled trials (RCT), all-or-none case series
B	2. Cohort studies, low-quality RCT, outcomes
	3. Case–control studies
C	4. Case series and poor-quality cohort studies

Further reading

1. Altman DG (2008). *Practical Statistics for Medical Research*. London: Chapman and Hall.
2. Friedman LM, Furberg CD, Demets DL (1998). *Fundamentals of Clinical Trials*. New York: Springer Science + Business Media, LLC.
3. Sackett DL, Straus S, Richardson WS, Rosenberg W, Haynes RB (2000). *Evidence-Based Medicine: How to Practice and Teach EBM*. London: Churchill Livingstone.

Clinical assessment

Communication skills

Communication skills are central to the practice of pediatrics. With experience and study, you will develop competencies in the following areas.

Personal

- *Courtesy* to families, colleagues, and members of the multidisciplinary team
- *Patience and sensitivity* in your communication with children and their families
- *Empathy* for children, young people, and their families experiencing difficulty and distress
- *Insight* into personal limitations and when help should be sought in managing sensitive and complex situations

Professional

- Understand how to manage consultations with infants, young children, adolescents, and their families effectively.
- Learn how to listen to children and young people, i.e., hear their needs, respect their views, and respond in an age-appropriate manner when the child is feeling vulnerable.
- Develop an effective way of communicating information about a diagnosis or prognosis or emotional issues to children, adolescents, and their families.
- Know when interpreters are required in your communication with those children and families unable to speak or understand English.
- Learn what information is appropriate to share with children, based on their physical and mental maturity.

Taking a pediatric history

This section will provide you with a framework for conducting the full pediatric medical history and examination. With experience, there may be shortcuts that can be made, but it is always advisable to be thorough and complete. As you become more skilled, you will develop your own style and process to ensure that you do not miss important information. When you write up your notes, it is standard to record the important positive and negative findings and observations. Remember that these notes are a form of communication between you and your colleagues, or for you at a later date. All written communications should be legible, clear, and logical.

Practice point

Always record the following:
• Date and time when you undertook the consultation
• Who was present, including chaperones
• Who gave the history

The presenting complaint

There are many ways in which the human body can respond to illness or disease. To the clinician, the presenting complaint may be a symptom, a sign, a finding, or a laboratory abnormality. If it is not clear to you what the problem is, ask yourself or the patient and/or caregiver, "Why has this child and family sought medical attention now?" Record the patient or parent's description of the problem.

Box 3.1 lists, in alphabetical order, a selection of common pediatric symptoms and problems that bring children to the hospital. Box 3.2 provides the most common complaints that result in telephone calls or clinic visits. A more detailed account of these complaints can be found throughout the book.

> **Box 3.1 Common pediatric symptoms and problems resulting in hospitalization**
>
> - Abdominal mass, p. 880
> - Abdominal pain, p. 364
> - Anemia, p. 628
> - Ataxia, p. 622
> - Apnea, p. 173
> - Asthma, p. 304
> - Bleeding, bruising, or purpura, p. 638
> - Croup, p. 295
> - Cyanosis, p. 275
> - Dehydration, p. 100
> - Developmental delay, p. 536
> - Diabetes, p. 482
> - Diarrhea, p. 358
> - Edema, p. 438
> - Fever, p. 702
> - Hypotonia, p. 608
> - Lymphadenitis, p. 652
> - Lymphadenopathy, p. 652
> - Pyelonephritis, p. 412
> - Rash, p. 836
> - Respiratory distress, p. 56
> - Seizure, p. 589
> - Shock, p. 77
> - Stridor, p. 295
> - Vertigo, p. 622
> - Weakness, p. 608
> - Wheeze, p. 304

Box 3.2 Common pediatric complaints resulting in telephone consultation

- Asthma, p. 304
- Constipation, p. 360
- Croup, p. 295
- Cough, p. 296
- Diarrhea, p. 358
- Earache, p. 936
- Fever, p. 702
- Hives, p. 942
- Immunization reaction, p. 746
- Rash, p. 836
- Sore throat, p. 712
- Trauma
- Vomiting, p. 356

History of present illness

Once you have established the presenting problem, you will need to answer the following questions:

- When did the current problem start—what was it like?
- Has the problem changed? If so, when and how?
- Has the patient sought medical attention before now? If so, what investigations have been done, and what treatments have been tried?
- Ask specifically about general health: activity level, alertness, eating, drinking, urination, stool patterns, and vomiting.

Past medical history

On reviewing the child's past medical history, there are six areas that should be covered by your questioning.

Prenatal history

- How many pregnancies has mother had; what were the outcomes?
- What was the length of pregnancy with this child?
- Were there any complications during the pregnancy, such as abnormal bleeding, illness, or infection?
- Did the mother take medications during pregnancy?

Birth history

- What was this child's length of gestation and what was the weight?
- How long was labor?
- Was there maternal fever or premature rupture of membranes?
- Was any intervention required at delivery?

Neonatal history

- Did the child have any neonatal problems—i.e., jaundice, cyanosis, or respiratory distress?
- Was vitamin K given?
- Was the baby treated in the neonatal intensive care unit?
- When did the baby and mother go home?

Child development

- When did the baby achieve key developmental milestones, e.g., smiling, rolling over, sitting unaided, standing, speaking, and toileting skills?
- Has the child grown normally in weight and length (height)?
- Have there been any concerns about physical or cognitive development, socialization, vision, hearing, or speech?
- Has the child lost physical or cognitive skills after they were obtained?
- How is the child performing in school?

Immunizations

- What immunizations has the child received? Start from birth and review the date when each was given. If any immunizations have been missed or omitted, identify any reasons (e.g., was the child unwell?)
- Did the child have any reactions to any of the immunizations?

Illnesses, hospitalizations, and procedures

In this part of the history you will need to find out about past visits to the doctor and any admissions to hospital that the child has had.

- Childhood illness and infections: What infections and illnesses has the child had? Does the child have any chronic conditions such as asthma, diabetes, or epilepsy?
- Is the child receiving any medication? Why?
- Are there any allergies to medications?
- Has the child been hospitalized? When and why?
- Surgical procedures and investigations: What, if anything, has been done in the past?
- Is the child seeing another clinician? Why?

Review of systems

An organized review of systems is an essential component of the physical examination and required for reimbursement for your encounter. The following list of questions can be used for further review, although it is not exhaustive. Some of these questions will have been covered in your assessment of the presenting problem, so there is no need to repeat them. However, it is important that you tailor this part of the history to issues you think are relevant to the child's condition, particularly when you suspect multisystem disease.

General health
• Is the child alert and responsive? Is there fatigue?

Head
• Is there a history of injury, headaches, or infection?

Eyes
• How good is visual acuity—are glasses needed?
• Is there a history of infection, injury, or surgery?
• Are there concerns about eyes crossing or eye movements?

Ear, nose, and throat
• Is there a problem with hearing or balance?
• Is there a history of ear infection or discharge?
• Is there any difficulty with breathing?
• Is there a history of nasal discharge, snoring, or bleeding?
• Are there any enlarged lumps or glands?
• Is there a history of sore throat, dental problems, or mouth ulcers?

Chest
• Is there any limitation to exercise?
• Is there a history of cough, wheeze, chest pain, or hemoptysis?
• Has there been any exposure to tuberculosis?
• Has the child ever had a chest X-ray?
• Does the child smoke? Are there any smokers in the family?

Heart
• Is there a history of heart murmur or rheumatic fever in the patient or family?
• Is there a history of dyspnea, orthopnea, chest pain, or cyanosis?

Gastrointestinal
• How is the child's appetite?
• Have there been any recent changes in weight, food tolerance, or bowel movements?
• Has there been any rectal bleeding?

Genitourinary

- Is there a history of infection?
- How frequent is urination?
- Is there any dysuria, or hematuria, or discharge?
- Is there a history of bedwetting?
- What was the age of menarche?
- (Adolescents) Is the child sexually active?

Joint, limbs, and tissue

- Is there any pain?
- Is there swelling or limitation in movement?
- Is there muscle weakness?
- Is there any difficulty walking or a limp?

Nervous system

- Is there a history of seizures, fainting or dizziness?
- Have there been headaches?
- Are there problems with balance?
- Are there any abnormal involuntary movements or tremors?
- How has the child being progressing at school? Has there been a recent change that has concerned the teachers or the family?
- Is there a history of hyperactivity?

Skin

- Is there a rash?
- Are there any birthmarks or unusual pigmentations on the skin?

Family history

In pediatrics, the family history is one of the most important components of the history.
- *Ages of parents and siblings*: You will need to be able to draw the family pedigree. Include the entire extended family with ages.
- *Illness in the family*: Does anyone have a history of seizures, asthma, cancer, heart disease, tuberculosis, or any other medical condition? What was the age of onset and what has been the medical advice so far?

Death in the family: Have there been any deaths in the family? What was the cause and age at death? Has anyone died during infancy or childhood?

> **Practice point**
>
> Draw a family pedigree to assist in your note-taking and identification of key family and social history information.

Social history
- Where does the family live?
- Who resides in the residence?
- What are the occupations of the family members?
- Are there any pets?
- How is the child performing at school?
- Does the child interact well with other children?

Examining a child

The physical examination of a child is one of the most difficult aspects of the doctor–patient interaction. You will need to have gained the confidence of the family and the child if you are to get the information you require. The way in which you approach the family (and how you communicate with them) throughout the interaction will be recognized by the child. A child may decide very early into the interview whether to trust you to examine them. No amount of coercing will improve the situation—the parent will often be your advocate and do the convincing for you. In order to provide the best medical care, it is very important to invest in the art of communication—how to talk with children, from toddlers to teenagers, and to parents of sick children.

The following description is not meant to be prescriptive. There is much overlap among the different systems and you will have to economize on when, and in what order, you do things. For example, the tongue is assessed in the respiratory, cardiovascular, and gastrointestinal systems—just look at it once and learn to do it quickly!

General condition

- *State of health*: Note the child's general appearance. Is there any evidence of chronic illness? Make an assessment of mental state: behavior, and interaction with the parents. Is the child alert, tired, lethargic, or agitated?
- *Height, weight, and head circumference*: These measurements are often made before you see the child. If these measurements are abnormal, repeat them yourself.
- *Hydration*: Examine capillary refill, mucous membranes, anterior fontanelle, sunken eyes, skin turgor, and pulse.

Practice point

- In children less than 2 years of age, obtain a length measurement using a table stadiometer. In older children, height can be measured in the standing position.
- Weigh the child unclothed.
- Measure the head occipitofrontal circumference (OFC) at the maximum point of the occipital protuberance and at the mid-forehead.
- Each of these measurements should be plotted on standard charts and the centiles recorded along with the raw data.

The body mass index (BMI) should be calculated.

Vital signs

See also p. 42.

- *Temperature*: There are various ways in which the body temperature can be measured. Different units use different methods:
  - an electronic thermometer in the axillary;
  - a chemical dot thermometer in the axillary; or
  - an infrared tympanic thermometer.

A sick child may have either a high or abnormally low temperature.

- *Pulse rate*: The pulse rate should be assessed from the radial pulse. (In the younger child, you may find it easier to use brachial pulse). Assess the rate, character, and rhythm at the radial pulse.
- *Respiratory rate*: In the older child, you can observe the chest and count the number of breaths per minute. Breaks or pauses in breathing that last longer than 15 seconds are abnormal. In the infant, count abdominal movements over 1 minute, if you find that it is easier to see diaphragmatic rather than chest wall movement (see Table 3.1).
- *Blood pressure (BP)*: Measurement is now commonly performed using an automated method (see Nephrology section). It is important that the size and width of the cuff is appropriate for the size of the limb in which pressure is being measured. Use a cuff that covers 50% to 75% of the upper arm or thigh. A single measurement is required in most instances, but if you suspect heart disease, then four limb measurements are needed. Plot the observations on BP centile charts.

Table 3.1 Normal values of respiratory rate and heart rate at different ages

Age	Respiratory rate (breaths per minute)	Heart rate (beats per minute)
0–6 months	30–50	120–140
6–12 months	20–40	95–120
1–5 years	20–30	90–110
6–10 years	18–25	80–100
>10 years	12–25	60–100

Respiratory system

See also p. 292.

- *Lips and buccal mucosa*: What is the color of the mucous membranes and lips? Is the tongue in good condition? What is its color? Are there any plaques, white patches, or spots?
- *Oropharynx*: What is the color and size of the tonsils? Is there an exudate? What is the shape of the palate, uvula, and posterior pharynx?
- *Chest*: What is the shape of the chest? Are there any scars or deformities? What is the position of the trachea? Is there dullness or hyper-resonance by percussion?
- *Breathing*: Are there any signs of respiratory distress: is there nasal flaring, intercostal, subcostal, and/or sternal retraction, use of accessory muscles, forced expiration, grunting, or tracheal tug? Is there an audible noise during inspiration or expiration?
- *Auscultation of the lungs*: Listen for breath sounds in all regions of the chest. Evaluate the length and ratio of inspiration and expiration. In the crying child you will still be able to listen during inspiration. Are there any fine crackles, rhonchi, or wheezes? Is there a pleural friction rub?
- *Ears*: The child will need to be positioned correctly for this part of the examination. It is often easier to have the child sit on the parent's lap; one of the parent's arms should be held around the upper body of the child, with hand of the other arm placed against the side of the child's head so that it is firm against the parent. Is there evidence of otitis externa? Is there a rash in the postauricular area (a feature of dermatitis, measles, and rubella)? On otoscopy check the state of the tympanic membrane: what is its color and degree of lucency? Is it perforated, or is there a myringotomy tube present?
- *Nose*: Is there discharge? Can the child breathe through each nostril?

> **Practice point**
>
> You should be able to recognize the following patterns of abnormal signs:
> - Consolidation
> - Collapse or removal of a lung
> - Pleural effusion
> - Pneumothorax
> - Airflow obstruction
> - Bronchiectasis

Cardiovascular system

- *Color and cyanosis* (see Respiratory system): Examine the color of the sclerae and conjunctivae.
- *Teeth*: Assess the number and condition of the teeth.
- *Clubbing*: Assess fingers and toes. Is there any peripheral edema?
- *Pulses and rhythm*: Compare the strength of the femoral and right brachial pulse. Pulse rate varies with the phase of respiration. It increases with inspiration and decreases with expiration.
- *Chest*: Identify the position of the apex beat and consider whether it is displaced. In young children (<7 years) it will be in the fourth intercostal space, to the left of the mid-clavicular line, on the left. In the child older than 7 years, it will be in the fifth to sixth intercostal spaces. If it is not palpable, check the right side to exclude dextrocardia. Are there any other pulsations, heaves, or vibrations that can be felt in the chest wall?
- *Murmurs* (see Box 3.3): Auscultate the heart with the child in the sitting and supine positions. Listen over the entire precordium: the apex, the second intercostal space to the left of the sternum (pulmonary valve area), the second intercostal space to the right of the sternum (aortic valve area), and the fourth intercostal space over the sternum (tricuspid valve area). Listen to the heart sounds in each of these areas. Are the sounds muffled and suggestive of pericardial fluid? In the pulmonary valve area, is the second heart sound split during inspiration? (Fixed splitting is found with atrial septal defect.) At the apex, is a third heart sound present, indicating mitral valve prolapse or atrial septal defect? Is there a gallop rhythm of congestive heart failure?

Box 3.3 Murmurs (see p. 260)

Now listen for added noises during the cardiac cycle. If there is one, then it should be described according to the following factors:
- Loudness—grade I to VI
- Timing in the cardiac cycle—diastolic or systolic; early, mid, or late
- Pitch—high or low
- Quality—blowing, musical, or rough
- Location where best heard—apex, pulmonary, aortic, or left sternal

Radiation—where, if anywhere, does the noise transmit across the chest? Listen to the back.

Gastrointestinal system

Make an assessment of whether the child is jaundiced.

Abdomen

The child needs to be relaxed and positioned supine, with the knees bent and hands by the sides.

- Look at the shape of the abdomen. Is it distended? Is the umbilicus everted?
- Does the abdominal wall move? Is the child in pain? Is peristalsis visible?
- Let the child know that you are going to touch the abdomen; they should be free to tell you if it hurts. Do not hurt the child. First auscultate for bowel sounds, and then percuss to assess for hepatomegaly and ascites. In the right midclavicular line an enlarged liver extends more than 2 cm below the costal margin. Table 3.2 describes the normal span of the liver—between its upper and lower margins.
- Palpate the abdomen and check for any tenderness before assessing rebound. Palpate for masses during inspiration and deep expiration. Can you feel an abnormal spleen, liver, or kidney?
- Watch the child feeding.

Rectum and anus

In most instances you will only need to observe the patency of the anus and to look for fissures and rectal prolapse. However, if the child has abdominal symptoms, then a digital examination may be required to check for sphincter tone, masses, and tenderness.

This examination should only be done once and you will need to decide whether this test is performed by a senior colleague or by a surgeon, if the child has an acute abdomen.

Table 3.2 Normal span of liver between upper and lower margins

At 6 months	2 cm below costal margin
At 3 years	4 cm span
At 10 years	6 cm span
In adults	10 cm span

Genitourinary system

See also p. 260.

The external genitalia are examined for any evidence of ambiguity, congenital abnormality, and size. For this examination you should have a chaperone present for both sexes. In the older child you must ensure privacy and preserve the child's dignity with appropriate use of covers, gloves, and gowns—only examine once.

- *In boys*: The development of the penis, testes, scrotum, and pubic hair can be staged using a standardized system (Tanner scale). Look at the state of the foreskin and whether there is evidence of infection or discharge. Locate the position of the penile meatus. Have both testes descended?
- *In girls*: Use the Tanner scale to stage the pubic hair. Is there evidence of fused labia, enlarged clitoris, or infection with discharge or bleeding?

Musculoskeletal system

See also p. 750.

- *Congenital anomalies*: Examine the fingers, toes, hands and feet, legs and arms. Look at the shape of the bones.
- *Deformities*: Are there deformities due to fracture? Are the lower limbs of equal length? What is the range of motion of each joint? Are the skin folds in the upper thigh symmetrical? In the infant under 6 months check for congenital hip dislocation. Inspect the full length of the spine, looking for tufts of hair, dimples, masses, or cysts at the base. Check for torticollis in the neck. Observe for any abnormal curvature or posture with the child standing and bending over, touching their toes.
- *Gait*: Watch the child walk and describe gait in light of your other findings.

Practice point (see also p. 582)

You should be able to recognize gaits associated with
- Myopathy (waddling)
- Hemiplegia
- Spastic diplegia
- Cerebellar ataxia
- Painful limb (antalgic gait)
- Foot drop
- Trendelenburg gait

Resuscitation

Cardiopulmonary arrest

Respiratory arrest is much more common in children than cardiac arrest and is associated with a survival rate of 80%. Cardiopulmonary arrest in children is often the end result of progressive deterioration in the lungs and heart. The outcome of cardiac arrest in children, both in the hospital (40%) and out of the hospital (5%), may best be improved by early recognition of impeding of arrest.

Children with any of the features in Table 4.1 warrant urgent medical review.

Table 4.1 Warning signs for impending acute deterioration

- Threatened airway obstruction
- Tachypnea

Age	Action respiratory rate
Term to 3 months	>60 breaths/minute
4–12 months	>50 breaths/minute
1–4 years	>40 breaths/minute
5–12 years	>30 breaths/minute
Above 12 years	>30 breaths/minute

- Bradycardia or tachycardia

Age	Bradycardia
Term to 3 months	<100 beats/minute
4–12 months	<100 beats/minute
1–4 years	<90 beats/minute
5–12 years	<80 beats/minute
Above 12 years	<60 beats/minute

- Hypotension

Age	Action systolic pressure
Term to 3 months	<50 mm Hg
4–12 months	<60 mm Hg
1–4 years	<70 mm Hg
5–12 years	<80 mm Hg
Above 12 years	<90 mm Hg

- Altered mental state or convulsion
- Low pulse oximetry values <90% (<60% if cyanotic heart disease)

Rapid cardiopulmonary assessment

The rapid cardiopulmonary assessment should take less than 1 minute.

Airway
- Is it patent?

Breathing
- What is the effort and work of breathing? Is there recession, nasal flaring, grunting, use of accessory muscles, stridor or wheeze?
- What is the air entry like in the chest?
- What is the respiratory rate: is it fast or slow?
- What is the skin color?

Circulation
- What is the heart rate?
- What is the systemic perfusion? Check pulse volume, capillary refill, skin temperature, level of consciousness, and urine output.
- What is the blood pressure?

Disability
- What is the level of consciousness?
- What are the pupils like—size and reaction?

Pediatric basic life support (BLS)

Cardiopulmonary arrest in children usually results from hypoxia due to respiratory or neurological failure or shock. If it occurs, irrespective of the cause, BLS must be started immediately (see Box 4.1).

Box 4.1 Pediatric basic life support algorithm

1. First things
- Assess the safety of the situation
- Stimulate the child and check responsiveness

2. Shout for help

3. Open the airway
- Give head tilt and chin lift, or jaw thrust

4. Assess breathing
- Look, listen, and feel

5. If no breathing: rescue breaths
- *Child*: 2 effective breaths mouth to mouth (5 attempts)
- *Infant*: 2 effective breaths mouth to mouth and nose (5 attempts)

6. Assess the pulse
- *Child*: at the carotid artery
- *Infant*: at the brachial artery

7. If heart rate <60/minute and poor perfusion: chest compressions
- *Child >8 years*: Use two-handed method for rate of 100/minute and ratio of 15 compressions to 2 breaths
- *Child 1–8 years*: Use heel of hand in the middle of the sternum for rate of 100/minute and ratio of 15 compressions to 2 breaths
- *Infant*: Use two fingers or the encircling chest technique if you have help, at rate of 100/minute and ratio of 15 compressions to 2 breaths

8. Provide 1 minute of life support

9. Contact emergency medical services

Conscious choking children

Box 4.2 is the algorithm to follow in the child or infant who is conscious. If the child becomes unconscious at any stage use the algorithm for unconscious choking children (Box 4.3).

> ## Box 4.2 Algorithm for conscious choking children
>
> *1. First things*
> - Assess the safety of the situation
> - Check the mouth and remove any visible object if safe to do so
>
> *2. Deliver 5 back blows*
> - *Child*: Follow this with 5 abdominal thrusts
> - *Infant*: Follow this with 5 chest thrusts
>
> *3. Are airway and breathing adequate?*
> - If not and the patient is conscious, return to step 2 and continue to follow this algorithm

Unconscious choking children

The algorithm in Box 4.3 should be followed:
- *Basic life support*: If the rescuer is unable to achieve ventilation despite 5 attempts with airway repositioning
- *Unconscious*: If following the conscious choking algorithm (Box 4.2) the child loses consciousness

---

Box 4.3 Algorithm for unconscious choking children

1. First things
- Assess the safety of the situation
- Check the mouth and remove any visible object if it is safe to do so

2. Deliver 5 back blows
- Follow this with 5 chest thrusts

3. Is the airway adequate?
- Check the mouth for visible obstructions
- Open the airway and if child is not breathing, attempt 5 rescue breaths

4. If airway and breathing are inadequate
- *Child*: Deliver 5 back blows and then 5 abdominal thrusts. Then check the mouth for visible obstructions, open the airway, and if not breathing, attempt 5 rescue breaths. If airway and breathing remain inadequate return to step 2 and continue to follow this algorithm
- *Infant*: Return to step 2 and continue to follow this algorithm

5. Object expelled or ventilation achieved
- Return to the BLS algorithm

Pediatric advanced life support

Box 4.4 Pediatric advanced life support algorithm

1. BLS algorithm

2. Ventilate and oxygenate
- For bag/mask ventilation, cycles of 15 compressions/2 breaths. ONCE stable airway is achieved, respiratory rate is 10–20

3. Check pulse (continuously if possible)
- Begin chest compressions for absent pulse or heart rate (HR) <60 with poor perfusion

4. Attach defibrillator and access cardiac rhythm
Ventricular fibrillation (VF)/pulseless tachycardia (VT)
- Defibrillate: 2 J/kg for initial shock, resume CPR for 2 minutes
- Reassess rhythm and pulse
- If VF/VT persists, then shock 4 J/kg, resume CPR for 2 minutes
- Reassess rhythm and pulse
- If VF/VT persists, then epinephrine (1:10,000: 0.1 mL/kg IV/IO), continue CPR for 2 minutes
- Reassess rhythm and pulse
- If VF/VT persists, then shock 4 J/kg, resume CPR for 2 minutes
- Reassess rhythm and pulse
- If VF/VT persists, then give amiodarone 5 mg/kg or lidocaine 1 mg/kg, consider magnesium 50 mg/kg

Asystole pulseless electrical activity
- Continue CPR, epinephrine 1:10,000: 0.1 mL/kg IV/IO, repeat every 3–5 minutes

5. During CPR
Ensure adequate compressions
- Central pulse should be palpable during compressions.

Relieve role of chest compressions every 3–5 minutes
Attempt and verify
- Tracheal intubation
- Intravenous (IV) or intraosseous (IO) access

Check
- Electrode or paddle placement: the position and contact, conducting gel

Give
- Epinephrine every 3 minutes: 0.1 mL/kg IV/IO (1:10,000 dilution)

Box 4.4 (Contd.)

Consider
- Anti-arrhythmics and buffers
- Potentially reversible causes: hypoxia, hypovolemia, hypokalemia, hyperkalemia, tension pneumothorax, cardiac tamponade, toxins, thromboemboli

6. Are there difficulties in ventilation?

Rule out the following potential problems:
- Is the endotracheal tube displaced?
- Is there an obstruction?
- Does the child have a pneumothorax?
- Is there equipment failure?
- Is there air in the stomach causing diaphragmatic splinting?

Box 4.5 Useful formula in children

Estimation of weight
- Under 1 year: Newborn = 3.5 kg; 6 months = 6.0 kg
- Over 1 year: Weight = [(Age in years + 4) × 2] kg

Endotracheal tube
- Size of cuffed tube = (Age in years/4) + 3
- Depth of insertion = tube internal diameter × 3

Rhythm disturbances

See p. 290.

Bradycardia
- Bradycardia is often the final response to hypoxia.
- A preterminal rhythm leading to asystole
- It is more important to treat in infants because of rate-dependent cardiac output.

Treatment
- Oxygen, with attention to airway and inflation
- May require atropine 20 µg/kg

Sinus tachycardia
- Heart rate can be as high as 220/minute in an infant but not higher
- Caused by fever, pain and shock, dehydration

Treatment
- Treat the cause.

Supraventricular tachycardia
- The most common primary arrhythmia in infancy and childhood
- Onset is sudden; HR: >220 infants, >180 children over 3 years
- Rhythm is regular and P waves may not be visible.
- Infants may present with shock, sweatiness, and poor feeding.

Treatment
- See algorithms in Box 4.6 and Box 4.7 on p. 51

Ventricular tachycardia
- Rare in children, caused by primary cardiac problem or overdose
- Heart rate: between 120 and 250 per minute
- Rhythm is almost regular but QRS is wide (>2 small squares)

Treatment
- Pulse present: amiodarone 5 mg/kg given slowly, synchronized shock
- Pulseless: treat as for ventricular fibrillation

Ventricular fibrillation
- Mainly caused by hypothermia and drug overdose
- 17% of all pediatric arrests

Treatment
- See algorithm in Box 4.4

Asystole
- Mainly caused by hypoxia and acidosis
- 60% of all pediatric arrests

Treatment
- See algorithm in Box 4.4

Pulseless electrical activity
- See algorithm in Box 4.4

Supraventricular tachycardia

Attach cardiac monitor and check blood pressure.

Box 4.6 Algorithm for treating a patient with supraventricular tachycardia but not in shock

1. Patient not in shock

2. Trial of vagal maneuvers

3. Adenosine
- 50 µg/kg given as a rapid IV push into the most central IV access available, followed by fast IV flush
- If no response, then 100 µg/kg
- If no response, then 250 µg/kg

4. Consider
- Synchronous DC shock
- Verapamil (IV bolus over 2–3 minutes)
  - Birth to 2 years: 100–200 µg/kg (maximum 2 mg)
  - 2–18 years: 100–300 µg/kg (maximum 5 mg)
- Amiodarone (IV bolus over 60 minutes)
  - 5 mg/kg
- Esmolol infusion
  - 50–300 µg/kg/min

Box 4.7 Algorithm for treating a patient with supraventricular tachycardia who is in shock

1. Patient in shock
- Attempt vagal maneuvers but do not delay progress to step 2.
- If IV access is available give adenosine (see Box 4.6) but do not delay progress to step 2.

2. Synchronous DC shock
- 0.5 J/kg
- If no response, then 1 J/kg
- If no response, then 2 J/kg

3. Consider using anti-arrhythmics

4. Synchronous DC shock
- Return to step 2 in the algorithm at 2 J/kg

Following unsuccessful resuscitation

The death of a child is distressing. The family or caregivers should be spoken to sympathetically and in private, in person, if at all possible. Most parents will want to see and hold their dead child and should be offered this opportunity. If available, services of pastoral care or social work should be extended.

Report to the medical examiner

In the United States, the coroner needs to be informed of the following:
- All unexpected deaths, deaths within 24 hours of discharge or admission to a hospital, and all deaths related to trauma
- Always call the medical examiner's office for clarification if you are uncertain of what needs to be done. The medical examiner will also dictate if any therapeutic devices may be removed, for example, the endotracheal tube. If the medical examiner declines the need for a postmortem exam, then the certificate of death needs to fully completed and signed.

Report to the organ procurement agency

In the United States, it is federal law to report all deaths, prior to death if possible, to the local organ procurement agency.

Follow-up

- Arrangements should be made for the family to discuss the results of the coroner's postmortem report and, when relevant, consider its implications for future pregnancies.
- Genetic counseling may be needed.
- Bereavement counseling should be offered. This may be provided by physicians or health professionals within the pediatric team or from other agencies.

Emergency and high-acuity care

The ABCs of high acuity

Providing effective emergency care requires a systematic approach to assessment and treatment that delivers potentially life-saving interventions in a timely manner. Graded intervention—tailoring your treatment to the degree of physiologic derangement—and anticipation of next steps are critical to successful life support. Always start with assessment and treatment of the ABCs (**A**irway, **B**reathing, and **C**irculation).

Establish an airway

Maintain airway and air movement

- Determine if the airway is clear, maintainable, or unmaintainable.
- Open the airway with a jaw thrust.
- Suction nasopharynx and mouth as needed.
- Provide oral or nasopharyngeal airway.
- Consider endotracheal intubation for an unmaintainable airway.
- Keep patient in a position of comfort: Do not force a distressed patient to lie down.

Use respiratory support for breathing

Provide oxygen

- Administer supplemental oxygen to maintain adequate arterial oxygen saturation (SaO_2) as measured by pulse oximetry (>94%).

Infants, toddlers
Nasal cannula (NC), face mask

Toddler, preschool
NC, face mask

School-age
NC, partial non-rebreathing mask

Support oxygenation and ventilation

- Identify the severity and anatomic or physiologic cause of respiratory distress—e.g., upper versus lower airway obstruction.
- Treat specific problems appropriately (e.g., with bronchodilators).
- Assist work of breathing with noninvasive support. This can be achieved with nasopharyngeal continuous positive airway pressure (CPAP) (see Bronchiolitis) or positive-pressure ventilation with a bag-mask resuscitator.
- If noninvasive interventions do not achieve a stable airway and adequate oxygenation and ventilation, consider endotracheal intubation and mechanical ventilation.

Assess circulation, establish IV access

- Start pulse oximetry and cardiac monitoring.
- Establish peripheral vascular access.
- If a peripheral IV line cannot be rapidly placed in a critically ill or injured patient, consider placement of an intraosseous (IO) line.
- Provide IV fluids: Administer crystalloid (normal saline or Ringer's lactate) in 20 cc/kg boluses to support circulation; reassess cardiorespiratory status after each bolus.
- Perform bedside glucose test—treat documented hypoglycemia.

Respiratory distress

Respiratory distress is defined as increased work of breathing with systemic compromise. The hallmarks are an increased respiratory rate (tachypnea) and respiratory effort (nasal flaring, retractions, use of accessory muscles). It can be associated with a change in airway sounds, skin color, or mental status. Distress can be caused by disorders of gas exchange (O_2 absorption, or CO_2 elimination), respiratory drive, neuromuscular disease, or infection.

The differential diagnosis for respiratory distress is provided in Box 5.1.

Box 5.1 Differential diagnoses for respiratory distress

Nasopharynx
- *Nose*: Choanal atresia, stenosis, foreign body, mass, trauma
- *Oropharynx*: Tonsillitis, trauma
- *Tongue*: Macroglossia, Ludwig's angina, trauma
- *Pharynx*: Peritonsillar abscess, retropharyngeal abscess, diphtheria, trauma

Upper airway obstruction
- *Larynx*: Croup, laryngomalacia, foreign body, thermal or chemical burn, vocal cord dysfunction, papilloma, hemangioma, trauma
- *Epiglottis*: Epiglottitis, foreign body

Lower airway disorder
- *Trachea*: Tracheitis, tracheomalacia, foreign body, trachoesophageal fistula
- *Bronchi*: Bronchomalacia, bronchitis, bronchogenic cyst, congenital malformation
- *Bronchioles*: Asthma, bronchiolitis, pertussis, allergy, aspiration, angioneurotic edema

Disordered gas exchange
- *Hemoglobin*: Anemia, carbon monoxide poisoning, methemoglobinemia, acidosis, loss, polycythemia
- *Shunt*: Pulmonary edema, hemorrhage, atelectasis, embolism
- *Dead space ventilation*: Asthma, bronchiolitis, pulmonary hypertension
- *Other*: Sickle chest syndrome, pneumonia, pneumothorax

Respiratory drive
- *Central nervous system*: Structural abnormality, immaturity, infection (meningitis, encephalitis, abscess), intoxication, seizure, trauma

Neuromuscular
- *Peripheral motor nerve*: Phrenic nerve injury, Guillain–Barre syndrome, multiple sclerosis, tick paralysis, porphyria
- *Neuromuscular junction*: Myasthenia gravis, botulism, organophosphates
Muscle: Muscular dystrophy, inborn error of metabolism, fatigue

Additional considerations
- *Pleural*: Pneumothorax, chylothorax, hemothorax, pleural effusion, empyema, diaphragmatic hernia
- *Chest wall*: Rib fractures, flail chest, burn
- *Cardiovascular*: Congenital (arrhythmia), acquired (myocarditis, infarction, pericardial effusion, aortic dissection, congestive heart failure, coronary aneurysm)

Respiratory distress: assessment

Clinical assessment

- *Work of breathing*: Nasal flaring, retractions, use of accessory muscles, body position of comfort
- *Airway sounds*: Upper airway obstruction produces stridor; lower airway obstruction leads to cough, wheeze, and a prolonged expiratory phase.
- *Respiratory drive*: Pattern and rate may reflect a central cause; bradypnea usually precedes impending failure.
- *Chest wall movement*: Chest and abdominal wall dynamics may indicate flail chest, diaphragmatic palsy, pneumothorax, or foreign body.
- *Appearance*: Tone, mental status
- *Circulation*: Color (pallor or cyanosis) and heart rate may reflect impending arrest.

Investigations

- *Pulse oximetry* to measure oxyhemoglobin saturation (SpO_2)
- *Arterial blood gas or capillary blood gas*: Assessment of acid base, PaO_2, $PaCO_2$. A capillary blood sample is a good alternative (for pH, PCO_2) if the extremity is warm and the blood flows freely.
- *Blood tests* may include complete blood count (CBC) and blood cultures (if concerned about infection, anemia), electrolytes, blood urea nitrogen (BUN), creatinine (Cr), and glucose (if concerned about metabolic or endocrine disease).
- *Chest X-ray* (anteroposterior [AP]/lateral) for diagnosis (e.g., severe pneumonia) or for assessment of complications (e.g., pneumothorax)
- *CT scan*: Head (if concerned about central mass, hydrocephalus), chest (if there is concern for congenital anomaly, tumor)

Monitoring

- Pulse oximetry
- Continuous electrocardiogram (ECG)
- Blood pressure
- Temperature
- Fluid balance
- Level of consciousness

Criteria for respiratory failure

Clinical

- Increasing fatigue, irregular respirations, tachypnea, bradypnea
- Altered mental status
- Poor or absent cough, gag, swallow
- Poor muscle tone

Laboratory
- Hypoxemia despite high fractional inspired oxygen (FiO_2): PaO_2 <60 mmHg in >60% O_2, previously healthy child
- Acidosis: pH <7.3
- Vital capacity <15 mL/kg
- Maximum inspiratory pressure <25 cm H_2O

Respiratory distress: management

Therapy

There are specific therapies for each condition listed in the differential diagnoses in Box 5.1 (see individual sections).

- For *all causes*, treatment should be initiated to restore ventilation and oxygenation.
- *Airway patency*: Position patient with chin lift (contraindicated if suspected neck trauma) or jaw thrust, clear oral cavity of fluids (secretions, blood, vomit). Unconscious patients may need nasopharyngeal, oral-airway, or endotracheal tubes (ETT).
- *Ventilation*: After patency has been established, support may include continuous positive airway pressure (CPAP), bag valve mask (BVM) ventilation, or endotracheal intubation, and placement of a nasogastric (NG) tube for stomach decompression.
- *Oxygenation*: Supplemental oxygen, 100% FiO_2
- *Consider overall fluid balance*: Additional fluid may be needed or excess fluid may impair ventilation and oxygenation.

Foreign-body inhalation

Foreign-body (FB) aspiration is more common in toddlers and infants, who tend to put objects in their mouths. FBs can be inhaled into the airway, or they may be retained in the esophagus and compress the trachea of a young child.

Symptoms

The symptoms of a FB in the respiratory/digestive tract range from no symptoms to complete airway obstruction.

- *Larynx*: Apnea and cyanosis due to complete obstruction; partial obstruction may present with stridor and increased work of breathing; hoarseness, cough, dysphonia
- *Trachea and bronchus*: Asymmetric breath sounds, wheezing, cough, increased work of breathing; may cause chest pain. After the initial coughing or choking episode, there may be a relatively asymptomatic period, followed by signs and symptoms of pneumonia (see p. 294).
- *Esophagus*: Drooling, dysphagia, vomiting. If the trachea is externally compressed, there is stridor and increased work of breathing.

Etiology

Inhaled FB should be considered in all previously well patients with a history of sudden onset of coughing, choking, or gagging, especially in the older infant or toddler age-group.

Diagnosis

- A monophonic *wheeze or absent breath sounds* on one side of the chest may be noted on examination.
- Chest and neck *radiographs*, with lateral views, may be helpful in identifying the location of a radio-opaque object, or demonstrate atelectasis. Inspiratory and expiratory films or lateral decubitus views may show unilateral hyperinflation due to air trapping.
- *Arterial blood gas analysis* is indicated when the patient is in severe distress.

Initial treatment

Follow standard protocols for foreign-body airway obstruction (FBAO):
- ABC
- FB removal
- If the child is calm, can cough, and make some sounds, do not interfere. Removal of the FB should take place under controlled circumstances in the operating room, as manipulation may change the position of the object and induce more severe obstruction.
- If the child is in severe distress and unable to make sounds, follow standard basic life support FBAO protocols:
  - For a *child*, perform subdiaphragmatic abdominal thrusts until the object is expelled or the patient loses consciousness.
  - For an *infant*, deliver 5 back blows followed by 5 chest thrusts repeatedly, until the object is expelled or the patient loses consciousness.

- Administer CPR if the child becomes unconscious; visualize the vocal cords using laryngoscopy, and remove a visible foreign body using Magill forceps.

Retained airway foreign bodies not expelled via BLS maneuvers are removed using rigid bronchoscopy under general anesthesia.

Drowning

Drowning results from submersion, usually in water, that results in respiratory impairment. Inadequate ventilation resulting in severe hypoxia leads to coma and cardiac arrest. Aspiration of water does not obstruct the airway; the type of water, sea versus freshwater, is of little consequence. Assess the duration of submersion, water temperature, and the time to establish a pulse and cardiac output. Early return of spontaneous circulation and alertness predict good outcome. Drowning in "very cold water," defined as ≤5°C, may allow survival despite long submersion and resuscitation durations.

Symptoms

- Altered mental status to coma denotes significant hypoxic insult and may lead to symptoms of cerebral edema and increased intracranial pressure, the usual cause of death or posthypoxic encephalopathy in survivors.
- Arrhythmias or cardiac arrest result from severe hypoxia.
- Mild respiratory distress to frothy pulmonary edema to full-blown acute respiratory distress syndrome (ARDS)

Etiology

The under-3-year-old and teenager are most at risk when unsupervised. Young children fall into pools; adolescents drown while swimming. Also consider the following:
- Alcohol or drug use
- Preexisting seizure disorder
- Head and neck injuries from diving or surfboard use
- Preexisting cardiac arrhythmia

Initial treatment

Follow standard basic and advanced life-support protocols:
- *AB*: Provide oxygen and ventilation as needed as soon as possible. If there is a history of possible trauma, immobilize the neck. If there are pink, frothy secretions or no gag or apnea, then intubate.
- *C*: Treat arrhythmias.
- *Temperature*: In the awake patient, remove all wet clothing at the scene. Warm the child to a core temperature >35°C (use a heating blanket). In the comatose patient, delay warming until arrival at the emergency department (ED), where mild hypothermia may be induced. For profound hypothermia, more invasive methods of warming may be used (e.g., heart-lung bypass, bladder or gastric lavage).

After resuscitation

- Assess and reassess frequently vital signs, lungs, heart, and central nervous system.
- Start pulse oximetry and cardiac monitoring.
- Blood glucose, blood gas, chest X-ray, social work consult, ECG
- Reassess frequently for worsening lower respiratory or cardiac dysfunction: use of accessory respiratory muscles, nasal flaring, tachypnea, cough, wheeze, and crackles.

Circulation: cardiovascular difficulty

The seven main categories of problems in the cardiovascular system (CVS) are described below.

1. Shock

Failure of the CVS to deliver an adequate amount of oxygen to the tissues and cells is caused by

- *Heart rate disturbance*: Bradycardia, dysrhythmias
- *Decreased stroke volume*: Hypovolemia, vasodilatation, poor contractility

2. Congestive heart failure

Excess cardiac work to maintain cardiac output produces cardiac fatigue. The causes are the following:

- *Excess volume load* from left-to-right cardiac lesions (ventricular septal defect [VSD], patent ductus arteriosus [PDA], arteriovenous [AV] canal), AV fistula, severe anemia, hypervolemia
- *Excess pressure load* from systemic vascular system (aortic stenosis, coarctation of the aorta, or hypertension), or pulmonary vascular system (pulmonary stenosis, advanced pulmonary hypertension, secondary pulmonary hypertension due to hypoxia, chronic hypoventilation, or severe upper airway obstruction)
- *Myocardial pathology* including cardiomyopathy, myocarditis, myocardial ischemia (anomalous coronary artery, coronary artery aneurysm secondary to Kawasaki), metabolic disorders (hypoglycemia, hypocalcemia, hypophosphatemia, acidosis)
- *Excess myocardial demand* due to fever, thyrotoxicosis, dysrhytmias

3. Dysrhythmia (see also p. 290)

These are uncommon, but there are two important dysrhythmias:

- Supraventricular tachycardia
- Congenital heart block

4. Hypertension (see p. 414)

5. Anaphylactic shock (see also p. 42)

Systemic anaphylactic shock can be the result of multiple causes:

- Food
- Medication
- Insect bites
- Environmental substances

The life-threatening problems are

- *Respiratory*: Airway narrowing of upper and lower airway
- *CVS*: Shock secondary to vasodilatation and increased vascular permeability

6. Pericarditis (see p. 286)

The causes include the following:

- Infection
- Rheumatologic disorders
- Trauma
- Malignancy
- Post-pericardiotomy syndrome

7. Congenital heart disease (see p. 266)

CVS difficulty: assessment

See also p. 260.

Shock

In early shock, findings can be subtle (see Box 5.2). Hypotension is a late sign signifying decompensated shock. Late shock is a pre-arrest phenomenon.

Box 5.2 Characteristics of shock

Early shock
- *Pulse*: Tachycardia
- *Blood pressure*: Normal or wide pulse pressure
- *Breathing*: Tachypnea
- *Limbs*: Cool and mottled
- *Central nervous system*: Agitated
- *Laboratory*: Mild metabolic acidosis

Classic shock
- *Pulse*: Tachycardia and weak pulses
- *Blood pressure*: Hypotension
- *Breathing*: Tachypnea and grunting
- *Limbs*: Cool, clammy, and pale
- *Central nervous system*: Depressed level of consciousness
- *Laboratory*: Metabolic acidosis

Late shock
- *Pulse*: Tachycardia and thready pulses; bradycardia is pre-arrest
- *Blood pressure*: Profound hypotension
- *Breathing*: Tachypnea or bradypnea (pre-arrest)
- *Limbs*: Cold (blue to white)
- *Central nervous system*: Coma
- *Laboratory*: Metabolic acidosis, multisystem organ failure

---

Congestive heart failure

Symptoms
- Sweating with feeds
- Generalized malaise
- Failure to thrive
- Poor exercise tolerance

Physical findings
- Tachycardia: ± gallop rhythm on auscultation
- Tachypnea: ± wheeze and crackles on auscultation
- Elevated jugular venous distension (JVD): ± hepatosplenomegaly and peripheral edema
- Pale or mottled and cool extremities
- Hypotension
- Features of underlying cause: e.g., murmur in VSD, or pallor in anemia
- Chest X-ray showing cardiomegaly and pulmonary vascular congestion to pulmonary edema

Arrhythmias

A 12-lead ECG and BP are needed for diagnosis.

Bradycardia

If there is hemodynamic instability (i.e., hypotension or poor perfusion), significant bradycardia is present if the heart rate is
- <80/minute in neonates
- <60/minute in children

Tachydysrhythmia

These may be
- *Narrow complex*: QRS duration <0.1 second in children, or <0.12 second in adolescents
- *Ventricular*: Prolonged QRS

Hypertension (see p. 414)

To diagnose hypertension, strict criteria should be followed: three measurements in nonstressful circumstances with values >95th percentile for age, height, and sex. Evaluate for the underlying cause and complications. Standard charts should be consulted, but by age, the 95th percentile of normal blood BP can be estimated by:

95% systolic BP = (100 + 2x age in years) + 4 mmHg

95% diastolic BP = (60 + 2x age in years) − 2 mmHg

until age 10 years; >80 mmHg thereafter

Pericarditis

The primary symptom will be chest pain. Evaluate for underlying cause. Physical exam findings include friction rub. ECG shows diffuse ST-segment elevation with PR depression. Complications of pericarditis are pericardial effusion and cardiac tamponade. Signs of tamponade are pulsus paradoxus (blood pressure drop of >10 mmHg during respiration), distended jugular veins, hypotension, and muffled heart sounds.

Congenital heart disease

In cyanotic babies the history and examination can be used to help exclude respiratory causes of cyanosis. The assessment also includes the hyperoxia test (measurement of PaO_2 after 15 minutes on FiO_2 100%):
- PaO_2 <100 mmHg: Likely cyanotic heart disease
- PaO_2 100–200 mmHg: Possible heart disease with complete mixing and increased pulmonary blood flow
- PaO_2 >250 mmHg: Cyanotic heart disease is unlikely

CVS difficulty: therapy

Shock

Initial therapy
- Airway: Ensure that it is appropriate.
Breathing: Provide supplemental oxygen, FiO_2 100%. Intubate if needed.
- Circulation: IV access for fluid resuscitation, medication administration (see Box 5.3)

Fluid volumes for shock
Hypovolemia
- IV bolus 20 mL/kg normal saline. Repeat as needed.

Stop resuscitation with volume
- When clinical improvement is achieved
- When clinical signs of improvement fail to appear
- If there are signs of volume overload: hepatosplenomegaly, JVD, S3 gallop, wheezing and crackles

Inotropes for shock
Start inotropes
When circulation remains unsatisfactory despite IV fluid and/or signs of congestive heart failure develop.

When central venous pressure (CVP) is >10–15 mmHg. Once initiated, titrate dose upward to produce the effect required.

Box 5.3 Intensive-care treatments for shock

- *Dopamine*: 1–20 µg/kg/min (start at 5–10 µg/kg/min). May cause tachycardia
- *Dobutamine*: 2–20 µg/kg/min (start at 5–10 µg/kg/min). May cause tachycardia, hypotension
- *Epinephrine*: 0.05–1 µg/kg/min (start at 0.05–0.10 µg/kg/min). Increases oxygen consumption
- *Norepinephrine*: 0.1–1 µg/kg/min (start at 0.1 µg/kg/min). May produce tachydysrhythmias
- *Amrinone*: Load 0.75 mg/kg IV over 3 minutes, then 5–10 µg/kg/min. May cause dysrhythmia, hypotension

Hypotension refractory to volume and single inotrope
- Seek intensive-care advice

Combinations of inotropes are used in this instance.

Diuresis for volume overload
- Start diuretics: After circulation is restored, expected urine volume is 1 mL/kg/hr.
- If there is oliguria or anuria, use furosemide 0.5–1 mg/kg IV

Dysrhythmias (see also p. 290)

Sinus bradycardia and heart block

- Do not treat if patient is hemodynamically stable
- If patient is symptomatic, give epinephrine (0.01 mg/kg to 1 mg), atropine (0.02 mg/kg to 1 mg), consider pacing
- Evaluate for underlying cause

Tachydysrhythmia

Treatment may require consultation with a cardiac specialist. If patient is hemodynamically unstable:

- *DC shock*: Synchronized cardioversion 0.5–1 J/kg. Give appropriate analgesia and sedation if time allows.

Supraventricular tachycardia

- *Vagal maneuvers*: Ice bag to face for 15–20 seconds or valsalva.
- *Adenosine*: 0.1–0.2 mg/kg as rapid IV push
- *Other drugs*: Diltiazem, esmolol, amiodarone. Synchronized cardioversion

Ventricular tachycardia

- *Amiodarone*: 5 mg/kg. Synchronized cardioversion.
- Pulseless ventricular tachycardia requires immediate CPR and defibrillation with 2 J/kg. If unsuccessful, repeat with 2–4 J/kg, then 4 J/kg (see Chapter 4, p. 50).

Congestive heart failure

Key treatments:

- Fluid support—use with caution
- Diuretics
- Adrenergic inotropic support
- Digoxin may be used for primary cardiac problem (TDD)

Hypertension (see p. 414)

For hypertensive emergency with end-organ dysfunction, especially hypertensive encephalopathy, the BP should be lowered by 25% during the first 8 hours and then normalizied over 1–2 days. Patients should be monitored closely. Rapid lowering of BP may lead to stroke. Short-acting antihypertensives are the treatment of choice.

- *Sodium nitroprusside*: 0.5–10 µg/kg/min
- *Labetalol*: 0.2–1.0 mg/kg load then 0.25–3 mg/kg/hr
- *Nicardipine*: 1–3 µg/kg/min

Congenital heart disease: prostaglandin E1 (see also p. 190)

In neonates, consider prostaglandin E1 (PGE1) infusion if:

- PaO_2 <3–40 mmHg
- Oxygen saturation <70% in FiO_2 100%
- Femoral pulses are diminished or absent with poor perfusion
- Pathologic murmur or other signs of cyanotic congenital heart disease
- Metabolic acidosis persists after volume and inotropes
- *PGE1*: 0.01–0.20 µg/kg/min (start at 0.05 µg/kg/min, and increase in 0.05 µg/kg/min increments if response is not adequate). Be aware that apnea may develop.

Cyanosis

Cyanosis is the result of deoxygenated hemoglobin or the presence of abnormal hemoglobin in the blood. Cyanosis is a clinical sign that is apparent when 4 g/dL of deoxygenated hemoglobin or 0.5 g/dL of methemoglobin is present. This means that patients with anemia may not demonstrate cyanosis even in the presence of marked arterial desaturation. In light-skinned patients, cyanosis is usually noted with oxygen saturations of less than 85%. In patients with darker complexions, cyanosis is more difficult to appreciate and saturations are generally lower.

Etiology
Pulmonary
- Alveolar hypoventilation
- Ventilation perfusion inequality
- Impaired oxygen diffusion across the alveolar membrane

Cardiovascular
- Right-to-left shunting

Hematologic
- Decreased affinity of the hemoglobin for oxygen

Differential diagnosis
Alveolar hypoventilation
Central nervous system insults
- Seizures
- Cerebral edema
- Cerebral hemorrhage with mass effect
- Infection
- Hypoxic ischemic encephalopathy
- Intoxication
- Environmental causes such as hypothermia
- Respiratory muscle dysfunction (muscular dystrophy, myasthenia gravis, Guillain–Barre syndrome)
- Tracheal compression, e.g., mediastinal mass

Ventilation perfusion inequality
Pulmonary
- Bronchiolitis
- Pneumonia
- Pneumothorax
- Pleural effusion
- Bronchopulmonary dysplasia
- Pulmonary hypoplasia
- Diaphragmatic hernia

Cardiac
- Decreased pulmonary blood flow, e.g., tricuspid atresia, pulmonary atresia, critical pulmonary stenosis, tetralogy of Fallot
- Decreased systemic perfusion, coarctation of the aorta

- Right-to-left shunting, congenital heart disease, Eisenmenger syndrome, arteriovenous fistula (pulmonary or systemic)

Decreased oxygen affinity of hemoglobin

- Methemoglobinemia: Aniline dyes, nitrobenzene, azo compounds and nitrites. Hereditary form is rare.
- Carboxyhemoglobinemia

Clinical assessment

It is essential to assess the respiratory and cardiovascular systems closely in patients with cyanosis.

Vital signs

- *Temperature*: Hypothermia and fever both have direct affects of respiratory rate.
- *Heart rate* is also influenced by temperature.
- *Blood pressure*: Check in all four extremities.

General appearance: Is there evidence of failure to thrive, atrophied lower extremities, etc?

Clubbing

- Fingers and toes should be examined for evidence of clubbing.
- Causes include the following:
  - Congenital heart disease
  - Chronic pulmonary conditions (e.g., cystic fibrosis)
  - Chronic gastrointestinal disease (e.g., Crohn's disease)
  - Ulcerative colitis
  - Cirrhosis
  - Hereditary and idiopathic

Respiratory

In the neonate it is helpful to note the degree of respiratory distress present—for example, a respiratory rate of 80 without apparent distress is more likely to be a result of cyanotic cardiac disease than a rate of 80 with tracheal tugging, retracting, etc. The infant with symptoms of respiratory distress is more likely to have a primary pulmonary process.

Cardiovascular

It is important to not limit the assessment to auscultation alone; evaluate for hepatomegaly.

Investigations

Laboratory evaluations

- CBC with differential
- Serum glucose
- If infection is a concern, blood cultures, urinary culture, and a lumbar puncture may be indicated.
- Carboxyhemoglobin and/or methemoglobin level
- Arterial blood gas (see Hyperoxia test for assessment of cyanotic heart disease in neonates, p. 229)

Radiologic evaluations

Chest X-ray (see also p. 275) is particularly helpful in the cyanotic neonate. Evaluation of lung fields for increased or decreased vascularity and pulmonary congestion aids in determining if this is a primarily cardiac or pulmonary process.

Characteristic radiographic findings of congenital heart disease include the following:

- Egg on a string: Transposition of the great arteries
- Boot-shaped heart: Tetralogy of Fallot, pulmonary atresia, ventriculoseptal defect
- Snowman sign: Supracardiac total anomalous pulmonary venous drainage

Electrocardiogram (see also p. 290)

Characteristic findings include the following:

- Superior left axis: Tricuspid atresia, endocardial cushion defect, primum atrial septal defect
- Left axis deviation: Pulmonary atresia +/- atrial atresia
- Marked right atrial hypertrophy: Ebstein's anomaly

Echocardiography

While chest X-ray and ECG findings can be suggestive of specific cardiac anomalies, echocardiography is the most helpful test for diagnosis of lesions and evaluation of cardiac function.

Monitoring

Patients with cyanosis should be placed on cardiac and respiratory monitoring with continuous pulse oximetry and cardiac monitors (see also p. 290).

Therapy

Therapy for specific cardiac, pulmonary, and toxicological causes of cyanosis are discussed elsewhere (see pp. 275).

Anaphylaxis

Anaphylaxis is a life-threatening allergic event. It is the extreme clinical example of an immediate hypersensitivity reaction.

Symptoms

The reaction includes involvement of the following:

- *Skin*: Urticaria and angioedema
- *Respiratory*: Acute airway obstruction with laryngeal edema and bronchospasm
- *Gastrointestinal*: Severe abdominal cramping and diarrhea
- *Systemic*: Hypotension and shock

Etiology

The symptoms of anaphylaxis are abrupt, often within minutes of exposure to an antigen. The causes include the following:

- *Drugs*: Penicillin, aspirin, other
- *Injections*: Radiographic contrast dyes
- *Stings*: Bites and envenomations
- *Foods*: Shellfish, nuts, peanuts, eggs

Diagnosis

Take a careful history and aim to determine the time between onset of symptoms and exposure to the potential precipitating cause.

Initial treatment

Follow a standard protocol

- ABC
- *Epinephrine*: Give intramuscularly (IM) 0.01 mg/kg (1:1000, maximum dose 0.5 mg). Repeat every 15 minutes if required.
- *Hypotension*: Put the patient head-down 30° (Trendelenberg position) and give IV normal saline (20 mL/kg bolus). IV epinephrine may be given every 2–5 minutes (0.1 mL/kg, 1:10,000) while an infusion is being prepared.
- *Albuterol*: Give nebulized albuterol 0.15–0.25 mg/kg in 3 mL normal saline; approximately 2.5 mg for child <30 kg, and 5 mg for child >30 kg, every 15 minutes if required.
- *Antihistamine*: H1 blocker: Give IV diphenhydramine (1 mg/kg). Repeat every 4–6 hours as needed. Consider H2 blocker: IV ranitidine (1 mg/kg) every 6–8 hours
- *Steroid*: Give IV bolus methylprednisolone (2 mg/kg). This dose should be followed by IV methylprednisolone 2 mg/kg/day (divided every 6 hours), or oral prednisolone 2 mg/kg (bolus once a day).

Hypovolemic shock

Shock is characterized by inadequate systemic perfusion. The most common type, hypovolemic shock, is related to abnormally low circulating blood volume.

Symptoms
See p. 66.

Etiology
The causes of hypovolemia include the following:
- Trauma
- Gastrointestinal bleeding
- Burns
- Sepsis
- Peritonitis
- Vomiting and diarrhea
- Diabetic ketoacidosis (osmotic diuresis)

Diagnosis
Perform a rapid clinical examination and direct your initial treatment toward the patient's vital signs.

Initial treatment
Follow a standard protocol
- Check airway, breathing, circulation, disability (ABCD)
- *Fluid*: Acutely, blood pressure and perfusion need to be restored with crystalloid infusion. IV bolus of normal saline, 20 mL/kg, can be given over 5–10 minutes and repeated if necessary. If patient is not improving clinically, airway and ventilatory support should be considered. In dehydrated patients, the water and electrolyte deficit needs to be replaced (see Diabetic ketoacidosis, p. 106).
- *Blood*: In patients with significant acute blood loss, transfusion of 10 mL/kg packed red blood cells will be required and repeated if necessary. (The patient may need O-negative unmatched blood in an emergency). Monitor the response with laboratory testing.
- *Refractory hypotension*: Intubation, inotropes, intensive-care monitoring and therapy are required (see p. 70).

Burns

There are different forms of thermal injury:
- Contact with fire
- Scalding fluids
- Chemicals
- Electricity
- Inhalation of flame, heated vapor, and toxic fumes
- Cold freezing injury

The severity of a burn to the skin is assessed according to its depth and total surface area.

Severity

Severity of the burn site is categorized according to the degree of involvement of the skin.
- *First degree*: Limited to epidermis; painful and erythematous
- *Second degree*: Epidermis and dermis; superficial layer is blistered and painful, and deep layer is white with erythematous areas
- *Third degree*: Epidermis and all of the dermis; stiff, dry, charred, leathery, and painless
- *Fourth degree*: Into underlying muscle or bone; stiff, charred, thrombosed vessels

Surface area

The extent of the burn, as a proportion of the body surface area (% body surface area [BSA]), can be calculated by making a sum of the individual areas involved in the injury (see Table 5.1).

One can also use the palmar method, which involves using the surface area of the patient's palm as an estimate of 1% BSA. Only second-degree and greater injuries are included in this calculation.

Symptoms

Hypovolemia, pain, and signs of inhalation injury may be present. Inhalation injury can affect the nasal and oral passages and the lungs, leading to impaired oxygenation and altered mental status.

Table 5.1 Contribution of different body parts to total body surface area at different ages

	<1 year	1–11 years	>11 years
Head	18%	13%	9%
Trunk (front)	18%	18%	18%
Trunk (back)	18%	18%	18%
Arm	9%	9%	9%
Leg	14%	16%	18%

Lung
- Tachypnea
- Respiratory distress
- Hoarseness
- Stridor
- Wheeze
- Cough
- Crackles
- Facial burns
- Singed nasal hairs
- Carbonaceous sputum

Brain
- Confusion
- Dizziness
- Headache
- Restlessness
- Coma
- Seizures

Skin
- Facial burns
- Nasal burn
Cherry-red color

Trauma
- Consider possibility of other traumatic injuries

Etiology
You should find out about the injury.
- The mechanism
- The duration of exposure
- Environmental factors (closed or open space)
- Loss of consciousness during the accident

Investigations
Minor burn
There is no need for burn center therapy in children with minor burns that are
- partial thickness and <5% body surface,
- or full thickness and <2 cm^2 (unless hands, face, genitals, joints involved)

Major burns
- Arterial blood gas
- Oximetry
- Carboxyhemoglobin level
- Blood count and cross-match
- Blood urea, creatinine, and electrolytes may be considered

Consider child protection issues.

Burns: treatment

Initial treatment
Follow a standard protocol
- Stop the burning process, remove smoldering clothes or burning material
- ABC. If there is evidence of inhalation, then respiratory stabilization and pulmonary toilet with endotracheal intubation may be needed. Rapidly forming airway and facial edema may complicate airway integrity and interventions.
- Assume that there is carbon monoxide poisoning and measure carboxyhemoglobin level and PaO_2. Give humidified 100% oxygen until results are available. Consider hyperbaric therapy for significant or symptomatic carbon monoxide exposure.
- Follow serial arterial blood gases and chest X-rays.
- Consider cyanide exposure and poisoning if the breath smells of almonds, if the accident is fire-related, or if there is metabolic acidosis with raised anion-gap.
- C. In infants with burns >10% of BSA, or children with >15%, consider IV placement (preferable in non-burn areas) and bolus of normal saline (20 mL/kg). Further fluid resuscitation should be directed toward maintaining a urine output of 0.5–2 mL/kg/hr. In patients with >25% of BSA, use Parkland's formula (Box 5.4) as a guide to fluid therapy. Other fluid estimation formulas are also available (i.e., Galveston formula, Mosteller formula). Inpatient fluid care, which may include colloid use, should be directed by a burn or intensive-care physician.

Box 5.4 Parkland formula

	Lactated Ringer's solution
0–24 hr	4 mL/kg per 1% burn (≥2nd-degree burn)
	Use 50% of this volume in the first 8 hr

- *Burns*: Cover initially with a clean dry sheet. Consider local antibiotic ointment after burns are cleaned and, if necessary, evaluated by the definitive care team
- *Analgesia*: Pain must be treated. First ensure that ventilation, oxygenation, and perfusion are adequate, and use IV analgesics (narcotics) as required.
- *Other injuries*: Do a full trauma evaluation looking for associated traumatic injuries. Assess for cardiac and skeletal muscle injury in electrical accidents. In chemical burn, wash and neutralize the chemical.
- Place a naso- or orogastric tube and urinary catheter: Follow outputs.
- Pulse oximetry and cardiac monitoring are useful, but remember pulse oximetry limitations in assessing carbon monoxide poisoning.
- *Eyes*: Examine the eyes for burn or abrasion and treat with topical antibiotics if required.

- *Transfer*: Patients with significant burns, mechanisms of injury, preexisting medical issues, and/or burns of critical body areas should be transferred to a center capable of managing burns and critically ill trauma/medical patients.
- *Discharge*: Those with minor burns can be discharged after wound care. Discharge instructions should include follow-up plans, wound care, analgesia, and preventative teaching as appropriate.
- Give tetanus immunoprophylaxis as required.

Sepsis

Sepsis is bacterial infection of the bloodstream accompanied by signs of systemic toxicity. In this section we will consider the recognition and specific treatment for sepsis. Shock and respiratory failure are covered elsewhere in the chapter (see p. 77 and p. 58).

Clinical assessment

Clinically there may be fever in the older child, but be aware that fever or hypothermia can be the presenting feature in the infant. Perfusion is usually poor and there may be evidence of shock and coagulopathy (i.e., petechiae or purpura).

Investigations

All organ systems may be involved in sepsis, so it is important to perform the following tests.

Blood
- Complete blood count with differential
- Coagulation state
- Serum electrolytes with BUN and creatinine
- Liver function tests
- Arterial or capillary blood gas
- Inflammatory markers (e.g., C-reactive protein and ESR)

Urine
- Urinalysis

Imaging
- Chest X-ray
- Abdominal X-ray

Sepsis screen
- *Blood culture*: Bacteria (aerobic and anaerobic), virus, fungi. (Remember that blood cultures may not be positive, so repeat when there is fever.)
- Urine culture
- Stool swab
- Cerebrospinal fluid (CSF)
- *Other cultures*: Respiratory, wound, and all ports of any indwelling catheters

Monitoring

Ensure the ABCs. After that, the form and type of monitoring will be dictated by the patient's condition. Start with the following:
- Continuous pulse oximetry
- ECG monitoring
- Intermittent BP monitoring
- Hourly urine output

Therapy
Antibiotics
- *When*: Do not delay the first dose because of tests, although it is worthwhile trying to get a blood culture first.
- Should I do a lumbar puncture (LP)? The LP can wait until you have stabilized the child. You may even have to defer it if there is any coagulopathy.
- *What*: The choice of antibiotics you should use will depend on the patient, as well as local microbial flora. In general, you can start with a third-generation cephalosporin and use the following antibiotics for specific groups of patients.

Age <30 days
- Consider *Escherichia coli*, group B streptococcus, *Staphylococcus aureus*, and *Listeria monocytogenes*
- Ampicillin-gentamicin

Age 31–60 days
- Also consider *Streptococcus pneumoniae*, *Neisseria meningitides*, and *Haemophilus influenzae*
- Ampicillin-ceftriaxone

Indwelling catheter
- Consider *Staphylococcus aureus*
- Anti-staphylococcal coverage that is appropriate in your institution

Intra-abdominal cause
- Consider gut anaerobes
- Piperacillin-tazobactam

Immunosuppressed or oncological patient
- *Pseudomonas*: Ceftazidime, gentamicin
- Fungi: Amphotericin B
- Herpes, varicella: Acyclovir

Cellulitis or fasciitis
- Consider group A streptococcus
- Penicillin

Altered level of consciousness (LOC)

The brain can be injured in many ways. Its responses to injury, however, are uniform and include any combination of the following:
- Altered level of consciousness
- Seizures
- Impaired respiratory function
- Loss of autoregulation
- Cerebral swelling
- Syndrome of inappropriate antidiuretic hormone secretion

Take note of the following:
- When symptoms started, and their progression (gradual vs. sudden)
- Possible ingestion or exposure to medication or toxins
- Possible recent trauma, illness, or exposure to infection
- History: Seizures, diabetes, allergies, chronic illness

Etiology

Infectious causes
- Meningitis, encephalitis (p. 836)
- Toxic shock
- Subdural empyema, cerebral abscess (p. 90)

Toxins
See Poisoning, p. 96.

Neoplastic causes
- Brain tumors (p. 664)

Trauma
- Head injury: concussion or contusion
- Hemorrhage: epidural, subdural, brain

Vascular causes
- Arteriovenous malformation
- Aneurysm, venous thrombosis

Metabolic causes
- Hypoglycemia (p. 104)
- Diabetic ketoacidosis (p. 106)
- Electrolyte abnormalities
- Inborn errors of metabolism (p. 979)
- Hepatic encephalopathy
- Hormonal abnormalities: thyroid, adrenal, pituitary (p. 498)
- Uremic encephalopathy

Other
- Hypothermia
- Hyperthermia
- Seizures and postictal state (p. 589)
- Hypertension (p. 414)
- Hydrocephalus (p. 602)
- Hypoxia–ischemia
- Sepsis (p. 828)
- Intussusception (p. 996)

Altered LOC: clinical assessment

Initial examination

General examination can provide an explanation for the patient's state.

General

- *Vital signs*: Make note of the adequacy and rate and depth of respiration, the pulse rate and rhythm, BP, and body temperature.
- *Medic-Alert bracelet*: Search for a bracelet or tag, or other information that may indicate a long-standing medical problem.
- *Skin*: Examine for evidence of trauma, rash, petechiae, jaundice, and needle tracks.
- *Breath*: Check for odors of alcohol, ketones, hydrocarbons, or toxins.

Head and neck

- *Head*: If the anterior fontanel is patent, a tense fontanel indicates raised intracranial pressure (ICP), whereas a sunken fontanel suggests dehydration.
- *Nose and ears*: Leakage of blood or CSF, "raccoon eyes" or Battle sign suggests basal skull fracture.

Pupils

- Small (2–3 mm) reactive pupils suggest a metabolic cause of coma.
- Midsize (4–5 mm) unreactive puils at midposition suggest a midbrain lesion.
- Pinpoint (1–2 mm) pupils indicate a pontine disorder, but are also commonly associated with opiates.
- Unequal pupils with one fixed and dilated suggest a brain disorder on the side of the dilated pupil.
- Bilateral fixed, dilated pupils imply a poor prognosis, although similar pupils may be produced by mydriatics, barbiturate intoxication, and hypothermia.

Fundi

- Examine for evidence of retinal hemorrhages and papilledema.

After checking ABCs, conduct a focused neurological assessment (see Box 5.5). Look for evidence of increased ICP and a potential site of an intracranial lesion.

Signs of raised intracranial pressure

The signs of increased ICP include the following:
- Abnormal respiratory pattern
- Unequal or unreactive pupils
- Impaired or absent oculocephalic or oculovestibular responses
- Systemic hypertension, bradycardia
- Tense fontanel
- Abnormal body posture or muscle flaccidity

Box 5.5 Detailed neurological examination

Pattern of respiration

- Cheyne-Stokes (alternating apnea and hyperpnea) can be seen with metabolic disturbance, bilateral cerebral hemisphere dysfunction, and insipient temporal lobe herniation.
- Central neurogenic hyperventilation (deep, rapid respiration) can occur with hypoxia–ischemia, hypoglycemia, or lesion between low midbrain and midpons.
- Ataxic respiration (irregular depth and rate) can be caused by abnormality of the medulla and impending respiratory arrest.
- Apneustic breathing (gasping, respiratory arrest in inspiration) indicates pontine involvement.

Eye movements

- Roving eye movements are seen in light coma without structural brain disease.
- Extraocular movements with coma suggest a metabolic disorder or a supratentorial disorder.
- Absent movements suggest an infratentorial disorder or drug intoxication.
- With an abnormality of lateral gaze, the eyes are deviated toward the side of a destructive cerebral lesion and away from an irritative cerebral lesion. In a brain-stem lesion the eyes are directed away from the side of the lesion.
- Skew deviation is seen with posterior fossa lesions.
- Ocular bobbing is seen in pontine lesions.

Lateral eye movement reflexes

Lateral eye movements, mediated by brain-stem structures, require an intact midbrain and pons and are assessed clinically by

- *Oculocephalic reflex* (doll's eye): Sudden turning of the head from one side to the other normally causes conjugate deviation of the eyes in the direction opposite to that in which the head is turned. **Do not test when the neck may be unstable**.
- *Oculovestibular reflex* (cold caloric): Cold water irrigated into the ear with the head held 30° above the horizontal plane normally causes conjugate deviation of the eyes toward the side of the irrigation.

Motor function and posture

- *Decorticate rigidity*: The arms are held in flexion and adduction, the legs in extension. This posture signifies a lesion in the cerebral white matter, internal capsule, or thalamus.
- *Decerebrate rigidity*: The arms are extended and internally rotated, and the legs are extended. This occurs with lesions from the midbrain to the midpons, and with bilateral anterior cerebral lesions. It can also be seen with metabolic abnormalities, hypoxia–ischemia, or hypoglycemia.

Altered LOC: Glasgow coma scale (GCS)

As a summary of conscious state, the GCS score should be used. It is also a useful tool for monitoring changes. The full score is calculated from the sum of E + V + M (see Tables 5.2 and 5.3). A score ≤8 is used as a criterion for endotracheal intubation in the head-injured patient.

Table 5.2 Response scoring in older children

Response	Score
Eye opening (E)	
Spontaneous	4
To verbal stimuli	3
To pain	2
None	1
Best verbal (V)	
Oriented	5
Confused speech	4
Inappropriate words	3
Nonspecific sounds	2
None	1
Best motor (M)	
Follows commands	6
Localizes pain	5
Withdraws to pain	4
Flexes to pain	3
Extends to pain	2
None	1

Table 5.3 Response scoring in infants

Response	Score
Eye opening (E)	
Spontaneous	4
To speech	3
To pain	2
None	1
Best verbal (V)	
Coos and babbles	5
Irritable cries	4
Cries to pain	3
Moans to pain	2
None	1
Best motor (M)	
Normal	6
Withdraws to touch	5
Withdraws to pain	4
Abnormal flexion	3
Abnormal extension	2
None	1

Altered LOC: management

Investigations

Consider the following tests if the cause of the coma is unknown.

Blood

- Complete blood count, clotting and bleeding time
- Glucose, electrolytes, urea, liver function tests, ammonia, and lactate
- Save two extra tubes of clotted blood for storage in the laboratory.

Toxicology

- Urine, blood, gastric aspirate for ingestions
- Serum lead and free erythrocyte protoporphyrin

Acid base

- Arterial blood gas

Microbiology

- Blood and urine cultures

Imaging

- Cranial computerized tomography (CT) scan
- Magnetic resonance imaging (MRI), particularly for posterior fossa, or white matter lesions

Electroencephalography

- Standard electroencephalogram (EEG)

Lumbar puncture

An LP should be deferred until a CT scan has been obtained if there are signs of raised ICP or focal neurology. The CSF can be examined for microscopy, culture, glucose, and protein.

Meningitis

- 200–20,000 white blood cells/mm^3 with a polymorphonuclear neutrophil leukocyte predominance
- An elevated protein level >100 mg/dL
- Low glucose <30 mg/dL (or <50% of plasma level)

Encephalitis

- 50–1000 cells/mm^3 with lymphocyte predominance
- Presence of red blood cells up to 500 cells/mm^3 suggests herpes simplex virus (HSV) infection.
- CSF protein can be normal or mildly elevated.
- Glucose is usually normal (~70% of plasma level).

Monitoring

The form and type of monitoring will be dictated by the underlying cause of the patient's state. Generally, after initial evaluation, monitor hourly:

- Vital signs, pupil reaction, fluid balance
- The GCS for neurological review: in those with GCS 9 to 11 a gastric tube and urinary catheter may be needed.

Treatment

Follow a standard protocol.

- *ABC*: The ABCs are the initial priority.
- *Glucose*: Whenever the cause of coma is not clearly obvious, glucose (0.5–1 g/kg) should be given intravenously after a blood sample has been taken for laboratory blood glucose testing.
- Specific therapies should be considered (see Box 5.6)

Box 5.6 Specific therapies of altered LOC

Meningitis
- Immediately begin the appropriate antibiotics (see Antibiotics, below)

Consider dexamethasone (0.15 mg/kg IV, qid for 4 days). Review potential use and optimal timing of steroids in relation to antibiotic administration with local experts.

Encephalitis
- In the presence of a compatible clinical history; treat for HSV encephalitis with acyclovir (10 mg/kg IV, tid for 14–21 days; 20 mg/kg IV tid for 21 days for neonates).

Suspected raised ICP
- GCS ≤8: rapid-sequence endotracheal intubation
- Ventilate to achieve normocapnia and normoxia
- Elevate the head of the bed to 30°
- Keep the head in the midline

Mannitol (0.25–1 g/kg IV) and/or furosemide (1 mg/kg IV)

Syndrome of inappropriate ADH secretion
- Limit the fluids to 67% maintenance

Antibiotics

Antimicrobial therapy is often given presumptively. The choice will depend on local epidemiology, public health, immunization, and antibiotic policy. In the comatose child, consider the following therapies.

Age <4 weeks
- Group B streptococcus
- Gram-negative bacteria
- *Listeria monocytogenes*
- *Recommend*: Ampicillin + aminoglycoside

Infants 1–3 months
- Group B streptococcus
- Gram-negative bacteria
- *Streptococcus pneumoniae*
- *Neisseria meningitides*
- *Recommend*: Ampicillin + aminoglycoside or third-generation cephalosporin

Older than 3 months
- *Streptococcus pneumoniae*
- *Neisseria meningitidis*
- *Recommend*: third-generation cephalosporin

In the comatose older child in whom no CSF is available, a combination of antimicrobials to cover HSV, *Streptococcus pneumoniae*, and *Mycoplasma pneumoniae* infection are often prescribed:
- Cefotaxime (50 mg/kg IV, qid; maximum 12 g/day)
- Erythromycin (10 mg/kg IV, qid)
- Acyclovir (10 mg/kg IV, tid)

Status epilepticus

Status epilepticus (SE) is a prolonged seizure lasting over 30 minutes, or recurrent seizures during which the patient does not fully regain consciousness within a 30-minute period. The success of treatment depends on prompt recognition and treatment.

Symptoms

SE is classified as convulsive (C) or nonconvulsive (NC). NCSE is diagnosed with an EEG, and should be considered in the unresponsive child with a history of seizures.

Etiology

The common causes of childhood seizures include the following:
- Known seizure disorder
- Fever
- Subtherapeutic anticonvulsant levels
- Acute infection (including meningitis and sepsis)
- Trauma
- Poisoning
- Tumor
- Metabolic abnormalities

Investigations

After emergency treatment, useful diagnostic tests may include the following:
- Brain imaging: CT, MRI
- EEG
- Lumbar puncture
- Serum glucose
- Other lab tests to consider include electrolytes, magnesium, calcium, phosphorus and creatinine levels (generally not useful in older children >1 year)
- Arterial blood gas or capillary blood gas
- Toxicology: blood and urine
- Anticonvulsant levels (for those on anticonvulsants)
- CBC and white blood cell differential (if infection is suspected)
- Blood culture (if infection is suspected)

Initial treatment

Box 5.7 summarizes a timeline for therapy. At any stage, if there is respiratory depression, support of breathing should be initiated with bag valve mask (BVM) ventilation and intubation if prolonged BVM is required. Vital signs should be obtained every 5 minutes and suction should be available in addition to airway equipment. Remember to check the glucose and consider administration of antibiotics if infection such as meningitis is suspected.

Box 5.7 Anticonvulsants in status epilepticus

0–5 minutes: ABC
- Establish intravenous access
- Monitor vital signs, especially pulse oximetry saturation
- Give 100% oxygen via mask
- Assess ventilation
- Assess circulation

5–15 minutes: start anticonvulsants
- Use IV lorazepam (0.05–0.1 mg/kg, up to 6 mg)
- Or rectal diazepam (0.5 mg/kg, up to 10 mg)
- If there is no response, repeat dosing every 5–10 minutes up to 3–4 doses (multiple doses may cause respiratory depression)

15–35 minutes: if seizure persists
- Load with IV fosphenytoin (15–20 mg/kg, at rate <3 mg/kg/min) or phenytoin (15–20 mg/kg, at rate <1 mg/kg/min)
- Or IV phenobarbitol (15–20 mg/kg, at rate <1 mg/kg/min) (causes respiratory depression)

45 minutes: refractory seizure
- Load with IV phenytoin or phenobarbitol (whichever was not given above)
- Additional fosphenytoin or phenytoin (5 mg/kg/dose)
- Additional phenobarbitol (5 mg/kg/dose, every 30 minutes to maximum of 30 mg/kg can be used)

Refractory seizure: intensive care
- If seizures persist, intensive care should be initiated.
- Intubate the trachea and support breathing.
- EEG monitoring

Poisoning

The peak incidence of childhood accidental poisoning is between the ages of 1 and 3 years. Most cases occur at home. In older children, self-poisoning should be suspected as a suicide gesture.

Etiology

Parents usually know the name of the material ingested and often have a good idea of the amount. If possible, obtain the bottle or container of the substance ingested. Get these details in the history:
- *Exact name* of the drug or chemical exposure
- *Preparation and concentration* of the drug exposure
- *Probable dose* (by history) of drug ingested in mg/kg, as well as maximum possible dose
- *Time* since ingestion or exposure
- *Contact the poison center* at 1-800-222-1222

Symptoms and signs

There are various signs and symptoms produced by poisoning. It is helpful to consider the constellation of clinical symptoms and think of potential causes (see Box 5.8). In addition, there are specific odors that may lead to diagnosis.

Odors
- Acetone
- Alcohol
- Bitter almonds (cyanide)
- Garlic (heavy metals)
- Oil of wintergreen (methyl salicylates)
- Pears (chloral hydrate)
- Carrots (water hemlock)

Diagnosis

The likely type of poisoning may be indicated by its clinical effect (see Box 5.8). Bedside or laboratory tests should also be considered:
- Urine toxicology screening
- Arterial blood gas
- Blood glucose
- Co-oximetry (carboxyhemoglobin level)
- Serum urea and electrolyte
- Osmolar gap: [Osmolality – (2 x Na) + Urea + Glucose]
- Drug levels
- ECG: 12-lead for assessment of rhythm, QRS duration and QT interval
- X-rays of abdomen to detect radio-opaque tablets (e.g., iron)

Box 5.8 Clinical effect and causative drugs or poisons

- *Depressed respiration*: Antipsychotics, carbamate pesticides, clonidine, cyclic antidepressants, alcohol, narcotics, nicotine
- *Tachycardia and hypertension*: Amphetamines, antihistamines, cocaine
- *Tachycardia and hypotension*: Carbon monoxide, tricyclic antidepressants, hydralazine, iron, phenothiazine, theophylline
- *Bradycardia and hypertension*: Clonidine, ergotamine, ephedrine
- *Bradycardia and hypotension*: Calcium-channel blockers, clonidine, digoxin, narcotics, organophosphates, phentolamine, propranolol, sedatives
- *Atrioventricular block*: β-adrenergic antagonists, calcium-channel blockers, clonidine, cyclic antidepressants, digoxin
- *Ventricular tachycardia*: Amphetamines, anti-arrhythmics (flecainide, quinidine, procainamide), carbamazepine, chloral hydrate, chlorinated hydrocarbons, cocaine, tricyclic antidepressants, digoxin, phenothiazine, theophylline
- *Torsade de pointes*: Amantadine, antihistamines (astemizole), cyclic antidepressants, lithium, phenothiazine, quinidine, sotalol
- *Coma with miosis*: Alcohol, barbiturates, bromide, chloral hydrate, clonidine, ketamine, narcotics, organophosphates, phenothiazines
- *Coma with mydriasis*: Atropine, carbon monoxide, cyanide, cyclic antidepressants, glutethimide
- *Hypoglycemia*: Alcohols, insulin, oral hypoglycemic agents, propranolol, salicylates
- *Seizures*: Amphetamines, anticonvulsants (carbamazepine, phenytoin), anticholinergic, antihistamines, camphor, carbon monoxide, chlorinated hydrocarbons, cocaine, cyanide, tricyclic antidepressants, isoniazid, ketamine, lead, lidocaine, meperidine, phenothiazine, phenylpropanolamine, propranolol, theophylline
- *High anion gap* ($Na - [Cl + HCO_3]$) *metabolic acidosis*: Alcohol, carbon monoxide, cyanide, ethylene glycol, iron, isoniazid, methanol, salicylate, theophylline
- *Low anion gap*: Bromide, lithium, hypermagnesemia, hypercalcemia

Fluid and electrolytes

Normal fluid requirements

Children with serious acute illnesses, admitted to the hospital, are usually given intravenous fluid and electrolyte solutions. It is important to match what you prescribe to what the child actually needs. There are a number of ways of calculating daily requirements, but the method we most commonly use is based on patient weight.

24-hour fluid requirements
- 100 mL/kg: for the first 10 kg of weight
- +50 mL/kg: for the second 10 kg of weight
- +20 mL/kg: for the remaining weight above 20 kg

24-hour electrolyte requirements
- Sodium: 2–4 mEq/kg
- Potassium: 1–2 mEq/kg

Normal fluid therapy is based on the above calculations. In the fasting patient, the type of fluid given should contain dextrose (usually 5%), sodium chloride, and added potassium chloride. Outside the neonatal period we use 0.45% or 0.25% saline with dextrose and additives. Do not use plain 5% dextrose in water or 5% dextrose 0.18% saline. The volume of fluid administered should be increased in dehydration (see p. 100), and restricted to 50%–75% of the usual maintenance volume in cases of the following:
- Syndrome of inappropriate antidiuretic hormone (SIADH) (p. 102)
- Fluid overload (p. 457)
- Congestive heart failure (p. 260)
- Renal failure with oliguria or anuria (p. 454)

Fluid and electrolytes: dehydration

Dehydration can lead to shock, severe metabolic acidosis, and death, particularly in infants. Its severity can be assessed using change in weight or the following physical signs.

Mild dehydration (0%–5%)

- *Weight loss*: 5% in infants and 3% children
- *Skin turgor*: May be decreased
- *Mucous membranes*: Dry
- *Urine*: May be low
- *Heart rate*: Increased
- *Blood pressure*: Normal
- *Perfusion*: Normal
- *Skin color*: Pale
- *Consciousness*: Irritable

Moderate dehydration (5%–10%)

- *Weight loss*: 10% in infants and 6% children
- *Skin turgor*: Decreased
- *Mucous membranes*: Very dry
- *Urine*: Oliguric
- *Heart rate*: Increased
- *Blood pressure*: May be normal
- *Perfusion*: Prolonged capillary refill time (CRT >2 seconds)
- *Skin color*: Gray
- *Consciousness*: Lethargic

Severe dehydration (10%–15%)

- *Weight loss*: 15% in infants and 9% children
- *Skin turgor*: Poor with tenting
- *Mucous membranes*: Parched
- *Urine*: Anuric
- *Heart rate*: Increased
- *Blood pressure*: Decreased
- *Perfusion*: Prolonged CRT
- *Skin color*: Mottled, blue or white
- *Consciousness*: Comatose

After you have assessed the degree of dehydration in the patient, two problems need to be addressed: water and electrolyte losses. In practice, our treatment is aimed at correcting both the water and electrolyte losses (see Table 5.4).

Table 5.4 Water and electrolyte losses in 10% dehydration

	Losses in 10% dehydration			
	Water ml/kg	Na mEq/kg	K mEq/kg	Cl mEq/kg
Isotonic Na 130–150 mEq/L	100–120	8–10	8–10	8–10
Hyponatremic Na <130 mEq/L	100–120	10–12	8–10	10–12
Hypernatremic Na >150 mEq/L	100–120	2–4	0–4	2–6

Isotonic and hyponatremic dehydration
- First assess the degree of dehydration (use weight change and signs)
- Calculate the fluid deficit
- Serum electrolytes (Na, K, Ca) with urea, creatinine, and glucose.
- Consider Complete blood count with differential

Emergency treatment is directed toward restoring any compromise in the circulation (see p. 77 on shock; use 20 mL/kg IV normal saline). Monitoring should include vital signs, losses (urine output, stool, vomitus, nasogastric), daily weights, and blood tests. After the initial phase, fluid administration should be calculated to correct deficits over 48 hours. Overall, take into account the deficit, maintenance requirements, and any ongoing losses:

Hourly rate = (24 hr maintenance + deficit − resuscitation fluids)/24

Hypernatremic
- Water losses exceed sodium loss
- Cerebral edema is a risk during rehydration. Correction of the deficit should be achieved slowly and evenly, over 48 hours.
- Emergency treatment of shock is treated with 10–20 mL/kg IV saline boluses. Thereafter, calculate the deficit and restore patient's needs over 48 hours.
- Monitor as above, with at least 8-hourly electrolyte studies and frequent exams of the patient's neurological status.
- Use 0.9% saline so that sodium correction occurs slowly.

Seizures and cerebral edema may complicate the rehydration phase of hypernatremic dehydration. If these occur, treat symptomatically and refer to an intensive care unit. There may be a number of causes of these problems: your initial role in this emergency is to do the ABCs. Further investigations and a CT scan may be needed.

Fluid and electrolytes: abnormalities

Hyponatremia (<130 mEq/L)

Assess the problem. Is the patient hypovolemic or fluid overloaded?

Sodium depletion

- *Associations*: Hypovolemia and low urine Na (<10 mEq/L)
- *Causes*: Inadequate Na intake, excessive Na losses
- *Treatment*: Restore circulation, replace water and salt deficits
- *Symptomatic therapy* (<120 mEq/L): If there are seizures, the serum Na level should be acutely raised by 5–10 mEq/L in about 1 hour. Use 3 mmol NaCl/kg IV over 30–60 minutes.

Dilution

- *Associations*: Normovolemia (occasionally overload), paradoxically high urine Na (usually >300 mEq/L), and sometimes cerebral edema
- *Causes*: Impaired water excretion, excess water given
- *Treatment*: Correct the volume-overloaded circulation with diuretics (furosemide 0.5–1.0 mg/kg IV). Provide oxygen and inotropes if required. Restrict fluids to less than maintenance.
- *Syndrome of inappropriate ADH secretion* (SIADH): There are many causes of SIADH. The features are low urine volume and high urine osmolality in the absence of hypovolemia; renal disease; and adrenal disease. Urine Na is paradoxically high (20–30 mEq/L) in the presence of hyponatremia secondary to volume overload.

Hypernatremia (>150 mEq/L)

Besides hypernatremic dehydration and salt poisoning, you will see hypernatremia in diabetes insipidus (DI), where there is excess renal water loss. The urine is 5 to 10 times the usual volume, with low osmolality (50–100 mosm/L), in the absence of glycosuria. So, assess the underlying problem, and restore compromised circulation.

ADH deficiency

- *Causes*: Severe asphyxia, and CNS trauma, surgery, or infection
- *Treatment*: Use two IV solutions: one at 30%–40% maintenance for replacement of insensible losses, the other for replacing urine losses. Check urine Na/K and prepare IV replacement solution to match.
- *Hormone replacement*: DI is sometimes transient and so initial fluid therapy is reasonable. However, if this problem is established, then hormonal replacement is needed: nasal DDAVP 1–40 µg/day in 1 or 2 doses; parenteral (IV) DDAVP 2–4 µg/day in 2 doses. You should see a response within 1 hour.

Hypokalemia (<3 mEq/L)

The critical problems that may occur are
- *ECG changes*: Flattened, prolonged or inverted T waves; prominent U waves; ST segment depression; atrioventricular block
- Dysrhythmias, hypotension

- *Neuromuscular*: Weakness, hypotonia, hyporeflexia, paraesthesias
- *Gastrointestinal*: Ileus, constipation

Correction
- *Urgent*: ECG changes, children on digoxin, or serum potassium <2.5 mEq/L

Treatment: Use 0.5 mmol KCl/kg IV over 1 hour via a central line. The bolus should not exceed 20 mmol, and should not be more concentrated that 60 mmol KCl/L. Monitor the procedure with continuous ECG and repeat serum K level 1–2 hours after the bolus.

Hyperkalemia (>5.5 mEq/L)
The critical problems that may occur are
- *ECG changes*: Peaked T waves, widened QRS, depressed ST segments progressing to increasingly aberrant ECG complexes
- *Dysrhythmias*: Bradycardia, VT, VF, cardiac arrest

Approach
- *Context*: Treatment is guided by the level, but first repeat the venous sample (hemolysis may produce elevated potassium levels). Stop all potassium administration and monitor the ECG while you wait for the result.

Symptomatic treatment (>8.0 mEq/L or ECG changes)
- *Protect the myocardium*: Calcium gluconate 10% (100 mg/kg/dose IV (maximum 100 mg/min, 1.5–3.3 mL/min, 50 mg/mL) and monitor for bradycardia and hypotension.
- *Increase intracellular K uptake*: NaHCO$_3$ (1–2 mmol/kg IV over 5–10 minutes); insulin with glucose (0.1 u/kg IV <u>with</u> dextrose 25% 0.5 g/kg IV over 30 minutes)
- *Induce kaluresis*: Albuterol nebulizer
- *Decrease total load of K*: Kayexalate (1 g/kg/dose PR 2 hourly with 5 mL 20% sorbitol)

Hypocalcemia (ionized calcium<1.1 mmol/L) (see also p. 532)
Low ionized values of Ca can result in the following:
- *ECG changes*: Prolonged QT, AV block
- Shock
- *CNS effects*: Seizures, tetany and weakness

Symptomatic therapy
Calcium gluconate 10% for seizures, tetany, hypotension, arrhythmias
Monitor heart rate and BP during treatment.

Refractory hypocalcemia
- Check magnesium level and serum albumin. If these levels are low, correct them (25–50 mg/kg IV magnesium sulfate over 30 minutes, 6 hourly for 3 doses)
- If these are normal, with raised phosphate, decrease phosphate intake and use phosphate binders. Check renal function.

See also Acute renal insufficiency, p. 456.

Glucose: hypoglycemia

In infants and children this emergency is defined as a blood value below 40–60 mg/dL (2.2–2.6 mmol/L) (see also p. 148).

Etiology

Hypoglycemia is a sign of an underlying disease process that interferes with carbohydrate intake or absorption, gluconeogenesis or glycogenolysis. These conditions are discussed in detail in Chapter 12, on endocrinology. Outside the neonatal period, in the acute setting, the causes of hypoglycemia can be grouped as follows.

Endocrine
- Hyperinsulinism
- Hypopituitarism
- Growth hormone deficiency
- Hypothyroidism
- Cortisol deficiency (caused by congenital adrenal hyperplasia, Addison's disease, ACTH deficiency)

Metabolic
- Glycogen storage disease
- Galactosemia
- Organic acidemia
- Ketotic hypoglycemia
- Carnitine deficiency
- Acyl CoA dehydrogenase deficiency

Toxic
- Salicylates
- Alcohol
- Insulin
- Valproate
- Oral hypoglycemics
- β-blockers

Hepatic
- Hepatitis
- Cirrhosis
- Reye syndrome

Systemic
- Starvation
- Malnutrition
- Sepsis
- Malabsorption

Clinical assessment

Take a thorough history and identify the timing of hypoglycemia in relation to feeding and medication. On examination assess for

- Short stature (p. 548)
- Failure to thrive (p. 362)
- Hepatomegaly (p. 980, in metabolic chapter)
- Congenital defects
- Features of any generalized disorder (p. 980, in Chapter 26)

Investigation

If possible, during an acute episode you should try to do the following:

- Save blood and urine for metabolic and endocrine testing
- Check blood glucose in the laboratory
- Check blood electrolytes, urea, liver function, and osmolality
- Check blood gas
- Get a toxicology screen
- Check urine ketones and reducing substances

Monitoring

Ensure ABCs. Then start with continuous pulse oximetry and ECG monitoring, and intermittent BP monitoring.

Treatment

Asymptomatic child

- Oral glucose drink or gel

Symptomatic child

- *Dextrose*: 10% 5–10 mL/kg IV, or 25% 2–4 mL/kg IV
- *Followed by*: Continuous infusion of salt solution with 5%–10% dextrose (6–8 mg/kg/min), e.g., 0.45% saline and 5% dextrose.
- If hypoglycemia persists, increase the dextrose to 10–12 mg/kg/min
- If there is no response, consider glucagons, hydrocortisone, or diazoxide. These patients will need advice from a specialist.

Diabetic ketoacidosis

Diabetic ketoacidosis (DKA) is a diabetic emergency and such patients can die from hypovolemic shock, cerebral edema, hypokalemia, or aspiration pneumonia. DKA is defined as:
- Hyperglycemia
- pH <7.3
- Bicarbonate <15 mEq/L
- Urinary ketones

Patients who meet the above criteria, who are more than 5% dehydrated, or who have altered level of consciousness require careful supervision and treatment. Some patients may need referral to an intensive care unit (e.g., those with pH <7.1, with severe dehydration with shock, or under 2 years of age).

Clinical assessment
- Degree of dehydration (p. 100)
- Level of consciousness (p. 84)
- Full examination for evidence of cerebral edema, infection, and ileus
- Weight

Investigations
The key tests are as follows.

Blood
- Full blood count with differential
- Serum electrolytes with urea and creatinine
- Glucose
- Liver function tests (transaminases)
- Arterial or capillary blood gas
- Lactate and ketone level

Urine
- Urinalysis
- Ketones
- Reducing substances
- Organic and amino acids
- Drug screen

Monitoring
- *Ensure the ABCs*: Afterwards, the form and type of monitoring will be dictated by the patient's condition.
- *CNS*: Follow the neurological state. If there is headache or altered consciousness treat as though raised ICP has developed.
- Continuous pulse oximetry and ECG monitoring: T-wave changes should alert you to hypokalemia or hyperkalemia.
- Intermittent BP monitoring
- Hourly urine output: Test for ketones

Diabetic ketoacidosis: treatment

Fluid therapy

We have already discussed the management of dehydration. Our therapy is similar in DKA, with the following caveats (p. 484).

Resuscitation fluid

- Use 0.9% saline for resuscitation of the circulation.
- This alone will bring down the glucose level.
- Remember to include the initial resuscitation volume in your calculation of total fluid replacement to be given in the 48 hours.

Calculation of deficit

- Never use more than 10% dehydration in the calculations.
- Restore deficit over 48 hours.

Type of fluid

- Use normal saline initially.
- When glucose has fallen to 250 mg/dL, add glucose to the fluid. If this fall occurs within 6 hours, the child may still be sodium depleted. In this instance add glucose to 0.9% saline. Usually the fall in glucose occurs after 6 hours and it is safe to change the fluid type to 0.45% saline with 5% dextrose.
- Potassium should be started with the rehydration fluids after the first 500 mL, provided the patient is passing urine. Add 40 mmol KCl/L (i.e., 20 mmol KCl to each 500 mL bag).

Bicarbonate and phosphate

- There is no evidence for using bicarbonate/phosphate in DKA (see consensus guidelines in *Archives of Disease in Childhood* 2004; **89**: 188–194).
- However, under extreme conditions and with critical illness these are sometimes considered.

Electrolytes

- Check glucose q1h, while on insulin infusion
- Check these q2h after resuscitation, and then q4h.

Oral fluids

- Initially NPO ± nasogastric tube
- Juices and rehydration solutions should only be given after substantial clinical improvement.
- These fluids should be added to the overall calculation of fluid intake.

Insulin therapy

Once the rehydration fluids and potassium have been started, insulin should be used to switch off ketogenesis and reverse DKA. There is no need for an initial bolus dose; continuous low-dose IV insulin is the preferred method of administration (see Box 5.9).

Box 5.9 Insulin treatment in diabetic ketoacidosis

Insulin infusion
- Make up a solution of 1 unit/mL of human-soluble insulin.
- Attach this to a second IV line or "piggy-back" to one line with the replacement fluids.
Give 0.1 unit/kg/hr (i.e., 0.1 mL/kg/hr).

Glucose fall
- If the blood glucose falls to around 250 mg/dL, then add dextrose (equivalent to 5%–10%) to the IV fluids.
Insulin dose needs to be maintained at 0.1 U/kg/hr in order to switch off ketogenesis—DO NOT STOP IT.

Recovery
- Once the pH is >7.3, the blood glucose <250 mg/dL, and a dextrose-containing fluid has been started, consider reducing the insulin infusion rate, but to no less than 0.05 U/kg/hr.
- Once the child is drinking well and able to tolerate food, IV fluids and insulin can be discontinued
- Subcutaneous insulin should be started in the newly diagnosed diabetic, according to local protocol. Resume usual insulin regimen in known diabetics.
Discontinue the insulin infusion 60 minutes after the first subcutaneous injection.

Treatment failure
- If blood glucose is uncontrolled or the pH worsens after 4–6 hours, check IV lines and insulin dose, and consider possible sepsis.

Complications

The most concerning complication of DKA is cerebral edema. The warning signs include the following:
- Headache, behavioral change with restlessness, drowsiness
- Body posturing, cranial nerve palsy, seizures
- Slowing of heart rate, hemodynamic instability
- Respiratory arrest

Once identified:
- Start ABCs
- Emergency mannitol (1.0 g/kg) IV
Transfer patient to the intensive care unit

Inborn error of metabolism

Inborn errors of metabolism are rare. If such conditions are suspected during the neonatal period, then there is a specific course of action that should be followed (see Chapter 6). Occasionally, infants or children present outside the neonatal period with a catabolic state induced by an intercurrent illness such as viral infection or fasting. The differential diagnosis at this time is broad and includes the following:

- *Infection*: Generalized sepsis, central nervous system infection
- *Gastrointestinal*: Pyloric stenosis, gastroenteritis
- *Cardiac*: Duct-dependent congenital heart disease
- *Metabolic*: Inborn error of metabolism

Clinical assessment

History
- Thorough history
- Assess whether there is any consanguinity or death of siblings from unknown or metabolic diseases.
- Identify developmental milestones.
- Has there been intermittent vomiting, sleepiness, or seizures?

Examination
- Full physical examination
- Think about abnormal odors (breath, skin)
- Check growth: failure to thrive
- Skin: dermatitis or alopecia
- Eyes: cataracts
- Breathing pattern: Kussmaul or central hyperventilation

Investigations

Until you know the diagnosis, consider the following blood and urine tests.

Blood
- Complete blood count with differential
- Serum electrolytes with urea and creatinine
- Glucose, liver function tests (transaminases)
- Arterial or capillary blood gas
- Lactate, pyruvate, ketones
- Plasma amino acids
- Ammonia
- Carnitine
- Drug screen

Urine
- Urinalysis
- Ketones
- Reducing substances
- Organic acids
- Amino acids
- Drug screen

Monitoring

Ensure ABCs. The form and type of monitoring will be dictated by the patient's condition. Start with continuous pulse oximetry and ECG monitoring, and intermittent BP monitoring. Follow hourly urine output.

Therapy

In the acute setting, treatment will be supportive. Treat any complicating metabolic acidosis or hypoglycemia. All protein intake and oral feeds should be discontinued until the diagnosis is confirmed. To avoid catabolism, give continuous dextrose infusion (10%–15%) during illness or periods of fasting. Consider transfer of patient to a hospital able to evaluate and treat pediatric metabolic diseases.

Supportive care

- The underlying or precipitating illness needs to be treated.
Ensure that immunizations are up to date to prevent future illnesses.

Acidosis

- Correct and optimize ventilation and circulation.
- Normal saline bolus 20 mL/kg
- After this, reevaluate acidosis: bicarbonate replacement may be needed.
- For more persistent problems, consider transfer of patient to pediatric metabolism centers.

Hypoglycemia

- Use dextrose 25% (2–4 mL/kg/dose IV) if central-line access is used or dextrose 10% (2–4 ml/kg/dose IV) if peripheral line access

Other acid–base problems

Since respiratory derangements in acid–base have already been discussed, we will restrict this section to metabolic acidosis (see Box 5.10 and p. 980). An acidotic pH (<7.30), with low bicarbonate (<20 mEq/L), suggests a primary metabolic acidosis. In an emergency, an alkalotic pH (>7.50) with raised bicarbonate (>30 mEq/L) is most usually seen when supportive ventilation has been started in a patient with chronic hypercapnia.

Box 5.10 Differential diagnosis of metabolic acidosis

Calculate the anion gap (AG)

$AG = [Na] - ([HCO_3] + [Cl])$ Normal AG = 10–12 mmol/L

Increased anion gap metabolic acidosis
This is due to the production of exogenous acid. Think of A MUDPILE:
- **A**lcohol or **A**spirin
- **M**ethanol
- **U**remia
- **D**KA
- **P**araldehyde
- **I**ngestion or **I**nborn error
- **L**actate
- **E**thylene glycol

Normal anion gap metabolic acidosis
This is commonly due to loss of bicarbonate from the gut or kidney, or impaired acid secretion by the kidney:
- Diarrhea
- Type I (distal) renal tubular acidosis (RTA)—inability to excrete hydrogen ion. Urine pH is always high (>6.5); it is caused by a variety of medications or is inherited, and often associated with hypokalemia and hypercalciuria.
- Type (proximal) II RTA—impaired reabsorption of bicarbonate from proximal tubule. It is usually associated with other proximal tubular dysfunctions such as phosphoturia or glycosuria (Fanconi syndrome).
- Type IV (hyperkalemic) RTA—inadequate aldosterone production or inability to respond to it, seen in acute pyelonephritis or obstructive uropathy.

Clinical assessment

History

A thorough history is important. You will need to identify any symptoms of fever, flank pain and vomiting (pyelonephritis), lethargy, or altered mental state (metabolic disease or poisoning). Then ask specific questions about the gastrointestinal and renal tracts and growth. Lastly, there may be a significant family history of renal disease, kidney stones, or early infant death.

Examination

A complete physical examination is needed. Assess
- Hydration
- Growth
- Respiratory state (compensation for metabolic acidosis)
- Abdomen
- CNS

Investigations

Until you know the diagnosis, consider the following:
- *Blood*: Complete blood count with differential, serum electrolytes with urea and creatinine, glucose, liver function tests (transaminases), arterial or capillary blood gas, lactate, pyruvate, ketones, plasma amino acids, ammonia, carnitine, and drug screen
- *Urine*: Urinalysis, ketones, reducing substances, organic and amino acids, and drug screen
- *Imaging*: Renal ultrasound scan, to look for nephrocalcinosis (type I RTA)

Monitoring

Ensure ABCs. Monitoring will be dictated by the patient's condition. Start with continuous pulse oximetry and ECG monitoring, and intermittent BP monitoring. Follow hourly urine output.

Therapy

If the patient is dehydrated, this problem should be treated with oral or IV replacement. This alone may improve serum bicarbonate level. However, for the specific metabolic disorders provide the following:
- *Increased AG*: Identify cause and treat
- *Distal or proximal RTA*: Bicarbonate supplementation (see also p. 470)
- *Hyperkalemic RTA*: Correct serum bicarbonate, and increase fluids to improve sodium delivery to the distal tubule (this will enhance potassium secretion).

Bicarbonate treatment

If you are using bicarbonate, then
- Estimate the deficit = $(20 - [HCO_3]) \times$ weight (kg) $\times 0.5$ mEq
- Replace over 24–48 hours with oral supplements

Neonatology

Perinatal definitions

Gestational age
The time elapsed between the first day of the last menstrual period and the day of delivery. Measured in completed weeks.

Chronological age
The time elapsed since birth.

Postnatal age
The same as chronological age.

Postmenstrual age
Gestational age + chronological age

Corrected age
Chronological age reduced by the number of weeks born before 40 weeks gestation (used only for children up to 3 years of age who were born preterm).
• *Postconceptual age* and *conceptual age* should not be used in clinical pediatrics.

Spontaneous abortion (miscarriage)
Spontaneous death of a fetus before the 20th week of gestation.

Live birth
A baby that displays any sign of life (i.e., breathing, heart beat, cord pulsation, or voluntary movement) after complete delivery from the mother, irrespective of gestation.

Fetal death
Death prior to the complete expulsion or extraction from its mother of a product of human conception, irrespective of the duration of pregnancy, and which is not an induced termination of pregnancy.

Late fetal death
Fetal death at 28 or more weeks gestation.

Fetal mortality rate (FMR)
Fetal deaths that occur at 20 or more weeks gestation, divided by the number of live births plus fetal deaths. U.S. rate ~6.23 per 1000 live births (2003).

Perinatal mortality
Late fetal deaths and infant deaths at <7 days of age.

Perinatal mortality rate (PMR)
Late fetal deaths and infant deaths at <7 days of age, divided by the number of live births plus fetal deaths. U.S. rate ~6.74 per 1000 live births (2003).

Infant mortality
Death of an infant <1 year old.

Infant mortality rate (IMR)
Number of infant deaths <1 year old divided by the number of live births in the same year. U.S. rate ~6.8 per 1000 live births (2004).

Neonatal mortality rate (NMR)
Death of infants aged 0–27 days. U.S. rate ~4.5 per 1000 live births (2004).

Neonatal period
From birth to 28 postnatal days in term infants. If preterm, from birth to 44 weeks postmenstrual age.

Postneonatal mortality rate (PNMR)
Infants who died between 28 days and 1 year of age. U.S. rate ~2.27 per 1000 live births (2004).

Preterm
Birth before 37 completed weeks gestation; ~12.5% of U.S. births.

Late preterm
Birth at 34–36 completed weeks gestation; ~8.9% of U.S. births.

Very preterm
Birth before 32 completed weeks gestation.

Term birth
Birth between 37 and 42 completed weeks gestation.

Post-term (postmature)
Birth after 42 completed weeks gestation; <5% of U.S. births.

Low birth weight (LBW)
Birth weight <2500 g; 8.1% of U.S. births.

Very low birth weight (VLBW)
Birth weight <1500 g; 1.5% of U.S. births.

Extremely low birth weight (ELBW)
Birth weight <1000 g.

Small for gestational age (SGA)
Birth weight <10th centile for gestational age.

Large for gestational age (LGA)
Birth weight >90th centile for gestational age.

References

Committee on the Fetus and Newborn (2004). Age terminology during the perinatal period. *Pediatrics* **114**(5):1362–1364.

Hamilton BE, Miniño AM, Martin JA, Kochanek KD. Strobino DM, Guyer B (2007). Annual summary of vital statistics: 2005. *Pediatrics* **119**:345–360.

Routine care of the newborn

Routine measurements

Measure within 1 hour of birth:
- Weight
- Head circumference
- Body length (Note: average length in centimeters x 0.8 = gestational age in weeks)
- *Babies should be weighed daily while in the nursery*. It is normal to lose weight after birth due to water loss, but this should not exceed 10% of birth weight. Birth weight should generally be regained by day 7. Subsequent mean growth is 20–30 g/day for first 3 months of life.

Vitamin K and eye prophylaxis

- *To prevent hemorrhagic disease* of the newborn, vitamin K1 is routinely given within 1 hour of birth.
- Dose: 1 mg IM.
- *To prevent gonococcal ophthalmia*: Erythromycin ointment is routinely placed in both eyes within 1 hour of birth.

Cord care

Immediately after birth, clamp the cord with a device specifically made for this purpose. Keep the umbilicus clean and dry. Antibiotic powders or sprays are not routinely required. The cord usually detaches after 7–10 days. If umbilical granulomas develop, chemically cauterize with a silver nitrate stick.

Thermal care

Babies should be delivered in a warm room, rapidly dried with a warm towel, and then wrapped or placed skin to skin on the mother's front and covered with a warm towel and/or blanket.

Feeding

Mothers should be encouraged to breast-feed their infants, or be supported in their choice to formula feed. Supportive and educational care regarding breast-feeding should be provided, and breast-feeding should take precedence over other routine care.

Vital signs

Record vital signs soon after birth and then at routine intervals during the nursery stay. Normal babies have a pulse of 100–160 beats/minute, respiratory rate of 35–60 breaths/minute, and temperature of 36.5°–37.5°C.

Bathing

Use tepid water for the initial bath. Genitalia should be cleaned superficially only. Do not retract the foreskin; it is attached to the glans.

Biochemical screening (see p. 1080)

In all 50 states, a heel blood sample is collected on newborns to screen for the following conditions:
- Phenylketonuria (PKU)
- Congenital hypothyroidism
- Congenital adrenal hyperplasia
- Galactosemia
- Sickle cell disease
- All states also screen for a variety of other metabolic diseases. In some states screening is done twice in the first month of life.
- Positive tests require follow-up and more detailed testing.

Neonatal immunization (see p. 846)
- Hepatitis B immunization of all term or near-term newborns is recommended.

Routine neonatal examination

Each baby should be examined at least once in the first 24 hours of life by a pediatrician, family physician, or pediatric nurse practitioner.

Purpose
- Maternal reassurance
- Health education; explaining common variations
- Detecting asymptomatic problems, e.g., congenital heart disease, developmental dysplasia of the hips (DDH)
- Screening for rare but serious conditions

Order of examination

Obstetrical record

Check prenatal problems, group B streptococcal status and intrapartum prophylaxis, hours of ruptured membranes, Apgar scores, and estimated gestational age.

Mother

Check maternal labs, including blood type, Rh status and antibody status, hepatitis B status, Venereal Disease Research Laboratory test (VDRL), and HIV. Review maternal medical and social history.

Baby

When the baby is quiet (use calming techniques such as having the baby suck on a clean gloved finger, examination after a feed), note the following (see also Box 6.1):
- General posture and movements
- Skin color
- Listen to the heart and note presence of murmurs, gallops, or irregular heart rates.
- Observe respirations, noting presence of symmetric chest movements, respiratory rate (normal 35–60 breaths/minute) retractions, and nasal flaring.
- Listen to the lungs, assessing equality of breath sounds bilaterally, and presence of grunting, stridor, or rales.

Box 6.1 Remainder of examination of the completely undressed baby, in head-to-toe order

- *Cranium*: Measure maximum occipital–frontal circumference (OFC; normal 33–37 cm at term); assess skull shape, fontanelle positions, tension and size (anterior may be up to 4 x 4 cm, posterior 1 cm). Check for presence of caput succedaneum, and cephalohematoma.
- *Eyes*: Assess for presence and size of subconjunctival hemorrhages (crescent-shaped hemorrhages adjacent to iris) and presence of red reflexes (to rule out cataracts and/or retinoblastoma).
- *Ears*: Assess position, size, and shape. Note preauricular pits and tags.
- *Face*: Assess any dysmorphism, nose, and chin size. Inspect the mouth. Visualize and palpate the palate for possible clefts.
- *Neck*: Inspect and assess movements; palpate clavicles.
- *Chest*: Assess shape, symmetry, and nipple position.
- *Abdomen*: Inspect shape, and umbilical stump. Check for inguinal hernias. Palpate for masses, liver (normal felt up to 2 cm below costal margin), spleen (normal up to 1 cm palpable), kidneys (sometimes palpable), and bladder.
- *Genitalia*: Girls—inspect (clitoris and labia are normally large). Boys—assess size (normal >2.5 cm), shape, and position of urinary meatus, palpate for descended testes (retractile testes are normal).
- Palpate the *femoral pulses* (absence or weakness may indicate aortic arch abnormalities).
- *Anus*: Assess position and patency.
- *Spine*: Inspect for deformity and sacral nevi, dimple, pit, hair patch, lipoma, and pigmentation (sacral dimples above the intergluteal cleft are worrisome).
- *Limbs*: Assess symmetry, shape, passive and active movements, and digit number and shape. Assess palmar creases. Examine hips for DDH (see p. 768).
- *CNS*: In addition to evaluation above, assess tone during handling, pulling the baby to sitting position by holding their wrists, and ventral suspension (the baby should be able to hold their head almost horizontally). Check Moro reflex by slightly dropping the head while supporting the infant's buttocks. If asymmetric, this may indicate brachial plexus injury).
- Consider a formal assessment of *gestational age* if dates or other estimates are uncertain.
- Assess *size for gestational age* by plotting weight, height, and OFC against gestational age using a standardized neonatal growth chart.
- Finally, check that *urine and meconium* are passed within the first 24 hours.

Normal variations and minor abnormalities

Skin

- *Vernix*: Normal "cheesy" white substance on skin at birth
- *Acrocyanosis*: Normal in first few days after birth
- *Postmature skin*: Dry, peeling skin, prone to cracking, common in postmature babies. Usually resolves spontaneously
- *Milia*: White papules at surface of sebaceous glands. Commonly seen on the nose of newborns
- *Salmon patch hemangioma*: Seen in up to 30% of newborns on eyelids, forehead or neck. Fades during infancy
- *Erythema toxicum*: Small pustules with surrounding erythema. Typically appear on second day of life; fades quickly

Head

- *Skull molding*: Overriding skull bones with palpable ridges are part of molding and are normal. This resolves within 2–3 days.
- *Preauricular pits, skin tags, or accessory auricles* are frequently isolated but can be associated with hearing loss or other abnormalities. Test hearing and consider surgical referral for cosmetic reasons.
- *Caput succedaneum, and cephalohematoma*: See p. 121.

Eyes

- *Blocked lacrimal duct*: Recurrent sticky eye, usually worse after sleeping. This may persist for months; consider surgery if >6–12 months.
- *Subconjunctival hemorrhage*: Associated with delivery. This is harmless and resolves within a few weeks.

Mouth

- *Epstein's pearls*: Self-resolving white inclusion cysts on palate and gums
- *Ranula*: Self-resolving bluish mouth floor swelling (mucous retention cyst)

Heart (see p. 260)

- *Transient murmurs* are frequently heard immediately after delivery. Murmurs that persist are likely innocent if they are grade I/VI in intensity, are of short duration during systole, are heard best at the left mid-sternal border, and have normal femoral pulses. The rest of the cardiovascular examination is normal.
- If murmur persists and does not satisfy the above criteria, a referral to a pediatric cardiologist and/or echocardiography as soon as possible should be strongly considered.

Umbilicus

- *Umbilical hernia*: Protuberant swelling involving the umbilicus. This rarely causes any problems and most cases spontaneously resolve within 24 months.
- *Single umbilical artery* is usually isolated and of no significance but can be associated with several syndromes and IUGR.

Genitalia

- *Undescended testes*: Differentiate from retractile testes (can be "persuaded" into the scrotum). Refer to pediatric urologist if condition doesn't resolve within 1–2 months.
- *Hydrocele* is common. Most cases resolve by a year. If it persists, refer to a surgeon (see p. 904).
- *Hernia*
- *Vaginal mucoid or bloody discharge* is due to maternal estrogen withdrawal. This spontaneously resolves.
- *Vaginal or hymenal skin tags*: Spontaneously shrink

Limbs

- *Single palmer crease*: Found in ~2% of normal babies. It may be associated with chromosomal abnormalities, e.g., trisomy 21.
- *Polydactyly*: Usually isolated, but may be associated with other abnormalities. Treatment is surgical.
- *Syndactyly*: Toes frequently require no treatment. For syndactyly of fingers refer to a surgeon.
- *Postural deformities* are common, especially after oligohydramnios or malpresentation (e.g., breech). Positional talipes is usually equinovarus or calcaneovalgus. If the affected joint can be easily massaged back to a normal neutral position the deformity will usually resolve. If it is difficult or impossible to get the foot into a neutral position, refer to an orthopedist.

Miscellaneous

- *Jaundice*: See pp. 144–147.
- *Sacral-coccygeal pits* require no action if they are within the intergluteal cleft. Higher pits require spinal imaging.
- *Breast swelling* is due to maternal hormones, and may lactate. This condition spontaneously resolves.

Infant feeding and nutrition

Breast milk

Breast milk is the "gold standard" for infant feeding. Manufacturers of formula attempt to duplicate the nutrient composition of breast milk.

Advantages of breast milk

- Decreased maternal postpartum hemorrhage
- Mild contraceptive effect
- Inexpensive
- Facilitates emergency preparedness when infant and mother remain together
- Associated with decreased infant morbidity and mortality (less in developed world)
- Decreased GI and respiratory illness
- Possible decreased risk for type 1 diabetes and atopic disease in at-risk populations
- Possible decreased risk of obesity

Contraindications

- Positive HIV status (developed countries)
- Certain maternal medications
- Maternal herpes lesion on breast
- Infantile galactosemia
- Infants with other inborn errors of metabolism may need modifications and/or limited to partial breast-feeding.

Infant formulas

Formulas are commercially available, substitute infant feedings when breast-feeding is not possible.

- *Formulas for infants born at term*: There are a large number of formulas available for the term infant. At 24–32 oz/day (usual intake for a healthy, appropriately growing infant) these products meet the nutrient recommendations for term infants. These products may differ in carbohydrate, fat, and protein composition (see Table 6.1).

Table 6.1 Formulas for infants born at term

Category	Examples	CHO Protein Fat	Comments	Indications
Cow's milk based standard infant formula	Enfamil Advance, Similac Advance, Good Start, Enfamil AR, Lactofree* (Enfamil and Similac), Generic Brands	Lactose Cow's milk Long chain	Lactofree formulas are prepared from cow's milk base and therefore may contain small residual amounts of lactose. Not recommended for individuals with galactosemia	Usual feeding for term, non breast fed infant * contraindicated for infants with galactosemia because of potential for lactose residuals
Soy Formula	Isomil, Prosobee	Corn syrup/sucroseSoy protein long chain		Family preference (eg vegetarian families), when lactose free diet indicated (ie galactosemia)
Hydrolysed Formulas	Alimentum, Pregestimil, Nutramigen*	Corn syrup/modified corn starch/maltodextrin hydrolyzed casein MCT and LCT	Nutramigen contains LCT and therefore would not be indicated for conditions of fat malabsorbtion	Used for infants with protein allergies. In some cases may be used in conditions of fat malabsorbtion because of the presence of medium chain fats (Nutramigen is an exception)
Amino Acid Based formulas	Neocate, Elecare	Amino acid based		Used for infants with extreme protein allergies who react to small peptides in above hydrolyzed formulas

Preterm infant feedings

Premature infants may receive either breast milk or formula during hospitalization (see Table 6.2). Products are available to increase the nutrient content or breast milk to meet current guidelines (fortifiers). Formulas designed to meet the nutrient requirements and address the maturational needs of the premature infant are also available (premature formula). Nutrient-enriched formulas with a protein mineral content between term and preterm formulas are available for post-discharge feeding (post-discharge formulas). There is inconsistent evidence to support routine use of these formulas, although they may benefit some infants.

After initial diuresis, both term and preterm infants should regain birth weight (6–10 days of life) and then show a consistent pattern of weight gain (20–30 g/day term, 15 g/kg/day preterm).

Supplement need guidelines

- Term infant formula fed: None needed
- Term infant breast fed: 200 IU vitamin D/day
- Preterm infant: Vitamins A, D, and C and iron

Table 6.2 Formulas for pre-term infants

	Example	Factors to consider in selection of fortifiers include:
Human Milk Fortifiers	Enfamil and Similac Human Milk Fortifier (powdered) Similac Special Care 30 may be used to fortify breastmilk (liquid)	Stage of lactation, product sterility, osmolality, CHO composition, milk supply
Premature Formula	Enfamil Premature, Similac Special Care	Lactose/glucose polymers Cows milk proteins LCT/MCT nutrient concentration higher than term formulas to meet preterm guidelines at lower volumes available at 20 and 24 kcal/oz Similac Special Care also available at 30 kcal/oz
Post discharge formulas	Enfacare and Neosure	22 kcal/oz, Lactose/corn syrup solids, cows milk protein, LCT/MCT, nutrient concentration between term and preterm formulas

Basic obstetrics

The aim of obstetrics is to monitor and promote fetal and maternal well-being during pregnancy, and to identify and manage high-risk pregnancies or complications. In the United States, obstetrician gynecologists, family physicians, and midwives typically care for low-risk pregnancies. Obstetricians, gynecologists, and maternal fetal specialists manage or consult on high-risk pregnancies.

Routine antenatal care of the low-risk pregnancy

In the United States a pre-conception visit is encouraged for patients with medical, genetic, or prior pregnancy complications. For low-risk patients, the first visit is encouraged at 6–10 weeks from the last menstrual period. Ultrasound may or may not be used to assess gestational age at that time. Nucal translucency is offered at 11–13 weeks as part of screening for trisomy 21, usually with serum metabolites (human chorionic gonadotrophin [hCG]) and pregnancy-associated protein A (PAP-A). This may be done alone or in combination with results of second-trimester blood tests (see Routine prenatal screening).

- Traditional prenatal care constitutes 13 visits—monthly until 28 weeks, every 2 weeks until 36 weeks, and weekly thereafter until delivery.
- At each visit routine assessments include
  - General health
  - Blood pressure
  - Urine glucose and albumin
  - Fetal growth, movements, heart rate, and position

Routine prenatal screening

Maternal testing is offered for the following:
- Blood group and antibodies (hemolytic disease)
- Serology for syphilis, rubella, hepatitis B, hepatitis C, and HIV
- Urine culture for bacteria
- Hemoglobin and hematocrit
- Cervical cultures for chlamydia and gonorrhea are usually done at the first prenatal visit.

Blood tests may be offered at 17–18 weeks to screen for chromosomal disorders and structural anomalies or may be included as part of integrated screening for trisomy 21. The "quad screen" is the most often used test and includes
- α-fetoprotein (AFP)
- Human chorionic gonadotrophin (hCG)
- Estriol
- Inhibin

A more detailed fetal ultrasound looking for abnormalities is usually done at ~18 weeks. A screen for gestational diabetes with a 50 g glucose load is done during the 24–28 week interval. Chorionic villus biopsy (>10 weeks' gestation) or amniocentesis (usually at 16–18 weeks') is offered for chromosomal, enzymatic, gene probe analysis if screening tests show significant risk for fetuses with suspected chromosomal or metabolic disorders.

Induction of labor

This is indicated when delivery is safer for either the mother or baby than the baby remaining in utero. Induction is carried out with vaginal prostaglandin, Cytotec, amniotomy, oxytocin, and an intracervical Foley balloon.

Normal labor

This occurs at >37 weeks and should result in delivery within 24 hours of starting.

- *First stage*: From the onset of labor to full cervical dilatation. Once the cervix is 4–5 cm dilated, dilatation should continue by at least 1 cm/hr.
- *Second stage*: Time from fully dilated cervix to birth of baby. Normal duration is 45–120 minutes in a primiparous woman, 15–45 minutes if she is multiparous, although the common use of epidural anesthesia can prolong these times.
- *Third stage*: Time from birth to placental delivery

Intrapartum fetus assessment

The aim of intrapartum fetal heart monitoring is to detect signs of fetal compromise.

It is performed using a fetal stethoscope between contractions in low-risk patients who decline continuous electronic fetal monitoring, or with intermittent or continuous electronic fetal heart rate monitoring (EFM) for the vast majority of normal- and high-risk patients.

Mode of delivery

Most term infants (60%) are delivered by spontaneous vaginal delivery. Common indications for cesarean section (CS; 30%) are the following:

- Antepartum hemorrhage
- Placenta previa
- Umbilical cord prolapse
- Labor disorders: Active phase arrest, and arrest of descent
- Failed induction
- Previous CS
- Fetal malpresentation (transverse lie and breech)
- Multiple pregnancy with non-vertex twin presenting first
- Severe pregnancy-induced hypertension
- Maternal HIV or HSV
- Non-reassuring fetal heart rate demonstrated by EFM

Instrumental delivery (10%) by forceps or vacuum extraction may be indicated when there is

- Maternal exhaustion
- Malpresentation, such as occipital–posterior
- Non-reassuring fetal heart rate pattern
- Arrest of descent at +2/5 station or below

Obstetric problems

A pediatrician is frequently requested to attend a birth if any of the following scenarios occur:

- Concerning fetal heart rate pattern
- Meconium-stained fluid
- Emergency CS
- Elective CS under general anesthesia (GA)
- Vaginal breech delivery
- Rotational forceps
- Multiple pregnancy
- Preterm delivery <37 weeks gestation
- Severe IUGR
- Maternal insulin-dependent diabetes mellitus (IDDM)
- Significant fetal structural abnormality
- Significant rhesus hemolytic disease

Intrauterine growth restriction (IUGR)

Serial detailed ultrasound scans are performed when fetal growth delay is suspected. In cases where the fetal growth is less than the 10% predicted for gestational age, Doppler evaluation of fetal umbilical and cerebral artery blood flow measurement can be performed to determine whether the growth failure is significant enough to cause alteration in either parameter. Fetal heart rate testing (non-stress test) can also be done, and together with Doppler studies can aid in determination of the appropriate timing of delivery of an SGA fetus.

Growth reduction can be symmetrical or asymmetrical. *Symmetrical IUGR is usually fetal in origin; asymmetrical suggests placental dysfunction.*

When the growth is <10% predicted, there is increased risk of fetal hypoxia or death, requiring close antenatal and intrapartum monitoring.

Macrosomia

This is usually clinically suspected when the fundal height in centimeters is significantly greater than the week's gestation. Ultrasound should be done to rule our uterine fibroid tumors, multiple gestation, or excess amniotic fluid. If these are normal, glucose tolerance tests should be performed to detect maternal diabetes if not previously done as a routine part of prenatal care.

If macrosomia is documented, growth should be monitored by either ultrasound or clinical examination. If the fetus is suspected to be extremely large, delivery management plans should be discussed with the mother prior to the onset of labor.

Multiple pregnancy

In multiple pregnancy there is an increased risk of the following:

- Perinatal mortality
- Prematurity
- Malformations
- Malpresentation
- Polyhydramnios

- Preeclampsia
- Antepartum hemorrhage
- Risk for adverse multiple adverse outcomes increases as the fetus number increases. If ≥3 fetuses, selective fetal reduction may offered to improve outcome for survivors.

Oligo- and polyhydramnios

Oligohydramnios

- Amniotic fluid Index <5 or 7 cm, depending on gestational age

Causes

- Placental insufficiency
- Preterm prolonged rupture of membranes (PPROM)
- Fetal urinary tract obstruction or renal disease

Polyhydramnios

- Amniotic fluid index (measured by ultrasound) >25 cm

Causes

- 50% secondary to fetal disease, e.g., upper GI tract obstruction
- 30% idiopathic
- 20% maternal diabetes mellitus

Risks

- Preterm labor
- Malpresentation
- Cord prolapse
- Antepartum hemorrhage (APH)

Indomethacin or amniotic fluid reduction may be beneficial.

Prolonged pregnancy

This is defined as longer than 42 weeks' gestation.

- Significant ↑perinatal mortality and morbidity (↑risk of perinatal hypoxia due to placental insufficiency, obstructed labor due to larger fetus, meconium aspiration).
- Induction of labor is usually considered after 41 weeks, especially when the cervix is favorable.

Antepartum hemorrhage (APH)

APH is bleeding after 24 weeks gestation.

Associations

- ↑Perinatal mortality and morbidity; preterm delivery

Major causes

- Placenta previa
- Vasa previa
- Placental abruption

An expectant-course or immediate delivery is performed depending on the severity and gestation.

Umbilical cord prolapse

This obstetric emergency, due to a high risk of cord compression and perinatal asphyxia, requires urgent delivery, usually by Cesarean section.

Preterm prelabor rupture of the membranes

- *In 80%:* Preterm labor rapidly follows.
- *Other 20%:* Significant risk of infection and neonatal pulmonary hypoplasia (if before 24 weeks)
- *Treatment:* Give mother antibiotics and corticosteroids.

Preterm labor

See p. 158.

Failure to progress

Labor progress can be delayed in both the first and second stage of labor. Active phase arrest of labor after 4 cm should be evaluated for adequacy of uterine activity. Oxytocin is used to correct inadequate uterine activity. Arrest of descent disorders in the second stage of labor can be due to uterine activity disorders, dense epidural anesthesia, or cephalopelvic disproportion. The latter is usually treated with cesarean section.

Disturbing fetal status in labor

This status may signify hypoxia. Fetal acidosis results if hypoxia is prolonged or repeated.

Signs
- Loss of variability in baseline fetal heart rate (<5 beats/minute)
- Late decelerations (symmetrical fetal heart rate deceleration, the nadir of which occurs after peak uterine contraction)
- Repetitive severe, variable decelerations
- Prolonged fetal deceleration (2–9 minutes below established baseline)
- Fetal bradycardia (>10 minutes below previously established fetal baseline)
- Persistent fetal tachycardia (>170/minute)

Tests
- *Fetal scalp stimulation test:* Tactile or sound stimulation resulting in fetal heart rate acceleration, the peak reaching 15 beats/minute above the baseline and remaining above the baseline for 15 seconds, is associated with fetal scalp pH >7.20 in 98% of patients.
- *Postnatal umbilical artery and venous sample* are used to determine the actual level of acidemia.

Malpresentation

The most common form is breech birth (3% at term).

Types

Types include frank (hips flexed and knees extended), complete (hips and knees flexed), and footling (feet are presenting apart). External cephalic version may be successful in turning the baby between 34 and 36 weeks. Vaginal breech delivery is associated with increased perinatal mortality and morbidity; CS is recommended.

Other malpresentations are associated with an increased risk of obstructed labor and CS rate (brow and transverse presentation).

Face presentation

In this instance, the baby will only deliver vaginally if the mentum (chin) rotates to the anterior position. Presenting position in labor is often predictive of whether the mentum will rotate to an anterior position at complete dilatation (most likely for anterior, least likely for mentum posterior). There is an increased incidence of non-reassuring fetal heart rate patterns. Increased risk of respiratory distress in vaginally delivered infants usually requires pediatric attendance at delivery.

Shoulder dystocia

Accessory delivery maneuvers are needed to deliver the body of the baby after the fetal head has emerged. The body is often preceded by the head retracting against the maternal perineum (turtle sign). Fetal compromise from umbilical cord compression is not usually significant in a previously healthy fetus until delivery delay exceeds 5–7 minutes.

- *Treatment*: Urgent delivery (<30–60 seconds) is not necessary.
- A logical sequence of maneuvers should be performed with emphasis being on avoidance of fetal injury.
- *Traditional maneuvers*: Maternal hip flexion, suprapubic pressure, and posterior fetal arm extraction
- *Other maneuvers*: Dorsal shoulder rotation (Rubin), ventral shoulder rotation (Woods), hands and knees (Gaskin), or cephalic replacement and cesarean section (Zavanelli)
- *Risks*: Clavicle fracture, Erb's palsy, humeral fracture. Perinatal asphyxia is a risk when delivery is prolonged >5–7 minutes.

Maternal disorders causing neonatal disease

Any maternal disease can affect adversely fetal and neonatal health. Certain maternal illnesses, e.g., congenital heart disease, also raise the risk of inheritance in the newborn.

The most common manifestations of maternal disease in the fetus are
- Spontaneous abortion
- Fetal death
- IUGR and preterm delivery

Maternal drug ingestion
Medications or substance abuse can affect the newborn (p. 218)
- Maternal anticonvulsants
- Alcohol abuse and fetal alcohol syndrome (p. 208)
- Tobacco (p. 218)

Hypertensive diseases
Pregnancy-induced hypertension (e.g., preeclampsia, eclampsia, HELLP syndrome—**H**emolytic anemia, **E**levated **L**iver enzymes, **L**ow **P**latelet count) is associated with increased fetal loss, need for preterm delivery, IUGR, and neonatal thrombocytopenia. Maternal drug treatment with magnesium sulfate may cause neonatal hypotonia.

Systemic lupus erythematosus (SLE)
SLE is associated with the following:
- ↑Risk of spontaneous abortion
- IUGR
- Preterm delivery
- Neonatal lupus syndrome (rare): Anti-Ro and -La antibodies or complete heart block, hemolytic anemia, leukopenia, thrombocytopenia, and discoid erythematosus skin rash

Antiphospholipid syndrome
Maternal antiphospholipid antibodies (e.g., lupus anticoagulant or anticardiolipin antibodies) are associated with spontaneous abortion, IUGR, fetal death, and need for preterm delivery.

Thyroid disease (see p. 469)
In ~10% of women with Graves' disease, TSH receptor–stimulator antibodies cross the placenta, causing neonatal thyrotoxicosis. The fetus is most likely to be affected if a high maternal IgG serum level develops and is not recognized. If the mother has severe disease and is treated with antithyroid medications (Tapazole or propothiouracil) the fetus may show signs of hypothyroidism or, in extreme cases, fetal goiter. Measure TFT at birth (cord blood) and at 2–7 days of life.

Myasthenia gravis

In ~10% of cases transplacental passage of IgG antibodies to motor end-plate acetylcholine receptors occurs and causes transient neonatal myasthenia gravis.

Diabetes mellitus (see p. 482)

Gestational diabetes

The incidence is rapidly increasing, secondary to maternal obesity. Infant risks include macrosomia with increased risks of birth trauma from failed vaginal delivery and successful but traumatic vaginal delivery.

Type 1 diabetes

Neonatal outcome is affected by pre-conception glucose control and Antepartum glucose control. Poor pre-conception control increases the risk of fetal birth defects in direct proportion to the variance of HgA1C from normal. Poor antepartum control results in increased risks of fetal macrosomia, preeclampsia, fetal compromise during labor, and intrauterine fetal demise.

Maternal infection

Genital herpes

Fetuses most likely to be affected are those whose mother acquires first herpes infection (type 1 or 1) during pregnancy and who deliver before the mother can mount an antibody response, which is passively passed to the fetus.

HIV

Effective antiviral therapy is not available to prevent fetal infection in most mothers infected with HIV. The challenge is identifying these patients in the antepartum period and enrolling them in effective treatment protocols to reduce transmission at birth.

Group B streptococcus (GBS)

Routine screening at 34–36 weeks is now standard practice and has significantly reduced the incidence of early-onset group B streptococcal disease in the newborn. In patients who deliver before routine screening can be performed, intrapartum antibiotics effective against GBS are indicated.

Hepatitis B

Routine prenatal screening for hepatitis B is now standard practice. At-risk infants should receive both passive and active immunization. Infants born to mothers with unknown HBAg status should be considered potentially infectious until serologic testing confirms otherwise.

Hepatitis C

Vertical transmission is less common than with hepatitis B, but increased with concomitant HIV positivity and high maternal viral load. Neither cesarean delivery nor immunoprophylaxis has been shown to be effective in preventing neonatal transmission in high-risk mothers.

Birth trauma

Risk factors

Risk factors include LGA, prematurity, cephalic–pelvic disproportion, malpresentation, precipitate deliveries, instrument delivery, and shoulder dystocia.

Head

- *Caput succedaneum*: Edema of the presenting scalp. Can be particularly large following vacuum extraction delivery. Rapidly resolves
- *Cephalohematoma*: Common fluctuant swelling(s), most often over parietal bones due to subperiosteal bleed. Resolves over weeks
- *Subgaleal (subaponeurotic) hematoma*: Rare. Bleeding is not confined by skull periosteum, so it can be large and life threatening. This presents as fluctuant scalp swelling, and can cross suture lines.

Skin

- *Traumatic injury*: Bruising and petechiae of presenting part
- *Lacerations*: Caused by forceps, vacuum extraction device, scalp electrodes, scalp pH sampling, or scalpel wounds during caesarean section. Close with Steri-Strips or suture.

Nerve palsies

Brachial plexus

The most common form is Erb's palsy (C5–C6 nerve routes), and it may result from difficult assisted delivery (e.g., shoulder dystocia). The arm is flaccid with pronated forearm and flexed wrist (waiter's tip position). Complete recovery occurs within 6 weeks in two-thirds of patients. X-ray the chest and spine to exclude fractures. Physiotherapy is of little or no value unless there is permanent nerve damage. Refer for specialist assessment.

Facial nerve palsy

This form of palsy follows pressure on the face, usually from maternal sacral promontory. It presents as facial asymmetry that becomes worse on crying (the affected side shows lack of eye closure and lower facial movement, and the mouth is drawn to the normal side). Most patients recover within 1–2 weeks. They may require eye care with methylcellulose and specialist referral.

Fractures

- *Clavicle* (most common)
- *Long bone fractures* are usually lower avulsion fractures of the femoral or tibial epiphyses, or mid-shaft fractures of the femur or humerus. The infant presents as unsettled, with affected limb pseudoparalysis, or obvious deformity or swelling. Confirm by X-ray.
- *Skull fracture* is associated with forceps delivery and usually requires no treatment unless depressed, requiring neurosurgical referral.

Treatment

Treatment includes analgesia, limb immobilization with a sling or splint until healed in a few weeks, or orthopedic referral. Rapid healing and remodeling usually occur.

Soft tissue trauma

Sternocleidomastoid tumor

Overstretching of the muscle leads to hematoma. Subsequent contraction of the muscle results in a non-tender "tumor" and torticollis (the head turns away from the affected muscle). Physiotherapy is almost always curative.

Fat necrosis

This is a tender, red, subcutaneous swelling caused by pressure over bony prominences or from forceps. It usually resolves spontaneously.

Neonatal life support

Every birth should be attended by a health professional who has been trained and has experience in administering the ABC's of resuscitation.

If meconium-stained newborns are not vigorous (heart rate <100 bpm, poor tone, or poor respiratory effort), do not stimulate the infant but intubate and suction the trachea. You may repeat this sequence if significant meconium is suctioned from the trachea, otherwise begin neonatal support algorithm from the beginning (see Fig. 6.1).

Ninety percent of neonates are perfectly healthy, and the best plan is to return these babies to the mother with no interference, to augment bonding. Mother-and-baby skin-to-skin contact is ideal, rather than swaddling or nursery cots, and is the best way to maintain temperature. A pediatrician or nurse trained in advanced neonatal resuscitation should attend the following births: emergency Caesarians, breeches, twins, forceps for fetal distress, intrapartum bleeding, prematurity, hydrops fetalis, and eclampsia.

Before birth

Check the equipment. Get a warm blanket. Heat the crib.

At birth

If pulse is <100 or there is poor color or respiratory effort, set a clock in motion, and see opposite. Be alert to the following:
- Hypothermia (use heat lamp)
- Hypoglycemia: Dextrose 10%, 5 mL/kg IV
- Pethidine toxicity: Naloxone, e.g., 200 µg IM. Contraindicated in opioid abuse
- Anemia (heavy fetal blood loss?)—give 20 mL/kg blood + 4.5% albumin
- Is there lung disease or congenital cyanotic heart disease? Transfer to NICU or SCBU for monitoring.
- Suck out the oropharynx only if meconium aspiration is suspected.
- 21% O_2 (air) is better than 100% O_2.

Endotracheal intubation is a key skill: use 3.5 mm uncuffed, unshouldered tubes on term infants; 3 if 1.25–2.5 kg (2.5 if smaller). Learn from experts. Have many sizes to hand. Practice on models.

Prognosis

Mortality for **premature infants** is 315/1000 if 5-minute Apgar score 0–3, vs. 5/1000 if score is > [3]7. Corresponding figures *at term* are 244/1000 and 0.2/1000. If a term infant with Apgar score ≥ has a low arterial pH ≥, the risk of neonatal death increases 8-fold. Survival in those needing CPR (cardiac resuscitation) is 63% for infants of 0.5–1.5 kg, compared with 88% in these weight groups if CPR is not needed. Severe intraventricular hemorrhage is seen in 15% of those needing CPR vs. 5% in those who don't.

Wrap (without drying) and place under radiant heat.

↓

Initial assessment; set a clock in motion; assess *color, tone, breathing* and *pulse*. If not breathing...

↓

Control the airway (head in the neutral position)

↓

Support breathing: 5 inflation breaths; 3 seconds long. Confirm response: visible chest movements or ↑ heart rate

↓

If there is no response, check *head position* and try a *jaw thrust*; then 5 inflation breaths. Confirm response: visible chest movements or ↑ heart rate.

↓

If there is still no response, get a second person to help with airway control and inflation breaths.
- Direct vision of oropharynx
- Repeat 5 inflation breaths
- Insert oropharyngeal airway
- Repeat inflation breaths

Consider intubation. Confirm response: visible chest movements or increased heart rate.

↓

When chest is moving, continue with ventilation breaths if there is no spontaneous breathing.

↓

Check heart rate; if absent or <60 (and not rising) *start chest compressions*. Do 3 chest compressions to 1 breath, for 30 seconds.

↓

Reassess pulse: If improving, stop chest compressions. If the infant is not breathing, go on ventilating. If heart rate is still, continue ventilation and chest compressions.

↓

Consider *IV or umbilical access* and *drugs*, e.g., adrenaline (epinephrine): 10 µg/kg (0.1 mL 1:10,000/kg) IV or 100 µg/kg via endotracheal tube.[1]

At all stages ask: *Do I need help?*

1 http://www.resus.org.uk/pages/pals.htm. 20UK resusc council accessed 2005. Give tracheal dose quickly down a narrow bore suction catheter beyond the tracheal end of the tube and then flushed in with 1 or 2 mls of normal saline.

Apgar	Pulse	Respirations	Muscle tone	Color	On suction
2	>100	Strong cry	Active	Pink	Coughs well
1	<100	Slow, irregular	Limb flexion	Blue limbs	Depressed cough
0	0	Nil	Absent	All blue or white	No response

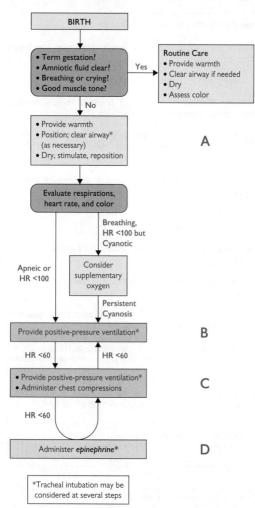

Figure 6.1 Neonatal Resuscitation Flow Algorithm. American Academy of Pediatrics, American Heart Association. *Textbook of Neonatal Resuscitation.* Kattwinkel J, ed. 5th ed. Elk Grove Village, IL: American Academy of Pediatrics; 2006. Reprinted with permission of the American Academy of Pediatrics.

Nonspecifically ill neonate

Early recognition of serious neonatal illness is an important skill. The nurse may say that the infant is just "not right." Listen to the nurse, examine the baby carefully, and act if in any doubt (see Box 6.2)! Any serious disease can present nonspecifically.

Major causes

- Infection (e.g., septicemia, meningitis) (p. 210)
- Hypothermia (p. 142)
- Metabolic (e.g., hypoglycemia, inborn errors of metabolism (IEM)) (p. 148)
- Cardiac (e.g., congenital heart disease, arrhythmias, p. 260)
- Gastrointestinal (e.g., NEC, p. 353)
- CNS (e.g., intracranial hemorrhage, seizures, p. 204).

Presentation

- *Skin*: Pallor, mottling, peripheral cyanosis, cool peripheries; capillary refill >2 seconds; rash; jaundice
- *Temperature*: ↑ or ↓, instability
- *CNS*: Lethargy, coma, weak or high-pitched cry, generalized hypotonic, irritability, jittery, seizures
- *Respiratory*: Apnea, expiratory grunting, flaring nostrils, tachypnea (>60 breaths/minute), intercostal or subcostal retractions, tracheal tug
- *Cardiovascular system*: Tachycardia (>160/minute), weak or absent pulses, bradycardia (<80/minute), hypotension
- *Gastrointestinal*: Vomiting, distended abdomen (ileus), diarrhea, bloody stools; abdominal tenderness
- *Metabolic*: ↑ or ↓blood glucose

Box 6.2 Management of nonspecifically ill neonates

- Quickly assess ABC. Secure airway, give oxygen, and provide ventilatory support if needed.
- Obtain vascular access and give bolus 0.9% saline or colloid (e.g., human albumin 5%) 10–20 mL/kg. Repeat if necessary.
- Monitor respiratory status, SaO_2, heart rate, BP, and temperature.
- Measure BP, blood glucose, CBC, and CRP. Consider clotting studies and blood gas. Ventilate early if there is respiratory failure.
- Full septic screen: Blood culture; chest X-ray; urine (suprapubic); lumbar puncture (LP; only postpone if baby is very unstable) for CSF culture and sensitivity, cell count and differential, protein, glucose; stool culture and virology
- Start antibiotics. If <48 hours old, give IV/IM ampillicin and an aminoglycoside (e.g., gentamicin). If >48 hours old, give cefotaxime and an aminoglycoside, unless indwelling lines were present before the illness, in which case consider vancomycin instead of cefotaxime. If all cultures are negative, and index of suspicion of sepsis is low, antibiotics can be stopped after 48 hours. If not, treat for 5–7 days, changing antibiotics according to sensitivities of significant identified pathogens. Treat for 14–21 days if meningitis is present. Consider viral disease, especially herpes virus, in an infant who does not improve rapidly with antibiotic treatment. If any doubt, consult infectious disease specialist.
- Give specific treatment as appropriate—e.g., correct hypoglycemia, give isotropic support if the infant is persistently hypotensive, blood transfusion if there is significant hemorrhage, clotting factors to correct DIC.

Neonatal jaundice

Jaundice (hyperbilirubinemia) is common in newborns, and significant jaundice may indicate underlying disease (see also p. 368). In addition, bilirubin is neurotoxic and can cause kernicterus (deafness, athetoid cerebral palsy, limitation of upward gaze) (see Fig. 6.2, Fig. 6.3, and Fig. 6.4).

Physiological jaundice

This type is common and appears after 24 hours, peaking around day 3 or 4, and typically resolving by 2 weeks. It is due to inadequate bilirubin conjugation and elimination by the immature newborn liver.

Pathologic causes of jaundice

Increased red blood cell destruction

- Isoimmunization (Rh incompatibility, ABO incompatibility, etc.)
- Red blood cell biochemical defects (G6PD deficiency, pyruvate kinase deficiency, etc.)
- Structural abnormalities of red cells (hereditary spherocytosis, etc.)
- Infection (bacteria or viral sepsis, etc.)
- Sequestered blood (cephalohematoma, bruising, subdural hematoma)

Disorders of conjugation of bilirubin (deficiency of hepatic enzymes)

- Crigler–Najjar syndrome
- Gilbert syndrome
- Hypothyroidism

Disorders of enterohepatic circulation

- Breast-feeding jaundice (due to poor intake at breast)
- Breast-milk jaundice (enhanced recirculation)

Major risk factors

- Pre-discharge total serum bilirubin level in the high-risk zone (see Fig. 6.2)
- Jaundice observed in the first 24 hours
- Blood group incompatibility with positive direct antiglobulin test (Coombs), other known hemolytic disease (e.g., G6PD deficiency), elevated end-tidal carbon monoxide (ETCO)
- Gestational age 35–36 weeks
- Previous sibling received phototherapy
- Cephalohematoma or significant bruising
- Exclusive breast-feeding, particularly if nursing is not going well and weight loss is excessive
- East Asian race (as defined by mother's description)

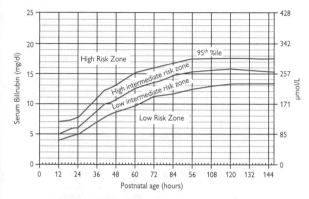

Figure 6.2 Risk of needing later treatment for hyperbilirubinemia. Reprinted with permission from Bhutani VK, Johnson L, Sivieri EM (1999). Predictive ability of a predischarge hour-specific serum bilirubin for subsequent significant hyper-bilirubinemia in healthy term and near-term newborns. *Pediatrics* **103**:6–14.

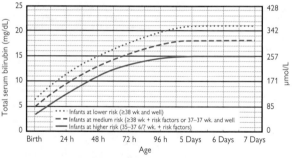

- Use total bilirubin. Do not subtract direct reacting or conjugated bilirubin.
- Risk factors = isoimmune hemolytic disease, G6PD deficiency, asphyxia, significant lethargy, temperature instability, sepsis, acidosis, or albumin <3.0g/dL (if measured)
- For well infants 35–37 6/7 wk can adjust TSB levels for intervention around risk line. It is an option to intervene at lower TSB levels for infants closer to 35 wks and at higher TSB levels for those closer to 37 6/7 wk.
- It is an option to provide conventional phototheraypy in hospital or at home at TSB levels 2–3 mg/dL (35–50mmol/L) below those shown but home phototherapy should not be used in any infant with risk factors.

Figure 6.3 Treatment of indirect hyperbilirubinemia: Guidelines for starting phototherapy. Reprinted with permission from American Academy of Pediatrics Subcommittee on Hyperbilirubinemia (2004). Management of hyperbilirubinemia in the newborn infant 35 or more weeks of gestation. *Pediatrics* **114**:297–316.

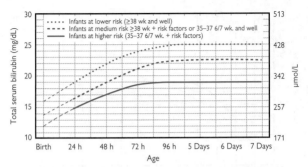

- The dashed lines for the first 24 hours indicate uncertainty due to a wide range of clinical circumstance and a range of responses to phototherapy.
- Immediate exchange transfusion is recommended if infant signs of acute bilirubin encephalopathy (hypertonia, arching, retrocollis, opisthotonos, fever, high pitched cry) or if TSB ≥5 mg/dL (85 μmol/L) above these lines.
- Risk factors - isoimmune hemolytic disease, G6PD deficiency, asphyxia, significant lethargy, temperature instability, sepsis, acidosis.
- Measure serum albumin and calculate B/A ratio (see legend)
- Use total bilirubin. Do not subtract direct reacting or conjugated bilirubin
- If infant is well and 35–37 6/7 wk (median risk) can individualize TSB levels for exchange based on actual gestational age.

Figure 6.4 Treatment of indirect hyperbilirubinemia: guidelines for doing an exchange transfusion. Reprinted with permission from American Academy of Pediatrics Subcommittee on Hyperbilirubinemia (2004). Management of hyperbilirubinemia in the newborn infant 35 or more weeks of gestation. *Pediatrics* **114**:297–316.

Prolonged jaundice

This is defined as >14 days in the term infant, >21 days in the preterm infant.

Causes

Causes include breast-feeding (benign, self-limiting, and usually resolves by 12 weeks), enclosed bleeding (e.g., cephalhematoma), prematurity, hemolysis, sepsis, hypothyroidism, conjugated jaundice (see below), and hepatic enzyme disorders (e.g., Crigler–Najjar syndrome, Lucy–Driscoll disease).

Treatment

Treatment depends on the cause. Rarely, phototherapy is beneficial, e.g., in Crigler–Najjar syndrome.

Conjugated jaundice

This is defined as conjugated serum bilirubin (SBR) >25 μmol/L. Stools may be clay colored in obstructive jaundice.

Causes

Causes include sepsis, TPN, biliary tract obstruction (e.g., biliary atresia, choledochal cyst), viral hepatitis; TORCH infections, α_1-antitrypsin deficiency, cystic fibrosis, inspissated bile syndrome after hemolytic disease, galactosemia, other IEM, and idiopathic giant cell hepatitis.

Treatment

Treatment depends on the cause.

Hypoglycemia in the newborn infant

- Hypoglycemia in the newborn infant is blood glucose <35–40 mg/dL.
- High-risk infants should be screened within 1 hour of birth—preterm, SGA, IDM, LGA—with or without symptoms.
- Confirm screening test with laboratory glucose measurement. Bedside glucose monitoring is inaccurate, especially in the low range.
- The target range for blood glucose concentration is 60–80 mg/dL in the first week of life.

Signs and symptoms

- Most commonly, hypoglycemia is asymptomatic or masked by concomitant illness (e.g., prematurity).
- Jitteriness, lethargy, apnea, seizures, poor feeding, irritability

Most common causes (see Table 6.3)

- Transitional immaturity of glucose regulation
  - SGA, preterm, and some otherwise normal-term infants
- Hyperinsulinemia in IDDM from excessive in utero glucose exposure

Table 6.3 The most common causes of hypoglycemia in newborns

Unusual causes	History and physical-exam findings
Hyperinsulinemia	
Beckwith–Wiedemann syndrome	Overgrowth, macroglossia, ear creases, omphalocele
Pancreatic islet cell hyperplasia, islet cell tumor	Overgrowth
Genetic defects in insulin secretion	Overgrowth
Pituitary insufficiency	Midline defects, optic dysplasia, microphallus
Inborn errors of carbohydrate metabolism	Hepatomegaly (rare at birth)
Adrenal insufficiency, CAH	Electrolyte abnormalities, hypotension, ambiguous genitalia
Maternal medication	History of β-agonist, sulfonylurea
Sepsis (usually hyperglycemic)	See Neonatal sepsis (p.210)

Initial approach

- Always consider sepsis and workup if appropriate.
- Confirm screening test with laboratory measurement of blood glucose.
- Treat (see Table 6.4) and reevaluate.
- History and physical examination for causes

Initial treatment (see Table 6.4)

Table 6.4 Initial treatment of hypoglycemia

Mg/dL	Treatment
35–45	Feed if appropriate, otherwise give IV glucose at 4–6 mg/kg/min
25–34	IV glucose at 4–6 mg/kg/min
<25	Minibolus = 2 mL/kg D10W IV over 1–2 minutes, then IV glucose at 4–6 mg/kg/min

IV rate in mg/kg/min equals

$$\left(\frac{\% \text{ glucose in I.V. solution} \times \text{I.V. rate in ml/hr} \times 0.167}{\text{weight in kg}} \right)$$

Follow-up

- Re-check blood glucose 30–60 minutes after each intervention.
- Re-bolus and increase infusion rate by 2 mg/kg/min as needed.

Further workup if hypoglycemia is prolonged or severe:
- Serum insulin concentration   } Draw while hypopoglycemic
- Serum cortisol concentration
- Serum growth hormone concentration
- Blood pH, lactate, pyruvate
- Metabolic screen
- Endocrine or metabolism specialist referral

Fluid and electrolyte management

Box 6.3 Fluid and electrolyte management

Purpose of intravenous fluid support for NPO infants
- Replace daily losses of water and electrolytes.
- Provide water and electrolytes for growth.
- Provide glucose (see Hypoglycemia, p. 148).
- Provide other nutrients (see Parenteral nutrition, p. 380).

Basic principles
- Intravascular volume deficit should be treated with crystalloid or blood products as appropriate.
- Monitor daily weight, I/O, electrolytes (q8–24h).
- Infants are born with ↑ total body weight (TBW) and Na, preterm > term
- Diuresis occurs in the first 1–2 days. Normal is 5%–10% weight loss in term infants, 15% in VLBW.
- Insensible water loss (IWL) = skin loss (↑↑ in VLBW infant) + respiratory loss (↓ on respirator). Must be estimated
- Sensible water loss (SWL) = urine + stool + other drainage. Can be measured
- Electrolyte needs: Amount lost in fluids + amount needed for growth (Na 1–3 meq/kg/day; K 1–2 meq/kg/day)
- Target U/O = 2–4 mL/kg/hr after initial diuresis
- Body weight for dosing may differ from actual weight
  - Use birth weight for dosing until infant regains, then use daily weight.
  - If there are abnormal fluid collections (edema, hydrocephalus, body cavity effusions) make birth weight inappropriately high, use 50% percentile for gestational age or weight percentile corresponding to length percentile.
- Calculate glucose infusion rate (GIR) daily. See Hypoglycemia (p. 148). At extremes of fluid administration, high or low, adjust dextrose concentration of fluid to achieve appropriate GIR.

Pre-diuresis fluid management

This is appropriate on the first day for most term infants. Ill and very preterm infants may have delayed diuresis (see Table 6.5).

Table 6.5 FLUID: D10W without electrolytes

Term or near-term infant, healthy, NPO	• Starting rate: 60–80 mL/kg/day
	• Likely to need post-diuresis fluids by second day
Very low birth weight infant, NPO	• Starting rate: 100–120 mL/kg/day
	• Increase rate as needed to meet IWL and prevent or correct hypernatremia
	• Reduce dextrose concentration as volume increases to prevent hyperglycemia
	• Add amino acids to D10W if possible and start PN within 24 hours
Renal failure (oliguric)	• Starting rate: 40–60 mL/kg/day
	• At 40 mL/kg/day need at least 15% dextrose to achieve adequate GIR

Post-diuresis fluid management

This occurs on the second day of life for most term infants. It is often delayed with severe illness or extreme prematurity (see Table 6.6 and Table 6.7).

Table 6.6 FLUID: D10W with electrolytes (often with parenteral nutrition components)

Term or near-term infant, healthy, NPO	• Add maintenance electrolytes: 2–3 mEq Na and 1–2 mEq K/kg/day • Advance volume by 20 mL/kg/day each day. A goal intake of 140–160 mL/kg/day provides maintenance fluids, allows adequate nutrition (with parenteral nutrition components), and can be handled by most neonatal kidneys.
Very low birth weight infant, NPO	• As skin keratinizes, IWL decreases, and intake volume can be reduced. Goal volume is similar to that of term infants. However, see below for conditions in which fluid restriction (100–120 mL/kg/day) may be helpful. The premature kidney is less capable of Na retention, so electrolyte requirements may be higher than at term (3–6 mEq/kg/day).
Renal failure	• Watch for diuretic phase with high urine volume. Replace losses of water and electrolytes guided by volume and composition of urine and serum electrolytes.
Neonatal illness considerations	• Lower fluid intakes may be helpful in RDS, PDA, and BPD, and may reduce risk for NEC in at-risk infants.
Infants with other sensible losses	• GI drainage, diarrhea, chylothorax drainage, surgical drainage, and abnormal skin integrity (e.g., epidermolysis bullosa) may produce substantial fluid losses. Replace cc/cc with solution of water, electrolytes, and albumin as appropriate, and follow serum concentrations closely. See Table 6.7 for typical composition of common body fluids.

Table 6.7 Common body fluids

Body fluid	Na (mEq/L)	K (mEq/L)	Protein
GI			
Gastric	20–80	5–20	Minimal
Small bowel	100–140	5–15	Minimal
Ileostomy	45–135	5–15	Minimal
Diarrhea	10–90	10–80	Minimal
Chylothorax	= serum	= serum	2–7 g/dL

Small for gestational age (SGA)

SGA is defined as birth weight <10 percentile or >2 standard deviations (SD) below the mean for gestational age. SGA is not synonymous with intrauterine growth restriction (IUGR). SGA is a postnatal description of weight that may or may not be caused by IUGR, whereas IUGR reflects failure of normal fetal growth that may or may not result in an SGA newborn.

IUGR infants can be subclassified into symmetric growth (weight, length, and head circumference all proportionally small) and asymmetric growth (weight relatively low for head circumference and length). Symmetric IGUR reflects either constitutional growth failure (e.g., chromosomal disorder, congenital infection) or early placental insufficiency, whereas asymmetric IUGR suggests placental problems later in pregnancy.

Causes of SGA
- Constitutional, i.e., small parents, chromosomal anomalies, other genetic syndromes
- Congenital anomalies (cardiac anomalies, gastrointestinal anomalies)
- Congenital infection (TORCH, syphilis, malaria) (p. 210)
- Inborn errors of metabolism
- Placental insufficiency (abruption, maternal hypertension, multiple pregnancy, maternal illness, maternal malnutrition, maternal blood dyscrasia or anemia, uterine abnormalities)
- Maternal substance use (alcohol, tobacco, cocaine, methamphetamines)

Complications
- Fetal death (SGA can be a marker of fetal compromise)
- Fetal asphyxia (SGA can be a marker of fetal compromise)
- Meconium aspiration syndrome (p. 168)
- Persistent pulmonary hypertension (PPHN; p. 174)
- Hypoglycemia (due to decreased glycogen stores; p. 148)
- Hyperglycemia (due to low resting insulin secretion; p. 469)
- Hypothermia (due to decreased subcutaneous fat)
- Polycythemia (due to chronic fetal hypoxia; p. 195)
- Feeding intolerance
- Necrotizing enterocolitis (increased risk compared with appropriately grown newborns; p. 216)
- Thrombocytopenia (p. 196)
- Neutropenia

Management
- Review maternal and prenatal history to identify risk factors and etiology.
- Establish gestational age as accurately as possible.
- Measure length and head circumference along with weight at admission
- Provide thermoregulatory support.
- Monitor blood sugar.
- If premature, use cautious feeding advancement.
- Consider further workup of etiology if SGA is unexplained by prenatal history (e.g., TORCH infection evaluation, karyotype)

Prognosis (see also p. 162)

Neurodevelopmental impairments are more common in SGA newborns. In general, symmetric IUGR/SGA infants have worse long-term neurological outcomes than those of asymmetric IUGR/SGA infants. SGA newborns who are born premature with a chromosomal anomaly or congenital infection have very high risk of neurocognitive impairments later in life. IUGR infants are at increased risk of developing cardiovascular disease, insulin resistance, cerebrovascular disease, and hypertension into adult life (Barker hypothesis).

Large for gestational age (LGA)

LGA is defined as birth weight >90th percentile or >2 SD above the mean for gestational age.

Causes of LGA

- Constitutional, i.e., large parents
- Infant of a diabetic mother (IDM) (see below)
- Beckwith–Wiedemann syndrome (BWS) (p. 1075)
- Other causes of fetal (congenital) hyperinsulinism: islet cell hyperplasia or adenoma, nesidioblastosis
- Hydrops fetalis (p. 192)

Complications

- Obstetric complications (perinatal asphyxia, shoulder dystocia, nerve palsies, fractures)
- Hypoglycemia (blood glucose level <35–40 mg/dL) is common with IDM, BWS, and hyperinsulinism
- Other problems associated with underlying cause of LGA (see below for IDDM)

Management

- Specialized obstetric management
- Examine for birth injuries and associated features (e.g., BWS, hydrops).
- Prevention and treatment of hypoglycemia (p. 148)
- Tailor management of other problems, depending on underlying cause of LGA

Prognosis

The prognosis depends on the cause and severity of complications. It is generally worse for LGA resulting from hydrops fetalis than that from other causes. Neurological impairments can result from severe or prolonged hypoglycemia.

Infant of a mother with diabetes mellitus (IDM)

Pathophysiology

Maternal hyperglycemia results in fetal hyperglycemia. Fetal hyperglycemia results in increased fetal pancreatic insulin secretion (in the fetus, insulin has a growth hormone–like function), resulting in macrosomia, organomegaly (particularly heart and liver), and polycythemia. Rarely, maternal diabetes-related vascular disease can lead to IUGR.

Associated complications

- *Obstetric complications* (see Complications): Increased risk of fetal loss and premature delivery. Additionally, there is an increased likelihood of operative delivery.
- *2–4x risk of congenital anomalies:* Caudal regression sequence, small left colon syndrome, neural tube defects
- *Hypertrophic cardiomyopathy* occurs in up to half of IDMs. It can lead to congestive heart failure.

- *Hypoglycemia* usually occurs within 1–2 hours of delivery and can be profound, but generally resolves as serum insulin levels fall over the first several days.
- *Perinatal asphyxia* occurs in up to 25% of IDMs.
- *Respiratory disease:* Increased risk of respiratory distress syndrome (RDS) (p. 166), transient tachypnea of the newborn (p. 168)
- *Polycythemia* increases the risk of thrombosis and hyperbilirubinemia.
- *Hyperbilirubinemia*
- *Hypocalcemia* (see p. 532) occurs in up to 50% of IDMs and can be symptomatic. Nadir calcium levels are at 24–72 hours of age.
- *Hypomagnesemia*

Management
Optimizing of maternal glycemic control during pregnancy will reduce the risk of complications. Specifically, elevated maternal hemoglobin A1C levels in the first trimester are associated with an increased risk of congenital anomalies. See p. 148 for management of hypoglycemia.

Prognosis
- Normoglycemia usually established within 48–72 hours
- Increased risk of diabetes mellitus later in life
- Increased risk of obesity later in life
- Increased risk of neurodevelopmental impairments (mitigated by optimal antenatal maternal glycemic control)

Prematurity

Prematurity is defined as birth prior to 37 completed weeks of gestation. It occurs among 5%–15% of all births in high-income countries. Approximately 2/3 of all preterm births are late preterm births (34–36 completed weeks).

Associated risk factors

- Prior preterm birth; poor maternal health or lower socioeconomic status; race (in the U.S., black mothers have higher rates of preterm birth); maternal substance use, including cocaine, methamphetamine, and tobacco; maternal use of assisted reproductive technologies; advanced maternal age or very young maternal age, short interpregnancy interval
- Preterm premature rupture of the membranes (PPROM)

Causes

- Iatrogenic (indicated) preterm delivery for fetal reasons
  - Growth failure
  - Fetal distress
  - Fetal anomalies
  - Multiple gestation
  - Severe oligohydramnios
- Preterm delivery associated with maternal reasons
  - Maternal preeclampsia, eclampsia, HELLP syndrome
  - Placental abruption
  - Abnormal placentation: previa, percreta, increta, acreta
  - Maternal infection (e.g., chorioamnionitis)
  - Maternal diabetes mellitus
  - Polyhydramnios
  - Cervical incompetence or uterine malformation

Associated problems

- Birth trauma (p. 136)
- Perinatal hypoxia or depression (p. 202)
- Respiratory distress syndrome (RDS) (p. 166)
- Apnea of prematurity (p. 173)
- Chronic lung disease (p. 186)
- Patent ductus arteriosus (p. 190)
- Hypothermia
- Hyperbilirubinemia (p. 144)
- Impaired fluid and electrolyte homeostasis (p. 150)
- Intracranial hemorrhage (intraventricular or intraparenchymal hemorrhage) and associated white matter disease (periventricular leukomalacia)
- Retinopathy of prematurity (p. 184)
- Anemia of prematurity (p. 192)
- Necrotizing enterocolitis (p. 216)
- Feeding intolerance
- Immunocompromised state leading to increased risk and severity of neonatal infections

- Increased risk of adverse long-term neuron-developmental impairments, behavioral problems, sudden infant death syndrome (SIDS), family stress and divorce

General management—antenatal

- Transfer mother to a regional center capable of managing a high-risk birth and newborn.
- Provide comprehensive counseling regarding risks and benefits to mother and fetus of preterm delivery, as well as survival and short-term and long-term sequelae of preterm birth.
- If there is sufficient time, administer corticosteroids (2 doses, 12 hours apart) to mother 24 hours prior to delivery if <34 weeks gestation; consider tocolysis until steroids are therapeutic. Steroids promote lung maturity and have been shown to improve postnatal outcomes.
- Prepare for delivery by having experienced delivery room staff present who are capable of performing neonatal resuscitation (this varies by the degree of prematurity; get senior-most staff for delivery of infant <28–30 weeks gestation).

General management—postnatal

- Provide immediate care per neonatal resuscitation algorithm (p. 130) with particular attention to thermoregulation and ensuring adequate ventilation.
- Consider prompt and routine intubation and administration of prophylactic surfactant for newborns <28 weeks gestation.
- Thermoregulatory support: Radiant warmer until infant can be placed in a double-walled, temperature-controlled isolette. Provide a thermo-neutral environment at all times. Minimize evaporative heat loss by keeping the baby dry.
- Minimize insensible water loss, especially for birth weight <1000 g, and consider using a humidified isolette.
- Maintain euglycemia with close monitoring of blood glucose levels.
- If there is an idiopathic preterm delivery or concern about infection, treat empirically with ampicillin and gentamicin after drawing a blood culture.
- Tailor treatments for specific prematurity-associated disease processes (e.g., apnea of prematurity, shock, respiratory distress syndrome).
- Minimize stimulation of the newborn (minimal handling, quiet room, minimize blood draws, etc.).
- Provide comprehensive psychosocial support for the family.

Prognosis

- Survival to discharge and long-term sequelae are inversely proportional to gestational age at delivery (and to lesser degree birth weight; p. 162).
- Preterm infants who also had IGUR are at higher risk of mortality and long-term sequelae than appropriately grown preterm infants.
- Although the mortality rate among late-preterm births (34–36 completed weeks) is only slightly increased compared with that of term newborns, in absolute numbers, deaths among late-preterm infants contribute significantly to neonatal mortality. Late-preterm infants have higher rates of short- and long-term sequelae than those of term newborns.

Birth of the extremely preterm-gestation infant

Ethical and operating principles (see Ethics, p. 1071)

- Parents are the primary decision makers.
  - They will always want the *right* to make difficult decisions, but occasionally will not want the *obligation*.
- The infant's *best interest* is the guiding decisional standard.
  - *Best interest* is an ill-defined, relative concept and will vary from parent to parent.
  - It is the physician's duty to confirm a *best-interest* decision.
- Physicians are obligated to provide information to parents in a manner that will facilitate decision making.
- Physicians are not required to provide interventions that have little or no chance of success and would cause suffering.

Predelivery counseling

Obstetric and pediatric counseling should be coordinated (i.e., use the same data and agree on interventions to be offered) and joint, when possible. If time permits, a tentative birth plan should be developed, incorporating the following:

- Current survival data (see Box 6.4)
- Estimated long-term morbidity (see Fig. 6.5; see p. 162)
- A realistic discussion of the anticipated clinical course expected
- A review of institutional policies, local customs, and individual physician attitudes

Delivery room management

Delivery of the extremely preterm infant requires the presence of a skilled resuscitation team familiar with and experienced in implementing the current AAP/AHA neonatal resuscitation program (NRP) algorithm (see p. 139).

It is important to remember that fetal estimates of gestational age and weight can be inaccurate.

There is no consensus among neonatologists on the limitations for withholding and/or requiring resuscitation between 22/0 days and 25 weeks gestation. Most are uncomfortable with initiating aggressive efforts below 23 weeks/0 days and with withholding resuscitation around 25 weeks/0 days. In most instances, parental preference should be of paramount consideration.

? Consensus guidelines (circa 2008)

Gestational age <23 weeks
- Comfort care

Gestational age 23–25 weeks
- Defer to parents

Gestational age >25 weeks
- Initiate resuscitation efforts

In the presence of ambiguity and absent agreement on a course of action among providers, and between providers and parents, resuscitation efforts should be initiated.

Box 6.4 Survival at threshold of viability

Gestational age (weeks)			
22	23	24	25
0–21%	17%–66%	44%–81%	72%–85%

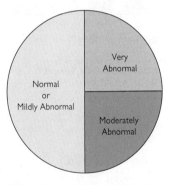

Figure 6.5 Morbidity summary 2007. Created by David Woodrum, MD, University of Washington, 2008.

Outcome following prematurity

In the United States, 12.7% of babies are born preterm. Very low birth weight (VLBW) infants constitute 1.49% of births, accounting for almost 62,000 infants with birth weights <1500 g. Risk of complications and associated morbidity and mortality steadily worsens as gestation age decreases; however, there is no gestational age, including term, that is exempt (see Table 6.8).

Survival rates for VLBW infants (<1500 g) in the Unites States are expressed in the following graphs by gestational age and birth weight (see Fig. 6.6 and Fig. 6.7).

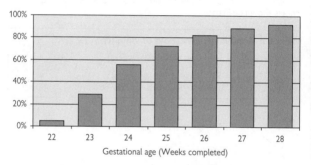

Figure 6.6 Survival by gestational age 22–28 weeks in the United States. Compiled from Vermont Oxford data for the years 2004–2006, Vermont Oxford Network Nightingale Database, 2007. Reprinted with permission.

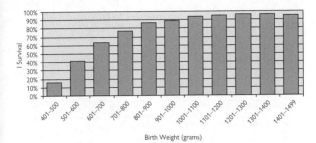

Figure 6.7 Survival of VLBW infants by birth weight in the United States. Compiled from Vermont Oxford data for the years 2004–2006, Vermont Oxford Network Nightingale Database, 2007. Reprinted with permission.

Table 6.8 Selected morbidity rates for VLBW infants

Respiratory distress syndrome	44%
Bronchopulmonary dysplasia	22%
Patent ductus arteriosus	29%
Necrotizing enterocolitis	7%
Late-onset septicemia	22%
Grade 1 intraventricular hemorrhage	11%
Grade 2 intraventricular hemorrhage	4%
Grade 3 intraventricular hemorrhage	7%
Grade 4 intraventricular hemorrhage	5%
Periventricular leukomalacia	3%

Adapted from Fanaroff AA, et al (2007). NICHD Neonatal Research Network. Trends in neonatal morbidity and mortality for very low birth weight infants, *Am J Obstet Gynecol* **196**:147.e1–8.

Table 6.9 Likelihood of disability for infants born at <26 weeks gestation

Overall disability	≤23 weeks	24 weeks	25 weeks	Total
None	12%	14%	24%	20%
Mild	25%	36%	35%	34%
Moderate	38%	22%	22%	24%

Infants in the EPICure study in the UK in 1995 were evaluated at 6 years of age. This study provides useful information regarding the likely neuro-developmental outcome of infants born at less than 26 weeks gestation (see Table 6.9).[1]

1 Marlow N, et al.; EPICureStudy Group (2005). Neurologic and developmental disability at six years of age after extremely preterm birth. *N Engl J Med* **352**:9–19.

Disability definitions
Severe
- If a child is likely to be highly dependent on caregivers; nonambulant cerebral palsy, IQ score >3 SD below mean, profound sensorineural hearing loss or blindness

Moderate
- Reasonable independence likely; ambulant cerebral palsy, IQ score 2–3 SD below mean, sensorineural hearing loss corrected with hearing aid, impaired vision without blindness

Mild
- Neurological signs with minimal functional consequences or other impairments such as strabismus or refractive errors

Neurodevelopmental outcomes steadily improve with increasing gestational age. Late preterm births (34–36 weeks gestation) are 4.5 times more common than births before 32 weeks gestation, and account for the largest increase in preterm births.

These infants have higher rates of respiratory distress, apnea, temperature instability, hypoglycemia, jaundice, kernicterus, feeding difficulties, and rehospitalization than those of term infants. They also have more problems in school than term infants.

Generally, morbidity and mortality have steadily improved, but exact figures vary between neonatal units. Know your own unit's figures and remember that many things influence outcome, including maternal health, fetal well-being and growth, infection, and adequate use of antenatal steroids.

Respiratory distress syndrome (RDS)

RDS and hyaline membrane disease (HMD) are the same entity. Respiratory distress begins shortly after birth, commonly occurring in premature infants with an incidence inversely proportional to gestational age. The use of maternal corticosteroid treatment to accelerate fetal lung development has reduced the incidence to ~35% in infants less than 30 weeks gestation. It is much less common after 32 weeks gestation.

Causes

Surfactant deficiency due to pulmonary immaturity results in increased surface tension in the terminal air sacs, leading to atelectasis. This causes increased work of breathing, and hypoxia occurs due to intrapulmonary shunting of blood (R → L) past collapsed alveoli.

Presentation

Onset of tachypnea, grunting respirations, chest wall retractions, nasal flaring, and cyanosis occur within the first 4 hours of life. Without treatment the baby's condition usually deteriorates over the next 48–72 hours. Depending on the severity it may resolve within 7 days.

Investigations

- Chest X-ray (PA and lateral) reveals a diffuse parenchymal "ground-glass" or granular appearance with air bronchograms and reduced lung volume. A chest X-ray will rule out pneumothorax, meconium aspiration, and congenital lung abnormalities (see Fig. 6.8).
- Assessment of gas exchange by arterial blood gas analysis and continuous pulse oximetry

Management

- Ensure adequate ventilation and oxygenation in the delivery room with appropriate resuscitative measures as indicated (p. 138).
- Respiratory support will depend on the severity of condition, beginning with nasal prong O_2, progressing to nasal CPAP (p. 138) or mechanical ventilation (pp. 138) according to the amount of supplemental O_2 required or inadequate ventilatory effort. Almost all extremely premature infants (e.g., <27 weeks gestation) with RDS will require either mechanical ventilation or CPAP if the FiO_2 exceeds 0.30. More mature infants (e.g., >30 weeks gestation) should have a higher threshold of oxygen requirement (e.g., >50%) prior to intubation.
- Surfactant administration requires intubation and a chest X-ray, unless prophylactically administered in the delivery room in extremely low birth weight (ELBW) infants. The dose may be repeated in 8–12 hours if $FiO_2 > 0.3$. There is questionable benefit from third or fourth doses.
- Nutrition: NPO, IV fluids, or peripherally inserted central catheter (PICC) if ELBW with parenteral nutrition until infant is stable, then incremental gastric tube feedings.

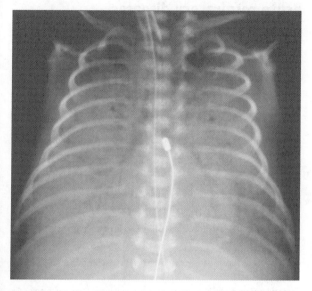

Figure 6.8 Respiratory distress syndrome (RDS), with bilateral, diffuse, "ground-glass" appearance (generalized atelectasis), airway bronchograms, and reduced lung volume.

Prognosis

- The majority have good recovery. Survival is greater than 90%–95% in infants >27 weeks. Bronchopulmonary dysplasia may ensue in approximately 15% of cases in inverse proportion to gestational age.
- Comorbidity may exist with intracranial hemorrhage, patent ductus arteriosis, and retinopathy of prematurity.

Prevention

- Corticosteroids (betamethasone/dexamethasone, 2 doses, 12 hourly) given to mother 1–7 days before birth decrease incidence and mortality by 40%. There is maximum benefit after 24 hours and it lasts 7 days. Tocolysis may be beneficial to gain time.
- Prevent coexisting morbidities, e.g., hypothermia, acidosis, hypoglycemia, and infection.

Acute respiratory diseases

All of the diseases presented below have signs of respiratory distress. Cerebral hypoxia, congenital heart disease, and metabolic acidosis can also induce respiratory distress and mimic respiratory disease (suspect these if the chest X-ray is normal).

Transient tachypnea of the newborn (TTN)

- Caused by delayed clearance or absorption of lung fluid after birth.
- Presents within 4 hours after birth. It is common after elective CS in the absence of labor.
- Chest X-ray shows streaky perihilar changes, fluid in horizontal fissure.
- Treatment: Supplemental O_2. Consider nasal CPAP and antibiotics if severity increases.
- Prognosis: TTN spontaneously resolves within 24 hours.

Congenital pneumonia

- Caused by aspiration of infected amniotic fluid
- Associated with prolonged rupture of membranes (PROM), chorioamnionitis, fetal hypoxia
- Usually group B streptococcus (GBS), *E. coli*, other gram-negative bacteria, *Listeria*, *Chlamydia*
- Presents in first 24 hours
- Chest X-ray shows patchy shadowing and consolidation.

Treatment
Treatment is with respiratory support; give antibiotics (begin with ampicillin and gentamycin) after septic screen.

Prognosis
Outcome is good unless condition is severe or associated with systemic sepsis and PPHN.

Meconium aspiration syndrome (MAS)

- 5% of term infants with meconium-stained liquor develop MAS (1–5/1000 live births).
- Hypoxia results in meconium passage in utero and associated gasping leads to aspiration. Meconium aspiration inhibits surfactant, obstructs the respiratory tract (sometimes resulting in pneumothorax), and induces pulmonary inflammation.
- MAS presents with respiratory distress soon after birth. It is associated with pulmonary air leaks and PPHN.
- Chest X-ray: Generalized overinflation with patchy collapse or consolidation, ± air leaks.

Prevention
If liquor is meconium stained, delivery should be expedited to prevent further hypoxia and gasping. If the baby is apneic at birth, visualize the larynx and suck out any meconium from larynx and trachea using a large-bore suction tube, followed by resuscitation as indicated.

Treatment

Treatment is supportive; give supplemental O_2; intermittent positive-pressure ventilation (IPPV) or HFOV if ventilation is required (to reduce air leak use high FiO_2, low PIP); surfactant; antibiotics (e.g., ampicillin and gentamicin); treat PPHN (p. 174); consider starting ECMO if condition is severe.

Prognosis

Mortality is <5%. Survivors do well; if ECMO is needed there are neurological sequelae.

Pulmonary air leaks

These are commonly secondary to other respiratory disease (e.g., RDS, MAS) or to assisted ventilation. Risk is reduced by surfactant treatment, reducing baby–ventilator asynchrony and avoidance of unnecessary high assisted ventilation pressures.

Pneumothorax

Spontaneous pneumothorax occurs in 1% of term infants. There is increased incidence in prematurity and respiratory disease.

Features

Most of these air leaks are small, asymptomatic, and resolve spontaneously. Larger ones present with respiratory distress. Tension pneumothorax is life threatening (signs: respiratory distress, cyanosis, mediastinal shift away from affected side, decreased chest movement and air entry on affected side, transillumination lights up affected side).

• Chest X-ray shows ipsilateral translucency, lack of peripheral lung markings, and collapsed lung (see Fig. 6.9).

Treatment

There is none if the patient is asymptomatic. If pneumothorax is larger, term infants may require only high supplemental FiO_2. If symptoms are severe or worsening, insert a chest drain (p. 244). In an emergency perform needle aspiration before inserting the chest drain.

Prognosis

Outcome is excellent in term infants. Mortality is doubled in infants with RDS. There is also an increased risk of periventricular hemorrhage in preterms.

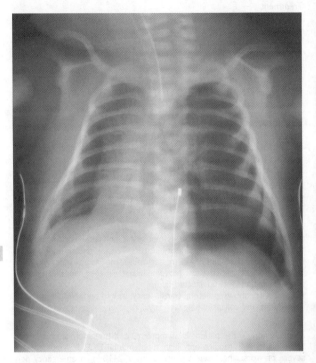

Figure 6.9 Left tension pneumothorax. Left chest hyperlucency and hyperinflation are evident, as well as a collapsed left lung (absence of peripheral lung markings), with the mediastinum shifted to the right.

Pulmonary interstitial emphysema (PIE)

Air leak into lung parenchyma results in small-airway and alveolar collapse. PIE follows high IPPV, particularly in preterm infants with severe RDS or MAS.

- *Signs*: Respiratory distress, chest hyperexpansion, poor air entry, coarse inspiratory crackles
- *Chest X-ray*: Hyperinflation, "honeycomb" pattern of cystic lucencies and bullae, generalized or local (see Fig. 6.10).
- *Treatment*: High FiO_2, low PIP, low PEEP, fast rate IPPV (low MAP), HFOV may be superior. In unilateral PIE, nurse infants with the affected side down, or administer selective intubation and ventilation of the healthier lung.
- *Prognosis:* Mortality 25%–50%. Chronic lung disease is likely (BPD).

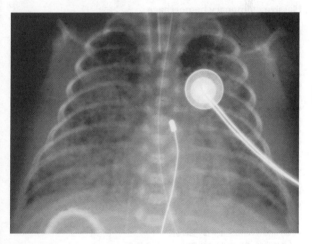

Figure 6.10 Pulmonary interstitial emphysema (PIE). There is bilateral lung hyperinflation (hyperlucency and downward displacement of diaphragm) with multiple radiolucent cystic areas. PIE may be unilateral. Isolated large bullae may appear. Cardiac compression may occur.

Pneumomediastinum

This is often preceded by pneumothorax or PIE. It is usually asymptomatic.
- *Chest X-ray*: Translucency around the heart extending superiorly, thymus is lifted and splayed from below ("sail" sign)
- *Treatment*: None if asymptomatic. Use high FiO_2 in term infants or drainage if they are symptomatic.

Pneumopericardium

This usually occurs with other air leaks with IPPV and can lead to cardiac tamponade (with quiet heart sounds, hypotension, bradycardia, cyanosis).
- *Chest X-ray*: Translucency around the borders of a small heart
- *Treatment*: Immediate insertion of drainage tube under the xyphisternum.
- *Prognosis*: High mortality if symptomatic

Massive pulmonary hemorrhage

This results in life-threatening hemorrhagic pulmonary edema. (Small bleeds are associated with tracheal trauma from the ETT or suction.) Incidence is ~1/1000 live births, almost always in VLBW infants.

Associations
- PIE
- Hydrops fetalis
- Perinatal hypoxia
- Sepsis
- Coagulopathy
- Fluid overload
- Surfactant therapy, rare

Signs
- Rapid systemic collapse
- Profuse, blood-stained fluid welling up from upper airway
- Respiratory crackles on auscultation
- *Chest X-ray*: Virtual "white-out"

Treatment
- O_2 and ↑ventilatory pressures
- Diuretics, e.g., furosemide 1–2 mg/kg stat
- Correct any hypovolemia and/or coagulopathy with fresh frozen plasma 10 mL/kg
- Consider blood transfusion
- Consider surfactant
- Treat known associations

Prognosis: Mortality is up to 50%.

Milk aspiration

Term infants can accidentally aspirate a feeding. The usual causes are
- Swallowing incoordination, e.g., in preterm, from neurological disease
- Structural upper airway or esophageal disorders, e.g., tracheo-esophageal fistula
- Gastroesophageal reflux

Presentation

Sudden choking or respiratory distress occurs during or after a feed, often with excessive milk in the mouth, or aspiration pneumonia. Chest X-ray is normal or shows patchy collapse or consolidation in the upper lobes.

Treatment

Observe in a well baby. If unwell, respiratory support and broad-spectrum antibiotics are needed. Investigate the cause and use nasojejunal tube feeding. A period of intravenous fluids or feeding may be necessary.

Prognosis depends on the cause.

Apnea

Apnea can result from any severe illness (asphyxia, hypoglycemia, sepsis) and the prognosis is dependent on the cause and degree of hypoxia.

Management

- Support respiration
- Investigate and correct primary cause

Apnea of prematurity

- Respiratory pauses of >15 seconds associated with bradycardia
- (<100 bpm) and oxygen desaturation (<85%)
- Apnea occurs in most infants <30 weeks gestation and usually abates by 34–35 weeks gestation, although it may persist beyond 40 weeks.

Cause

- May be central (40%), obstructive (10%), or mixed (50%)
- Onset within 1–3 days of life
- Consider and exclude other causes of CNS depression or airway obstruction (see p. 204). Infants are obligate nose breathers.

Treatment

- Depends on frequency and severity of condition and requires continuous cardiopulmonary and pulse oximetry monitoring to determine progression from tactile stimulation, caffeine or theophylline, nasal CPAP, to occasionally mechanical ventilation.
- Monitoring is usually required for around 5 days after the last episode requiring intervention.

Prognosis No adverse long-term effects have been reported.

Neonatal hypotension

Neonatal hypotension is mean arterial blood pressure (MAP) 1–2 SD below the mean for gestational and chronological age.

Causes
- Hypovolemia or acute bleed (e.g., vaso previa)
- Septic shock
- Maternal vasodilatory medications (e.g., atenolol)
- Cardiomyopathy (e.g., IDDM; viral myocarditis)
- Perinatal asphyxia resulting in myocardial dysfunction
- Adrenal insufficiency

Management
Depends on cause
- *Hypovolemia*: Fluid boluses; blood transfusion if bleeding
- *Septic shock*: Fluid and pressors (dopamine, epinephrine)
- *Cardiomyopathy*: Pressors (dobutamine)
- *Adrenal insufficiency*: Hydrocortisone

Persistent pulmonary hypertension of the newborn (PPHN)

PPHN is increased pulmonary vascular resistance (similar to fetal circulation). Decreased pulmonary blood flow and shunting of deoxygenated blood from right side of circulation to the left results in hypoxemia.

Causes
Rarely, PPHN is primary or idiopathic. More commonly, PPHN is associated with the following:
- Perinatal hypoxia–ischemia
- Meconium aspiration syndrome
- Pulmonary hypoplasia (e.g., Potter syndrome)
- Congenital diaphragmatic hernia
- Severe illness (e.g., GBS sepsis)

Presentation
- Cyanosis in term or near-term infant without heart defect
- Preductal (right hand) oxygen saturations > postductal (foot), only if ductus is still open
- Loud, single second heart sound; may have high-pitched murmur at left upper sternal border (tricuspid regurgitation)
- Echocardiogram
  - High pulmonary artery pressures
  - Right-to-left shunting at foramen ovale and ductus arteriosus
  - Right ventricular hypertrophy

Management
- Treat underlying cause or illness.
- Correct acidosis, hypotension, severe hypoxemia, polycythemia, if present.
- Optimize ventilation if there is parenchymal lung disease, including high-frequency ventilation, surfactant if indicated.
- Use minimal handling; sedate infant if agitated.
- Treatments known to lower pulmonary vascular resistance (reverse right-to-left shunt):
  - Alkalosis (metabolic or respiratory)
  - Inhaled nitric oxide (start at 20 ppm)
- Treatments designed to raise systemic vascular resistance (reverse right-to-left shunt)
  - Pressors (dopamine, epinephrine)
  - Fluid boluses
- Extracorporeal membrane oxygenation (ECMO) is used when medical management has failed.
  - Oxygenation index (OI) >40
  - $OI = \dfrac{FiO_2 \times MAP \times 100}{PaO_2}$, where MAP = mean airway pressure

Neonatal respiratory support

Supplemental oxygen

Inspired O_2 >80% is toxic and predisposes to alveolar collapse. In infants <32 weeks gestation and/or <1500 g, maintain PaO_2 in the 50–80 mmHg range with corresponding SaO_2 (usually 89%–93%) as much as possible to lower the risk of retinopathy of prematurity.

Supplemental oxygen is given via the following means:

- Head box (concentration is easily monitored, prevents sudden changes, is comfortable)
- Nasal cannula, usually at <2 L/min (allows parents to hold infant but can't monitor inspired O_2 easily—inhaled oxygen concentration depends on the infant's tidal volume and the cannula's flow rate and FiO_2)
- High-flow nasal cannula with humidified gas, usually at 2–6 L/min (provides back-pressure similar to CPAP with less discomfort and risk of nasal trauma, but the amount of pressure is difficult to measure and thus may cause pulmonary air leak, gastric distension, etc.)

Continuous positive airway pressure (CPAP)

CPAP is intended to prevent alveolar and airway collapse. Maintenance of functional residual capacity above closing volume reduces the work of breathing.

Uses

- Mild RDS and other respiratory diseases characterized by atelectasis; recurrent apnea, e.g., in preterm infants
- Ventilation weaning
- Upper airway obstruction such as tracheomalacia

Method

- Given via nasal prongs or nasal mask
- Usual pressure is 4–6 cmH₂O. Probable safe upper level is 8 cmH₂O but ↑risk of pneumothorax as pressure ↑

Complications

- Baby struggling, leading to hypoxia (use sedation judiciously)
- ↑Airway resistance and effort of breathing
- Pulmonary air leaks, e.g., pneumothorax
- Nasal trauma
- Upper GI distension or perforation (insert gastric tube and leave open to air to reduce risk)

Positive-pressure ventilation

- Pressure support ventilation alone (pressure support with every breath through endotracheal tube)
- Time-cycled, positive-pressure ventilation (IPPV), including synchronized ventilation modes
- Pressure-regulated, volume control (PRVC) and volume guarantee modes: See p. 178.
- High-frequency oscillatory ventilation (HFOV): See p. 182.

Extracorporeal membrane oxygenation (ECMO)

ECMO reduces mortality in severe respiratory disease, e.g., meconium aspiration syndrome, persistent pulmonary hypertension of the newborn.

Eligible criteria

These include severe but reversible cardiac or respiratory disease and oxygenation index* >30–40 for 2–4 hours.

Contraindications

- Weight <1.8 kg (because catheters large enough for ECMO to work don't fit well in small vessels)
- Gestation <33–34 weeks (because of high risk of intracranial hemorrhage in premature infants)
- Severe congenital malformation or poor CNS prognosis, e.g., severe HIE (because of poor outcome and intracranial hemorrhage)
- Intracranial hemorrhage beyond subependymal (because of risk of extension of hemorrhage from heparinization)

Technique

Blood draw continuously from a major vein is pumped through a membrane oxygenator and then returned to the body. Blood is heparinized and low-level conventional ventilation is maintained in the event that ECMO must be discontinued abruptly. ECMO is maintained until disease recovery. It may be

- *Venous–venous*: Double-lumen cannula in superior vena cava via right jugular vein
- *Venous–arterial*: Drawing from right jugular vein and returned to right carotid artery

Outcome

Approximately 10%–20% of ECMO survivors suffer major long-term problems. Complications include neurological brain injury (secondary to neck vessel trauma, thromboembolism, CNS hemorrhage) and peripheral thromboembolic phenomena to other organs.

$$* \text{ Oxygenation index} = \frac{\text{Mean airway pressure} \times FiO_2 \times 100}{PaO_2}$$

Conventional positive pressure ventilation

Intermittent positive pressure ventilation via endotracheal tube (ETT) with continuous flow of heated and humidified gas allows the non-paralyzed baby to breathe spontaneously. Inflation is time cycled and pressure limited because neonatal lungs are often noncompliant and there is a leak around the ETT (see Table 6.10).

Indications

- Worsening respiratory failure, e.g., RDS
- Impending or actual respiratory arrest from any cause
- Recurrent apnea, bradycardia, and cyanosis events, e.g., apnea of prematurity
- Severe pulmonary hemorrhage
- Severe cardiac failure
- Persistent pulmonary hypertension of the newborn
- Severe congenital lung malformation, e.g., diaphragmatic hernia

Table 6.10 Ventilation parameters

Parameter	Abbr.	Typical starting settings for RDS	Comments
Fraction of inspired oxygen	FiO_2	0.21–0.60	Depends on nature of lung disease
Peak inspiratory pressure	PIP	16–22 cmH_2O	Higher for more mature or sicker patients
Positive end-expiratory pressure	PEEP	4–6 cmH_2O	Beware of auto-PEEP if f >60
Pressure support	PS	4–8 cmH_2O	Used with synchronized modes
Tidal volume	V_t	4–5 mL/kg	Used with volume-targeted modes
Inspiratory time	T_i	0.3 seconds	Depends on mode of ventilation
Expiratory time	T_e	Depends on f	Beware of auto-PEEP if T_e <1 sec
Frequency of breathing	f	20–40/minute	Depends on spontaneous rate and $PaCO_2$
Gas flow	Flow	5–8 L/min	Depends on mode of ventilation

Monitoring ventilation
- Review and adjust ventilation settings soon after commencement.
- Blood gas normal range is PaO_2 50–80 mmHg, $PaCO_2$ 35–55 mmHg), pH 7.25–7.4.

Time-limited pressure-cycled ventilation (e.g., pressure support, pressure control)
- If PaO_2 is too low: ↑FiO_2, or ↑mean airway pressure (see Fig. 6.11)
- If $PaCO_2$ is too high: ↑alveolar ventilation by increasing minute ventilation (by one or more of these: ↑PIP, ↑PS, ↓PEEP, ↑f, ↑ gas flow, better synchronization)

Volume-controlled ventilation (e.g., "volume-guarantee" mode)
- If PaO_2 is too low: ↑FiO_2, or ↑mean airway pressure (by ↑V_t or ↑PEEP)
- If $PaCO_2$ is too high: ↑ alveolar ventilation by increasing tidal volume or rate (by one or more of these: ↑V_t, ↑f if not breathing above backup vent rate, ↑gas flow, better synchronization)

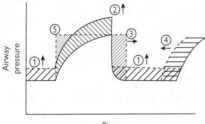

Figure 6.11 Methods to increase mean airway pressure. From Peter Tarczy-Hornoch, MD, University of Washington, 2008.

1. Increase PEEP
2. Increase PIP
3. Increase T$_i$
4. Increase f
5. Increase flow

Acute deterioration during ventilation

This may present as systemic collapse, hypoxemia, or hypercarbia. Ventilate with a manual system, e.g., self-inflating bag, and 100% O$_2$. Rapid improvement suggests a ventilator problem. Otherwise consider ETT obstruction from secretions or kinked tubing, hidden extubation, pneumothorax, or non-respiratory disease, e.g., intraventricular hemorrhage (IVH).

Slow deterioration during ventilation

This may present as slow deterioration in overall clinical condition, hypercarbia, or hypoxemia. Consider worsening respiratory disease, partial ETT obstruction, airway circuit leak, or non-respiratory disease.

Ventilator weaning

Wean O$_2$ to lowest amount needed to maintain adequate PaO$_2$ (↓retinopathy risk). As lung compliance improves, wean PIP in 2 cmH$_2$O steps until in the 12–14 cmH$_2$O range, and wean rate until 10–20 breaths/minute, for pressure-cycled ventilator.

For volume-controlled ventilation, reduce V$_t$ to 3.5 mL/kg and reduce backup ventilator rate to 25 or lower. Consider caffeine if at patient is at high risk for apnea of prematurity, and consider CPAP if lung compliance remains poor or significant retractions are observed.

Respiratory patterns under different modes of ventilation

See Figure 6.12.

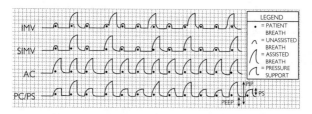

Figure 6.12 IMV = intermittent mandatory ventilation; SIMV = synchronized intermittent mandatory ventilation; AC = assist control; PC/PS = pressure control/pressure support. Dot = patient breath; lowest curve = unassisted breath; highest peak = assisted breath; mid-sized curve = pressure support. From Peter Tarczy-Hornoch, MD. University of Washington, 2008.

High-frequency oscillatory ventilation (HFOV)

A continuous positive distending pressure (mean airway pressure) is applied for oxygenation, and ventilation is achieved by oscillating by a diaphragm or an interrupter device in the ventilator circuit (see Table 6.11). It can be used as a rescue mode for patients failing conventional ventilation, or as a primary mode for respiratory distress syndrome, pulmonary hypoplasia, etc., in hopes of reducing barotrauma or to prevent or reduce the severity of pneumothorax. Data about its superiority against low-volume conventional ventilation for routine patients are scanty, but it can be highly effective in the rescue mode.

Table 6.11 Ventilation parameters

Parameter	Abbr.	Typical starting settings for RDS	Comments
Fraction of inspired oxygen	FiO_2	0.21–0.60	Depends on nature of lung disease
Mean airway pressure	MAP	10–18 cmH_2O	Usually set 2 cmH_2O higher than conventional ventilation; higher for more mature or sicker patients; avoid over-distension of lungs
Amplitude (delta pressure)	δP	25–40	Look for adequate "shake" of chest
Frequency per second, Hertz	Hz	6–15/second	15 for <1 kg, 12 for 1–3 kg, 10 for term
Bias flow	Flow	20 L/min	Usually not adjusted

Oxygenation (PaO_2) is dependent on both MAP and FiO_2. As MAP↑, PaO_2 will improve as functional residual capacity (FRC)↑. At some point, because of overdistension, further ↑FRC will ↓PaO_2. Inadequate MAP leads to repetitive opening and closing of alveoli, and thus can cause worse lung injury.

CO_2 removal ($PaCO_2$) is dependent on alveolar ventilation and thus on both the frequency and amplitude. Unlike conventional ventilation, ventilator constraints make tidal volume inversely proportional to the frequency. It is normal for generated tidal volumes to be less than physiological, yet adequate ventilation occurs. This apparent paradox is explained by complicated air flow physics of HFOV that augment CO_2 diffusion. Once the frequency is set, CO_2 removal is increased by ↑amplitude.

Monitoring ventilation

- Upon initiation, observe the infant's chest oscillation, and alter amplitude settings as required.
- Follow PaO_2 and SaO_2 carefully; if desaturation is prolonged, consider IV fluid bolus to help overcome impaired thoracic venous return. Follow $PaCO_2$ carefully, and consider continuous monitoring with transcutaneous device.
- Perform a chest X-ray after 1 hour, at 8–12 hours, and then daily to assess chest expansion: 8–9 posterior ribs visible above the diaphragm is appropriate.
- *If PaO_2 is too low*: ↑ either the FiO_2 or MAP by 1–2 cmH_2O every 30–60 minutes (avoid chest overexpansion).
- *If $PaCO_2$ is too high*: ↑ amplitude by 2 cmH_2O increments every 30–60 minutes. <u>Decrease</u> Hz if $PaCO_2$ is still high after reaching a δ P of about 50 (lower Hz leads to larger tidal volume and thus better ventilation, but at the cost of more barotrauma).

Weaning ventilation

As clinical status improves, ↓FiO_2 to 0.5 and then MAP by 2 cmH_2O steps until 6–7 cmH_2O is tolerated. Also progressively ↓ amplitude to the minimum required to maintain normal CO_2. Wean MAP according to location of diaphragms on chest films. Some babies will tolerate weaning to what is essentially CPAP prior to extubation. However, it may be more practical to change to conventional ventilator settings prior to extubation.

Complications

Severe and prolonged hypocarbia from high-frequency ventilation of any type may lead to periventricular leukomalacia, probably from hypocarbia-induced reduction in cerebral blood flow. Infrequent suctioning is necessary with HFOV to avoid derecruitment of alveoli, but that may lead to obstruction of the airway with dried secretions. Excessively high MAP may interfere with cardiac output and cause hypotension and desaturation.

Retinopathy of prematurity (ROP)

ROP is a pathological condition that occurs as a result of abnormal vascularization of the retina in premature infants. Its prevalence increases with decreasing gestational age at birth. Its pathogenesis is multifactorial. The two most important risk factors are thought to be extreme prematurity and a relative retinal hyperoxia in the early neonatal period.

Retinopathy of prematurity – screening guidelines

Infants with a birth weight of <1500 g or gestational age of 32 weeks or less (as defined by the attending neonatologist) and selected infants with a birth weight between 1500 and 2000 g or gestational age of more than 32 weeks with an unstable clinical course, including those requiring cardiorespiratory support and who are believed by their attending pediatrician or neonatologist to be at high risk, should have retinal screening examinations performed after pupillary dilation using binocular indirect ophthalmoscopy to detect ROP (see Table 6.12).

Table 6.12 Timing of first eye examination based on gestational age at birth

Gestational age at birth (weeks)	Age at initial examination (weeks)	
	Postmenstrual	Chronologic
22	31	9
23	31	8
24	31	7
25	31	6
26	31	5
27	31	4
28	31	4
29	32	4
30	33	4
Above 30	34	4

From: Section on Ophthalmology American Academy of Pediatrics, American Academy of Ophthalmology, American Association for Pediatric Ophthalmology and Strabismus (2006). Screening examination of premature infants for retinopathy of prematurity. *Pediatrics* **117**: 572–576.

The international classification of ROP is based on the following considerations:

1. The location of the area of abnormal vascular growth on the retina in relation to the optic disc.

- **Zone I** is the most posterior and intimately related area of the retina to the optic disc. Abnormal vascular proliferation in this area is associated with worrisome prognosis.
- **Zone II** involves the more peripheral area of the retina, extending from the edge of zone I nasally to the ora serrata. Abnormal vascular proliferation involving zone II is associated with a variable prognosis, less serious than zone I, but still of concern.
- **Zone III** This area of the retina is anterior and even more peripheral to zone II. It is the last portion of the retina to be vascularized normally. Vascular proliferation noted in zone III is usually associated with a benign prognosis.

2. The second component of the international classification of ROP is the *extent* of the problem circumferentially, recorded in clock hours. The more extensive the involvement, the worse the prognosis.

3. The final component of the international classification is based on the *stage* of the problem.

- **Stage I** The appearance of the demarcation line, a structure that separates the avascularized retina from the vascularized retina, is altered in stage I ROP. Vessels are seen to branch into abnormal arcades leading up to the demarcation line. The prognosis associated with ROP limited to stage I is benign.
- **Stage II** The determination of stage II ROP is made when the height, width, and the volume of the demarcation line is increased. Once again, stage II ROP is usually associated with a benign prognosis and the problem regresses.
- **Stage III** A determination of stage III ROP is based on extraretinal proliferation of vascular material along the demarcation line. A determination of stage III ROP is associated with an increasingly worrisome prognosis.
- **Stage IV** ROP is a catastrophic determination indicating retinal detachment and possible severe visual loss.

Plus disease
Determination of plus disease is made by the ophthalmologist at the time of retinal examination showing increased vascular engorgement in the posterior pole of the fundus. Such a determination is ominous in terms of progression of ROP; it is indicative of the development of vascular shunts and may be an indication for treatment.

Threshold disease
This is an indicator for treatment with laser or cryotherapy, and is based on the presence of any stage with plus disease in zone II or any disease in zone I. The risk of retinal detachment and blindness is 50% in the absence of appropriate treatment.

Bronchopulmonary dysplasia (BPD)

BPD, also known as chronic lung disease (CLD) of prematurity, is a persistent or prolonged respiratory disease characterized by irregular and scattered parenchymal densities, or consolidated areas of the lung, or focal areas of hyperinflation, or all of these seen on chest X-ray (see Fig. 6.13). Infants are dependent on supplemental oxygen and demonstrate increased work of breathing, which may persist for a few weeks or months.

The classification based on severity and gestational age has been devised for epidemiological purposes and is described in Table 6.13.

Table 6.13 Classification of BPD

Mild	<32 weeks at birth* >0.21 FiO_2 for at least 28 days plus: Room Air (RA) at 36 weeks or discharge
Moderate	Need for <0.3 FiO_2 at 36 weeks or discharge
Severe	Need for >0.3 FiO_2 and or positive pressure (PPV or CPAP) at 36 weeks or discharge

*Infants born ≥32 weeks are assessed at 56 days of postnatal age or discharge, whichever comes first, using the same criteria.

Incidence

↑ incidence with ↓ gestation and ↑ length of ventilation is ~50%–60% at <26 weeks gestation; 25% at 27–29 weeks gestation; and <10% at 30–32 weeks gestation. Using the above classification, BPD occurs in 15%–20% of all premature infants <32 weeks.

Cause

BPD is primarily due to immaturity of the lung in addition to putative factors, such as barotrauma, O_2 toxicity, infection, inflammation, ↓ vitamin A, RDS, and PDA.

Management

- Supplemental O_2 to maintain SaO_2 >90%
- Assisted ventilation (minimize barotrauma)
- Optimize nutrition
- Assess possible contribution of PDA and medication
- Antibiotics if there is superimposed pulmonary infection
- Diuretics: Short-term use may ↓ FiO_2 needs, long-term use has unproven benefit.
- Bronchodilators have unproven efficacy.
- Glucocorticoids: Over the short term they may improve gas exchange in critically ill infants; long-term use is associated with adverse side effects and unproven benefit.
- Home O_2 when FiO_2 <0.3 and infant is otherwise stable.
- Monoclonal antibody prophylaxis against respiratory syncitial virus (RSV) infection

Prognosis

- Mortality is <10%.
- Lung function: Increased risk of recurrent lower respiratory tract infection and reactive airway disease until 2 years of age
- Survivors are usually clinically well by 3–4 years, depending on the severity at discharge.
- Some infants will have growth retardation by 1 year.
- Neurodevelopmental abnormalities are increased over gestational age–matched controls

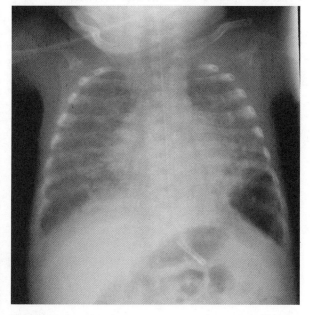

Figure 6.13 Chronic lung disease. Hyperexpansion, diffuse, patchy collapse, and fibrosis interspersed by radiolucent cystic areas are apparent, as well as an area of emphysema in the left lower lung.

Circulatory adaptation at birth

See Figure 6.14.

Transitional circulation
- There is no more placenta; oxygenated blood now comes only from the lungs.
- Pulmonary vascular resistance falls (as soon as the lungs are inflated) → increased pulmonary blood flow.
- Most of the right ventricular output now goes to the lungs.
- Systemic vascular resistance rises.
- The ductus venosus closes (1–7 days).
- The ductus arteriosus closes (1–3 days term; later in preterm).
- The foramen ovale closes (1–3 weeks).

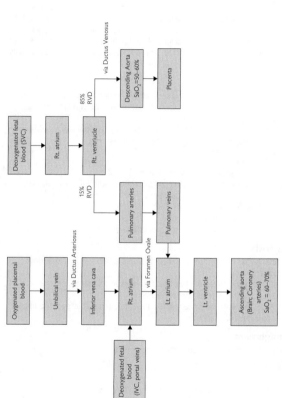

Figure 6.14 Fetal circulation. Figure created by Christine Gleason, MD, University of Washington, 2008.

Patent ductus arteriosus (PDA)

The ductus arteriosus is a normal fetal blood vessel that connects the pulmonary artery with the descending aorta. In the fetus, the ductus allows deoxygenated right ventricular blood to shunt away from the high vascular resistance lungs to the descending aorta and then to the placenta. In healthy term infants, the ductus functionally closes within 1–3 days after birth. PDA refers to a ductus arteriosus that does not close normally after birth.

Causes
- Prematurity: Incidence is inversely related to gestational age.
- Congenital heart defect may be associated with certain syndromes (e.g., congenital rubella, trisomy 18, trisomy 21).
- Pharmacologic maintenance of ductal patency (prostaglandin infusion for ductal-dependent congenital heart defects)

Presentation
- Systolic heart murmur, upper left sternal border
- Widening pulse pressure (due to "diastolic runoff" of left ventricular output into pulmonary vascular bed). The result is "bounding" peripheral pulses; hypotension.
- Hyperactive precordium
- Respiratory deterioration due to pulmonary edema

Diagnosis
- Chest X-ray: Increased heart size and pulmonary vascular markings
- Echocardiogram
  - Directly visualizes ductus; assesses degree and direction of ductal shunting (right → left or left → right)
  - Assessment of secondary effects, i.e., left atrial enlargement, left ventricular dysfunction

Management
You must weigh risks vs. benefits of treatment.

Medical
- Supportive
  - Modest fluid restriction (~120 mL/kg/day)
  - Diuretic therapy if fluid "overloaded"
  - Ventilatory support, as indicated
  - Circulatory or cardiac support: Pressors (e.g., dopamine, dobutamine)

Pharmacologic
This treatment is not likely to be effective in term babies and those with syndrome-associated PDA.
- Prostaglandin synthetase inhibitors
  - Indomethacin (0.1–0.2 mg/kg/dose IV q12–24h x 3–6 doses)
  - Ibuprofen (10 mg/kg IV then 5 mg/kg q24h x 2 doses)

Risks and complications
- Decreased renal function/urine output is less significant with ibuprofen than with indomethacin.
- Impaired platelet function
- Decreased cerebral blood flow response to hypoxia
- Decreased intestinal blood flow: Indomethacin is associated with increased risk of spontaneous intestinal perforation and NEC in preterm infants.
- GI hemorrhage

Contraindications
- Severe renal dysfunction (creatinine >1.8 mg/dL)
- Thrombocytopenia (but can transfuse platelets prior to treating)
- NEC

Surgical ligation
- Failed (or contraindicated) medical management

Hydrops fetalis

This condition consists of abnormal accumulation of fluid in the skin and one or more body compartments: pleural, pericardial, peritoneal cavity, or placenta.

Incidence

It occurs in 1 in 2500 to 1 in 4000 pregnancies, but varies with ethnic population and etiology.

Etiology

Hydrops fetalis occurs when the production of interstitial fluid exceeds its rate of reabsorption and removal by the capillary and lymphatic channels. The production of interstitial fluid is a function of capillary hydrostatic and oncotic pressure and endothelial integrity.

Box 6.5 Causes of hydrops fetalis

Immune
- *Hemolytic disease* of newborn: Alloimmune, Rh, Kell, C

Nonimmune
- *Cardiac*
  - *Structural*: Ebstein's, premature ductal closure, hypoplastic left or right heart
  - *Arrhythmias*: SVT, atrial flutter
  - *Cardiomyopathies*: Viral infection (TORCH, Coxsackie virus), endocardial
- *Genetic disorders*: Turner syndrome, trisomy 21, 18, 13, 15, 16
- *Malformations and tumors*: Congenital diaphragmatic hernia, congenital cystic adenomatoid, malformation of lung, bronchopulmonary sequestration
- *Neonatal anemias*: α-chain hemoglobinopathies, G6PD deficiency, twin–twin transfusion, fetomaternal hemorrhage
- *Infections*: CMV, toxoplasmosis, syphilis, human parvovirus B19, *Listeria monocytogenes*
- *Idiopathic*

Diagnosis

Hydrops fetalis is prenatally diagnosed by ultrasound findings (skin edema, pleural, pericardial, peritoneal effusion, large placenta, polyhydramnios).

Management

In utero management of cause
- *Fetal tachycardia*: Maternal medication (e.g., digoxin, β-blockers); fetal drug administration via umbilical vein (experimental)
- *Anemia*: Packed red cell transfusion in fetal umbilical vein during percutaneous umbilical blood sampling (PUBS)

- *Twin–twin transfusion*: Amnioreduction of polyhydraminos; laser ablation of fetal vessels (experimental)
- *Fetal pleural effusions*: Intrauterine centesis; pigtail pleuroamniotic drain placement
- *Fetal tumors*: Fetal surgery of sacrococcygeal taratomas or CCAMs

Neonatal management

- Resuscitation
    - Ventilation, intubation
    - Paracentesis, thoracentesis
    - Blood transfusion or partial exchange transfusion
- Supportive management
    - Cardiac support: pressors, ionotropes
    - Respiratory support: mechanical ventilation
    - Chest tube placement, drainage of ascites
    - Fluid and electrolyte management
    - Treatment of anemia: blood transfusion or partial exchange transfusion
    - Treatment of infections
    - Octreotide to treat chylothorax and ascites

Prognosis

For fetuses or infants with nonimmune hydrops, the survival rates are variable, in the range of 50%. Higher survival is reported in infants with SVT, chylothorax, and parvovirus infections, and lower rates in those with chromosomal abnormalities.

Neonatal hematology

Neonatal anemia

Causes (see Table 6.14)

Table 6.14 Causes of neonatal anemia

	Blood loss	Increased destruction	Decreased production
Perinatal causes	Fetal: maternal hemorrhage	Immune hemolysis (Rh incompatibility)	Congenital infection (CMV, toxoplasmosis, syphilis parvovirus B19)
	Donor of twin–twin transfusion	AVM or vascular tumors	
	Vasa previa		Congenital bone marrow dysfunction
Neonatal causes	Repeated blood sampling	DIC	Anemia of prematurity
	Subgaleal hematoma	Infection	Iron deficiency
	Intracranial hemorrhage	Hemoglobinopathies	Chronic illness
		RBC enzyme disorders	
		Membranopathies	

Presentation

This depends on the cause and timing of presentation:
- Acute anemia: Clinical shock
- Chronic anemia: Subtle or none, pallor, O_2 requirement, poor feeding, growth failure, apnea, tachycardia
- May see jaundice, stigmata of congenital infections, hepatosplenomegaly

History and labs

- Pregnancy history, birth complications, family history, neonatal medical course
- CBC, indices, reticulocyte count, peripheral smear
- Consider bilirubin, direct Coombs test, iron studies

Treatment considerations

Treatment depends on the cause.
- Iron supplementation
- Erythropoietin
- Blood transfusion
  - 15 mL/kg once or 10 mL/kg twice (separated 12 hours apart)
  - CMV negative, irradiated
  - For volume-sensitive patients, consider furosemide following transfusion.

Polycythemia

Table 6.15 Causes of neonatal polycythemia

Increased erythropoiesis	Transfusion
Placental insufficiency	Delayed cord clamping
Maternal DM	Maternal–fetal transfusion
Down syndrome	Twin–twin transfusion
Hyper- or hypothyroidism	
CAH	
Chromosomal anomaly	
Beckwith–Weidemann syndrome	

Definition
- Arterial/venous hematocrit (Hct) >65%
- Capillary heelstick samples are often greater than central ones.

Presentation
- Plethora, cyanosis, jaundice
- Lethargy, hypotonia, irritability, jitteriness, poor suck, poor feeding

Potential complications
- Increased blood viscosity leading to decreased blood flow and tissue perfusion
- Hypoglycemia (RBC dependant on glycolysis) and hypocalcemia
- Cardiorespiratory distress and CHF
- Seizures, stroke
- NEC
- Renal failure
- Priapism
- Hyperbilirubinemia

Treatment
- Consider if symptomatic and Hct >60% or asymptomatic and Hct >65–70%
- Partial exchange transfusion
  - Goal is to reduce Hct to <55%
  - Replacement of blood with isotonic normal saline in 10–20 mL increments
  - Exchange volume =

$$\frac{\text{Observed Hct} - \text{Desired Hct} \times \text{BV (100 mL/kg)} \times \text{Wt (kg)}}{\text{Observed Hct}}$$

Thrombocytopenia

Table 6.16 Causes of neonatal thrombocytopenia

Decreased production	Increased destruction	Combination
Congenital thrombocyto-penia (TAR, etc.)	Neonatal alloimmune (NAIT)	TORCH infections
Marrow disorders	Maternal ITP	Polycythemia
Congenital malignancies	Drug-induced	Exchange transfusion
Viral infections	Hypoxic–ischemic encephalopathy (HIE)	Down syndrome
	Microangiopathy (DIC, Kasabach–Merritt syndrome)	Chromosomal anomaly
		Hypothermic injury
	Infections or sepsis	Placental insufficiency

Presentation
- Petechia
- Intracranial hemorrhage
- Mucosal hemorrhage

Treatment
- Consider platelet transfusion if:
  - Symptomatic (bleeding, intracranial hemorrhage)
  - Platelet count <50,000 and high risk of intracranial hemorrhage
  - Platelet count <20,000
- Platelet transfusion
  - 10–15 mL/kg of platelets
- NAIT-specific
  - Platelet transfusion—use PLA1-negative or maternal platelets

Coagulopathy
Causes of bleeding
- DIC from sepsis or HIE
- Hemorrhagic disease of newborn (vitamin K deficiency)
- Hemophilia
- Liver failure
- Renal failure
- Medications
- Platelet abnormalities (see Thrombocytopenia section)

Presentation
- Bleeding from mucous membranes, umbilicus, or IV puncture sites
- Petechiae, ecchymoses
- Intracranial hemorrhage
- Pulmonary hemorrhage
- Hematuria
- Hematochezia or hematemesis

Depending on the duration and cause, you may see
- Shock
- Sepsis

Evaluation
- CBC with platelets
- PT, PTT, thrombin time, fibrinogen—will suggest cause of coagulopathy

Management
This depends on the severity and cause.
- Management of hemorrhage, ICH, shock, and sepsis, and PRBC volume replacement as clinically indicated
- Consider vitamin K therapy if clinically indicated
- Replacement therapy depends on deficiency:
  - Platelet (20 mL/kg) for thrombocytopenia
  - FFP (10–30 mL/kg) for clotting factor deficiency, vitamin K deficiency, or DIC
- Cryoprecipitate (6–15 mL) for deficiency in factor VIII, von Willebrand's factor (vWF), or fibrinogen

CNS malformations

Neural tube defects

- Result from failure of primary neural tube closure during fourth week of gestation
- One of the most common CNS malformations but decreasing prevalence due to
  - Prenatal diagnosis (increased AFP; ultrasound) resulting in pregnancy termination
  - Maternal periconceptional folate therapy
- High risk of latex allergies in patients with neural tube defects (NTDs)

Anencephaly

- Lethal condition. Absence of skull bones, forebrain, and upper brainstem

Encephalocele

- Midline skull defect through which brain protrudes; defect is skin covered. Most cases are occipital; 50% have other defects. Most require early neurosurgical management. There is a high risk for neurodevelopmental impairments, but variable severity.

Myelomeningocele

- Spinal cord malformation due to failure of posterior neuropore closure
- May be covered by meninges or skin or be "open" (exposed neural tissues)
- Usually at thoracolumbar, lumbar, or lumbosacral level
- Arnold–Chiari malformation is a constellation of hindbrain abnormalities resulting in downward displacement of the brainstem and cerebellum, with two major complications, hydrocephalus and brainstem dysfunction.
- *Presentation*: Decreased movement below lesion; clubfeet; urinary dribbling; hydronephrosis; hydrocephalus; bulbar paresis
- *Treatment*: Surgical closure or coverage of defect; ventricular drainage; monitoring and management of brainstem dysfunction.
- *Prognosis*: Related to severity of associated problems. Very large or high lesions have a worse prognosis.

Occult spinal dysraphisms

- Defects of caudal neural tube formation. Usually these have an intact skin covering. The majority have an associated lumbosacral midline cutaneous lesion (dimple, lipoma, hair tuft, dermal sinus).
- Associated spinal cord defects may include meningocele, lipoma, dermal sinus, or tethered cord.
- Spine ultrasound and MRI are helpful in diagnostic evaluation.

Congenital hydrocephalus

- *Causes*: Aqueductal stenosis; Dandy–Walker malformation; intracranial hemorrhage in utero; brain atrophy (hydrocephalus ex vacuo)
- *Presentation*: Usually patients have OFC >97th percentile, split sutures; they may have "sun-setting" of eyes.
- Cranial ultrasound is diagnostic.

- *Treatment*: In-dwelling ventricular drainage device.
- *Prognosis* depends on etiology and severity of cortical compression.

Dandy–Walker malformation

- Cerebellar vermis hypoplasia associated with hydrocephalus and significant posterior fossa CSF collection ("cyst") that expands into the fourth ventricle
- Associated with a variety of syndromes, including fetal alcohol syndrome and trisomy 13 and 18
- *Prognosis* depends on associated abnormalities.

Agenesis of the corpus callosum

- Nonspecific feature of numerous conditions; associated with wide variety of CNS malformations
- May be total or partial (splenium is involved but genu is intact)
- May be an incidental finding at autopsy
- *Prognosis* depends on associated syndromes and/or CNS malformations.

Hydrancephaly

- Absence of cerebral hemispheres; cranial cavity is filled with CSF. Brainstem, midbrain are usually intact.
- *Cause*: Severe vascular insult causing extensive cortical necrosis—brain "meltdown"
- *Presentation*: May have macrocephaly or normal head size. Patients usually do not have split sutures. They may behave normally in the neonatal period.
- *Prognosis*: Severe neurodevelopmental impairment; usually fatal

Microcephaly

- Small cranial vault (OFC <3rd percentile).
- Primary defect is marked reduction in brain size.
- *Causes*: Congenital infection; fetal alcohol or drug exposure; various syndromes; may occur postnatally due to severe brain injury
- *Prognosis*: Generally poor neurodevelopmental prognosis

Holoprosencephaly

- This is the most common human brain malformation. It is due to incomplete cleavage of the forebrain (prosencephalon). There is a single, central ventricular cavity.
- Three types: Alobar (single ventricle with no separate hemispheres), lobar, and semilobar (partially formed hemispheres)
- This condition may have associated craniofacial abnormalities such as cyclopia (single central eye) or median cleft lip and is associated with certain genetic syndromes (e.g., trisomy 13).
- *Prognosis* depends on the severity of brain malformations and associated syndromes.

Neuronal migration disorders

- These consist of failure of developing neurons to migrate to the appropriate positions in the six layers of the cerebral cortex.
- Lissencephaly (smooth brain; absence of gyri) is the most severe form.
- Pachygyria (very few gyri)
- Schizencephaly (deep cerebral cleft) may be bilateral or unilateral.
- Polymicrogyria (excess number of small convolutions on cortical surface)
- Neuronal heterotopia (displaced collections of neurons, usually in periventricular white matter)
- Associated problems include hydrocephalus and seizure disorders.
- *Prognosis* depends on the type of disorder and associated problems and CNS malformations.

Hypoxic-ischemic encephalopathy

Hypoxic–ischemic encephalopathy

There are many mechanisms by which the neonatal brain can sustain injury. One common cause is perinatal asphyxia, defined as a critical and severe lack of oxygen to the fetus during labor and delivery. This occurs in 2–4 of every 1000 live-born term infants, and more frequently in preterm births. Without treatment, up to 60% of affected infants either do not survive, or sustain severe and lifelong neurodevelopmental handicaps that include mental retardation, cerebral palsy, seizures, deafness, blindness, and learning disabilities.

Diagnostic criteria

Infants at highest risk for poor outcome are identified by a combination of markers that includes evidence of a sentinel intrapartum event (e.g., fetal bradycardia), the need for delivery room resuscitation, a 5-minute Apgar score of ≤5, cord arterial pH level of ≤7.00, and/or base deficit ≥16 mEq/L, and postnatal evidence of moderate to severe encephalopathy as indicated by both an abnormal clinical examination and an abnormal EEG (see Table 6.17).

Table 6.17 Clinical grading system for neonatal encephalopathy

Clinical feature	Grade I (mild)	Grade II (moderate)	Grade III (severe)
Level of consciousness	Hyper alert	Lethargic	Stuporous
Muscle tone	Normal	Mild hypertonia	Flaccid
Posture	Mild distal flexion	Strong distal flexion	Intermittent decerebration
Tendon reflexes	Overactive	Overactive	Decreased or absent
Suck	Weak	Weak/absent	Absent
Moro	Strong (low threshold)	Weak, incomplete (high threshold)	Absent
Autonomic dysfunction	Generalized sympathetic dysfunction	Generalized parasympathetic dysfunction	Both sympathetic and parasympathetic dysfunction
Heart rate	Tachycardia	Bradycardia	Variable
Seizures	None	Common: focal or multifocal	Absent or difficult to control

Adapted from Sarnat HB, Sarnat MS (1976) Neonatal encephalopathy following fetal distress. A clinical and electroencephalographic study. *Arch Neurol* **33**: 696–705.

Differential diagnosis

- Intrauterine insult (cord accident, placental abruption, maternal hypoxia)
- Maternal drugs (e.g., anesthesia)
- Acute blood loss
- Intracranial hemorrhage (ICH)
- CNS malformation
- Cardiopulmonary disease
- Infection
- Acidosis

Management

- Establish airway and circulation, insert IV ± arterial lines.
- Maintain head of bed slightly elevated.
- Keep O_2 and CO_2 in normal range. Hyperoxia should be avoided (oxidative damage). Hyper- or hypocarbia should also be avoided as this affects cerebral blood flow.
- Maintain mean blood pressure at >30mm/Hg using pressors if needed.
- Fluid management: Restrict total fluid intake to <60 mL/kg for first 1–3 days, watch for evidence of SIADH (low serum Na, low urine output); keep glucose and calcium in a normal range. Follow urine output carefully.
- For moderate to severe HIE, keep patient NPO for 3–5 days until bowel function is established (passing gas and stool).
- Monitor for associated abnormalities, including disseminated intravascular coagulopathy, cardiogenic shock, and liver and/or renal damage.
- Assess history and physical exam for cause of distress. Treat associated or causative conditions appropriately.
- Assess degree of encephalopathy (see Table 6.17).
- Treat clinical seizures (load with 20 mg/kg phenobarbital). Consider obtaining an early EEG.
- Consider brain imaging to diagnose possible malformations, bleeding, and stroke, and to evaluate the extent of injury.
- Some centers are practicing total body cooling or head cooling under experimental protocols.
- Consult neurology.

Prognosis

Apgar scores correlate poorly with outcome. The best guide is the worst Sarnat grade and clinical evolution, e.g., normalization of physical exam and EEG within 1 week is a good prognostic sign.

Risk of later disability or death is grade I, <2%; grade II, 24%; and grade III, 78%. Additional poor prognostic features include poor interictal EEG (discontinuous, burst suppression, or persistent low-voltage activities), status epilepticus, and diffuse changes in cerebral hemispheres or basal ganglia on MRI or CT from 5–14 days.

CNS injury

Intracranial hemorrhage (ICH)

Incidence and severity of ICH is inversely proportional to gestational age. Other risk factors include pneumothorax, hypotension, bleeding disorder, and severity of illness.

Cause

Most intraventricular hemorrhage (IVH) begins in the highly vascularized germinal matrix and extends to ventricles and further to the parenchyma. The cause is unknown.

Classification

- Grade I: Germinal matrix (subependymal) hemorrhage
- Grade II: Clot in ventricle, without ventricular dilation
- Grade III: Extensive clot in ventricle, enough to dilate it
- Grade IV: Parenchymal hemorrhage (alone or in combination with blood in ventricles)

Diagnosis

Diagnosis is usually by ultrasound. Clinical presentation may be catastrophic (cardiovascular collapse; acute drop in hematocrit; bulging fontanelle; seizures). More commonly ICH is discovered on screening ultrasound (within first week; rarely at second week or 1 month).

Complications and prognosis

- Posthemorrhagic hydrocephalus has a higher risk with grade III.
- Neurodevelopmental impairments depend on the severity of hemorrhage and associated conditions.

Term intracranial hemorrhage

- *Subdural*: Risk factor is difficult extraction
- *Subgaleal*: Presentation is shock; risk factor is vacuum extraction
- *Subarachnoid*: Presentation is irritability; seizures
- *Parenchymal or intraventricular* form is usually hemorrhagic infarction; seizures
- Cephalhematoma is subperiosteal hemorrhage; it does not cross suture lines.
- *Prognosis* depends on associated conditions and severity, etc.

Ischemic injury

Periventricular leukomalacia (PVL)

- Periventricular white matter lesions: ↑ echogenicity; cysts
- *Cause*: Poor cerebral perfusion or ischemia
- *Risk factors*: Extreme prematurity; hypotension; severe illness
- May not be apparent for several weeks after birth
- *Diagnosis*: Periventricular echodensities or cysts seen on ultrasound
- *Prognosis*: Higher risk of cerebral palsy (usually spastic diplegia), especially if there is cyst formation

Cerebral infarction (stroke)
- *Cause*:
  - Preterm infants: due to venous infarction associated with ICH
  - Term infants: Usually due to arterial ischemia involving middle cerebral artery distribution
  - Stroke may be associated with thrombophilic disorder (e.g., factor V Leyden deficiency)
- *Presentation*: Focal seizures
- *Diagnosis*: CT scan or MRI
- *Management*: Control seizures
- *Prognosis*: Most case series report approximately 50% with abnormal neurological outcome.

Skull fractures
- These are usually associated with operative delivery (e.g., forceps assisted) but can also occur from pressure of the head next to sacral promontory during forceful uterine contractions.
- They may be linear or depressed, usually in the frontal or parietal region, and often associated with cephalohematoma.
- *Diagnosis*: Skull X-ray and/or CT scan
- *Treatment*: Linear fractures need no treatment. Depressed fractures may need surgical elevation if they cause brain compression, seizure focus.

Peripheral nerve injury: brachial plexus
Risk factors
- Difficult delivery; macrosomia; shoulder dystocia

Cause
- Traction or stretching of brachial plexus, usually involving C5 and C6. In severe cases, it may be avulsion of nerve from the spinal cord.

Presentation
This injury is usually unilateral and more common on the right.
- *Erb palsy*: Injury is to the upper brachial plexus involving C5, C6. The arm is held in tight adduction and internal shoulder rotation with extension and pronation of the elbow. Asymmetric Moro reflex. Grasp relax is present.
- *Klumpke palsy*: Less common injury to lower brachial plexus. There is weakness of wrist flexion and hand muscles; grasp reflex is absent
- May be associated with fractured clavicle
- Injury to C4 can lead to phrenic nerve paralysis or diaphragm eventration.
- Injury to T1 → Horner syndrome (ptosis, anydrosis, miosis)

Management
Place arm in "natural" position; physical therapy is needed to avoid development of contractures.

Prognosis
- Erb palsy: Complete recovery by 1–18 months
- Klumpke palsy: Poor prognosis for recovery

Neonatal seizures

The true incidence of neonatal seizures (defined clinically as a paroxysmal alteration in neurological function, i.e., behavioral, motor, and/or autonomic function in an infant <28 days of life) is unknown, but is estimated at 2/1000 live births in the United States.

Clinically recognized seizures do not always have EEG correlates and, conversely, EEG-documented seizures may be unrecognized clinically. Some common, benign conditions that may mimic seizures include startle or Moro reflexes, normal "jitteriness" (fast, fine limb movements abated by holding the limb), and REM sleep movements.

In neonates seizures are classified as subtle (eye deviation, eyelid fluttering, apnea, limb cycling or swimming motions, mouthing, lip smacking, sucking), tonic, clonic (repetitive jerks 1–4/second), or myoclonic (repetitive jerks affecting flexor muscle groups).

Differential diagnosis

- Idiopathic (most common)
- Brain injury
  - Hypoxic–ischemic encephalopathy (HIE)
  - Intracranial hemorrhage (germinal matrix, intraventricular, intraparenchymal, subdural, subarachnoid)
  - Cerebral infarction (hemorrhagic or ischemic)
  - Birth trauma
- Infection
  - Meningitis: Common bacterial pathogens include *Escherichia coli* and group B streptococcus
  - Encephalitis: Herpes encephalitis (HSV), cytomegalovirus (CMV), and toxoplasmosis
- Cerebral malformation: Lissencephaly, pachygyria, polymicrogyria, and linear sebaceous nevus syndrome
  - Metabolic: Hypoglycemia, hypocalcemia, hypomagnesemia, pyridoxine-dependent seizures, nonketotic hyperglycinemia
  - Inborn errors of metabolism most commonly present in infants >72 hours of age, after the infant starts feeding.
- Toxins: Neonatal withdrawal, hyperbilirubinemia
- Other: Benign familial neonatal seizures, benign deep-sleep myoclonus, "fifth-day" fits, hypertension, and drug reaction

Evaluation

This should include a complete physical exam, family history, history of pregnancy and delivery, evaluation for infection, serum electrolytes, calcium, magnesium, and glucose and an EEG. If appropriate, further investigation may include radiological evaluation (head CT or MRI), toxicology screening, serum ammonia, urine organic acids, serum amino acids, karyotype, and TORCH screening.

Box 6.6 Treatment of neonatal seizures

Immediate

O_2, maintain airway, insert IV, treat underlying cause. When to start anticonvulsants is controversial; usual indication is >3 seizures/hour or single seizure >3–5 minutes.

First-line anticonvulsant
- IV phenobarbital (10–20 mg/kg bolus, give additional 10 mg/kg if seizures persist after 30 minutes, maintenance dose 5 mg/day)

Second-line
- IV phosphenytoin

For intractable seizures, consider therapeutic trial of parenteral pyridoxine (50 mg).

Duration of therapy

Depending on the cause, it is probably safe to stop treatment after a few days of no seizures, but many clinicians prefer to wait until several months are seizure-free before ceasing.

Prognosis

Prognosis varies with the cause of seizures, but is generally good for idiopathic seizures, sleep myoclonus, fifth-day fits, hypocalcemia, and benign familial neonatal seizures. There is a significant risk of adverse neurodevelopmental outcome after meningitis, HIE, hypoglycemia, cerebral infarction, hyper- or hypo-Na^+, cerebral malformations, kernicterus, and some inborn errors of metabolism.

The floppy infant

Generalized hypotonia, "frog-leg" posture, respiratory failure, and obstetric problems (e.g., polyhydramnios due to impaired swallowing, breech presentation) are common to the floppy infant. A physical examination can help distinguish the site of the disorder: upper motor neuron lesion (central) vs. lower motor neuron lesion.

- *Central conditions*: Encephalopathy, dysmorphism, reasonable muscle strength, ↑ or normal tendon reflexes
- *Lower motor neuron* causes include normal level of consciousness, muscle signs (weakness, myotonia, fasciculations, or fatiguing), ↓ or normal tendon reflexes, flat facies, micrognathia, high arched palate, ptosis, undescended testes, limb contracture/ deformities (arthrogryposis multiplex congenital), hip dislocation

Differential diagnosis

Upper motor neuron causes (central)
- *Chromosomal*: Turner syndrome, trisomy 21, Prader–Willi syndrome
- *Infection*: Sepsis, meningitis, encephalitis
- *Metabolic*: Hypocalcemia, hyponatremia, hypermagnesemia, hypoglycemia, hypothyroidism, aminoaciduria, gangliosidoses, hepatic encephalopathy
- *Toxin*: Drug intoxication (e.g., alcohol, narcotics), heavy metal poisoning, organophosphate poisoning, anticholinergic exposure
- *Perinatal trauma*: Perinatal asphyxia (HIE), hemorrhage, stroke

Lower motor neuron causes
- *Brainstem or spine*: Spinal muscular atrophy (anterior horn cell disorder), infection (poliomyelitis, Coxsackie)
- *Neuromuscular junction*: Congenital myasthenia gravis, myasthenic syndrome, Guillain–Barre syndrome, botulism
- *Muscle*: Muscular dystrophy, congenital myopathy, inflammatory myopathy
- *Other*: Benign congenital hypotonia

Evaluation

This should include a complete physical exam, family history, history of pregnancy, evaluation for infection, serum electrolytes, calcium, glucose, creatine phosphokinase (CPK), and thyroid function tests.

If appropriate, further investigation may include radiological evaluation (head CT or MRI), electromyogram, nerve conduction studies, muscle or sural nerve biopsy, toxicology screening, serum ammonia, urine organic acids, serum amino acids, karyotype, specific cytogenetics (e.g., myotonic dystrophy, SMA), and TORCH screening.

Prognosis

Prognosis varies with the cause of hypotonia.

Neonatal infection

Neonatal infection can be acquired transplacentally (congenital), by ascent from the vagina or during birth (intrapartum infection), or postnatally from the environment, staff, parents, or other infants. In the developed world, blood culture or serology confirmed sepsis occurs in up to 1% live births.

Infections are categorized as early-onset vs. late-onset sepsis. Preterm infants are at greater risk for both types of infections. In some studies, 21% of very low birth weight Infants (<1500 g) had late-onset, culture-proven sepsis.

Risk factors for early-onset neonatal sepsis
- Prolonged rupture of membranes >18 hours, especially if preterm
- Signs of maternal infection, e.g., maternal fever, chorioamnionitis, UTI
- Vaginal carriage or previous infant with group B streptococcal (GBS) infection
- Preterm labor; fetal distress
- Skin and mucosal breaks

Risk factors for late-onset sepsis
- Central lines and catheters
- Congenital malformations, e.g., spina bifida
- Severe illness, malnutrition, or immunodeficiency

Early-onset neonatal infection
Infection presents within 48 hours of birth. Incidence is ~2–5/1000 live births. Infection is caused by organisms acquired from the mother at or after birth, usually GBS, *E. coli*, or *Listeria*. Other possibilities include herpes virus, *H. influenza*, anaerobes, *Candida*, and *Chlamydia trachomatis*.

Presentation (symptomatic)
Possible clinical signs include temperature instability, lethargy, poor feeding, respiratory distress, systemic collapse, DIC, and limb pseudoparalysis due to osteomyelitis or septic arthritis.

Initial investigations
These include blood culture, cerebrospinal fluid (CSF) glucose, protein, cell count and culture, CBC with differential, and CRP at 24 and 48 hours (if mother was treated with antibiotics). If the patient has fever, liver failure, or seizures, or bacterial blood cultures continue to be negative after 24 hours with the infant worsening, consider workup for herpes simples virus (HSV), which includes serum HSV PCR, CSF HSV PCR, and swabs of nasopharynx, conjunctiva (eyes), and rectum.

Treatment
- Supportive
- Broad-spectrum antibiotics, e.g., ampicillin (100 mg/kg/dose IV bid) and gentamicin (4 mg/kg q36h if GA <37 weeks or q24h if >37 weeks), for 48 hours until blood culture results are final. If positive, treat for 10 days from date of a negative culture.

- If meningitis is present, treat for 14 days with ampicillin and cefotaxime (100 mg/kg/day divided q12h if <7 days, q8h if 8–30 days), or if gram-negative culture positive, treat for 21 days, and repeat the lumbar puncture at the end of treatment to evaluate if bacteria has cleared and WBC is normalized.
- For herpes viremia, treat with IV acyclovir 60 mg/kg/day divided bid for 2 weeks. For meningitis or encephalitis treat with the same dose for 21 days.
- If patient is asymptomatic but has risk factors for sepsis (e.g., maternal fever, chorioamnionitis, prematurity without other cause), treat with ampicillin and gentamicin for 48 hours until cultures are negative, unless infant has elevated CRP and mother was pretreated with antibiotics prior to delivery.
- The value of routinely including an LP with CSF examination and culture in the early workup for the asymptomatic infant has not been established.

Prognosis
- Up to 15% mortality (up to 30% if VLBW)

Late-onset neonatal infection

This infection presents later than 48 hours after birth. Incidence is ~4–5/1000 live births. Infection is caused by environmental organisms such as coagulase-negative staphylococci (CONS), *Staph. aureus*, *E. coli*, and other gram-negative bacilli, *Candida* species, and GBS.

Investigation
Obtain CBC with differential, blood culture, urinalysis (catheterized specimen) and urine culture, CSF glucose, protein, cell count and culture.

Treatment
Give broad-spectrum antibiotics, e.g., ampicillin and cefotaxime (dosing as in early sepsis) for 7 days. If there is a high suspicion related to an indwelling central catheter, treat with vancomycin (30–45 mg/kg/day divided q12h; treat 10–14 days for confirmed MRSA bacteremia) and cefotaxime (as above). For fungal infection use fluconazole IV 12 mg/kg loading dose, then 5 mg/kg q24–48h depending on post-menstrual age.

Transplacental (congenital infections)

Causes
- TORCH infections (*Toxoplasma gondii*, rubella, CMV, herpes simplex)
- Herpes zoster
- Parvovirus B19
- Syphilis
- Enterovirus
- HIV
- Hepatitis B
- Rarely, bacterial, e.g., GBS, *Listeria monocytogenes*, *N. gonococcus*

Presentation
- *TORCH infection*: SGA, jaundice, hepatitis, hepatosplenomegaly, purpura, chorioretinitis, micro-ophthalmos, cerebral calcification, micro- or macrocephaly, hydrocephalus
- *Rubella and CMV*: Deafness, cataracts, congenital heart disease, osteitis (rubella only)
- *Parvovirus B19*: Rubella-like rash, hemolytic anemia ± hydrops
- *H. zoster*: Cutaneous scarring, limb defects, multiple structural defects
- *Congenital syphilis*: SGA, jaundice, hepatomegaly, rash, rhinitis, bleeding mucous membranes, osteochondritis, meningitis
- *Gonorrhea*: Purulent conjunctivitis (ophthalmia)
- *Listeriosis*: Preterm labor and/or meconium-stained amniotic fluid

Investigation
Consider:
- Blood culture
- Pathogen-specific IgM and IgG (paired for H. zoster, toxoplasma)
- VDRL
- Maternal-specific serology
- Urine CMV shell vial and/or culture
- Throat swab viral culture
- CSF culture
- Stool viral culture
- Skin vesicle viral culture and electron microscopy

Treatment
- Most congenital infections have no specific treatment.
- General treatment is supportive and involves careful follow-up to identify sequelae, e.g., deafness and CMV.
- Syphilis: Penicillin G (50,000 units/kg/dose q12h x 7 days then q8h for 7 additional days)
- Symptomatic CMV: Genciclovir (6 mg/kg/dose of 12 hours every 6 weeks)
- Treatment of asymptomatic CMV infection is controversial but it can include ganciclovir, evaluated on a case-by-case basis.
- Toxoplasma: Pyrimethamine plus sulfadiazine for 1 year, dose to be determined by a specialist

Prognosis
- Variable and depends on disease, severity, and timing of infection.

Prevention of neonatal infection

General measures
- Hand washing before and after each patient contact
- Avoidance of overcrowding
- Low nurse-to-patient ratio
- Isolation measures appropriate to patient signs and symptoms
- Minimal handling
- Rational antibiotic use
- Minimize indwelling vascular access

Group B streptococcal (GBS) disease
The American College of Obstetrics and Gynecology recommends that intrapartum antibiotic prophylaxis be offered to women with
- A previous baby with neonatal GBS disease
- GBS bacteriuria in current pregnancy
- Positive GBS screen during current pregnancy

Hepatitis B
Hepatitis B is usually contracted at birth. Routine antenatal screening detects maternal carrier state (HBsAg+). Transmission risk is ~10% if the mother is a low-risk carrier (i.e., anti-HBe+).

To prevent vertical transmission, give Hep B vaccine to the infant within 24 hours of birth. Also give specific Hep B immunoglobulin (IG) 200 IU IM if the mother is a high-risk carrier (i.e., HBeAg+, or anti-HBe-, or antibody/antigen status unknown), since the untreated transmission risk is 90%. In both groups subsequent Hep B vaccine is required at 1 and 6 months.

If the infant is <2000 g and the mother is HBsAg+, administer Hep B vaccine and Hep B IG within 12 hours of birth. Repeat vaccine at 1, 2–3, and 6–7 months of chronologic age.

Human immunodeficiency virus (HIV) (see p. 744)
The vertical transmission rate is ~15%–25%. Risk is decreased by
- Maternal antiretroviral drug zidovudine (AZT) during third trimester and labor and postnatally to the baby for 6 weeks
- Elective CS
- Avoidance of breast-feeding (in the developed world). Infants are usually asymptomatic at birth.

Test at birth, and 1–2 and 2–4 months for
- HIV viral DNA PCR

Infection is very unlikely if all tests are negative at 6 months and the baby is well.

Herpes simplex

In infants, 85% of neonatal HSV is contracted at birth from the mother. Elective C-section reduces transmission if the mother has active genital herpes. Treat the infant with prophylactic IV acyclovir if born by vaginal delivery and there is primary maternal herpes (transmission risk is 50% compared with 3% in secondary herpes). To prevent infection from caregivers with cold sores, cover the lesions with a mask and treat the sores with topical acyclovir.

Herpes zoster

Perinatal infection can cause severe disseminated disease with high mortality (30%) if

- Maternal rash occurs between 5 days antenatally and 2 days postnatally
- A LBW infant (under 1 month old) has contact with varicella whose mother is nonimmune (i.e., check maternal antibody status if unsure)

Prevention

- Specific immunoglobulin (ZIG) 125 u IM given soon after delivery.

Necrotizing enterocolitis

Necrotizing enterocolitis (NEC) is a severe inflammatory disorder of the intestine. Preterm infants are at highest risk, with an incidence of 7%–10% in infants <1500 g. Ten percent of cases occur in term infants. While typically sporadic, NEC can be epidemic. Mortality is 25%–30%.

Prenatal steroids and human milk feedings are protective. The most common site of involvement is the terminal ileum.

The spectrum of pathology ranges from an isolated perforation with little inflammation (most common in extremely low birth weight infants) to NEC totalis, involving the entire small bowel (see Table 6.18). Time of presentation is inversely correlated to gestational age.

Cause

NEC is multifactorial. Necrosis is the end result of intestinal compromise (ischemia) and local invasion of bacterial pathogens. The most important predisposing factor is prematurity. Others include IUGR (chronic bowel ischemia), hypoxia, hypotension, PDA, polycythemia, exchange transfusion, and hyperosmolar feeds. There is no evidence that umbilical lines increase the incidence or severity of NEC.

Management

- Systemic support as needed, broad-spectrum antibiotics, and bowel rest with decompression (NPO, Replogle to low intermittent suction) are the mainstays of treatment.
- If NEC is advanced, surgical intervention may be required. Indications for surgery include GI perforation, deterioration despite medical treatment (necrotic bowel likely), and GI obstruction secondary to stricture formation (late).
- Acute surgical intervention may include drain placement, resection of involved bowel with primary repair, or a two-stage repair with bowel resection(s) and enterostomy, followed by later intestinal reanastomosis.

Prognosis

Mortality is 25%–30%. It is associated with extreme prematurity, extensive intestinal involvement, multi-organ failure, and intrahepatic portal gas. Long-term sequelae can include short bowel syndrome, strictures, and neurodevelopmental delay.

Table 6.18 Classification: Modified Bell's Staging Criteria for Necrotizing Enterocolitis

Stage	Systemic signs	Abdominal signs	Radiographic signs	Treatment
I—Suspected	Temperature instability, apnea, bradycardia, lethargy	Abdominal distension, emesis, heme-positive stool	Normal or intestinal dilation, mild ileus	NPO, bowel decompression, antibiotics x 3 days
IIA—Definite Mildly ill	Same as above	Same as above, plus absent bowel sounds with or without abdominal tenderness	Intestinal dilation, ileus, pneumatosis intestinalis	NPO, bowel decompression, antibiotics x 7–10 days
IIB—Definite Moderately ill	Same as above, plus mild metabolic acidosis and thrombocytopenia	Same as above, plus absent bowel sounds, definite tenderness, with or without abdominal cellulitis or right lower quadrant mass	Same as IIA, plus ascites	NPO, bowel decompression, fluid resuscitation, antibiotics x 10–14 days
IIIA—Advanced Severely ill, intact bowel	Same as IIB, plus hypotension, bradycardia, severe apnea, combined respiratory and metabolic acidosis, DIC, and neutropenia	Same as above, plus signs of peritonitis, marked tenderness, and abdominal distension	Same as IIA, plus ascites	NPO, bowel decompression, antibiotics x 14 days, fluid resuscitation, inotropic support, ventilator therapy

The substance-exposed newborn

The use of illicit substances during pregnancy is a common problem.

Estimated prevalence
- Illicit drugs (opioid, cocaine, amphetamines) ± 3% of pregnancies
- Alcohol ± 10%
- Tobacco ± 20%

Neonatal abstinence syndrome (NAS)

NAS is a term descriptive of a constellation of signs most often, but not always, attributable to a newborn infant's withdrawal from fetal exposure to opioid-type substances used during pregnancy.

Neonatal abstinence score

Formerly the Finnegan Scale, the neonatal abstinence score is a semi-quantitative observational assessment too used to determine the severity of withdrawal symptoms and ascertain the necessity for pharmacologic intervention (see Fig. 6.15). Serial scores of >8 indicate the need for treatment. If at all possible, treatment decisions should be based on daily average scores, or 24-hour trends.

Common substances of abuse during pregnancy

See Table 6.19.

Table 6.19 Common substances of abuse during pregnancy

	NAS	Early symptoms	Infection (Esp. sexually transmitted diseases)	Congenital abnormalities	Breast feeding contra-indications
Opioids	High	?	Yes	Rare	No
Ampheta-mines	No	High	Yes	Rare	Yes
Cocaine	No	Yes	Yes	Rare	Yes
Alcohol	No	Rare	Rare	High	No
Nicotine (Tobacco)	No	Yes	No	No	No

* Tremulous, irritable, poor feeding, disordered sleep, lethargic.

NEONATAL ABSTINENCE SCORE

Date:_____   Weight:_____

System	Signs & Symptoms	Score	Time AM PM	Comments
Central Nervous System Disturbances	Excessive high pitched cry	2		
	Continuous high pitched cry	3		
	Sleeps <1 Hour after feeding	3		
	Sleeps <2 Hours after feeding	2		
	Sleeps <3 Hours after feeding	1		
	Hyperactive moro reflex	2		
	Markedly Hyperacive Moro Reflex	3		
	Mild Tremors Disturbed	1		
	Moderate-Severe Tremors Disturbed	2		
	Mild Tremors Undisturbed	3		
	Moderate-Severe Tremors Undisturbed	4		
	Increased Muscle Tone	2		
	Excoriation (Specific Area)	1		
	Myoclonic Jerks	3		
	Generalized Convulsions	5		
Metabolic/Vasomotor/ Respiratory Disturbances	Sweating	1		
	Fever < 101° F(37.2-38.2° C)	1		
	Fever < 101° F(> 38.4° C)	2		
	Frequent Yawning (>3-4 Times/Interval)	1		
	Mottling	1		
	Nasal Stuffiness	1		
	Sneezing (> 3-4 Times/Interval)	1		
	Nasal Flaring	2		
	Respiratory Rate-60/min	1		
	Respiratory Rate-60/min with Retractions	2		
Gastrointestinal Disturbances	Excessive Sucking	1		
	Poor Feeding	2		
	Regurgitation	2		
	Projectile Vorniting	3		
	Loose Stools	2		
	Watery Stools	3		
	Total Score			
	Intials of Scorer			

Figure 6.15 Neonatal abstinence score. Adapted from Finnegan LP, Kaltenbach K (1992). The assessment and management of neonatal abstinence syndrome. In Hoeckelman RA, Nelson NM (eds.) *Neonatal Abstinence Syndrome*, 2nd ed. St. Louis: Mosby, p. 1367. Reprinted with permission.

Possible interventions

NAS

- *General and supportive*: Swaddling, low stimulus, dark, quiet environment, frequent low-volume feedings
- Specific pharmacologic treatment to be initiated if the neonatal abstinence score is consistently >8:
  - Treat with a morphine preparation, tincture of opium or solution of morphine sulfate in a concentration of 0.4 mg/mL
  - Initial dose, 0.1–0.15 mL/kg q3h; may be slowly increased, 0.1 mL/kg at a time, once or twice per 24 hours to control symptoms
  - When symptoms are well controlled, i.e., NAS scores are consistently <8, wean daily as tolerated by 10% increments.
  - Some infants, especially if they are premature or require large doses, should be placed on an apnea monitor.
  - Seizures should be controlled with phenobarbital.

Early symptoms

These include difficult feeding, disoriented sleep, etc.

- Patient and careful nursing with emphasis on maternal education before discharge

Infection

- Consider ruling out HIV/AIDS.

Congenital anomalies

- Careful physical examination and selective use of noninvasive studies (e.g., ultrasound) where appropriate

Appropriateness of breast-feeding

- With the exception of active abuse of amphetamines and/or cocaine, and HIV positivity, the benefit of breast-feeding outweighs the risk. For those mothers who must use tobacco and/or alcohol, use should be avoided for several hours prior to a feed.

Long-term issues

Intrauterine exposure to the type of substances discussed in this section has been repeatedly in the literature associated with a number of adverse outcomes. Such associations include an increased risk for premature delivery, IUGR, congenital malformations, SIDS, and long-term neurodevelopmental and/or behavioral problems. Accordingly, it seems reasonable to strongly support comprehensive follow-up for both the mother (to prevent problems with future pregnancies) and the infant (to optimize development).

Orofacial clefts

- Birth prevalence is 1/700 to 1/1000 live births

Classification (descriptive)

1. Median cleft lip
2. Unilateral and bilateral cleft lip
3. Oblique facial clefts
4. Lateral facial clefts
5. Median mandibular cleft

Etiology

The cause of orofacial clefts is multifactorial and includes genetic and environmental factors (especially folic acid deficiency, maternal use of alcohol, tobacco, steroids, anticonvulsants, and retinoic acid).

Thirty percent of orofacial clefts are syndromic and 70% are nonsyndromic. Isolated clefts are more common and constitute 66% of all orofacial clefts.

Embryology

There is failure of the medial nasal process to either contact or maintain contact with the lateral nasal and maxillary processes.

Associated complications

1. Feeding problems
2. Infections—ear (secretory otitis media), aspiration pneumonia
3. Speech difficulties
4. Dental problems

Treatment

Team approach

Refer patient to a craniofacial team consisting of a surgeon, geneticist, otolaryngologist, audiologist, orthodontist, speech pathologist, dentist, psychologist, and social worker.

Surgery

- Done in stages
- Cleft lip is repaired by 2–3 months of age.
- Cleft palate is repaired by 6–9 months of age.

Feeding

Feeding is by means of special devices, nipples (Haberman feeder), devices to help breast-feeding, and use of a prosthetic palate (obturator).

Neonatal dermatology

Development and function

Term
The infant has well-developed stratum corneum and is covered with vernix caseosa—both provide water and barrier protection.

Preterm
The infant has very thin stratum corneum and minimal vernix. Thus, there is increased insensible water loss, increased absorption of drugs, and reduced resistance to infection.

Basic skin care
- Limit use of adhesives.
- Limit bathing; avoid cleansing agents.
- Use short-contact chlorhexidine for antimicrobial skin preparation.
- Avoid excessive thermal, light exposure, especially in preterm infants.
- Protect skin injury sites with appropriate occlusive dressings.
- Know the composition of any topical creams, ointments, and emollients.

Colorful findings
- Plethora (deep red) may indicate polycythemia.
- Jaundice (yellow) is usually seen with bilirubin level >5 mg/dL.
- Pallor (white) may be due to anemia, birth depression, or shock.
- Cyanosis (blue)
  - *Central*: Due to arterial oxygen desaturation; may be due to congenital heart disease or lung disease
  - *Peripheral*: Acrocyanosis is a normal finding; if severe, suspect methemoglobinemia.
- Harlequin (clear line of demarcation between red area and normal color) is usually benign and transient but may also indicate shunting due to PPHN or aortic coarctation.

Benign skin conditions
- *Milia*: Tiny yellowish-white spots on the face; due to blocked sebaceous glands
- *Erythema toxicum*: Multiple, discrete red macular-papular lesions, usually with a white center. Wright's stain → eosinophils
- *Neonatal pustular melanosis*: There are three stages of lesions over the entire body: 1) pustules, 2) ruptured pustules or vesicles with scaling, and 3) hyperpigmented macules. More common in black infants
- *Mongolian spots*: Dark blue or purple bruise-like macular spots usually seen over the sacrum. Common in Asian, black infants
- *Acne neonatorum*: Comedones and pustules seen over the cheeks, chin, forehead
- Superficial capillary hemangiomas (salmon patches; stork bites)
- Erythematous, macular lesions seen on eyelids, midline face, posterior scalp

- *Sucking blisters*: Common on hand, wrist, upper lip
- *Strawberry hemangiomas*: Flat, bright red, sharply demarcated lesions commonly found on the trunk. Usually regress over years
- *Diaper rash*: Contact dermatitis; it may be associated with candida.

Nonbenign skin conditions

Infectious lesions

- Herpes (vesicles); *Staph.* "scalded skin" or bullous impetigo; disseminated candida; congenital viral infections—blueberry muffin spots

Congenital skin disorders

- Epidermolysis bullosa (blisters)
- Neurofibromatosis (cafe-au-lait spots)
- Neuroblastoma (raised bluish papules)
- Incontinentia pigmenti
- Cavernous hemangioma: Large red, cystic-appearing, firm, ill-defined mass found anywhere on the body. May be associated with platelet consumption or thrombocytopenia (Kassabach–Merritt syndrome)
- Port wine stain (nevus flammeus): Does not blanch with pressure; does not disappear over time. If it is on the forehead or upper lip, consider Sturge–Weber syndrome.

Purpura/petechiae

- Suspect thrombocytopenia; bleeding disorder (including DIC)

Practical procedures

Capillary blood sampling

Capillary blood sampling is used when small volumes of blood are necessary for analysis, e.g., CBC, blood gas, blood glucose territory. An automated device pierces the skin and causes less pain. It also punctures to a predetermined limit depth, which should prevent underlying bone damage or infection. Gloves should always be worn when testing or sampling body fluids.

Equipment
- Alcohol-impregnated swab
- Automated device or sterile lancet
- Appropriate sample bottles or capillary tubes
- Cotton ball or gauze pad

Site
- Plantar heel surface outside the medial and lateral limits of calcaneous bone in the young infant (see Fig. 7.1)
- Finger site in the child

Procedure
- Warm the heel or finger.
- In the case of the foot, hold dorsiflexed.
- Clean with an alcohol-impregnated swab.
- Gently massage area to improve blood flow and use your hand as a tourniquet.
- Puncture skin with an automated device or a sterile lancet.
- "Scoop" droplets of blood into an appropriate sample container or onto blood glucose-measuring strip. (Excessive squeezing results in falsely high serum potassium and hematocrit levels, as well as painful bruising.)
- Once sample is collected, stop any residual bleeding by local pressure with a cotton ball.

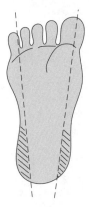

Figure 7.1 Site for capillary blood sampling on plantar surface of foot. Sampling area is indicated by shaded area.

Venipuncture

When a significant volume of blood is needed for testing (e.g., coagulation studies), or when sterility of sample is important (i.e., blood culture), venipuncture is preferable to capillary blood sampling.

Equipment

- In older children, as in adults, a 21–23G needle and syringe should be used.
- In infants and small children use either a 23G butterfly needle and syringe or 21–23G butterfly needle without the normal tubing.
- Alcohol-impregnated swab
- Appropriate sample bottles or capillary tubes
- Cotton ball or gauze pad

Procedure

- Suitable sites include antecubital fossa, dorsum of the hand, and dorsum of the foot. Sometimes other sites such as the scalp are used, particularly in infants.
- Identify suitable vein and warm limb if necessary.
- Topical local-anesthetic cream applied under an occlusive dressing for 30–60 minutes reduces pain and may be appropriate for young children.
- Apply a tourniquet. In infants this is best done using gloved fingers. Stretch the overlying skin to stabilize the vein. In young children an assistant is often required to keep the child's limb stationary.
- Clean overlying skin with an alcohol-impregnated swab.
- Along the line of the vein and in a proximal direction insert needle through overlying skin at 15°–30° into the vein until blood flashes back into the needle.
- Stabilize needle/butterfly with your fingers and then aspirate into the syringe, or if using a butterfly with no tubing, allow blood to drip into sample bottles. Gentle release with retightening of the tourniquet often increases blood flow.
- Once blood has been collected, release the tourniquet and then apply gentle pressure to the puncture site for a few minutes with a cotton ball. Once bleeding has stopped, an occlusive bandage is optional.

Intravenous cannulation

Intravenous cannulation is required for the infusion of fluids or drugs. At the time of admission it might be possible to plan blood sampling at the time of cannulation. This "combined" technique will save puncturing the child twice.

Equipment
- Alcohol-impregnated swab
- IV cannula: 24G in newborns, 21G in older children
- IV extension set and three-way tap with Luer lock flushed with 0.9% saline
- Tourniquet (older children)
- Tape or transparent occlusive dressing to secure cannula in site

Procedure
- Carefully identify a suitable vein. The dorsum of the hand or foot or antecubital fossa is ideal. Other suitable sites include anatomical snuff-box, volar aspect of the forearm, great saphenous vein at the medial malleolus, or knee. Avoid larger veins if a percutaneous central-line insertion is likely to be needed later. (Scalp veins can be used, but hair may need to be shaved.)
- *Tip*: Transillumination with a "cold" light of the hand or foot can be very useful for locating "hidden" veins, particularly in the newborn. In emergency, or if one or more normal sites have been used, scour the whole body and use whatever vein you can find!
- Consider at least 45 minutes of local anesthetic cream applied under an occlusive dressing over the intended vein before starting. Remove cream before starting.
- Ensure good vein perfusion—e.g., warm extremity before cannulation.
- If needed, ask an assistant to help with keeping the child's limb steady. This may require wrapping the child in a towel or sheet.
- In older children apply tourniquet proximal to the vein. In infants, if attempting the hand dorsum, apply compression and immobilization by flexing the wrist and then grasp with the index and middle fingers over the dorsum while your thumb is over the child's fingers.
- Clean site with alcohol-impregnated swab.
- Insert cannula at an angle of 10°–15° to the skin with the bevel upright, just distal and along the line of the vein.
- When the vein is entered, blood will flash back (not always if the vein is small!).
- Once the vein is entered, advance cannula 1–2 mm (to ensure cannula is also in vein) and then advance cannula over stylet into the vein.
- Remove stylet, collect any blood that is required from the cannula hub.
- Flush cannula with 0.9% saline to confirm IV placement and to prevent clotting, then connect IV line.
- Secure cannula with appropriate adhesive tape or dressing, leaving the cannula tip visible in case of extravasation.
- Splint extremity to prevent cannula from kinking.

Peripheral arterial blood sampling

This procedure is used for determination of blood gases or acid–base status, or when large volumes of blood are required and venous access is difficult.

Equipment
- As for venipuncture
- Heparinized arterial blood syringe, if intending blood gas analysis

Procedure
- In descending order of appropriateness the suitable sites are the radial artery, posterior tibial artery (in newborns), dorsalis pedis artery (newborns), and ulna artery (only if Allen's test confirms patent adjacent radial artery). If the femoral artery is to be used in the older child, cannulation is preferable before sampling. The brachial artery should rarely, if ever, be used because of its "end arterial" distribution.
- Identify artery position by palpation of pulse or using a suitable "cold" light source to transilluminate area.
- Partially extend limb (e.g., extend wrist for radial artery sampling), and with a finger, slightly stretch skin over artery to stabilize its position.
- Clean overlying skin using an alcohol-impregnated swab.
- Insert needle through overlying skin at a 15°–30° angle into the artery until blood flashes back. If after inserting the needle there is still no flashback, withdraw it slowly, as often blood will then appear.
- Collect blood by aspirating into the syringe or direct into a heparinized capillary tube.
- Remove needle and apply pressure with a cotton ball to puncture wound for at least 5 minutes.

Peripheral arterial cannulation

This procedure is indicated when repeated arterial blood sampling or pressure monitoring is required. The most common arteries used are those used for peripheral arterial sampling. Remember to perform an Allen test before attempting to cannulate the radial or ulnar artery.

Equipment
As for intravenous cannulation (see p. 228).

Procedure
- Identify selected artery by method described for peripheral blood sampling.
- Partially extend relevant limb joint.
- Clean site with an alcohol-impregnated swab.
- Insert cannula in a proximal direction at an angle of 25°–30° to the skin and in the same line as the artery.
- When blood flashes back into the hub, advance the cannula smoothly over the needle and into the artery.
- Remove the needle and immediately stop the bleeding by applying pressure over the artery and the tip of the catheter with your gloved finger.
- Connect a three-way tap that has been previously flushed with heparinized saline. Samples can be obtained from the unused port of the three-way tap.
- Flush the arterial line with heparinized saline (1 unit/mL).
- Connect the infusion line and run at 1–2 mL/hr with heparinized saline.
- A transducer may be attached to continuously monitor blood pressure.

Umbilical arterial catheter

This catheter is placed in neonates up to 48 hours old for invasive blood pressure and continuous blood gas monitoring. It is also used for blood sampling for blood gas analysis or other frequent blood tests, fluid infusion, and exchange transfusion. The catheter may reside in the neonate for up to 10 days.

Site

To avoid the origins of the celiac, mesenteric, and renal arteries, the tip of the catheter should be positioned in the aorta and above the diaphragm at T8–T10 vertebral level or, alternatively, in the distal aorta at L3–L4 level.

Equipment

- Antiseptic solution, e.g., 0.5% chlorhexidine
- Surgical instruments, including fine forceps, blunt-ended dilator probe, scalpel, artery forceps, scissors, suture forceps, sutures
- Sterile drapes
- Umbilical catheters: 3.5 Fr if birth weight <1500 g, 5.0 Fr for babies ≥1500 g. Catheters with a terminal electrode can be used for continuous measurement of arterial O_2 and CO_2 concentrations.
- Three-way taps, IV extension sets, syringes, cord ligature
- 5- to 10-mL syringes, one containing heparinized saline (1 unit/mL)
- Blood pressure transducer if monitoring is intended

Procedure

- Monitor baby closely during procedure—e.g., O_2 saturation monitoring.
- An assistant should hold the baby's legs down with the infant supine, or leg restraints should be used.
- Calculate the distance (cm) to insert the catheter from the umbilicus to the aorta at T8–10 level using the formula:

    $3 \times$ weight in kg + 9 + stump length

- To control possible bleeding, tie a cord ligature around the umbilicus stump.
- Connect a three-way tap to catheter and prime with heparinized 0.9% saline (do not use heparinized saline if coagulation testing is required).
- Catheter insertion should be performed using strict aseptic technique.
- Clean cord and periumbilical area with antiseptic solution.
- Surround periumbilical area with sterile towels to create sterile field.
- Clamp the umbilical cord horizontally with artery forceps 0.5–1 cm above umbilical skin. Using the artery forceps as a guide, cut the umbilical cord horizontally and immediately below with the scalpel.
- Identify the two umbilical arteries and umbilical vein (see Fig. 7.2).
- Dilate the end of one of the arteries with fine forceps or probe until wide enough for the catheter tip to be easily introduced.
- Gently advance catheter the calculated distance. If resistance is met, put gentle traction on the umbilicus using artery forceps, as this often eases insertion down the spiral umbilical artery.

- Aspirate blood to confirm position and take required samples. *Note*: arterial blood should pulsate and still bleed if the catheter hub is held above the infant.
- Secure catheter with a purse-string suture, taking care not to puncture the catheter. Remove cord ligature and check for bleeding.
- Connect catheter to three-way tap and IV infusion set. Blood pressure monitoring can be performed by connecting an appropriate transducer.
- Confirm correct placement with a chest or abdominal X-ray. The catheter should loop initially downward as it traverses the iliac arteries before ascending up the aorta.
- Check perfusion of the perineum and lower limbs. If ischemia occurs, this may be corrected by an IV bolus of 0.9% saline or albumin. If ischemia remains, remove the catheter immediately.
- Following insertion, the abdomen should remain exposed to allow immediate observation of any hemorrhage, e.g., from accidental removal of catheter.
- When no longer required, the catheter should be removed. Cut the surrounding suture, then slowly withdraw it, taking several minutes to remove the final few centimeters from the artery. Then apply pressure or suture to limit any bleeding.

Umbilical vein: single, thin walled, large opening, large diameter

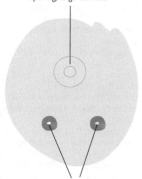

Umbilical arteries: paired, thick walled, small opening, spiral down cord, small diameter

Figure 7.2 Cut surface of umbilical cord.

Umbilical venous catheter

This catheter is indicated in neonates up to 14 days of age. It is used for frequent blood draws, total parenteral nutrition (TPN), frequent medication drips, or continuous infusions.

Equipment
- 3.5 or 5Fr umbilical venous catheter
- The remaining equipment is as for umbilical arterial catheter (p. 232).

Procedure
- Measure umbilicus (including stump) to acromoclavicular joint and subtract 4 cm.
- Clean and prepare umbilical stump as detailed on page 232 for insertion of umbilical artery catheter.
- Identify umbilical vein (see p. 233) and then dilate, opening with fine forceps or dilating probe.
- Insert catheter the measured distance (see p. 232).
- Aspirate blood to confirm insertion. Blood from the umbilical vein should not pulsate. When the catheter hub is held open to the air above the infant, blood will slowly fall back to the infant. Do not do this for long, or an air embolus will result!
- If blood will not aspirate or resistance is felt before catheter is inserted the measured distance, it is likely that the catheter tip has wedged in the hepatic portal veins or sinus. Withdraw the catheter and then reinsert as far as it will go while still allowing blood to be aspirated.
- Flush umbilical catheter with heparinized saline.
- Secure catheter with a purse-string suture, taking care not to puncture the catheter.
- Remove cord ligature and check for bleeding.
- Confirm correct position by combined chest and abdominal X-ray. A venous catheter should only follow a direct course proximally through the liver (unlike an umbilical arterial catheter); ideally, the tip should lie just above the diaphragm in the inferior vena cava.
- The catheter can then be used for blood sampling, fluid or drug administration, or central venous pressure monitoring (if the catheter tip is above the diaphragm).
- Remove catheter slowly as soon as it is not needed and then gently compress the umbilical stump until bleeding stops.
- In an emergency (e.g., resuscitation at birth), simply cut the umbilical cord with a scalpel blade 1–2 cm above distal to the skin and rapidly insert the umbilical catheter until blood can be aspirated. Don't worry about hemorrhage, as cardiac output will be minimal or absent in such an emergency. Any bleeding can be controlled by squeezing the base of the umbilicus between the thumb and index finger. Resuscitation drugs and fluids can then be given safely. Use caution to avoid an air embolism.

Central venous catheterization via a peripheral vein

Indications
This procedure is used for administration of prolonged or concentrated IV fluids or drugs.

Sites
Suitable sites include the veins of the antecubital fossa or long saphenous vein anterior to the medial malleolus or inferior-medial to the knee. Less preferred sites include the axillary scalp veins.

Equipment
- Sterile surgical instruments, including fine forceps and scissors
- Sterile gloves, gauze swabs, gown and drapes
- Antiseptic solution, e.g., 0.5% chlorhexidine
- 23 or 27G silastic long-line catheter. 27G should only be used when a 23G line cannot be inserted.
- 2- to 5-mL syringe and heparinized (1 unit/mL) saline solution
- Introducer, e.g., 19G butterfly needle, 20G IV cannula
- Sterile adhesive tape and transparent occlusive dressing

Procedure
- Measure distance from insertion site to just above the right atrium. Placement of the catheter tip in the right atrium risks pericardial tamponade.
- Use strict aseptic technique.
- Set out equipment and prime catheter with sterile heparinized saline.
- Immobilize relevant limb and then clean insertion site with antiseptic.
- Place sterile drapes around insertion point to create sterile field.
- Apply tourniquet proximal to the selected insertion point.
- Insert introducer needle into the vein until blood flashes back. If using a cannula, remove stylet.
- With fine forceps advance the catheter through the introducer needle.
- Continue to advance catheter into the vein until the desired distance is reached. Often the catheter will meet resistance as it becomes wedged against a kinked vein or valve. Milking in a proximal direction with a finger over the catheter tip may facilitate further advancement.
- Remove tourniquet and then flush catheter with heparinized saline.
- Once fully inserted, withdraw the introducer needle and remove it from the line after unscrewing the catheter hub. Then reconnect hub to the catheter.
- Ensure hemostasis at puncture site by applying gentle pressure with a sterile gauze swab. This may take considerable time!
- Secure line in place by using thin strips of sterile adhesive tape and sterile transparent occlusive dressing.

- Start infusion of heparinized saline to keep line patent.
- Confirm catheter tip placement with a chest X-ray. This may be aided by injection of 0.5 mL of contrast solution into the line immediately before taking the X-ray. Ideally, the catheter tip should lie just proximal to the right atrium. Withdraw it before use if in the right atrium.

Airway management

Before effective ventilation can take place, the airway must be patent. This can be ensured, alone or in combination, in various ways:

- *Head tilt*: Tilt the head back gently to a neutral position in newborns, slightly extended in older children.
- *Chin lift*: Using one or two fingers, apply forward pressure to just under the chin to pull the tongue forward.
- *Jaw thrust*: Apply forward pressure behind one or both angles of the jaw to pull the tongue forward.
- *Oropharynged airway*. Slip airway over the tongue until flange reaches the lips. Be careful not to push the tongue back. To determine size, hold airway along the line of the jaw with the flange in the middle of the lips. The end of the correct-sized airway should be level with the angle of the jaw.
- *Endotracheal intubation*: See p. 240.
- *Tracheotomy* is used to bypasses upper airway obstruction and when oral/nasal endotracheal intubation fails or is contraindicated. This is performed by an experienced surgeon.

Mask ventilation

This procedure is useful during resuscitation or for short periods of assisted ventilation. It can be performed using a self-inflating bag and face mask with an appropriate-sized reservoir bag or, alternatively, by using a mask, "T" piece, a continuous supply of gas, and a pressure-limiting device. In the latter situation a breath is given by occluding the open aperture of the T piece.

Procedure

- Ensure patent airway: See Airway management (p. 238).
- Select appropriate-sized mask: It should be big enough to cover the face from the bridge of the nose to below the mouth, but not extend over the edge of the chin or over the orbits.
- Connect face mask to appropriate self-inflating bag or tubing with a T piece to an oxygen or air supply at an adequate flow rate, e.g., 5–8 L/min in the newborn.
- In newborns a pressure-limiting valve should initially be set at ~30 cmH$_2$O.
- Apply mask to face over the mouth and nose and apply enough downward pressure to make an effective seal.
- Give inflation breath by either compressing self-inflating bag or occluding open aperture of T piece.
- Observe and auscultate chest wall for adequate inflation. Note whether the condition of the child is improving or deteriorating.
- If inflation is poor or the child is deteriorating, check that the airway is not obstructed and use one or more of above techniques to ensure a patent airway.

Prolonged mask ventilation is likely to lead to a distended stomach. Insert an orogastric tube on free drainage to decompress the stomach and prevent diaphragmatic splinting.

Endotracheal intubation

Indications

This procedure is used as part of advanced resuscitation to remove harmful airway substances (e.g., blood or meconium), protect the airway (e.g., epiglottitis), allow prolonged artificial ventilation (e.g., respiratory failure or during general anesthetic), or administer drugs (e.g., surfactant).

Equipment

- Appropriate-sized laryngoscope. Neonatal laryngoscopes are straight, the blade size starts at 0 (7.5 cm long) for use in preterm infants; use size 1 (10 cm) in term infants. In older children use curved-blade laryngoscopes (Macintosh).
- Endotracheal tube (ETT). The appropriate size is 2–2.5 mm (internal diameter) in an infant weighing <1000 g, 3 mm in an infant of 1000–3000 g, and 3.5 mm in neonates >3000 g. The appropriate size then increases progressively as child size increases up to the male adult size of 8–9 mm. Generally, child endotracheal tubes are uncuffed. Cole (shouldered) endotracheal tubes are suitable for oral intubation in the neonatal unit. Straight (non-shouldered) tubes can be used for oral or nasal intubation.
- Appropriate-sized introducer if required
- Lubricating jelly if attempting nasal intubation
- Magill forceps if attempting nasal intubation
- Suction catheter and tubing connected to suction source
- Appropriate endotracheal connection adaptors, tubing, and oxygen source
- Fixation device and tape

Procedure

- Oral intubation is preferred during short-term intubation or during resuscitation. Nasal intubation has advantages if ventilation is prolonged.
- Check all equipment, laryngoscope light, suction, and oxygen supply.
- If electively intubating, connect the child to a pulse oximeter and cardiac monitor.
- Sedation or anesthesia should be given prior to elective intubation.
- Preoxygenate the child by hyperventilation with 85% O_2 for 15–30 seconds.
- Place the child in a supine position with the head in the neutral position and the neck slightly extended.
- Stand immediately behind the head.
- If nasal intubation is being performed, a prelubricated ETT should be passed into one nostril as far as the nasopharynx prior to insertion of the laryngoscope. If the ETT will not pass easily, do not try force, as this may penetrate the cribriform plate.
- Open the mouth and perform suction to clear the airway of any secretions.
- Holding the laryngoscope in the left hand, insert the blade to the right side of the mouth and advance to the base of the tongue.

- Advance the blade further until the epiglottis is seen and then insert blade tip into the vallecula (space between the base of tongue and epiglottis).
- Vertically lift up the whole blade, thereby exposing the vocal cords (see Fig. 7.3). Cricoid pressure with the little finger of the left hand may assist in visualizing the vocal cords. Perform suction if secretions obstruct vision.
- If the vocal cords cannot be seen after 30 seconds, do not attempt blind intubation. Abandon the attempt, maintain patent airway (p. 238), and, if required, perform mask ventilation (p. 239) before trying again.
- Once vocal cords are visualized, insert the ETT between vocal cords (via the mouth if orally intubating). If this is difficult or you are performing nasal intubation, use the Magill forceps with the right hand to advance the ETT tip.
- If using a straight tube, the ETT should be advanced until the proximal end of the thick black line is level with the vocal cords. If using a Cole ETT, advance it until the shoulder just reaches the vocal cords.
- If using a cuffed tube, advance it until the cuff is just below the vocal cords and no further. Then inflate the cuff with air using a syringe.
- Once intubation is successful, connect tubing and ventilate.
- Visually check chest movement and auscultate over each lung to ensure appropriate and equal bilateral air entry. Oxygenation and heart rate should improve.
- Fix ETT in place appropriately, following institutional guidelines.
- Perform a chest X-ray to confirm position of the ETT, which should be 1–2 cm above the carina.
- Causes of failure to intubate include poor visualization of vocal cords from overextension of the neck or advancement of the laryngoscope too far into the esophagus; spasm of the vocal cords (wait, as almost certainly the vocal cords will open eventually—do not attempt to force ETT through, as this may cause damage); and anatomical abnormalities, e.g., laryngeal atresia; vocal cord edema.
- Conditions that may give the impression of failed intubation include thoracic pathology (e.g., tension pneumothorax, diaphragmatic hernia); intubation of the right main bronchus (detected by diminished air entry on left-pull back tube until there is air entry in both lungs); and obstruction of the airway or ETT, e.g., very thick meconium (suction of the ETT may be successful).

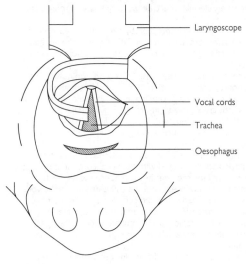

Figure 7.3 Anatomy of laryngeal intubation.

Insertion of a chest drain

Indications

This procedure is used to drain a pneumothorax, pleural effusion, or chylothorax. In an emergency (i.e., tension pneumothorax), drainage should first be performed by inserting a 21–23G butterfly into the affected side at the second intercostal space in the midclavicular line. The butterfly tubing can be placed underwater following insertion; alternatively, a three-way tap can be attached, allowing aspiration with a syringe. Once the patient is stable, a formal chest drain should be inserted.

Equipment

- Antiseptic solution, e.g., 0.5% chlorhexidine
- Local anesthetic, e.g., 1% lidocaine, needle and 10 mL syringe
- Intercostal drain, size 8–12 Fr for newborns, up to 18 Fr for young adults
- Straight surgical scalpel blade, artery forceps and suture
- Sterile dressing pack (including gauze, gloves, drapes)
- Underwater drainage system and suction pump
- Steristrips and plastic transparent dressing, e.g., Tegaderm

Procedure

- Position child supine with the affected side raised 30°–45° with a towel.
- Raise the arm toward the head.
- Suitable sites are the fourth intercostal space in the midaxillary line (be careful to avoid the nipple), and second intercostal space in the midclavicular line.
- Clean the skin over the insertion site with antiseptic solution and then infiltrate a small amount of local anesthetic into the tissues down to the pleura.
- Wait 1–2 minutes, then make a small skin incision with the scalpel just above and parallel to the rib. Blood vessels lie just below each rib.
- Using artery forceps, make a blunt dissection down to and through the parietal pleura.
- Using forceps, clamp chest drain and then insert into the pleural space. Most clinicians remove the trocar before insertion.
- Aim to push the chest drain tip toward the lung apex. In the event of a smaller pneumothorax aim the tip in the direction of the pneumothorax, remembering to aim anteriorly (air rises in the ill child lying supine).
- Connect the drain tightly to the underwater drainage system, unclamp drain, and apply negative pressure of 5–10 cmH$_2$O. Bubbling should start to occur.
- Using single sutures, close skin wound closely around the chest drain. Do not use purse-string suture, as this will increase scarring.
- Suture chest drain in place.
- Perform a chest X-ray to check drain position and effusion or pneumothorax drainage.

- Remove the drain when no longer required (e.g., pneumothorax has resolved and there has been no bubbling for over 24 hours.) Rapidly remove drain, followed by immediate pressure and gentle rubbing with gauze swab to close underlying tissues. Apply Steristrips across the skin incision to provide an airtight seal. Perform a chest X-ray to confirm that a significant pneumothorax has not reaccumulated.
- *Note*: If pleural fluid is required for diagnostic purposes only, then simple needle aspiration at the above sites is the technique of choice.

Intraosseous infusion

Indication
This procedure is used for emergency vascular access to give resuscitation drugs, fluids, or allow blood sampling.

Equipment
- 22G intraosseous (IO) needle or 1.5G spinal needle in neonates
- Alcohol-impregnated swab
- 5 mL syringe
- Local anesthetic, e.g., 1% lidocaine and 2 mL syringe and small-gauge needle if patient is conscious and local anesthetic appropriate

Sites
- ≤3 years old: Antromedial proximal aspect of tibia, 1–2 cm below tibial tuberosity or anterolateral surface of femur, 2–3 cm above lateral condyle
- Any age: Medial malleolus of the tibia above the ankle

Procedure
- Identify site and inject local anesthetic if the patient is conscious.
- Clean skin with an alcohol-impregnated swab.
- Insert at 90° to the skin and advance needle into bone using a rotary action.
- Advance trocar until bone cortex is reached, when a give will be felt.
- Remove stylet, attach syringe, and aspirate to confirm position. Obtain any required blood samples.
- Flush needle with 0.9% saline to again confirm position. Swelling outside the bone indicates needle displacement.
- Infuse any required fluids (any fluid that can be given IV can be used).
- Obtain conventional vascular access as soon as possible and then remove IO needle.

Intracardiac injection

This is indicated only during resuscitation when all other attempts at securing vascular access have failed.

Equipment

- Alcohol-impregnated swab
- 21G needle and syringe containing resuscitation drug

Procedure

- Attach needle and syringe. Flush needle with drug to expel air.
- Locate site: fourth intercostal space immediately lateral to the left sternal edge (immediately below the line joining the nipples).
- Clean site with an alcohol-impregnated swab.
- Insert needle and aspirate syringe as needle is inserted.
- Once blood flashes back, stop advancing needle.
- Inject resuscitation drug(s).

Pericardiocentesis

Indications

This procedure is used for therapeutic drainage of a pericardial effusion or for diagnostic purposes under supervision of an experienced senior physician.

Equipment

- Alcohol-impregnated swab/antiseptic solution, e.g., 0.5% chlorhexidine
- 21G needle or intravenous cannula and 10–20 mL syringe
- Sterile gloves, drapes and gown
- Sterile sample containers if pericardial fluid analysis is intended

Procedure

- Lay child on a 30° slope to cause effusion to pool inferiorly.
- Locate insertion site, which lies just below the angle between the sternum and the left costal margin.
- Use sterile gloves and gown. Clean the site with antiseptic and place sterile drapes around insertion site.
- Local-anesthetic infiltration may be appropriate.
- Insert needle connected to syringe at an angle 30° to the skin and advance slowly, aiming toward the left shoulder. Gently aspirate the syringe as the needle is inserted.
- Stop when the pericardial fluid (usually straw colored) is aspirated and remove desired amount as indicated.
- Once drainage is complete, remove needle and apply sterile plaster.

Abdominal paracentesis

Indications
- This is used for drainage of ascites when it compromises breathing (e.g., hydrops fetalis), or for diagnostic purposes, (e.g., following trauma).

Equipment
Equipment is as for pericardiocentesis.

Procedure
- In infants the left iliac fossa is the preferred site (which avoids the liver and spleen). In older children a midline site between the symphysis pubis and the umbilicus is preferred because of less vascularity.
- Lay the child supine. If ascites is minimal, also tilt them toward the left side.
- Except in emergencies, clean and prepare the site as described for pericardiocentesis.
- Attach needle to the syringe and carefully insert it at 90° to the skin.
- Aspirate fluid and place it in sample containers. If large amounts of fluid are to be drained, use an intravenous cannula. Once inserted, remove the needle, and leave the catheter in place to reduce the risk of bowel perforation. If prolonged drainage is needed, attach the canister.
- Once complete, remove the needle and apply a sterile bandage to the site.
- If a large amount of fluid is withdrawn, drainage should be followed by intravenous infusion of albumin.

Suprapubic aspiration of urine

This is the optimal method for obtaining urine for bacteriology in a child <2 years of age.

Equipment
- 21–23G needle
- 2- to 5-mL syringe
- Alcohol-impregnated swab
- Sterile urine sample container
- Gauze pad
- Adhesive bandage

Procedure
- Wait at least 30 minutes from last urination.
- Perform bladder ultrasound to confirm that it contains urine, if in doubt.
- Place child supine (with assistant holding hips abducted) and then identify site: midline anterior lower abdominal wall 1 cm above the pubic bone.
- Clean site with an alcohol-impregnated swab.
- Insert needle connected to the syringe perpendicular to the skin, aspirating continuously until urine is obtained.
- Insert to almost the depth of the needle; if no urine is obtained, partially withdraw it before inserting again at a different angle.
- Once required urine is aspirated, remove the needle, press on the puncture site with a gauze pad, and apply an adhesive bandage.
- Place urine in a sterile container.
- If unsuccessful, repeat the procedure 30–60 minutes later.

Urethral bladder catheterization

Indication

This procedure is used for bladder decompression (e.g., potential obstruction), accurate measurement of urine output, and collection of urine for bacteriological investigation in suspected urinary tract infection.

Equipment

- 3–8 Fr urinary catheter (depending on child's size)
- Anesthetic lubricating gel, e.g., 0.1% lidocaine gel
- Water-based antiseptic solution, e.g., 0.5% chlorhexidine
- Sterile urine sample container
- Sterile gloves and adhesive tape

Procedure

- Place child in supine position with hips abducted (with an assistant holding the child).
- Clean penile tip or vulval area with antiseptic solution.
- Apply anesthetic lubricating gel to catheter tip and urethral opening.
- Partially withdraw foreskin in males.
- Insert and advance catheter into urethra in a posterior manner until urine is obtained, indicating that the bladder has been entered.
- Once in the bladder, inflate the catheter balloon with saline if the catheter is intended to be indwelling.
- Use adhesive tape to secure the catheter to the thigh.
- Connect catheter to the urine collection bag or aspirate urine for analysis.

Lumbar puncture

Indication

A lumbar puncture is used to obtain a sample of CSF for microbiological, biochemical, or metabolic analysis, and to therapeutically drain CSF in communicating hydrocephalus.

Contraindications

These include thrombocytopenia or coagulation defect, raised intracranial pressure, and significant cardiorespiratory compromise, as positioning may risk cardiorespiratory arrest (see also p. 42).

Site

L3–L4 intervertebral space (spinal cord is as low as L2 in neonates).

Equipment

- 24–22 G 1.5 inch spinal needle
- Antiseptic solution, e.g., 0.5% chlorhexidine
- Sterile dressing and sterile drapes
- Sterile sample containers—usually three are needed for culture, cell count, protein, and glucose, but sometimes they are also needed for virology, cytology, or immunology.
- Adhesive bandage
- Pressure manometer and three-way tap if measuring CSF opening pressure.

Procedure

- Apply topical local anesthetic cream to site under an occlusive dressing for 45 minutes before the procedure.
- Place patient on their side with their back along an edge of a firm surface.
- Ask an experienced assistant to firmly, but gently, hold the child with the spine maximally flexed. Beware of compromising respiration!
- Locate the site: The L4 spinous process lies on a line joining the iliac crests.
- Using strict aseptic technique, clean the site with antiseptic solution and then create a sterile field by surrounding it with sterile drapes.
- Inject local anesthetic into the site if desired.
- Insert spinal needle into the intervertebral space slowly at 90° to the skin and aim in the direction of the umbilicus, i.e., slightly cephaled.
- Advance needle slowly until there is a sudden give, which occurs as the dura is penetrated.
- Remove stylet and wait for CSF to drain. If no CSF drains, advance needle very slowly and withdraw stylet every 1–2 mm to check for drainage. If bone is struck or the needle is fully inserted and no CSF is obtained, remove the stylet and withdraw the cannula very slowly in case CSF appears.
- Allow 10 drops or 1 mL of CSF to drain into each sample bottle.

- If measuring CSF pressure, connect three-way tap before collecting samples and direct fluid up attached manometer. Once opening pressure is measured, turn three-way tap to allow CSF to drain.
- If therapeutic CSF drainage is required, drain required amount.
- Once drainage is complete, remove the needle and rub the puncture site with a sterile gauze swab while applying pressure.
- Cover site with an adhesive bandage.
- The child should lie flat for the next 6 hours and have hourly neurological observations and blood pressure measurement.

Cerebral ventricular tap

Indications

This procedure is done for drainage of CSF in non-communicating hydrocephalus, to obtain CSF for microbiological testing (e.g., to diagnose ventriculitis), and to administer intraventricular antibiotics. It should be performed with experienced senior physicians.

Equipment

Equipment is as for lumber puncture (p. 252).

Procedure

- Before the procedure is undertaken, lateral ventriculomegaly must be confirmed by ultrasound.
- Full aseptic technique should be used.
- Place the baby supine, with an assistant firmly holding the baby's head.
- Measure the necessary depth required for needle insertion.
- Palpate and locate the lateral corner of the anterior fontanelle on the intended side to drain.
- Shave a small area of the scalp at the needle insertion point if required.
- Set out sample containers ± CSF pressure manometer if needed.
- Clean area with antiseptic solution and create a sterile field with sterile drapes.
- Insert needle into the lateral corner of the fontanelle in a direction slightly forward and inward, aiming toward the inner canthus of the ipsilateral eye.
- After the needle is inserted to the predetermined distance, remove stylet; CSF should drip out.
- If CSF pressure measurement is required, attach manometer and allow it to fill until measurement is complete.
- If CSF drainage or sample is required, then allow fluid to drip out spontaneously into containers until the required amount is drained.
- Once required CSF has been drained, remove the needle and adhesive bandage.
- The child should lie flat for the next 6 hours and have hourly neurological observations and blood pressure measurement.

Exchange transfusion

Exchange transfusion is indicated for the following conditions:
- Severe or rapidly rising hyperbilirubinemia, (e.g., due to severe rhesus or other hemolytic disease; see p. 194)
- Cardiac failure secondary to severe anemia (with normal or increased plasma volume), e.g., hydrops fetalis due to rhesus hemolytic disease
- Disseminated intravascular coagulation
- Polycythemia with a venous hematocrit >70% and/or symptomatic
- Acute poisoning, including that due to metabolic disease

Exchange is achieved by sequentially removing 10–15 mL of blood from the child and then infusing warmed (37°), cross-matched, fresh (<72 hours old), rhesus-negative, cytomegalovirus (CMV)-negative, irradiated or leukocyte-filtered (to prevent graft versus host disease) partially packed or whole blood. Exchange transfusion can be performed by either withdrawing and then infusing blood via a single central venous catheter (e.g., umbilicus venous catheter) or withdrawing blood via a central catheter (arterial or venous) or peripheral arterial catheter and replacing it through a central or peripheral venous catheter.

Blood volume (mL) to remove and then replace (i.e., exchange):
- Severe anemia with hydrops requires a single volume exchange, i.e., 80 mL/kg body weight. This should be performed over a minimum of 1 hour.
- Removal of toxins, e.g., bilirubin or ammonia, requires a two-volume exchange, i.e., 160 mL/kg. This replaces ~90% of total blood volume and should be performed over a minimum of 2 hours.
- A dilutional exchange transfusion, to treat polycythemia, volume depends on hematocrit (Hct) and can be calculated using the formula:

$$\text{Volume} = \left(\frac{\text{measured Hct} - \text{desired Hct}}{\text{measured Hct}} \right) \times \text{blood volume}$$

In dilutional exchange, blood is replaced with 0.9% saline or albumin.

Equipment
- Venous and arterial catheters, either central or peripheral
- Two 20 mL syringes and three-way taps
- Blood administration set and warming coils
- Calibrated waste blood container
- ± High-flow rate infusion pump
- Cross-matched blood (see above)
- ECG and BP monitor

Procedure
- Ensure that all equipment, including blood, is available.
- Insert central or peripheral venous/arterial catheters.
- Start continuous ECG and frequent BP monitoring.
- As a baseline, measure CBC and serum, electrolytes, BUN, creatinine, Ca^{2+}, glucose, and blood gases.

- Use a full aseptic technique throughout the procedure.
- Prime blood administration set and warm blood to 37°.
- Connect three-way taps into the system (exact arrangement depends on choice of method—see below).
- Arrange for an assistant to keep a constant accurate log of volumes removed and replaced throughout the procedure.
- If using a single central venous catheter, e.g., umbilical venous catheter, use three-way taps to perform the following in order:
    1. Withdraw 5–20 mL blood from the baby using a syringe over a few minutes.
    2. Turn tap to allow blood to be syringed into the waste bag.
    3. Turn tap to allow 5–20 mL fresh, warmed blood to be drawn from the pack.
    4. Turn tap and syringe fresh blood slowly into the baby over a few minutes.
- If using two catheters together, remove 5–20 mL aliquots of blood from the central or arterial catheter over 5–10 minutes and then turn three-way tap to allow blood to be pushed into the waste bag. Simultaneously, the same volume of fresh, warmed blood is infused into the patient via the other venous catheter using a high-rate flow infusion pump.
- A safe volume of aliquot to remove varies according to the size of the infant. Remove 5 mL aliquots for extremely low birth weight (ELBW) infants, increasing up to 20 mL for full-term infants.
- Apart from continuously monitoring pulse, ECG, BP, and temperature, measure every 30–60 minutes during the procedure the blood gases, CBC, electrolytes, BUN, creatinine, serum Ca^{2+}, and glucose. Measure again at the end of the procedure and get a coagulation profile. Correct any abnormality found.
- Once the procedure is completed, leave catheters in place in case repeat exchange transfusion is required.

Complications of exchange transfusion

- Catheter-induced thrombotic or embolic phenomenon, e.g., portal vein thrombosis or necrotizing enterocolitis (NEC)
- Hemodynamic compromise, e.g., cardiac arrhythmia or hypotension
- Metabolic, e.g., hypoglycemia (transfused plasma often has a low blood sugar concentration due to red cell consumption), hypokalemia, hypocalcemia, hypomagnesemia, acidemia
- Coagulopathy or thrombocytopenia
- Hypothermia
- Infection: Bacteremia, HIV, CMV, hepatitis B or C. Blood must be screened prior to transfusion.
- Graft-versus-host disease (GVHD). Risk is reduced by irradiation or leukocyte reduction.

Cardiovascular issues

Common presentations

The cardiovascular examination in children is described on page 37. The majority of children with cardiovascular disease will present with one or more of the following three clinical problems:

- Cyanosis
- Murmur
- Heart failure

Cyanosis

Distinguishing between respiratory and cardiac causes of cyanosis is important (see pp. 42–43).

Murmur

Heart murmurs should be characterized in terms of type, location, radiation, and quality of sound. In young children this may not be easy because of their relatively fast heart rates.

Murmurs are classified as follows:

- *Systolic*: Holosystolic, systolic ejection
- *Diastolic*: Early diastolic, mid-diastolic

The location where a murmur is best heard may give a clue to the underlying etiology:

- *Lower sternal border*: Ventricular septal defect, innocent heart murmur
- *Upper sternal border*: Aortic or pulmonary valve stenosis
- *Base of neck*: Aortic valve stenosis
- *Posterior or back*: Pulmonary valve stenosis, patent ductus arteriosus

Innocent heart murmur

This is the most common cause of a heart murmur in children and is noted in the majority at some point during childhood.

It arises from the rapid flow of blood through the great vessels and across normal heart valves. It does <u>not</u> signify the presence of any underlying cardiac abnormality or any other pathology.

Characteristics of an innocent heart murmur

- Systolic in timing—always. Never diastolic
- Short duration, low-intensity sound
- Intensifies with increased cardiac output (e.g., exercise and fever)
- May change in intensity with change in posture and head position
- No associated cardiac thrill or heave
- No radiation
- Asymptomatic patient

Types of innocent heart murmurs

- Vibratory murmur: "Still's murmur"
  Midsystolic murmur. Twanging sound. Lower left sternal edge
- Flow murmur (pulmonary): Systolic ejection murmur. Nl S2 and no ejection click. Upper left sternal edge. Due to rapid blood flow across the pulmonary valve

- Peripheral pulmonary stenosis (PPS): Systolic ejection murmur radiating to the axilla. Commonly present in newborns, resolves by 6–9 months of age. Due to the relatively hypoplastic branch pulmonary arteries at birth
- Venous hum: "Machinery"-quality sound. Right > left infraclavicular region. Only heard in the upright position (disappears when child is supine) and can be obliterated by turning the head. Sound is due to turbulence in the jugular venous system.

Distinguishing an innocent from a pathologic heart murmur can be difficult, so investigation with echocardiography may be indicated.

Pathological heart murmur

Characteristic features of pathological heart murmurs:

- All diastolic murmurs
- All holosystolic murmurs
- Late systolic murmurs
- Loud murmurs >3/6
- Continuous murmurs
- Associated cardiac abnormalities (ECG and/or chest X-ray)
- Abnormal clinical features:
  - Shortness of breath (SOB)
  - Tiredness, easy fatigue
  - Failure to thrive (FTT)
  - Cyanosis
  - Finger clubbing
  - Hepatomegaly

Investigation: clinical features

A likely diagnosis can be made by combining the clinical examination and features from the chest X-ray and ECG (see Table 8.1).

Table 8.1 Likely diagnoses based on clinical features of murmurs

Murmur character	Diagnoses	Clinical features
Continuous		
Left infraclavicular (machinery) Pulmonary area	PDA (p. 190)	Acyanotic, bounding pulses, fixed split S2
	TAPVD (p. 278)	
Systolic		
Lower LSB (holosystolic) ± parasternal thrill	VSD (p. 268)	Acyanotic
LSB and apex + prominent LV heave	HCM (p. 273)	Acyanotic, brisk pulse
LSB	ToF (p. 275)	Cyanotic, single S2
Systolic ejection		
Second IC space (PV) ± parasternal thrill	ASD secundum (p. 267)	Acyantoic, fixed wide split S2, mid-diastolic murmur (lower LSE)
	ASD primum (p. 267)	Acyantoic, fixed wide split S2, ± loud S1, ± pulmonary click, pan-diastolic murmur (apical radiates to L axilla)
Second IC space (PV) + radiates to back + parasternal heave	PS (p. 269)	Acyanotic, ejection click over LSE
Maximum between the shoulder blades	CoA (p. 270)	Acyanotic, weak or absent femoral pulses, BP arms >> legs
Harsh at the RUSB; radiating to neck and back	AS (p. 271)	Acyanotic, carotid thrill, delayed soft S2, ejection click, small volume and slow rising pulse

AS, aortic stenosis; ASD, atrial septal defect; BP, blood pressure; CoA, coarctation of the aorta; HCM, hypertrophic cardiomyopathy; IC, intercostal; JVP, jugular venous pulse; LSB, left sternal border; LSE, left sternal edge; LV, left ventricle; PDA, patent ductus arteriosus; PS, pulmonary stenosis; PV, pulmonary valve; RUSB, right upper sternal border; S1 first heart sound; S2, second heart sound; TAPVD, total anomalous pulmonary venous drainage; ToF, tetralogy of Fallot; VSD, ventricular septal defect.

Chest x-ray and ECG (see Table 8.2)

Table 8.2 Likely diagnoses based on chest X-ray and ECG findings

Chest X-ray	ECG	Diagnosis
Normal	Normal ECG	Normal or small VSD (p. 268)
Mild cardiomegaly		
+ ↑ pulmonary markings	LVH	VSD (p. 268)
	+ RAD ± RBBB	ASD secundum (p. 267)
	+ LAD + RBBB	ASD priumum (p. 267)
	± prolonged PR	
	Normal ECG or LVH	PDA (p. 190)
Cardiomegaly	Normal ECG	HLHS (p. 272)
	LVH ± RVH	HCM (p. 273)
	LVH	AS (p. 271)
Other features		
Small, boot-shaped heart + oligemic lung fields	RAD + RVH	ToF (p. 275)
Narrow mediastinum, heart "egg on side," + pulmonary vascular markings	Normal	TGA (p. 276)
Rib notching	LVH	CoA (p. 270)
PA post-stenotic dilatation	Normal or RVH	PS (p. 269)

CoA, coarctation of the aorta; HLHS; hypoplastic left heart syndrome, LAD; left axis deviation, LV left ventricle; LVH; left ventricular hypertrophy; PA, pulmonary artery; PS, pulmonary stenosis; RAD, right axis deviation; RBBB right bundle branch block; RVH, right ventricular hypertrophy; TGA, transposition of great arteries; ToF, tetralogy of Fallot.

Heart failure

Heart failure may be manifested by symptoms of poor tissue perfusion (e.g., fatigue, poor exercise tolerance, confusion) and/or by symptoms of circulatory congestion (e.g., dyspnea, pleural effusion, pulmonary edema, hepatomegaly, peripheral edema).

The underlying mechanisms that lead to the compromise of cardiac stroke volume, cardiac decompensation, and heart failure include the following:

- Increased afterload (pressure work)
- Increased preload (volume work)
- Myocardial abnormalities
- Tachyarrhythmias

Causes of heart failure

In children the most common cause of heart failure is congenital structural defects of the heart.
- Large left-to-right intracardiac shunts: Large VSD
- Left-sided obstructive cardiac lesions: Coarctation of aorta, aortic stenosis
- Cardiomyopathy: Hypertrophic, dilated, restrictive
- Myocarditis: Viral, rheumatic fever
- Endocarditis
- Myocardial ischemia: Anomalous origin of the left coronary artery (ALCAPA), Kawasaki disease
- Tachyarrhythmias: Supraventricuar tachycardia
- Acute hypertension
- High-output: Severe anemia, thyrotoxicosis, arteriovenous malformations

Clinical features

The clinical features of heart failure depend on the degree of cardiac reserve. The most common symptoms and signs are those in keeping with increased compensatory sympathetic drive:
- Diaphoresis
- Breathlessness, tachypnea, grunting, coughing
- Poor feeding (infant), poor weight gain and failure to thrive
- Hepatomegaly
- Cardiomegaly
- Tachycardia, "gallop" heart rhythm

In contrast to adults, there may be few signs of systemic congestion. Children or adolescents with chronic heart failure may exhibit "adult" signs such as edema, orthopnea, paroxysmal nocturnal dyspnea, and elevated jugular venous pressure (JVP).

Investigations

These are directed at finding a cause and quantifying cardiac function.
- Chest x-ray   Cardiac enlargement
                       Lungs—oligemic, edema
- Echocardiography   Congenital heart defects, ventricular function
- Arterial blood gas   Reduced PO_2, metabolic acidosis
- ECG   Often not diagnostic
- Serum electrolytes   Hyponatremia due to water retention

Management

Treat the underlying cause of heart failure if possible.

General measures
- Supplemental oxygen
- Diet—sufficient calorie intake
- Diuretics
- Inotropic agents, e.g., digoxin, dobutamine, dopamine
- Vasodilators, e.g., angiotensin-converting enzyme (ACE) inhibitors, phosphodiesterase inhibitors

Useful resource
Rosenthal D, Chrisant MR, Edens E, et al. (2004) International Society for Heart and Lung Transplantation: Practice guidelines for management of heart failure in children. *J Heart Lung Transplant* **23**(12):1313–1333.

Diseases and conditions: congenital heart disease

Definition

Congenital heart disease (CHD) is the failure of normal cardiac development or persistence of the fetal circulation after birth.

Incidence

- 7–9 per 1000 live births
- 10%–15% are complex cardiovascular lesions
- High incidence with identified syndromes and malformations of other organ systems

Causes

The cause is unknown in most cases. CHD is commonly associated with the following conditions:

- Chromosomal defects—e.g., Down syndrome, Turner syndrome
- Gene defects—e.g., 22q deletion, Di George syndrome
- Congenital infections—e.g., rubella
- Teratogenic drugs—e.g., phenytoin, warfarin, alcohol

Classification

Congenital heart disease can be classified into acyanotic or cyanotic types depending on whether the predominant presentation is with or without central cyanosis. The latter is caused by deoxygenated blood gaining abnormal access to the systemic side of the circulation via the left side of the heart or the aorta.

Acyanotic CHD

- Ventricular septal defect
- Atrial septal defect
- Patent ductus arteriosus
- Pulmonary valve stenosis
- Coarctation of the aorta
- Aortic valve stenosis
- Hypoplastic left heart syndrome
- Hypertrophic cardiomyopathy

Cyanotic CHD: the "5 T's"

- Tetralology of Fallot (ToF)
- Transposition of the great arteries (TGA)
- Tricuspid atresia
- Truncus arteriosus
- Total anomalous pulmonary drainage

The diagnosis of a specific lesion is made after clinical examination, chest X-ray, ECG, and echocardiography (see p. 264).

Acyanotic: atrial septal defect (ASD)

ASD may be subtyped as secundum, primum, or sinus venosus defects.

Secundum atrial septal defect

This defect is in the region of the foramen ovale. The atrioventricular (AV) valves are normal. The defect is usually isolated and often found incidentally.

Clinical features

Most children are asymptomatic. Infrequently, large ASDs may result in clinically apparent heart failure.

Prognosis

Ostium secundum defects are typically well tolerated. Symptoms and complications usually only present in the third decade or later.

Treatment

ASD closure is frequently advised, even if asymptomatic. This is achieved by placement of an occluding device at cardiac catheterization or, less commonly, by open-heart surgery.

Primium atral septal defect

This defect is located in the lower atrial septum and is associated with a cleft in the anterior leaflet of the mitral valve. Ostium primium defects are often seen with Down syndrome and are one of the endocardial cushion defects, which also include atrioventricular canal defects (ASD + VSD + a common AV valve).

Clinical features

Most children with small defects are asymptomatic. Those with larger defects are predisposed to recurrent pneumonia and heart failure.

Prognosis

The prognosis depends on the degree of left-to-right shunt, pulmonary hypertension, and severity of mitral regurgitation. Without surgical repair, congestive cardiac failure may develop in infancy and early childhood.

Management

Surgical closure of the defect is indicated.

Ventricular septal defect (VSD)

VSDs account for 25% of all CHD (2 per 1000 live births). They may occur in isolation or as part of complex malformations. The clinical features depend on the size and location of the defect.

Subtypes
- Large or small VSD
- Perimembranous
- Muscular
- Multiple small defects

Clinical features
- Asymptomatic (small defects)
- Heart failure (large defects)
- Recurrent pneumonia
- Cyanosis (rare, late)—secondary to pulmonary hypertension—i.e. Eisenmenger's complex

Examination
- Holosystolic murmur
  - Lower left sternal edge
  - +/– parasternal thrill

Prognosis
Many cases of VSD will close spontaneously with time. Long-term prognosis is excellent even if surgery is required.

Management
- Medical: Treat heart failure if present.
- Surgery is indicated if there is severe heart failure.

Pulmonary stenosis

This form of CHD is due to the following:
- Thickened pulmonary valve with fused commissures: valvar pulmonary stenosis
- Subvalvar (infundibular) or supravalvar pulmonary stenosis
- Peripheral branch pulmonary artery stenosis
- Suparvalvar pulmonary stenosis (PS) is commonly seen in Noonan syndrome (p. 966)

Clinical features
- Asymptomatic (mild to moderate stenosis)
- Poor exercise tolerance (severe stenosis)
- Right ventricular failure or cyanosis (severe stenosis)

Prognosis
Mild to moderate stenosis is compatible with normal activities, but patients require monitoring because worsening obstruction and significant pressure gradients may develop, which will predispose to heart failure.

Treatment
Moderate to severe pulmonary valve stenosis requires treatment with transvenous catheter balloon dilatation. Moderate to severe subvalvar or supravalvar pulmonary stenosis requires surgical intervention for obstruction relief.

See also Patent ductus arteriosus (p. 190).

Coarctation of the aorta

Constrictions of the aorta may occur at any point. In the majority (98%) of cases, it is usually distal to the origin of the left subclavian artery at the level of the ductus arterious. Blood pressure (BP) is elevated in blood vessels proximal to the obstruction and, with time, an extensive collateral circulation develops.

Coarctation of the aorta is seen in boys (2:1), although it is common in Turner syndrome (page 551). In ~70% of cases an abnormal bicuspid aortic valve is present, but it does not produce signs unless stenosis is significant.

Clinical features

Coarctation of the aorta results in a disparity in pulse volume and BP between the arms and legs. Coarctation of the aorta recognized after infancy is rarely associated with any significant symptoms.

Mild defects may present with hypertension and heart failure in adulthood. In severe defects a PDA is required to maintain the systemic circulation; heart failure and collapse may occur in the neonatal period.

Prognosis

If untreated, morbidity from untreated hypertension is high, usually arising in the third to fourth decades of life. Complications include premature coronary artery disease, congestive cardiac failure, hypertensive encephalopathy, and intracranial hemorrhage.

Treatment

Early treatment with catheter balloon dilatation or stenting or surgical resection is usual.

Aortic stenosis

Congenital aortic stenosis accounts for about 5% of all causes of CHD and is the most common cause of left ventricular outflow obstruction. It is due to thickening of the aortic valves, although subvalvular (subaortic) stenosis is also an important form of obstruction.

Congenital aortic stenosis is more common in boys (3:1). A supravalvular form of aortic stenosis is also recognized, which may be sporadic or familial. Supravalvular aortic stenosis is associated with Williams syndrome (p. 1067).

Clinical features

These are dependent on the severity of obstruction and age at presentation. Mild stenosis is usually asymptomatic and found on routine examination. Severe defects in the neonate may present with heart failure and cardiovascular collapse. In the older child sudden, unexpected syncope and chest pain on exertion may occur.

Prognosis

The prognosis is good in the majority of patients with mild or moderate stenosis. In severe stenosis sudden death is a risk.

Management

Surgical or balloon dilation is indicated if symptoms develop or if a high resting pressure gradient of >50 mmHg is present. Avoidance of competitive sports recommended.

Hypoplastic left heart syndrome

This term is used to describe a group of disorders associated with underdevelopment of the left-sided heart structures. The left ventricle is small and nonfunctional and the right ventricle maintains both pulmonary and systemic circulations. The latter is achieved by pulmonary venous blood passing through an atrial septal defect (ASD) or patent foramen ovale.

Clinical features

HLHS presents early (days of life) with cyanosis and heart failure, which, if unrecognized, leads to cardiovascular collapse. Most infants will appear sick (grayish blue in color) with poor peripheral perfusion and weak peripheral pulses. Central cyanosis and evidence of heart failure will be present.

Treatment

Medical management (intravenous prostaglandin) is necessary to maintain patency of the ductus and support systemic blood flow. Surgery is typically palliative, involving three staged surgeries over the first few years of life; occasionally an infant is listed for heart transplantation.

Hypertrophic cardiomyopathy

This condition is characterized by massive ventricular hypertrophy. All portions of the left ventricle can be affected, although the ventricular septum may be more so, and the right ventricle may also be involved.

Myocardial fibrosis results in a stiff muscle with decreased distensibility. Ventricular filling is decreased, but systolic pumping is maintained until late in the course of disease.

HCM has been recognized in all age groups and may occur in members of the same family. A dominant pattern of inheritance is sometimes observed.

Clinical features

Most children with HCM are frequently asymptomatic and only detected following routine clinical examination and the discovery of an incidental heart murmur. Symptoms, when present, include fatigue and dyspnea, chest pain, and syncope on exertion. HCM is an important cause of sudden, unexpected death.

Prognosis

The prognosis is unpredictable, especially in those patients without symptoms.

Treatment

Avoidance of competitive sports and strenuous activity is encouraged. Therapy is aimed at reducing the outflow obstruction.
- Medical therapy: Beta-blocking agents, calcium antagonists
- Surgical therapy: Ventricular septal myotomy

The right-sided heart

This is an abnormal position of the heart, with the heart located on the right side of the chest. This condition includes both *mirror-image* dextrocardia, in which the heart appears to have pivoted or rotated to the right, as well as dextroposition, in which the heart has shifted into the right chest due to external forces (severe scoliosis, pneumothorax, and others).

In mirror-image dextrocardia, the cardiac apex points to the right. Conversely, in dextroposition the apex points leftward. In mirror-image dextrocardia, which may be seen with complete situs inversus, normal cardiac chamber and great vessel relationships are retained.

Cyanotic CHD: tetralogy of Fallot (ToF)

ToF, the most common cyanotic CHD, is characterized by four anatomic features:
- Large VSD
- Overriding aorta
- Right ventricular outflow obstruction (infundibular and valvular pulmonary stenosis)
- Right ventricular hypertrophy

Systemic venous return to the right side of the heart is normal. In the presence of pulmonary stenosis, however, blood is shunted across the VSD into the aorta and persistent arterial desaturation and cyanosis result. The severity of cyanosis depends on the degree of right ventricular outflow obstruction; when this is moderate a balanced shunt across the VSD occurs and cyanosis may be mild or absent.

Clinical features

Tetralogy of Fallot presents in early infancy with the following features:
- Cyanosis, progressive
- Murmur
- Heart failure and failure to thrive
- Paroxysmal hypercyanotic spells (late infancy): Spontaneous and unpredictable onset, tachypnea, restlessness and increasing cyanosis, duration from a few minutes to hours. ToF is commonly viewed as an indication to proceed with surgical repair.

Management of hypercyanotic spells (see p. 275)

Treatment

Tetralogy of Fallot with severe cyanosis in early infancy requires medical palliation (prostagladin E1 infusion; see p. 190) and surgery (e.g., modified Blalock–Taussig shunt) to maintain pulmonary blood flow and oxygenation. Corrective surgery to repair the underlying heart defect is carried out by 6 months of life.

Prognosis

Untreated, the combination of right-to-left shunt, chronic cyanosis, and polycythemia predispose to
- Cerebral thrombosis and ischemia
- Brain abscess
- Bacterial endocarditis
- Congestive cardiac failure

Patients generally do very well after surgical corrections. Long-term follow-up suggests that this quality of life is maintained and most patients are able to lead unrestricted lives.

Transposition of the great arteries

The normal systemic and pulmonary blood flow circuit is replaced by two separate parallel circuits—i.e., systemic venous blood passing through the right side of heart returns directly to the systemic circulation via a connecting aorta. Pulmonary venous blood returning to the left side of the heart is returned directly to the pulmonary circulation via a connecting pulmonary artery. This condition is not compatible with life unless there is adequate mixing of the blood from both circulations via an ASD/VSD or PDA.

Clinical features

Infants usually present in the first few hours or days with severe cyanosis. Hypoxia is usually severe, but heart failure is not a feature. This is a medical emergency, thus early diagnosis and intervention are required to avoid severe hypoxia.

Treatment

Once diagnosed, arterial oxygenation can often be improved with prostaglandin E1 infusion and balloon atrial septostomy. Careful monitoring and prompt correction of acidosis, hypothermia, and hypoglycemia are essential. Corrective arterial switch operation is performed in the first few weeks of life.

Tricuspid atresia

In tricuspid atresia (TA) there is no connection between the right atrium and the right ventricle. Venous blood is diverted to left side via a widely patent foramen ovale. Pulmonary blood flow is dependent on either an associated VSD or PDA. The right ventricle is variably hypoplastic.

Clinical features

Most patients with TA present in the first few days to early months of life with increasing cyanosis. The clinical features will vary depending on other associated cardiac abnormalities.

Treatment

In emergency, duct patency is achieved with prostaglandin E1 infusion (see p. 190). Surgical palliation and procedures include the following:

- Blalock–Taussig shunt
- Pulmonary artery banding
- Bidirectional Glenn followed by a Fontan procedure

Total anomalous pulmonary venous drainage

All blood retuning to the heart (systemic and pulmonary) returns to the right atrium, and an obligatory patent foramen ovale or ASD is necessary for survival. The pulmonary veins most frequently form a single confluence and join the systemic venous circulation through a supracardiac (SVC), cardiac, or infracardiac (IVC) connection. Supracardiac TAPVD is most common.

Clinical features

Infants usually present in the first few days of life with varying degrees of duct-dependent cyanosis and congestive cardiac failure. Presentation will depend on the degree of obstruction of the pulmonary venous return.

Treatment

Palliative prostaglandin E1 infusion may be required preoperatively (see p. 190). Surgical anastomosis of the confluence to the left atrium, with closure of ASD, and interruption of connections to the systemic venous circuit is required.

Acquired heart disease: infective endocarditis

Infective endocarditis (IE) is uncommon; however, it can be life threatening and may be associated with high morbidity. The majority of cases of IE are believed to be the result of randomly occurring bacteremia from routine daily activities in susceptible patients.

There are both acute and subacute forms of IE. Children at increased risk are those in whom turbulent blood flow exists secondary to certain types of congenital or acquired heart disease, including flow from a high- to a low-pressure chamber (VSD and PDA) or across a narrowed valve orifice (aortic stenosis), and those in whom prosthetic material has been used during corrective or palliative surgery.

The most common pathogens associated with infective endocarditis are the following:

- *Streptococcus viridans*: normal flora of the skin, oral, and respiratory tract
- *Staphylococcus aureus*: Frequently in the setting of central venous catheters
- Group D streptococcus: normal flora of the gastrointestinal (GI) tract

The causative organism is not identified in up to 10% of cases.

Clinical features

In the early stage, symptoms are varied and often subtle. Prolonged fever persisting over several months may be the only feature. Alternatively, rapid onset of high, intermittent fever can occur. Nonspecific symptoms include the following:

- Myalgia
- Arthalgia,
- Headache
- Weight loss
- Night sweats

Examination

Examination is highly variable; classic signs include the following:

- Pallor/anemia
- Nail bed: Splinter hemorrhages
- Tender nodules: Fingers and toes (Osler's nodes)
- Erythematous rash: Palms and soles of feet (Janeway lesions)
- Necrotic skin lesions
- Splenomegaly
- Hematuria (microscopic)
- Retinal infarcts (Roth's spots)
- Heart murmurs (change in character with time)

Diagnosis

A high index of suspicion is required. Blood tests, including CBC (elevated WBC), ESR, and CRP (both elevated), should be taken as well as repeated blood cultures. Echocardiography is performed to look for visible vegetations.

Prognosis

Even with antibiotic treatment morbidity and mortality may be high. Systemic emboli from left-sided vegetations may result in brain abscess and stroke.

Treatment

- *Antibiotic therapy*: Broad-spectrum antibiotics should be started as soon as possible after blood cultures are drawn. Delays may result in progressive endocardial damage and deterioration in cardiac function. Coverage can be narrowed once an organism is identified. Intravenous antibiotics (e.g., penicillin/vancomycin) are required for a minimum of 6 weeks.
- *Bed rest* is recommended and heart failure should be treated.
- *Surgery* may be necessary for removal of infected prosthetic material.

Prophylaxis

Prophylaxis is no longer recommended solely on an increased lifetime risk of acquisition of IE. Prophylaxis is now recommended for only those patients with the highest risk of adverse outcome following endocarditis:

- Prosthetic cardiac valve
- Previous IE
- Congenital heart disease
  - Unrepaired cyanotic CHD, including palliative shunts and conduits
  - Completely repaired CHD with prosthetic material or device, whether placed by surgery or catheter intervention, during the first 6 months after the procedure
  - Repaired CHD with residual defects at or adjacent to the site of a prosthetic patch or device
- Cardiac transplantation recipients with valvulopathy

Prophylaxis is recommended for any dental procedure involving manipulation of the gingival tissue or the periapical region of the teeth, or perforation of the oral mucosa. Only in very limited circumstances do procedures involving the respiratory, GI, or genitourinary (GU) tracts require prophylaxis.

Useful resource

American Heart Association (AHA) guidelines:

Wilson W, Taubert KA, Gewitx M, et al. (2007) Prevention of infective endocarditis, guidelines from the American Heart Association. *Circulation* **116**(15):1736–1754.

Kawasaki disease

Kawasaki disease is an acute vasculitis with predilection for the small arteries, including the coronary arteries (see p. 730 for clinical features and treatment). The pericardium, myocardium, endocardium, valves, and coronary arteries may all be involved.

Cardiovascular manifestations, including coronary artery aneurysms or ectasia, decreased left ventricular (LV) function, mitral regurgitation, and/or pericardial effusion, can be prominent in the acute phase and are the leading cause of long-term morbidity and mortality.

Kawasaki disease has surpassed acute rheumatic fever as the leading cause of acquired heart disease in children.

Cardiovascular evaluation

Echocardiography should be performed at the time of diagnosis, at 2 weeks, and at 6–8 weeks after the onset of symptoms.

Low-dose aspirin (3–5 mg/kg per day) is continued until there is no evidence of coronary artery changes by 6–8 weeks after the onset of illness. In those who develop coronary artery abnormalities, aspirin is continued indefinitely.

Of note, the concomitant use of ibuprofen antagonizes the platelet inhibition induced by aspirin; thus, in general, ibuprofen should be avoided in children with coronary artery aneurysms who are taking aspirin for its antiplatelet effect.

Useful resource

American Academy of Pediatrics (AAP)/AHA guidelines:

Newburger JW, Takahashi M, Gerber MA, et al. (2004) Diagnosis, treatment, and long-term management of Kawasaki disease: A statement for health professionals from the Committee on Rheumatic Fever, Endocarditis, and Kawasaki Disease, Council on Cardiovascular Disease in the Young, and the American Heart Association. *Pediatrics* **114**(6):1708–1733.

Acute rheumatic fever

This disease remains an important cause of acquired heart disease worldwide. It is infrequently seen in children from developed countries.

Acute rheumatic fever develops in susceptible children following infection with the group A, β-hemolytic streptococcus. It is most frequently seen in children aged 5–15 years. Incidence patterns mirror those for group A streptococcal respiratory tract infections.

Clinical features

There is usually a latent period of 2–6 weeks between the onset of symptoms and previous streptococcal infection (e.g., pharyngitis). Symptoms are nonspecific and variable. There is no single manifestation or laboratory test that unequivocally establishes the diagnosis. Rather, the grouping together of a number of clinical features in the setting of a previous strep. infection makes the diagnosis more likely (Jones criteria; see Box 8.1). These can be categorized into major or minor features.

Box 8.1 Jones criteria

Major features
- Carditis (50%)
  - Endocarditis, myocarditis, pericarditis
- Polyarthritis (80%)
  - Migratory—to other joints over 1–2 months
  - Joints—knees, ankles, wrists
- Erythema marginatum (<5%)
  - Early, trunk and limbs
  - Pink border, fading center
- Subcutaneous nodules (rare)
  - Pea-sized, hard, extensor surfaces
- Sydenhams chorea (10%)
  - Late feature: 2–6 months post-infection
  - Involuntary movements—choreathetoid
  - Emotional lability

Minor features
- Fever
- Arthralgia
- Abnormal ECG—prolonged P-R interval
- Elevated ESR, CRP
- Evidence of preceding streptococcal infection, e.g., raised ASO titer
- History of previous rheumatic fever

Diagnosis

To establish a diagnosis of acute rheumatic fever the following conditions must be met:

- Evidence of previous group A streptococcal infection

AND

- Two major features

OR

- One major + two minor features

Complications

The major complication is the development of valvular disease, most commonly affecting the mitral valve and resulting in regurgitation.

Management

In the *acute phase* treatment includes the following:

- Bed rest
- Anti-inflammatory drugs (e.g., aspirin)
- Corticosteroids (2–3 weeks)
- Diuretics, ACE inhibitors if there is heart failure
- Antibiotics for concurrent streptococcal infection (e.g., penicillin V for 10 days)

Long-term therapy is aimed at secondary prevention of further attacks of acute rheumatic fever and the development of chronic rheumatic heart disease. Antibiotic prophylaxis in the form of daily oral penicillin therapy or monthly intramuscular (IM) penicillin G depot injections is recommended.

Chronic rheumatic heart disease

Recurrent bouts of rheumatic fever with associated carditis resulting in scarring and fibrosis of the heart valves (most commonly, mitral valve) may result in severe valve dysfunction requiring replacement.

Pericarditis

Pericardial inflammation may be primary, or a secondary manifestation of a generalized reactive process. The principle causes of pericardial inflammation include the following:

- Infectious
  - Viral (e.g., Coxsackie B, Epstein–Barr virus [EBV])
  - Bacterial (e.g., streptococcus, mycoplasma)
  - Tuberculosis
  - Fungal (e.g., histoplasmosis)
  - Parasitic (e.g., toxoplasmosis)
- Connective tissue
  - Rheumatoid arthritis
  - Rheumatic fever
  - Systemic lupus erythematosus (SLE)
  - Sarcoidoisis
- Metabolic
  - Uremia
  - Hypothyroidism
- Malignancy
- Radiotherapy

Clinical features

Features depend on the extent of pericardial involvement. The predominant symptom is typically sharp, precordial pain that is exacerbated and exaggerated by lying down and relieved by sitting or leaning forward. The pain may be referred to the left shoulder. Other symptoms include cough, dyspnea, and fever.

Pericardial inflammation is frequently accompanied by excessive accumulation of pericardial fluid. The accumulation of sufficient fluid to cause cardiac tamponade and impair cardiac output is rare.

Examination

The signs and symptoms are determined by the amount and rapidity of fluid accumulation, the compliance of the pericardium, and competence of the myocardium. Findings on physical examination can include *pulsus paradoxus,* pericardial rub, and quiet or distant heart sounds.

Investigations

The following are directed at confirming the diagnosis:
- ECG (typically low-voltage QRS complexes or diffuse ST segment elevation)
- Echocardiogram

Other investigations are directed at identifying the underlying cause and may include pericardiocentesis and/or rarely pericardial biopsy, serology related to specific diagnoses, cardiac troponin, WBC, and ESR.

Management

Treatment is directed at both the underlying cause and symptoms:

- Analgesia for pain relief
- Anti-inflammatory drugs to reduce pericardial inflammation
- Pericardiocentesis for pericardial effusion causing cardiac tamponade and low cardiac output

Constrictive pericarditis

Constrictive pericarditis is rare in children. The fibrotic, thickened pericardium impairs cardiac filling. Clinical features resemble those of congested right heart failure: hepatomegaly with ascites, peripheral edema and neck vein distention. On auscultation there is typically tachycardia and may be a diastolic knock. Echocardiography demonstrates a thickened pericardium and enlarged atria and vena cava. Treatment requires pericardiectomy.

Myocarditis

Myocarditis severe enough to be clinically recognized is rare; the prevalence of subclinical mild cases is probably much higher. Myocarditis may be due to the following:
- Infections: Viral (e.g., Coxsackie B, EBV)
- Kawasaki disease (see p. 830)
- Drugs: Adriamycin
- *Connective tissue disease*: SLE (see p. 904), rheumatoid arthritis (see p. 890), rheumatic fever (see p. 284), sarcoidoisis

Clinical features

Features are variable and dependent on the age of the patient and the time course of the underlying disease. Symptoms include lethargy and anorexia, pallor, tachypnea, and dyspnea. Ventricular arrhythmias may occur.

Examination

Typical cardiovascular examination includes
- Weak pulses
- Tachycardia
- Gallop heart rhythm
- Distant heart sounds

Diagnosis

Chest X-ray shows cardiomegaly and ECG shows tachycardia with reduced QRS voltages. Echocardiography reveals cardiac-chamber enlargement and poor ventricular function. A definitive histological diagnosis is made after percutaneous endomyocardial biopsy.

Treatment

This is directed at the underlying cause and at controlling symptoms. Cardiac transplantation may be recommended in patients with refractory heart failure.

Cardiomyopathy

A cardiomyopathy may be primary, or secondary to systemic or metabolic disease (see p. 1090). Primary cardiomyopathies are classified as
- Hypertrophic (see p. 273)
- Dilated
- Restrictive (see p. 286)

Dilated cardiomyopathy

This condition is rare and characterized by cardiomegaly and massive dilatation of the ventricles. The cause is unknown in most cases, although it can be seen in association with other conditions:
- Post-viral infection phenomenon
- Metabolic disorders (e.g., mitochondrial disease, p. 1104)

Clinical features

Insidious onset of progressive congestive cardiac failure is common.

Management

This is mainly directed at treating heart failure and, where possible, any underlying cause. Heart transplantation may be recommended.

Restrictive cardiomyopathy

This condition is rare and characterized by poor ventricular compliance and inadequate ventricular filling. The clinical features are similar to those seen in constrictive pericarditis (p. 286). Prognosis is poor and cardiac transplantation is often required.

Arrhythmias

Sinus arrhythmia (i.e., acceleration on inspiration and vice versa) is normal in children and adolescents. Other types of cardiac arrhythmia are rare in childhood. Cardiac arrhythmias may be transient or permanent.

Cardiac arrhythmias may occur in structurally normal or abnormal hearts. They may be secondary to myocardial disease (e.g., rhematic fever, myocarditis) or occur following exposure to toxins and drugs, or occur following cardiac surgery.

Children with suspected cardiac arrhythmias require evaluation, including detailed history and examination (see also p. 260). The arrhythmia should be identified and characterized by ECG. Intermittent cardiac arrhythmias may be identified by 24-hour ECG.

Supraventricular tachycardia (SVT)

SVT is the most common arrhythmia seen in childhood. Re-entry within the AV node is the most common mechanism of SVT. It may occur in association with the Wolf–Parkinson–White pre-excitation syndrome.

Clinical features

Features include sudden onset (and cessation) lasting from a few seconds to hours, and heart rate between 250 and 300 beats per minute. It is well tolerated in older children, but heart failure may occur in young infants if it is unrecognized. SVT is often precipitated by intercurrent (febrile) illnesses.

Management

Vagal stimulatory maneuvers may be effective. IV adenosine transiently blocks conduction at the AV node and interrupts the circuit. Alternatively or if the patient is hemodynamically unstable, cardioversion may be performed.

Congenital complete heart block

Congenital complete heart block is rare. Mothers of affected children are usually positive for serum anti-Ro antibodies and have evidence of an underlying connective tissue disorder. Alternatively, complex structural heart disease is found in association.

Clinical features

- Fetal hydrops
- Neonate: Heart failure
- Childhood: Asymptomatic, syncope

Management

Treatment depends on ventricular rate and symptoms. A transvenous or epicardial pacemaker may be required.

Respiratory issues

Introduction

Disorders of the respiratory system account for a major part of pediatric medicine. Several of the most common clinical presentations are addressed here, as are commonly used assessment methods for evaluating respiratory complaints. Lastly, a summary of disorders that you will encounter and manage is listed.

Using the history, physical findings, and radiographs of the chest, clinicians should be able to identify which of the six compartments of the respiratory system or combinations thereof are abnormal in a patient and provide a rapid, rational approach to supportive care while investigating specific diagnoses. The six compartments are 1) central nervous system/respiratory drive, 2) upper airways (extrathoracic), 3) lower airways (intrathoracic), 4) parenchyma (including intersitital and vascular structures), 5) pleurae, and 6) surrounding structures (thorax, respiratory muscles, abdomen).

History

History of present illness (HPI)
- Age of onset of symptoms or problem
- Patterns of persistence or recurrence, seasonality of symptoms, trends of improvement or worsening over time
- Antecedent events or illnesses prior to the current problem
- Severity of disease (exercise, school attendance, emergency department or hospital care)
- Exacerbating factors, e.g., exercise, sleep, environmental irritants (tobacco smoke, allergens) and exposures (e.g., daycare, travel)
- Responses to previous therapies (e.g., antibiotics, bronchodilators)

Review of systems
- Symptoms related to the upper airways (noisy breathing, congestion), and swallowing difficulties (choking, emesis)
- Muscle weakness, developmental delay
- Symptoms of gastroesophageal reflux, swallowing problems, nutritional state

Past medical history
- Illnesses involving other organs, e.g., heart disease, connective tissue disease, primary or acquired immunodeficiency
- Family history
- Atopy, asthma, genetic lung disease, or other breathing problems

Examination (see also p. 36)
- General information: Vital signs, state of nutrition, neurological state, respiratory distress or lack thereof, oxyhemoglobin saturation by oximetry
- Rate, pattern of breathing (periodic, apnea), duration of inspiration and expiration, use of accessory muscles to do inspiratory and/or expiratory work (e.g., subcostal, intercostal, or suprasternal retractions, use of abdominal muscles to exhale)

- Character to breath sounds on inspiration and expiration as separate findings, symmetry of breath sounds, including reduced or absent sounds, monophonic vs. polyphonic sounds (location[s] of abnormal sounds)
- Sounds loudest at the nose or mouth compared to those in the chest (central or upper airway narrowing); voice quality
- Chest wall shape and size (pectus profundum, pectus excavatum, sternal bowing, Harrison's grooves)
- Nasal, aural, and oral findings (polyps, nasal mucus, tympanic membrane scarring, tonsil enlargement, pharyngeal size, macroglossia, dental caries and gingivitis, mouth breathing, nasal flaring, micrognathia)
- Digital clubbing
- Truncal tone, abdominal muscle strength, hepatosplenomegaly, abdominal distension, scoliosis
- Character of sputum if expectorated
- Character of witnessed cough (paroxysms, barking, honking, wet, wheezy, brassy, throat clearing)

Clinical pearls

- Expiratory work suggests intrathoracic lower airway narrowing.
- Upper airway noises suggest nasopharyngeal, supraglottic, glottic, or subglottic airway narrowing.
- Tachypnea with or without retractions suggests restrictive disease of the lung parenchyma, pleural disease (e.g., pneumothorax or effusion), muscle weakness, or compression of the lungs by surrounding structures (abdomen or chest wall).
- Airflow through terminal bronchioles and into alveoli does not make sound. Crackles represent turbulent airflow through small bronchi as they reopen, the result of mucous plugging (e.g., cystic fibrosis, bronchiolitis) or loss of integrity.
- Alveolar disease (e.g., pneumonia) produces absent or diminished sounds.

Wheeze

Wheeze is a continuous high-pitched sound produced by apposition of airway surfaces, e.g., airway walls or walls with mucus, heard during inspiration and expiration. Expiratory wheezes reflect intrathoracic airway disease (narrowing or inflammation). Inspiratory and expiratory wheeze together suggest a fixed airway narrowing.

Wheezes can be from one site with a singular sound (monophonic) or multiple sites with multiple sounds (polyphonic). Wheezing can be associated with a prolonged expiratory phase. Wheeze may be present at rest but is elicited more easily with exercise or a forced expiratory maneuver.

Differential diagnosis

The differential diagnosis depends on site(s) of airway narrowing and mechanism of narrowing:

- Extrinsic airway compression by lymph nodes, aberrant or engorged vessels, heart enlargement, tumors, cysts
- Intralumenal occlusion
- Aspirated liquids (hypopharyngeal contents or vomitus) or solids (foreign body)
- Airway mucus (asthma, cystic fibrosis) and endobronchial debris (infection or inhalation injury)
- Airway edema or blood
- Intralumenal growths (hemangiomas) and webs
- Granulation tissue (tuberculosis, trauma)

Airway wall abnormalities

- Bronchoconstriction (asthma)
- Bronchial edema (inflammation, i.e., asthma, bronchitis, bronchiolitis)
- Lack of integrity (tracheo- or bronchomalacia)
- Loss of integrity (bronchiectasis)
- Fibrosis (bronchiolitis obliterans, chronic lung disease of prematurity)
- Airway hypoplasia or restriction (choanal and tracheal stenosis)
- Bronchial cellular infiltration (neutrophils/eosinophils) or storage disease (bronchiolitis, asthma)

More than one mechanism may be at play in certain diseases, e.g., asthma. Therapeutic trials, such as bronchodilator treatment, may help to identify a mechanism for wheeze.

Upper airway noises: stertor, stridor, and percolation

Noisy breathing results from narrowing or partial occlusion in the upper airway, usually above the thoracic inlet and sometimes above the carina. It is a short continuous inspiratory sound that may be long or short in duration. It may come and go, being more prominent in certain states, e.g., sleep, position, or with agitation.

Stertor is a coarse, inspiratory sound produced by vibration or collapse of the palate or tongue on the posterior pharynx, akin to snoring.

Stridor is an inspiratory whistling noise resulting from narrowing in the periglottic region of the upper airway. It indicates either dynamic or fixed extrathoracic airway obstruction (at or above the thoracic inlet). It can be acute, recurrent, or chronic.

Hypopharyngeal pooling of secretions occurs in children with dysphagia and swallowing disorders. It has been described as bubbling, purring, or *percolation* by parents. Children with this finding should be considered at risk for aspiration-related symptoms.

The differential diagnosis of stridor and stertor depends on the upper airway site of narrowing. Lateral neck radiographs may identify a source of narrowing above and/or below the larynx. Laryngeal etiologies may require direct visualization with a laryngoscope, nasopharyngoscope, or flexible bronchoscope to evaluate structures and movement of the glottis.

Nose and nasopharynx
- Congenital obstruction, e.g., choanal atresia or stenosis
- Inflammation, e.g., rhinitis and sinusitis
- Adenoidal hypertrophy

Mouth, oropharynx, and hypopharynx
- Congenital obstruction, e.g., macroglossia with micrognathia
- Midface hypoplasia with small pharyngeal dimensions
- Tonsillar hypertrophy
- Spasticity of the tongue with posterior placement
- Masses, e.g., cystic hygroma, retropharyngeal abscess
- Foreign body

Larynx
- Congenital obstruction, e.g., laryngomalacia, laryngeal web or cleft, vocal cord paralysis
- Inflammation, e.g., gastroesophageal reflux
- Infection, e.g., epiglottitis, laryngotracheobronchitis or croup
- Masses, e.g., hemangiomas
- Trauma, e.g., subglottic stenosis, foreign body inhalation

Trachea
- Congenital obstruction, e.g., vascular ring, subglottic stenosis
- Infection, e.g., bacterial tracheitis

Cough

Cough is a protective response for removing secretions and particulate matter from the airway. It is a normal host defense called into play when primary pulmonary host defense, e.g., mucociliary clearance, is over-whelmed or deficient. Cough is achieved by first increasing intrathoracic pressure against a closed glottis, which has the effect of compressing the major airways, and then expelling air at high velocity through the narrowed large airways.

Differential diagnosis of acute cough (<3 weeks duration)

Upper airway disease
- Upper respiratory tract viral infections, e.g., rhinovirus, coronavirus
- Other infections, e.g., sinusitis, croup (barky cough and stridor)
- Postnasal drip from allergic rhinitis, nasal irritants (tobacco smoke)

Lower airway disease
- Asthma (common)
- Infection, e.g., bronchiolitis due to respiratory syncytial, adenovirus, influenza, human metapneumovirus, and parainfluenza viruses
- Acute foreign-body aspiration

Lung parenchymal disease
- Infection, e.g., viral and bacterial (pneumococcus is most common) pneumonia
- Atypical pneumonia, e.g., *Mycoplasma* or *Chlamydia pneumoniae* infection, tuberculosis

Focus on treating the underlying cause of the cough rather than simply treating the cough alone.

Differential diagnosis of chronic cough (≥3 weeks duration)

A chronic cough is defined as one lasting more than 3 weeks. It differs from recurrent cough, which may be related to recurrent respiratory infections. Chronic cough may be "wet," indicating stasis of secretions in the airways, or dry.

Chronic cough may be due to persistent stimulus for a cough, e.g., ongoing aspiration, environmental irritants, or a foreign body. It can also occur because the cough itself is ineffective or inefficient and hence persistent, due to airway narrowing or collapse (e.g., trachomalacia), insufficient glottic closure due to vocal cord disease, or insufficient force generation with neuromuscular weakness.

Cough may lead to poor sleep, tussive emesis, or tussive syncope and merit therapy for these reasons. Chronic cough is a nonspecific symptom and may or may not reflect serious underlying disease.

Following are the causes of chronic cough.

Upper airway disease
- Infection, e.g., chronic sinusitis and tonsillitis, *Bordetella pertussis*
- Edema and inflammation, e.g., gastroesophageal reflux

Lower airway distension, distortion, or irritation
- Congenital abnormalities, e.g., tracheoesophageal fistula, cleft larynx, pulmonary artery sling
- Asthma
- Infection, e.g., post-bronchiolitis symptoms, atypical infections
- Foreign body
- Bronchiectasis, e.g., damage to the airway from chronic infection and tuberculosis, or immunodeficiency
- Cystic fibrosis

Lung parenchymal and pleural disease
- Infection, e.g., pneumonia
- Pulmonary fibrosis
- Pulmonary edema
- Atelectasis
- Pneumothorax, hemothorax, empyema

Central causes
- Psychogenic, habit cough
- Tourette disease with a tic involving throat clearing or cough

Snoring

Snoring in children may or may not adversely affect sleep quality and breathing, It may indicate children likely to have complete intermittent complete upper airway obstructions during sleep, known as obstructive sleep apnea (OSA).

Snoring is associated with breathing pauses of any duration, gasping for air, mouth breathing, restless sleep, unusual sleep position, and daytime sleepiness. The most common cause of OSA in young children is adenotonsillar hypertrophy. The other causes or risk factors are as follows.

Differential diagnosis

Congenital anatomical
- Midface, e.g., hypoplasia

Choanal atresia or stenosis
- Tongue, e.g., macroglossia in Beckwith syndrome (p. 1075), trisomy 21
- Lower jaw, e.g., retro- and micrognathia

Laryngomalacia
- Syndromes with craniofacial anomalies, e.g., Pierre Robin sequence, Treacher Collins, Goldenhar, Apert, Crouzon's

Inflammation
- Adenotonsillar hypertrophy
- Allergic rhinosinusitis
- Nasal polyposis
- Midface, e.g., hypoplasia

Choanal atresia or stenosis
- Tongue, e.g., macroglossia in Beckwith syndrome (p. 1075), trisomy 21
- Lower jaw, e.g., retro- and micrognathia
- Syndromes with craniofacial anomalies, e.g., Pierre Robin sequence, Treacher Collins, Goldenhar, Apert, Crouzon's

Masses
- Gastroesophageal reflux
- Encephalocele
- Nasal gliomas
- Hemangioma
- Congenital cyst
- Obesity

Central causes of pharyngeal hypotonia during sleep
- Cerebral palsy
- Seizures
- Hydrocephalus
- Arnold–Chiari malformation
- Prader–Willi syndrome

Hypotonia
- Neuromuscular (Duchenne muscular dystrophy [DMD])
- Myasthenia gravis
- Mitochondrial cytopathy

When snoring is associated with OSA and/or sleep fragmentation, the underlying cause should be treated.

Investigations

Chest radiograph

A chest X-ray is a useful diagnostic technique in respiratory medicine. It provides information about spine and thoracic cage characteristics, general and regional lung volumes, hemidiaphragm positions, cardiac size and shape, perihilar masses and adenopathy, location and nature of lung parenchymal densities, and pleural features.

Lung parenchymal densities are most often of water density and represent blood, water, pus, or tissue. Tissue density occurs with infiltration of inflammatory cells, storage cells, fibrosis, or when air is absent, e.g., in atelectasis.

The chest radiographic findings of airway disease are indirect, as one does not see lumens of airways lower than lobar or segmental airways. Indirect evidence of airway disease, such as hyperinflation, atelectasis, and bronchial wall thickening, correlates poorly with lung function and severity of disease.

A chest radiograph does not replace pulmonary function testing (PFT), e.g., spirometry when airway disease is suspected. Chest radiographs are also insensitive to bronchiectasis, interstitial lung disease, and pulmonary vascular disease. These entities must be assessed by alternative means, e.g., high-resolution computerized tomography (CT).

Review of serial radiographs can be useful to determine if an abnormality is persistent or recurrent and whether abnormalities are extending or worsening over time. A chest radiograph is designed to be used with the clinical examination, not as a replacement for it.

Wheeze

- A chest X-ray is not needed every time a patient presents with asthma or bronchiolitis. However, tachypnea and significant hypoxemia in the presence of these presentations indicates that additional problems, e.g., air leak, atelectasis, or pneumonia, may also be present. Similarly, asymmetric auscultatory findings may be an indication for a chest radiograph in the presence of wheezing, i.e., to rule out a foreign body.
- Monophonic wheezing may prompt a chest radiograph to rule out etiologies for a localized external airway compression, i.e., hilar lymph nodes, a large left atrium, or mediastinal mass.

Stridor

- Suspected supraglottic or subglottic central-airway narrowing due to compression can sometimes be identified with a chest radiograph. A normal film does not rule out most diagnoses.

Cough

- Cough can occur from a diffuse condition (e.g., asthma) or a localized process (pneumonia or lung abscess). The chest radiograph identifies region(s) that may be abnormal within the thorax related to coughing. A normal chest radiograph dose not rule out airway pathology.

Other imaging techniques

- *Chest computed tomography* is more useful to assess the nature and distribution of parenchymal, pleural, and, sometimes, airway disease than a chest radiograph. CT scans also depict mediastinal structures (heart, great vessels, lymph nodes) and pleural disease adjacent to lung parenchyma (e.g., empyema). CT angiograms are used to diagnose pulmonary emboli. High-resolution CT scans at maximum inspiration and expiration are performed to assess interstitial lung disease and peripheral airway disease, e.g., bronchiolitis obliterans.
- *Thoracic magnetic resonance imaging (MRI)* is useful to evaluate vascular and mediastinal anatomy.
- *Nuclear imaging* is useful for assessing regional ventilation (V) and perfusion (Q), and matching of regions of ventilation to regions of perfusion.

Common respiratory function tests

Respiratory function tests are used to characterize and quantify the nature and degree of respiratory disorders on initial assessment and serially over time to assess progression or resolution of disease or response to treatment.

Laboratory tests

Pulse oximetry

- This is the most commonly used outpatient test, measuring the degree to which hemoglobin is saturated with oxygen (SpO_2). It has replaced arterial blood gas measurements in the non-ICU setting.

Blood gases

- *Sampling of arterialized capillary blood* for CO_2 and pH has largely replaced arterial blood sampling due to ease and reasonable correlation of capillary CO_2 with arterial CO_2. Venous CO_2 measurements are convenient but much less reflective of lung function.
- *Respiratory failure* is defined as PCO_2 >50 and/or a SpO_2 <88%. Use of PCO_2 and pH values in conjunction with a serum bicarbonate or total CO_2 from serum electrolytes allows one to assess whether acidosis or alkalosis exists, and whether it is due to a respiratory disease with metabolic compensation or a metabolic disease with respiratory compensation.

Pulmonary function tests

Spirometry

The most underused outpatient test of lung function is spirometry, which tests the mechanical features of the lung, particularly the airways. It measures the amount of air a child can inhale and subsequently exhale with maximal force and effort and how quickly air moves through the airways.

- *Forced vital capacity (FVC)* is the total amount of air exhaled.
- FEV_1 is the amount of air exhaled in the first second, a measure of the caliber of both central and smaller airways together.
- FEV_1/FVC ratio is a useful index of airway obstruction, reflective of obstructive lung disease if <85%, independent of norms.
- *FEF 25%–75%* indicates flow in the mid-half of the effort, which reflects bronchial obstruction when the central airway effects have been deleted. It measures smaller bronchi but not small airways, e.g., bronchioli.
- *Peak expiratory flow rate (PEFR)* is useful for monitoring but not diagnosing airway obstruction, as the measurement is very effort dependent.
- *Spirometry* measures only vital capacity, not all lung volumes—e.g., total lung capacity (TLC) or functional residual capacity (FRC).
- For *diagnosis of reversible airway obstruction* (e.g., asthma), spirometry can be repeated after an inhaled short-acting bronchodilator. An improvement in FEV_1 >12% suggests reversible airway obstruction.

Measurements are normalized for height and gender; weight and age have much less effect. Results are expressed as a % of predicted, based on published norms.

Spirometry testing can be achieved in ≥5-year-olds, but varies with the maturity of the child. Inspection of a volume-time trace or, better yet, a flow-volume loop will differentiate true abnormalities from suboptimal test performance by a child.

Further investigations

There are multiple additional tests to measure respiratory function, usually available in pediatric referral centers.

- *Body plethysmography* or *gas dilution techniques* are used to measure air-trapping, restrictive lung disease, and lung diffusion capacity (alveolar–capillary surface area).
- *Bronchial provocation testing* is used to evaluate response to exercise, inhaled allergens, or bronchoconstrictors.
- *Exercise testing* is used to evaluate cardiopulmonary adaptation to exercise.
- *Polysomnography (sleep study)* is used to measure sleep-related changes in breathing, including obstructive sleep apnea.
- *Maximal inspiratory and expiratory pressures (MIPs and MEPs)* are used to measure respiratory muscle strength.

Flexible bronchoscopy

This procedure is used in all ages of children to safely evaluate airway anatomy and size, mucosal inflammation, secretions, and to sample distal portions of the lung for cells and microbial pathogens using broncho-alveolar lavage (BAL). It is commonly used in children who are suspected of having infection but cannot expectorate and those who are immuno-compromised.

The technique is not used for distal airway manipulation (e.g., foreign-body removal or laser surgery) but can be used for airway biopsies and scrapings (for cilia) in older children.

Asthma

Asthma is a disease characterized by airways inflammation, bronchial hyperreactivity, and reversible airway obstruction. Increased airway secretions and structural adaptation (remodeling) can also occur. The prevalence in children is approximately 10%. It can present at any age, although most children present with it before 5 years of age. There is often a family history of asthma and a strong association with other atopic diseases (allergic rhinitis/conjunctivitis, eczema).

Diagnosis

History
- Cough, especially with exercise or early morning; persistent cough after upper respiratory infections
- Shortness of breath, especially with exercise
- Wheezing, chest tightness
- Exercise limitation
- Chest pain or discomfort

Examination
- Wheezing, prolonged expiratory phase
- Increase anteroposterior (AP) chest diameter, due to hyperinflation
- Increased work of breathing (chest retractions, tachypnea)

Diagnostic tests
Chest X-ray
This is not routinely necessary. If one is obtained, it may show the following:
- Hyperinflation, flattened hemidiaphragms
- Peribronchial cuffing
- Atelectasis, due to mucous plugging

Spirometry
- Measurement of airways obstruction
- FEV_1 <80% of the predicted value (based primarily on patient height)
- FEV_1/FVC <0.8 is abnormal and suggests airways obstruction
- PEFR can be obtained with a handheld meter, but PEFR is less sensitive than FEV_1 and is more effort-dependent.
- Bronchodilator response with beta-agonist therapy, >12% increase in FEV_1 or PEFR
- Airway challenge tests with exercise, methocholine inhalation, or cold air inhalation to test airway reactivity

Asthma medications

Asthma medications can be separated into short-term relievers, e.g., the bronchodilators (relax smooth muscle) and controller medications, used to prevent or suppress airway inflammation, and oral corticosteroids for management of asthma exacerbations. The use of controller therapy is determined by the severity and persistence of a patient's asthma.

Bronchodilators

- Short-acting β_2-agonists (for quick relief): Albuterol, levalbuterol, terbutaline
- Long-acting β_2-agonists (used in conjunction with inhaled corticosteroids) for long-term asthma control: Salmeterol, formoterol
- Short-acting anticholinergic: Ipratropium bromide

For treatment of persistent asthma

- Inhaled corticosteroids: Fluticasone, mometasone, budesonide, beclomethasone
- Fixed combinations of inhaled corticosteroids and long-acting beta-agonists: Fluticasone/salmeterol, budesonide/formoterol
- Leukotriene inhibitors: Montelukast
- Oral corticosteroids: Prednisone
- Sodium cromoglycate and theophylline (rarely used)

Adverse effects of asthma medications

Oral corticosteroids

When long-term oral corticosteroids are used, adverse effects include the following:

- Linear growth suppression
- Osteoporosis
- Adrenal suppression
- Posterior subcapsular cataracts
- Weight gain

Inhaled corticosteroids (doses >800 µg/day)

- Linear growth suppression
- Hoarseness
- Possibly adrenal suppression

Beta-agonists

- High doses can result in hypokalemia
- Tremors, increased heart rate

Asthma: inhaled drug delivery methods

Inhaled medications can be delivered to patients by several methods using technology that is continuously changing, with new devices being developed annually. Inhaled medications are used for children with asthma, but also children with cystic fibrosis or bronchiectasis, and with tracheostomies.

Inhaled medications include bronchodilators, anti-inflammatory agents, compounds that alter sputum rheology and clearance, and antibiotics. Some medications can only be used with specific delivery devices to maintain efficacy and avoid degradation. All delivery devices depend on an effective interface with the patient (e.g., mask or mouthpiece). The main delivery methods are itemized below.

Metered dose inhaler (MDI) (with spacer)

One actuation of the device delivers a metered dose of drug. For children, the MDI is attached to a spacer and mask interface used to overcome difficulties with timing of a patient's inspiration with actuation of the MDI.

With proper use, drug delivery with an MDI and spacer is equal to that with a nebulizer, even in infants and small children. The devices are portable and quick to use. The technique needs to be demonstrated and reinforced with each visit.

Older children and adults
- Shake MDI before each actuation.
- Place MDI into spacer (optional with HFA preparations).
- Position spacer or MDI at the lips with mouth open.
- Exhale slowly and deeply.
- With actuation of the MDI, inhale fully and hold breath for 10 seconds.

Child >6 months
- Shake MDI before each actuation.
- Place MDI into spacer attached to face mask.
- Place face mask gently on the face, without it leaking.
- During quiet breathing with mask in place, actuate the MDI once.
- Hold MDI, spacer, and mask in place for 10 breaths.

Important tips for use
- Crying children may receive less drug from an MDI, as the drug impacts on the posterior hypopharynx with greater inspiratory flows. Quiet breathing at rest is preferred, including during sleep.
- If an MDI has not been used on a regular basis, it may need to be primed (four actuations before delivering drug to the child).
- Double pumping an MDI into a spacer does not deliver twice the dose. Avoid this practice.

Nebulizer delivery

In this procedure, compressed gas (air or oxygen) is used from hospital sources or portable gas compressors to generate flow through the nebulizer cup filled with liquid medications or solutions. Nebulizers are often used in emergency departments and hospital settings and among children <2 years old. Their drawback is the time (10 minutes or more) needed to deliver medication (until the nebulizer runs dry).

Dry powder inhaler (DPI)

DPIs are breath actuated. They require sufficient inspiratory flow by the patient to deliver the predicted drug amount. Children <4 years of age (and sometimes older) cannot generate adequate flow, precluding use of DPIs in this age group.

Bronchodilators, inhaled corticosteroids, and combinations of these drugs are available in DPI devices. They come in various shapes, and spacers are not used with them. As with MDIs, inhalation should be followed by a 10-second breath hold to enhance drug delivery, and proper technique should be reinforced at each visit.

Asthma outpatient management (1)

Asthma management is a long-term partnership with the family and child to provide proactive preventive strategies, pharmacotherapy at the lowest doses that achieve complete asthma control, as well as education and empowerment of the family to master self-assessment and management of chronic asthma and acute exacerbations. Families need ready access to resources.

Treatment is aimed at helping the child lead a normal life without symptoms and with a minimal burden of care to reduce the risk of future exacerbations and progression of disease.

Patients with persistent, incompletely controlled asthma should be managed in consultation with an asthma specialist.

Asthma severity is assessed at initial encounter or diagnosis prior to use of anti-inflammatory medication. This assessment will dictate the initial intensity of asthma care and medication. After daily asthma controller medication has been initiated, asthma control is determined.

Intermittent asthma

Characteristics

- Most children with asthma have this type of asthma.
- Less than two acute episodes per year
- Symptom-free between acute episodes
- Normal exercise levels compared to peers, and normal sleep, uninterrupted by asthma symptoms
- No regular treatment is needed.

Management strategy

- Treat acute episodes with inhaled short-acting β_2-bronchodilators
- Use a 4- to 6-day course of prednisolone for acute, severe asthma.
- Reassess for persistent asthma if there are more than two acute asthma events per year.

Persistent asthma (mild, moderate, or severe)

Characteristics

- More than 2 days of symptoms/week or use of short-acting beta-agonist more than twice per week to prevent or reduce symptoms
- More than two acute exacerbations requiring oral corticosteroids or unscheduled use of medical care (office, emergency department or hospitalization) per year

Management strategy

- Use daily or twice-daily inhaled corticosteroids as a first option.
- An alternative second option is a trial of a leukotriene receptor antagonist.
- Long-acting β_2-bronchodilator in combination with an inhaled corticosteroid may be helpful if daily-inhaled corticosteroids (ICS) provide incomplete control.

- The ideal dose of ICS may be high, and the choice of increasing inhaled steroid dosing vs. using a combination of asthma-controller medications is patient-specific.
- Oral steroids may be needed for acute exacerbations but often reflects suboptimal chronic asthma control. Chronic oral corticosteroid use for asthma care should be managed by an asthma specialist.

Exercise-induced asthma (EIA)

Most EIA is due to poorly controlled asthma with exercise as a trigger, rather than being a unique form of asthma.

Management strategy

- *Mild*: Use β_2-bronchodilator before exercise
- *Severe*: Low-dose inhaled steroid or leukotriene receptor antagonist in addition to as-needed albuterol

Once asthma severity or degree of control is established, patients with asthma should be reevaluated regularly (every 1–6 months, more often if poorly controlled [every 2–6 weeks]) to achieve optimal asthma outcomes. When control is achieved for 2–3 months, the patient should be evaluated to reduce the asthma therapy to maintain control. A step up or down in asthma treatment has been devised by multiple national asthma guidelines. Box 9.1 depicts the current recommended approach to escalating therapy when asthma is not optimally controlled.

Box 9.1 Stepwise approach to asthma drug therapy

At each visit, assess asthma symptom control, limitations to activity, relief-medication use, and changes to environment and triggers.

• STEP UP if symptom control is POOR
• STEP DOWN if symptoms are well controlled >2 months

Before altering treatment, ensure that medication is being taking in an effective manner, prescriptions are filled in a timely way and available when needed, and reasons for not taking medicines are explored.

Step 1: Occasional use of relief bronchodilators
(intermittent asthma or exercise-induced asthma)
• Short-acting β_2-bronchodilator for relief of symptoms or prevention of exercise-related asthma

Step 2: Low-dose controller (anti-inflammatory) therapy
(mild persistent asthma)
• *Preferred*: Low-dose inhaled corticosteroid
• *Alternative:* leukotriene receptor antagonist + short-acting β_2-bronchodilator as needed

Step 3: Medium-dose controller therapy (moderate persistent asthma)
• *Preferred*: Medium-dose inhaled corticosteroid
• *Alternative*: Low-dose inhaled steroid + long-acting bronchodilator (LABA) or leukotriene receptor antagonist (LTRA) + short-acting β_2-bronchodilator as needed

Step 4: Medium-dose controller therapy
(moderate persistent asthma, inadequate control)
• *Preferred*: Medium-dose inhaled corticosteroid + LABA
• *Alternative*: Medium-dose inhaled steroid + LABA or LTRA + short-acting β_2-bronchodilator as needed

Step 5: High-dose inhaled controller therapy
(severe persistent asthma, controlled)
• *Preferred*: High-dose inhaled steroid + LABA
• *Alternative*: High-dose inhaled steroid + LRTA or theophylline + short-acting β_2-bronchodilator as needed

Step 6: High-dose inhaled + oral controller therapy
(severe persistent asthma, inadequate control)
• *Preferred*: High-dose inhaled steroid + LABA + oral corticosteroid at lowest dose to effect control (daily or every other day) + short-acting β_2-bronchodilator as needed

Asthma outpatient management (2)

0–4 years

Inhaled medications should be delivered by MDI via a valve-holding chamber with the appropriately sized mask or by small-volume nebulizer (and not by dry powdered inhalers).

Quick-relief medications

Bronchodilators (reliever medications)

- Albuterol HFA MDI (90 µg/puff) 2 puffs every 4–6 hours
- Levalbuterol HFA MDI (45 µg/puff) 2 puffs up to every 4–6 hours
- Ipratropium is not recommended in this age group.

Long-term control medications

- *Mild persistent asthma*: Low-dose ICS is first-line; second-line is montelukast 4 mg orally once daily; cromolyn 20 mg by nebulizer 3 times daily
- *Moderate persistent asthma*: Medium-dose ICS or medium dose ICS + either a long-acting beta-agonist (salmeterol, formoterol) or montelukast
- *Severe persistent asthma*: High-dose ICS + either a long-acting beta-agonist or montelukast

5–11 years

Quick-relief medications

Bronchodilators (reliever medications)

- Albuterol HFA MDI (90 µg/puff) 2 puffs every 4–6 hours
- Levalbuterol HFA MDI (45 µg/puff) 2 puffs up to every 4–6 hours
- Ipratropium is not recommended in this age group

Long-term control medications

- *Mild persistent asthma*: Low-dose ICS is first-line; second-line is montelukast 4 mg orally once daily; cromolyn 20 mg by nebulizer 3 times daily
- *Moderate persistent asthma*: Medium-dose ICS or low-medium dose ICS + either a long-acting beta-agonist (salmeterol, formoterol) or montelukast
- *Severe persistent asthma*: High-dose ICS + a long-acting beta-agonist or montelukast

≥12 years

Quick-relief medications

Bronchodilators (reliever medications)

- Albuterol HFA MDI (90 µg/puff) 2 puffs or 2.5 mg by nebulizer every 4–6 hours
- Levalbuterol HFA MDI (45 µg/puff) 2 puffs or 1.25 mg by nebulizer up to every 4–6 hours
- Ipratropium MDI (18 µg/puff) 2–3 puffs or 500 µg by nebulizer every 6 hours as needed

Long-term control medications

- *Mild persistent asthma*: Low-dose ICS is first-line; second-line is montelukast 4 mg orally once daily; cromolyn 20 mg by nebulizer 3 times daily is rarely used.
- *Moderate persistent asthma*: Medium-dose ICS or low–medium dose ICS + either a long-acting beta-agonist (salmeterol, formoterol) or montelukast
- *Severe persistent asthma*: High-dose ICS + a long-acting beta-agonist or montelukast

Box 9.2 Useful clinic guides to asthma treatment

Inhaled corticosteroids

- Fluticasone, budesonide, and mometasone have fewer adverse effects than beclomethasone on a dosage-equivalent basis. All have more adverse effects at higher dosages.
- Patients on doses of ICS >440 µg/day of fluticasone, >1200 µg/day of budesonide, or >480 µg/day of beclomethasone should be under the supervision of a specialist clinic (these are the new National Heart, Lung, and Blood Institute [NHLBI] "high doses").

Long-acting β_2-agonists (LABA)

- Salmeterol and formoterol, used in conjunction with an inhaled corticosteroid, can help to reduce symptom frequency and changes in FEV_1. Long-acting beta-agonists should not be used alone for asthma treatment.
- Consider in patients on inhaled beclomethasone or budesonide 400 µg/day, or fluticasone 200 µg/day.

Allergen avoidance

- Removal of feather or woolen bedding
- Plastic mattress encasements to reduce dust mite exposure
- Reduce cloth surface areas, drapes, stuffed toys, carpets
- Use HEPA filter on vacuum cleaner
- No pets in the bedroom if they need to be indoors
- No smoking in the house or car
- Reduce odors in the home, i.e., woodstove, perfumes, candles, air fresheners

Education

Families and children should be empowered and educated to assume self-management of asthma, including the following:

- Accurate self-assessment of asthma control, using peak flow meters if needed
- Which medication to use and when
- Best drug delivery device and technique
- What to do when asthma worsens
- Avoid active and passive tobacco smoke exposure
- Environmental precautions that are realistic for the family
- An asthma management plan with patient-specific goals of care
- Long-term partnership with a care provider to manage asthma

Cystic fibrosis

Cystic fibrosis (CF) is the most common life-shortening genetic disease in Caucasians (incidence of 1/2000 to 1/4000 live births). CF is an autosomal recessive disorder caused by mutations in the CF transmembrane conductance regulator (CFTR) protein, which results in defective ion transport in exocrine glands (i.e., primarily reduced chloride secretion and secondary increased sodium absorption). There are over 1000 disease-causing mutations in the *CFTR* gene; the most common is the ▶F508 deletion.

CF is a multisystem disease affecting the lungs and upper respiratory tract, gastrointestinal (GI) tract, pancreas, liver, sweat glands, and genitourinary (GU) tract. In the lung, the abnormal sodium and chloride ion transport results in reduced airway surface liquid volume and thickened mucus, with resultant reduced mucociliary clearance and chronic endobronchial infection.

Chronic bacterial infection of the airways with progressive obstructive lung disease and bronchiectasis accounts for >90% of all CF deaths. The median survival is currently ~37 years and is gradually increasing with emerging supportive therapies.

Diagnosis
Screening
Cystic fibrosis can be identified by newborn screening with abnormally elevated immunoreactive trypsinogen (IRT) and/or detection of *CFTR* mutations from blood-spot analysis (e.g., Guthrie card). Perinatal screening via *CFTR* mutational analyses is also offered to all pregnant women.

Clinical features
- Chronic sinopulmonary disease with recurrent or persistent infections of the airways with CF pathogens (i.e., *Staphylococcus aureus, Hemophilus influenzae, Pseudomonas aeruginosa*). Respiratory tract disease may include recurrent or chronic cough, wheeze, and/or sputum production, obstructive lung disease, and nasal polyps, and be associated with digital clubbing.
- Gastrointestinal abnormalities include meconium ileus (~10%–20% of newborns), pancreatic insufficiency (~85% of patients), distal intestinal obstruction syndrome (DIOS), rectal prolapse, failure to thrive, focal biliary cirrhosis, hypoproteinemia/edema, and fat-soluble vitamin deficiencies.
- Salt-loss syndromes due to excessive NaCL losses from the sweat glands, resulting in a hypochloremic metabolic alkalosis
- Obstructive azospermia due to congenital abnormalities or obstruction of the vas deferens, resulting in infertility
- CF in a first-degree relative or a positive newborn screening in a clinically normal infant

Laboratory criteria
- Two abnormal sweat chloride values (>60 meq/L) via quantitative pilocarpine iontophoresis. A sweat chloride value of 40–60 meq/L needs follow-up at a CF center. For children less than 2 months old, any patient with a sweat chloride value >30 meq/L should be referred to a CF center.

OR
- Two disease-causing *CFTR* mutations

OR
- An abnormal nasal potential difference pattern

History
The following presenting clinical features should prompt investigation of possible cystic fibrosis:
- Cough and wheeze
- Recurrent sinus and lower respiratory tract infections
- Nasal polyps
- Shortness of breath and exercise intolerance
- Sputum production or hemoptysis
- Malabsorption, steatorrhea, rectal prolapse
- Failure to thrive, weight loss

For diagnosed CF patients, focus on nutrition and signs and symptoms of pulmonary exacerbation:
- Increased cough or change in sputum production
- Reduced exercise tolerance or dyspnea
- Weight loss or malabsorbtion symptoms (e.g., post-prandial abdominal pain, steatorrhea)
- School or work absenteeism in past week
- Acute and chronic sinus complaints (e.g., congestion, pain, drainage)

Examination
Full assessment of the following:
- Respiratory system
- Liver and GI system
- Growth and development

Investigations
- *Chest X-ray*: Hyperinflation, increased anteroposterior diameter, bronchial dilatation, cysts, linear shadows and infiltrates
- *High-resolution chest CT scan*: Bronchiectasis, bronchial wall thickening, mucus plugging, regional air trapping
- *Lung function*: Obstructive pattern with reduced FEV_1 and FEF 25%–75%, air trapping with decreased FVC

Cystic fibrosis: problems

Lifelong therapy and quarterly visits at a CF center are required to optimize health in patients with CF. There are a variety of problems that can be expected at different ages.

Infancy
- Meconium ileus
- Anemia, hypoproteinemia (rare)
- Neonatal jaundice (prolonged)

Childhood
- Recurrent lower respiratory tract infections, bronchiectasis
- Sinusitis
- Nasal polyps (rare)
- Malabsorption, DIOS
- Rectal prolapse (rare)

Adolescence
- Recurrent lower respiratory tract infections, bronchiectasis
- Chronic *Pseudomonas* endobronchial infection
- Cirrhosis and portal hypertension (rare)
- Diabetes mellitus
- DIOS
- Pneumothorax (rare)
- Hemoptysis
- Allergic bronchopulmonary aspergillosis (ABPA)
- Medical adherence issues, coping with chronic disease

Cystic fibrosis: management

Management of the child with CF requires close cooperation between the primary-care provider, local hospitals, and regional CF centers. Effective management requires a multidisciplinary team approach, which should include the following:

- Pediatric pulmonologist
- Respiratory therapist
- Nutritionist or dietician
- Social worker
- Nurse or nurse practitioner in CF
- Genetic counselor
- Primary-care team

All patients with CF should have quarterly visits to a CF center with a multisystem review and annual full laboratory assessment. Table 9.1 summarizes the information to be monitored. These data are helpful to assess clinical trends or disease progression.

Pulmonary care

Pulmonary exacerbation

There are no accepted standards for diagnosis of exacerbation, but presence of 3 of these 11 criteria should raise clinical concern:

- Increased cough
- Change in sputum production
- Reduced exercise tolerance or dyspnea
- Increased respiratory rate or work of breathing
- Weight loss >5%
- School or work absenteeism in past week
- Fever
- New finding on chest physical exam
- New finding on chest X-ray
- Decreased in FEV_1 by >10% from baseline
- Decreased SaO_2 (oximetry) from baseline

Respiratory therapy

All symptomatic children with CF should have physiotherapy at least twice a day; treatments are increased to 3 to 4 times a day with pulmonary exacerbation. The frequency for healthy infants is controversial. Parents and older children are taught how to do age-appropriate airway mucus clearance techniques:

- Chest percussion and postural drainage
- Deep-breathing exercises
- Handheld devices (i.e., Acapella or Flutter)
- Oscillating vests

Table 9.1 Information needed for annual multisystem review of a CF patient

Blood tests (annual)

Hematology	CBC, PT/INR
Biochemistry	Cr, BUN, Na, K, Cl, HCO_3 , vitamin A, E, D
Liver function	AST, ALT, GGT
Glucose control	Random glucose, fasting glucose/oral glucose tolerance test (>13 years)
Immunology	Total IgE; if IgE >500, then RAST to aspergillus, and aspergillus precipitins

Radiology

X-rays (annual)	Chest x-ray; consider chest HRCT less frequently
Ultrasound (as indicated)	Liver
Dexa scan	Consider annually in children >16 years, or those on increasing doses of steroids, or those who have fractures

Lung function

Spirometry quarterly, consider annual plethysmography	FVC, FEV_1, FEF 25%–75%, RV, TLC
	Resting SpO_2
Oximetry	

Bacteriology (quarterly)

Sputum	Send for CF pathogens, including *Staphylococcus aureus*, *Hemophilus influenzae*, *Pseudomonas aeruginosa*, *Stenotrophomonas maltophilia*, *Burkholderia cepacia* spp., and acid-fast bacteria
Cough swab (non-expectorators)	Requires special media and lab expertise

Morbidity (annually)

Hospitalizations	Number of pulmonary exacerbations and admissions
	Number of courses of IV antibiotics

Reviews

Medications	Requirements (dose)/new maintenance therapies
Lung function/imaging	Review trends with patient and family
Physiotherapy	Technique, education, equipment
Nutrition	Review weight, height, BMI; education; enzymes, supplements
Social	Family support, genetics, housing, school, statement of special needs
Psychology	Is an assessment needed?

Antimicrobial therapy
- Oral during minor acute illnesses for *Staphylococcus aureus* and *Haemophilus influenzae* infections
- Inhaled (maintenance) for patients with chronic *Pseudomonas aeruginosa* infection (i.e., tobramycin, colistin)
- Inhaled plus oral for those colonized with *Pseudomonas aeruginosa* and minor acute illnesses (i.e., inhaled tobramycin with or without oral quinolone)
- Intravenous for acute exacerbations: Two antibiotics of different classes (i.e., β-lactam and an aminoglycoside) are administered via an indwelling long-line for 10–21 days. If exacerbations become more frequent, a more permanent form of IV access (such as an indwelling Portacath) can be placed.

Other therapies
- Annual influenza immunization, pneumococcal vaccine
- Bronchodilators for those with reversible airway obstruction
- Mucolytics: Nebulized recombinant human DNAase qd to bid
- Airway hydration: Nebulized hypertonic saline (7%) bid

Gastrointestinal management
Distal intestinal obstruction (meconium ileus equivalent)
- Clinical assessment and abdominal X-rays; suggest surgical consultation if there is significant abdominal pain, distention, or bowel obstruction.
- If safe for oral therapy, use Miralax PO bid or Go-Lytely by mouth or, more likely, via nasogastric tube.
- If unable to tolerate oral therapy, consult radiology department for isomolar contrast enemas (i.e., Gastrograffin)
- Fluid/volume status needs to be monitored during this treatment; most patients will need supplemental IV fluids.
- At discharge, review enzyme compliance, hydration issues, and need for continued Miralax or Lactulose use for several weeks.

Nutritional support
- *Pancreatic insufficiency* is treated with oral enteric-coated pancreatic supplements taken with all meals and snacks. Ranitidine or proton-pump inhibitors may be useful if the response to standard enzyme doses is unsatisfactory.
- *High-calorie diet*: Children with CF require 130%–150% of normal energy intake. This may require night feedings via gastrostomy tube.
- *Salt supplements*: Salt depletion is a risk in CF patients during the first year of life and in the summer months in older patients. For newborns through age 2 years, give 1/8th teaspoon of sodium chloride (i.e., table salt) per day. For older pediatric patients in summer months or with athletics, increase salt by mouth by adding salt to meals, eating salty snacks, and hydrating with electrolyte drinks.
- *Fat-soluble vitamin supplements*
  - *Multivitamins*: CF-specific multivitamin drops high in fat-soluble vitamins A, D, E, and K (e.g., Aquadeks, Source CF, or Vitamax)

Chronic lung disease of infancy

As the quality of care for low birth-weight preterm infants improves, more and more infants are surviving into childhood with chronic lung disease (CLD) and other pulmonary complications. Infants at highest risk are those born at ≤30 weeks' gestation and/or weighing ≤1200 g. A variety of lung conditions affect premature and full-term newborns that necessitate mechanical ventilation; these are discussed in Chapter 6 (Neonatology). CLD can be the end result of many primary processes:

• Meconium aspiration syndrome
• Pulmonary hypoplasia
• Persistent pulmonary hypertension of the newborn (PPHN)
• Chronic aspiration
• Congenital or neonatal infection, specifically pneumonia
• Congenital heart disease
• Congenital disorders of the lungs, chest wall, and airways

Diagnosis

Patients have an abnormal chest X-ray and require supplemental O_2 >28 days after birth or >36 weeks corrected gestational age. Severity is graded by oxygen/respiratory support required at >36 weeks corrected gestational age.

• *Mild* = FiO_2 <23%
• *Moderate* = FiO_2 23%–29%
• *Severe* = FiO_2 >30% and/or CPAP or mechanical ventilation

Management

Complications of CLD

• Growth impairment due to chronic increased work of breathing
• Obstructive airway disease and recurrent wheezing
• Air-trapping and carbon dioxide retention
• Increased susceptibility to lower respiratory tract infections
• Pulmonary arterial hypertension
• Gastroesophageal reflux and aspiration
• Glottic scarring or subglottic stenosis with fixed airway obstruction
• Tracheobronchomalacia

CLD of infancy improves as infants grow. New, healthy lung tissue is generated until the preschool years, and airway length and caliber increases so long as height increases. The main long-term consequence of CLD is obstructive lung disease ± asthma.

Nutrition

Weight gain and linear growth should be monitored closely. High-calorie formulas and/or involvement of a pediatric nutritionist are often needed, and gastrostomy or transpyloric tubes to safely administer feedings are sometimes required.

Oxygen therapy

Oxygen therapy should be targeted for hemoglobin saturations >92%, with minimal tachypnea and work of breathing. Weaning is appropriate when the infant is clinically well and gaining weight. It should be done in conjunction with home pulse-oximetry monitoring, with a goal of incremental weans first during the day, then at night. Supplemental oxygen therapy requirements are higher for children with pulmonary hypertension and cor pulmonale.

Obstructive airway disease

Long-term therapies include inhaled corticosteroids and bronchodilators, as well as diuretics (hydrochlorothiazide and spironolactone) in some patients. Exacerbations of wheeze often require pulse systemic corticosteroids and increased bronchodilator therapy. For infants with chronic respiratory failure (pCO$_2$ >50 mmHg), one should have a low threshold for hospital admission during exacerbations.

Gastroesophageal reflux disease (GERD)

Long-standing lung hyperinflation and increased work of breathing put patients with CLD at risk for GERD. Aspiration of gastric contents worsens underlying obstructive airway disease. Medical therapy should be tried first, but some infants may require transpyloric enteral feeding or surgical fundoplication.

Immunizations

All infants with CLD should receive routine childhood immunizations. During viral respiratory season, all infants born at <32 weeks who are ≤6 months of age, OR <2 years of age with persistent oxygen requirement and/or ventilator support should receive respiratory syncytial virus (RSV) monoclonal antibody (palivizumab or Synagis) monthly.

Sleep apnea

Apnea is defined as a lack of airflow at the nose and mouth. *Central apnea* occurs when there is no effort made to breathe. *Obstructive apnea* refers to a lack of airflow despite respiratory efforts during sleep.

The obstructive sleep apnea syndrome (OSAS) may be due to tonsillar/adenoidal hypertrophy, macroglossia, and micrognathia, The risk of sleep apnea is increased in any condition that compromises the size of the upper airway or conditions that cause the upper airway to be floppy.

Diagnosis

History
- Snoring
- Restless sleep, bedwetting, unusual position, multiple nocturnal arousals
- Mouth breathing, sweating, morning sleepiness, morning headaches
- Excessive daytime sleepiness, behavioral problems such as hyperactivity, inattention, mood swings, poor school performance
- Only about 15% of snoring children have significant airway obstruction
  About 15% of children have primary snoring; 2%–3% have obstructive sleep apnea and hypopnea syndrome.

Examination
An examination should include the following:
- Height and weight, BMI, BP
- Examination of the nose, mouth, and throat
- Middle ear infection and chronic effusion (features associated with adenoidal hypertrophy)
- Mouth breathing leads to dry mouth and arched palate.

Investigation
One cannot depend on history and a physical exam to diagnose sleep apnea, since a normal physical exam does not rule out sleep apnea. If it is suspected, then more definitive testing is recommended.
- *Sleep study*: An extensive overnight polysomnography is needed. A polysomnography is a diagnostic tool that outlines sleep architecture, and show details about breathing pattern (apnea, hypopnea), movements, oxygen saturations, carbon dioxide levels, arousals, and limb movements.
- *Actigraphy*: Sleep–wake pattern.
- *Multiple sleep latency testing* (objective measure of sleepiness) as an adjunct to an overnight polysomnography.
- *Chest radiograph* if hypoxemia occurs at night.
- *Electrocardiogram*: To screen secondary right heart consequences of airway obstruction, e.g., pulmonary hypertension
- *Echocardiogram*: To diagnose pulmonary hypertension or right ventricular hypertrophy (RVH) associated with severe sleep apnea.

Treatment of obstructive sleep apnea

- Continuous positive airway pressure (CPAP) or bilevel positive airway pressure (BiPAP) if surgery is not indicated or if there is residual disease after tonsillectomy and adenoidectomy (T&A).
- Oxygen supplementation as a bridge to other forms of therapy
- Weight loss
- Treatment of nasal inflammation, e.g., topical steroids for allergic rhinitis

Surgery is indicated when the following criteria are met:
- Adenotonsillectomy for
  - Airway obstruction or obstructive sleep apnea documented by an overnight sleep study
  - History of recurrent tonsillitis (more than 7 episodes in 1 year, or more than 10 episodes in 2 years)
  - History of two episodes of peritonsillar abscess
- Adenoidectomy for
  - Airway obstruction
  - Recurrent or chronic middle ear infection
  - Recurrent or chronic nasopharyngitis
  - Chronic mouth breathing
- Mid-face advancement surgery (congenital anomalies)
- Uvulopalatoplasty (rarely used in children)
- Tracheostomy (last resort)

Allergic rhinitis

Up to 20% of children have symptoms of allergic rhinitis, characterized by rhinorrhea, nasal congestion, sneezing, and itching of the nose and palate. In children, it is also frequently associated with cough, irritability, poor sleep, and fatigue.

Allergic rhinitis is classified as *seasonal* if symptoms occur at particular times of year due to outdoor environmental triggers, or *perennial* if symptoms occur year round due to indoor allergens.

Diagnosis

History

- Identify seasonality of the symptoms and explore both indoor and outdoor environmental exposures such as mold, pets, cockroaches and dust mite vectors (e.g., stuffed toys, carpet, bedding etc), grasses, trees, and weeds.
- Explore associated symptoms: Eczema, urticaria, upper airway congestion
- Narrowing, wheezing and/or asthma, snoring at night, history of anaphylaxis

Examination

- Conjunctival erythema, cobblestoning, tearing
- Suborbital venous congestion ("allergic shiners") and skin creases ("Denny's lines")
- Nasal congestion, mucosal pallor (or erythema) and edema, polyps, purulent discharge
- Transverse nasal skin crease from repeated wiping of nose
- Mouth breathing, postnasal drip, throat clearing
- Cough, wheezing
- Epidermal xerosis, eczema, urticaria

Investigation

- *Skin tests* for common and specific antigens (based on history), including dust mite, cockroach, dog and cat dander, tree and grass pollens, household molds
- *Serum IgE radioallergosorbent tests (RASTs)* to specific antigens as an alternative to skin testing
- *Spirometry* if history and/or physical exam findings suggest recurrent wheezing to evaluate for asthma
- *Nasal smear* for eosinophila

Treatment

- Allergen avoidance
- Intranasal steroids
- Intranasal or oral antihistamines
- Immunotherapy

Upper airway infections (URI)

Ear, sinus, nose, and throat infections account for 80% of respiratory infections, most of which are viral infections. The diagnosis URI may include any of the following:

- *Rhinitis or rhinosinustis (common cold)*: Commonly due to rhinoviruses, coronaviruses, and respiratory syncytial virus (RSV)
- *Pharyngitis and tonsillitis*: Pharyngitis is usually due to viral infection with adenovirus, enterovirus, and rhinovirus. Bacterial infection with group A β-hemolytic streptococcus may be present in the older child. Tonsillitis associated with purulent exudates may be due to group A β-hemolytic streptococcus or the Epstein–Barr virus (EBV).
- *Acute otitis media*: Common pathogens include viruses, *Pneumococcus*, group A β-hemolytic streptococcus, *Haemophilus influenzae*, and *Moraxella catarrhalis*.
- *Sinusitis* may occur with viral or bacterial infection.

Diagnosis

History

Children often present with a combination of the following:

- Painful throat, difficulty swallowing, poor oral intake
- Fever and irritability or malaise
- Blocked nose (that may lead to feeding difficulty in infants)
- Nasal discharge (clear to purulent)
- Earache with or without drainage
- Headaches in sinus areas
- Conjunctivitis, depending on the pathogen

Examination

In infants, inadequate oral hydration and intake may reflect difficulty breathing due to nasal congestion. In all ages it may be difficult to determine those children who should receive and respond to antibiotics. Due to emergence of drug resistance in community-acquired bacterial pathogens, e.g., *Pneumococcus*, common practice is to delay antibiotic use for 48–72 hours if viral infection is suspected.

- *Ears.* Otitis media is likely if there is discharge, if the tympanic membrane is not intact, and if the eardrums are bright red and bulging with loss of normal light reflection.
- *Nose and sinuses.* Acute sinusitis is likely if there is persistent purulent nasal discharge, headache and/or sinus tenderness, fever, and malaise in combination.
- *Pharynx.* Tonsillitis exists if there are purulent exudates on inflamed tonsils with tender cervical lymphadenopathy. Petechiae on the palate also suggest bacterial pharyngitis.
- Displacement of a tonsil medially should raise concern for a peritonsillar abscess.

Treatment

Symptom relief

- Acetaminophen (paracetamol) or ibuprofen for fever and discomfort associated with pharyngitis, sinusitis, and otitis
- Over-the-counter (OTC) antitussives and decongestants are not recommended in the pediatric population and may be dangerous.

Antibiotics

Virus infection causes the majority of URIs and antibiotics should not be prescribed. However, if bacterial tonsillitis or pharyngitis due to group A β-hemolytic streptococcus is suspected, they should be given after a throat swab has been taken for bacterial culture.

- *Tonsillitis and pharyngitis*: Use penicillin V, amoxicillin, or erythromycin in allergic patients, for 7 days.
- *Acute otitis media*: If treatment is indicated, treat initially with amoxicillin or macrolide. If resistant organisms are suspected, amoxicicllin-clavulanate will be effective against β-lactamase-producing *H. influenzae* and *M. catarrhalis*.

Laryngeal and tracheal inflammation

There are multiple causes of laryngeal and tracheal inflammation and obstruction. In the acute setting, the following conditions should be considered:

- *Viral laryngotracheobronchitis (croup)*: Mucosal inflammation of the glottis, which is commonly due to parainfluenza, influenza, metapneumovirus and respiratory syncytial virus in children aged 6 months to 6 years, with peak age 18–36 months
- *Spasmodic croup*: Barking cough and hyperreactive upper airways with no apparent URI symptoms, can have an allergic trigger, may be transient and recurrent
- *Acute epiglottitis*: Life-threatening swelling of the epiglottis and septicemia, classically due to *Haemophilus influenzae* type b infection in children aged 2–7 years; uncommon in immunized children
- *Bacterial tracheitis*: Uncommon but severe bacterial infection of the trachea associated with inflammation and copious secretions, most commonly due to *Staph. aureus*, *Moraxella*, or *H. influenzae*; often follows a viral lower respiratory tract infection.
- Angioedema, anaphylaxis
- Acute or chronic foreign-body aspiration

Diagnosis (see Table 9.2)

History
- Time course, severity, and prodromal symptoms
- Contact with sick persons or known allergic triggers
- Potential for foreign-body aspiration
- Immunization history, especially for *Haemophilus influenzae* type b

Table 9.2 Differentiating between viral croup, acute epiglottis, and bacterial tracheitis

	Croup	**Epiglottitis**	**Tracheitis**
Age of patient	**6 months to 4 years**	**2–7 years**	**6 months to 8 years**
Time course	Days	Hours	Hours
Prodrome	Coryza	Sore throat	Neck pain
Cough	Barking	Slight, if any	Brassy/barky
Toxic	No	Yes	Yes
Fever	<38.5°C	>38.5°C	>38.5°C
Voice	Hoarse	Weak or silent	Hoarse

Examination
- Level of consciousness, fatigue
- Temperature, respiratory rate, pulse oximetry
- Timing and degree of stridor (inspiratory and/or expiratory) (may diminish when fatigue develops—a concerning sign)
- Suprasternal and subcostal retractions
- Expiratory work of breathing or wheeze.
- Avoid direct exam of the throat, as it may precipitate acute upper airway obstruction (epiglottitis)
- Associated findings: Rhinnorhea, urticaria
- Immunization status is important data

Treatment

Priority

The main priority in the emergency setting is to differentiate between viral croup and life-threatening epiglottitis or tracheitis. In any child who is toxic appearing or in marked respiratory distress, focus on stabilization, keeping the child calm by avoiding unnecessary noxious stimuli that may precipitate airway obstruction. Provide supplemental oxygen by the least bothersome method and be prepared for possible emergency intubation.

Viral croup

Children with mild illness (e.g., barky cough and stridor only when agitated) can be managed at home, but advise parents that if there is worsening work of breathing and/or stridor at rest, they should return to the hospital.
  Treatments include the following:
- *Moist or humidified air*: Although widely used to ease breathing, the benefit of these physical measures is unproven.
- *Steroids*: Oral prednisolone (2 mg/kg for 3 days) or dexamethasone (0.6 mg/kg single IM or oral dose) reduces the severity and duration of croup. They are also likely to reduce the need for endotracheal intubation
- *Nebulized epinephrine* can provide transient relief of symptoms. Because effects wear off quickly (~2 hours), patients should be observed for hours after administration and hospital admission should be considered if it is used.

In cases that require endotracheal intubation, steroids should be given, and if there is evidence of epiglotitts on direct visualization or bacterial tracheitis, antibiotics should be added.

Acute epiglottitis
- Second- or third-generation cephalosporin (e.g., cefuroxime, ceftriaxone, or cefotaxime) IV for 7–10 days
- Rifampicin prophylaxis to close contacts

Bacterial tracheitis
- Broad-spectrum antibiotics to cover upper airway pathogens and Staph. aureus

Bronchial disease

Bronchitis can be acute, persistent, or recurrent. Acute bronchitis is caused most often by viruses and can last 3 weeks. A cough lasting >4 weeks, or acute symptoms more than twice per year should raise questions of underlying lung disease or persistent stimulus for airway secretions, e.g., of inhaled irritants. Bronchitis is a clinical diagnosis without pathognomonic laboratory or radiographic findings.

Important underlying conditions include those with altered host defense (cystic fibrosis, ciliary dyskinisia, primary immunodeficiencies) or those that stimulate secretions (environmental irritants, GERD, aspiration syndromes). Other considerations should include conditions that render cough ineffective and therefore protracted, e.g., neuromuscular weakness disorders, underlying structural narrowing of the central airway.

Diagnosis
History
- Cough productive of mucous, often lasting >4 weeks.
- Exposure history: Daycare, tobacco smoke, wood-burning stoves, strong odors (e.g., perfumes, incense, cleaners, spices)
- Feeding history, technique, and risk of aspiration

Examination
- Productive or "wet" cough
- Coarse, sometimes asymmetric breath sounds with inspiratory pops and squeaks (air moving past mucous) and expiratory wheeze

Investigation
- A chest radiograph is often unhelpful, as airways are not clearly seen.
- Sputum culture, if able
- In chronic, recurrent, or unresponsive cases, consider further workup:
  - Sweat chloride test
  - Immunodeficiency evaluation
  - Chest CT to rule out bronchiectasis, airway anomaly
  - Bronchoscopy and bronchoalveolar lavage for culture
  - Fluoroscopic swallowing evaluation

Treatment
- Acute bronchitis is most often due to a respiratory virus rather than bacteria, and does not require antibiotics. Treatment is supportive with focus on adequate hydration.
- Exceptions to keep in mind are *Bordetella pertussis* and *Mycoplasma pneumoniae*, which can produce symptoms for weeks (the "100-day cough").
- Antitussives are not indicated unless there is significant weight loss due to tussive emesis.

- Persistent or protracted bronchitis in children is often due to bacterial infections that warrant a 2- to 4-week trial of oral antibiotic treatment. Common pathogens include *Moraxella*, *Haemophilus influenzae* non-type b, and *Pneumococcus*.
- Chest physiotherapy may be of use in chronic bronchitis depending on the reason for poor airway secretion clearance.
- Removal of environmental irritants can be helpful in chronic cases.

Pertussis and whooping cough

Bordetella pertussis infection typically induces three stages of illness:
- *Catarrhal* (1–2 weeks): Mild symptoms with fever, cough, and coryza
- *Paroxysmal* (2–6 weeks): Severe paroxysmal cough, followed by inspiratory whoop and vomiting
- *Convalescent* (2–4 weeks): Less frequent and severe coughing paroxysms over time

A pertussoid syndrome may be caused by *Bordetella parapertussis*, *Mycoplasma pneumoniae*, *Chlamydia*, or adenovirus.

Diagnosis

There may be a typical history. In young infants, acute pertussis infection may present with apnea. In older children there may be a history of persistent forceful cough. Previous childhood immunizations may not protect adolescents.

Examination and investigation

- *Eyes.* Subconjunctival hemorrhages due to coughing
- *Chest X-ray* to rule out pneumonia and/or atelectasis, especially in infants.
- *Blood count*: Leukocytosis and lymphocytosis
- *Nasal swab*: Polymerase chain reaction (PCR) for pertussis and fluorescent antibody (FA) for adenovirus and other respiratory viruses

Treatment

Hospital care

- *Infants.* Admission is required for those with a history of apnea, hypoxemia, or significant paroxysms preventing adequate hydration or caloric intake. Close monitoring is required, particularly of infants, due to risk of seizures and encephalopathy.
- *Isolation.* Patients should be isolated for 5 days after starting treatment with macrolide antibiotics.

Contacts

- Immunization is recommended for children <7 years of age who have been in close contact if they are not protected. Immunization reduces the risk of an individual developing infection by 90%, but the level of protection declines steadily throughout childhood.
- Prophylactic antibiotics should be given to close contacts.

Antibiotics

- Give azithromycin or other macrolide antibiotic to reduce contagion, but realize that this has little effect on the course of the cough.

Bronchiolitis

Bronchiolitis, most commonly due to respiratory syncytial virus (RSV), affects 60%–70% of infants in the first year of life, with a peak incidence at 2 months of age. Some 1%–2% of previously well infants born at full term require hospitalization with RSV, and 2% of those hospitalized require intubation and mechanical ventilation. Metapneumovirus accounts for a significant portion of RSV-negative bronchiolitis later in the viral season, but any respiratory virus can produce the syndrome. RSV invades the nasopharyngeal epithelium and spreads to the lower airways where it causes increased mucous production, desquamation, and then bronchiolar obstruction. The net effect is airway obstruction with mucous plugging, wheezing, hyperinflation, tachypnea, atelectasis, and hypoxemia. Hypercapnic respiratory failure occurs with severe disease.

The following children are predisposed to severe bronchiolitis:
- Premature birth <32 weeks gestation
- Age <2 years with chronic lung disease
- Age <2 years with hemodynamically significant congenital heart disease
- Congenital or acquired immunodeficiencies
- Infants and toddlers with neuromuscular weakness
- Children with congenital abnormalities of the lungs and airways

RSV immunoprophylaxis is indicated in these groups of patients.

Diagnosis
History
Infants have a history of 3–5 days of coryza with rhinnorhea and cough, followed by acute onset of tachypnea and increased work of breathing. Other features in the history include
- Wheeze
- Low-grade fever
- Feeding difficulty, with or without dehydration
- Episodes of apnea and cyanosis
- Contact with other ill children or adults (often siblings or through daycare)

Examination and investigation
Physical findings:
- Cyanosis, alertness or lethargy
- Tachypnea (often respiratory rate >60 breaths/minute)
- Subcostal and intercostal retractions
- Prolonged expiration
- Chest wall hyperinflation with sternal bowing
- Pauses in breathing or apnea
- Diffuse, polyphonic wheeze and/or crackles

Investigations are used to assess the severity of illness:
- *Pulse oximetry* in room air and on oxygen to assess hypoxemia
- *Capillary blood gas* to evaluate CO_2 retention and pH in patients with significant distress or fatigue

- *Chest radiograph* is not necessary in mild–moderate cases. Generally it shows patchy bilateral perihilar infiltrates and/or atelectasis, airway thickening, and hyperinflation with diaphragm flattening. It may be indicated with severe hypoxemia.
- *Nasopharyngeal swab*: Immunofluorescent antibody testing for RSV and other viral pathogens is optional. This may be of use in cohorting infants with similar viral infections during winter months. Results do not alter treatment, which is supportive.

Hospital treatment

The usual course of RSV infection is 7–9 days, with peak symptoms occurring at day 4–5. Patients presenting with moderate to severe illness on day 1–2 should be observed closely, as they will likely worsen before improving. Average hospital length of stay is 3–4 days.

The treatment of RSV bronchiolitis is supportive and anticipatory:

- Oxygen to achieve goal saturation of 90%–94%
- Adequate hydration with oral or IV fluids
- Antipyretics in the presence of hypoxemia or hypercapnia to reduce the body's rate of oxygen consumption and CO_2 production
- If tachypnea limits the ability to orally feed for longer than 24–48 hours, consider a nasogastric or transpyloric feeding tube. Infants with bronchiolitis are at risk of aspiration of oral contents and GERD aggravating bronchiolitis.
- Mechanical ventilation for severe respiratory distress, apnea, or respiratory failure
- Bronchodilators may be indicated on a therapeutic trial basis, but are not helpful routinely.
- Nebulized racemic epinephrine may improve work of breathing transiently but does not alter length of hospital stay.
- Systemic corticosteroids in previously healthy infants provide no predictable benefit. However, consider therapy in patients with a history of chronic lung disease of prematurity or asthma.
- Antibiotics are not indicated.
- Antiviral therapy with ribavirin should be reserved for immunodeficient patients.

Prophylaxis

Palivizumab is a monoclonal antibody to RSV, used for passive immunoprophylaxis. It does not prevent RSV infection, but reduces severity of lower respiratory tract disease. It is administered with monthly IM injections begun before the RSV season begins to reduce the risk of hospitalization.

Follow-up

Recurrent wheezing is common after RSV bronchiolitis, particularly within the first several years after illness. Recurrent wheezing after RSV bronchiolitis is often precipitated by viral URIs and is bronchodilator and corticosteroid responsive.

Whether RSV causes asthma or predisposes to subsequent atopy is controversial. Wheezing that does not resolve between infections should raise concern for other etiologies (e.g., aspiration or bronchiolitis obliterans).

Bronchiolitis obliterans

Bronchiolitis obliterans (BO) is an uncommon consequence of acute viral lower respiratory infection, most commonly with adenovirus. It is characterized by fixed small-airway narrowing, persistent wheeze (unresponsive to bronchodilators), and hyperinflation from air trapping.

A CT scan is diagnostic when patchy "mosaic" areas of hyperinflation are seen intermixed with normal lung on expiratory views.

Pneumonia

Pneumonia is an infection of the lower respiratory tract and lung parenchyma that leads to consolidation of air spaces. Viruses alone account for 14%–35% of all community-acquired pneumonia in childhood. In 20%–60% of children a pathogen is not found. Common infecting bacterial agents by age are the following:

- Neonates (birth to 1 month): Group B streptococcus, *Escherichia coli*, *Klebsiella*, *Staphylococcus aureus*
- Infants (1–4 months): *Streptococcus pneumoniae*, *Chlamydia trachomatis*, *Staphylococcus aureus*, *Bordetella pertussis*
- Toddlers (6–24 months): *Streptococcus pneumoniae*, *Haemophilus influenzae*, *Moraxella catarrhalis*.
- School age: *Streptococcus pneumoniae*, group A streptococcus, *Mycoplasma pneumoniae*, *Chlamydia pneumoniae*.
- In general, anaerobic pathogens are uncommon in children, unless poor oral health or recurrent aspiration is present.

Existing pulmonary pathology places children at risk of pneumonia:
- Congenital lung or airway malformations
- Acquired or congenital immunodeficiencies
- Recurrent aspiration
- Neuromuscular weakness and inability to clear secretions (e.g., Duchenne muscular dystrophy)
- Bronchiectasis
- Sickle cell disease
- Tracheostomy in situ

Diagnosis

History
- Preceding URI is common
- Pleuritic chest pain, splinting or abdominal pain
- Abdominal pain
- Temperature ≥38.5°C
- Tachypnea and increased work of breathing
- Cough (can be productive or nonproductive)
- Malaise, lethargy, anorexia, and low-grade fever are more commonly seen with atypical pathogens.

Examination
- General health, vital signs, and mental status
- *Signs of respiratory distress*: Tachypnea, grunting, intercostal retractions, use of accessory muscles for breathing
- *Desaturation and cyanosis*: Pulse oximetry should be performed in every child with pneumonia. A resting SpO_2 ≤92% in room air indicates severe illness that should be observed in the hospital.
- *Auscultation signs of lobar pneumonia*: Asymmetric breath sounds depending on distribution of the infection in the lungs. One should note chest wall expansion, decreased or absent breath sounds, bronchial breath sounds, and airway crackles and pops. Wheezing is occasionally heard with atypical pathogens.

Investigations

- *Chest radiograph* can be deferred in patients who are nontoxic appearing with a characteristic physical exam, but should not be deferred in patients with a history of recurrent pneumonia.
- *Sputum*: Culture may be of limited value, composed of oral flora.
- *Nasopharyngeal aspirate*: Viral immunofluorescence assay or polymerase chain reaction (PCR) assay
- *Blood*: Culture should be drawn in all children hospitalized with severe bacterial pneumonia. CBC is not routine, but should be considered because of the risk of hemolytic anemia and marrow suppression with pneumococcal disease.

Chest radiograph

Abnormalities range from lobar consolidation to multifocal patchy infiltrates in community-acquired pneumonia. In addition to consolidation, look for pleural effusions, air-fluid levels suggestive of lung abscess, apparent round pneumonia, cavitation, hilar adenopathy, and any calcification.

Expansile, round pneumonias are seen in infections with pneumococcus, anaerobes or *Klebsiella pneumoniae*. Areas of cavitation or abscess with fluid levels should also raise clinical suspicion for anaerobes and *Staph aureus*. Reactive pleural effusions and empyema are not uncommon in children infected with common respiratory pathogens, including *Staph. aureus* and *Strep. pneumoniae*, but are rare and small with viral pneumonia.

At follow-up, patients with history of significant, acute X-ray change (e.g., lobar collapse, apparent round pneumonia, empyema) or continuing symptoms will require a repeat X-ray; however, resolution should not be expected until 3–6 months after acute illness.

Treatment

Oral antibiotics are safe and effective in the treatment of community-acquired pneumonia. Intravenous antibiotics are used in children who cannot absorb oral antibiotics or in those with severe symptoms. The specific choice of antibiotic is based on the following:

- Age of the age of the child (see Box 9.3)
- Host factors (e.g., tracheostomy, aspiration)
- Severity of illness
- Information about cultures if known
- Chest X-ray findings
- Community resistance patterns of common pathogens

Box 9.3 Antibiotic therapy

Neonates (0-21 days)

Group B streptococcus and gram-negative enterics are most likely pathogens.
- *First-line treatment*: Ampicillin and gentamicin

1-4 months

Streptococcus pneumoniae is most likely, but consider *Chlamydia trachomatis* with neonatal exposure risk or interstitial infiltrates on X-ray. For severe illness, empyema or cavitation, cover for *Staph. aureus*.
- *First-line treatment*: Amoxicillin or macrolide
- *Alternatives*: Co-amoxiclav, cefuroxime or cefaclor

Less than 5 years

Again, *Strep. pneumoniae* is most likely, but consider atypical pathogens such as *Chlamydia* and *Mycoplasma pneumoniae*. Consider *Staph. aureus* if patient is unresponsive to initial outpatient therapy or has severe illness or characteristic X-ray findings.
- *First-line treatment*: Amoxicillin or macrolide
- *Alternatives*: Co-amoxiclav, cefuroxime or cefaclor

Over 5 years

Mycoplasma pneumoniae is more common in this age group.
- *First-line treatment*: Macrolide or amoxicillin if more focal infiltrate
- *Alternatives*: Co-amoxiclav, cefuroxime or cefaclor, ciprofloxacin

Pneumonia requiring hospitalization
- Co-amoxiclav, cefotaxime, or cefuroxime IV

Clindamycin should be added if a patient is not improving on single antibiotic coverage in order to augment tissue penetration, or for anaerobic coverage in patients with acute or recurrent aspiration.

Vancomycin should be considered in patients in whom *Staph. aureus* is suspected for coverage of methicillin-resistant strains.

Other therapies

Supportive
- Antipyretics for fever
- Ibuprofen, acetaminophen, or low-dose narcotics for pain control, will allow for ambulation, cough, and deep breathing
- Intravenous fluids: Consider if patient is dehydrated or not drinking, to assure perfusion and minimize airway mucus plugging
- Nutritional supplements (enteral or, rarely, parenteral)
- Supplemental oxygen: Administer oxygen via nasal cannulae or mask to maintain SpO_2 92%–95%

Physiotherapy

Chest physiotherapy is generally not beneficial in children with pneumonia and is limited by patient discomfort. Deep breathing exercises (e.g., blowing bubbles), ambulation, and incentive spirometry help to prevent atelectasis.

Chronic or recurrent pneumonia

Potential pathology

- Congenital lung malformations: Cystic adenomatous malformation, lobar emphysema, or lobar sequestration
- Congenital or acquired airway anomalies that compromise effective cough, leading to mucous plugging: Stenosis, bronchiectasis, compression, foreign body or mass
- Abnormal secretion clearance: cystic fibrosis, ciliary dyskinesia
- Acquired or congenital immunodeficiencies: HIV, etc.
- Recurrent aspiration

Box 9.4 Investigation of chronic, recurrent pneumonia

Initial tests

- *Hematology*: CBC with differential, complement screen, ESR, CRP
- *Immunology*: Quantitative IgA, IgG, IgE and IgM, IgG subclasses, antibody response to immunizations (tetanus and pneumococcus)
- Sweat chloride test
- *Microbiology*: Sputum culture (if able)
- *Lung function*: Spirometry, lung volumes and reversibility
- *Radiology*: Chest X-ray, barium swallow

Further investigations

- *Hematology*: Neutrophil and monocyte function, lymphocyte subsets, and cellular immune function
- *Imaging*: High-resolution CT scan of the chest
- *Ciliary biopsy*: Microscopy and function, sampled from the posterior nasopharynx or lower airway
- *Bronchoscopy*: Visualization of dynamic airway function as well as microbiological sample collection

---

Parapneumonic effusion and empyema

Pneumonias often produce an inflammatory pleural reaction, called a *parapneumonic effusion*. Some effusions become infected and purulent and are then called *empyemas*. Pleural disease due to pneumonia evolves from initial straw-colored, thin exudates, to thick, purulent material (pea-soup consistency), to an organizing peel that changes from a chicken fat quality to a rind. After treatment, the rind resolves radiographically.

Effusions that mature (loculated or organized) are not easily drained with chest tubes alone and are called *complicated parapneumonic effusions*. The course and outcome of these effusions differ between adults and children; children usually heal without long-term sequelae (e.g., fibrothorax) within 3–6 months of the pneumonia.

Diagnostic assessments

- *General appearance*: Fatigue, tachypnea and distress, pain
- *Pulse oximetry* to assess for degree of hypoxemia
- *Auscultation*: Decreased or absent breath sounds on affected side
- *Chest radiograph*: Extent of associated pneumonia, unilateral or bilateral pleural involvement, size of effusion and mediastinal shift, evidence of lung abscess or pyopneumothorax
- *Ultrasound* of the chest to identify loculations and ideal location for thoracentesis if this procedure is considered
- *CT scan of the chest*: If degree of pneumonia vs. pleural effusion is questioned as the primary pathogenic condition
- *Blood culture*, complete blood count (for leukocytosis and anemia) and inflammatory markers (CRP, sedimentation rate)

Not all parapneumonic effusions need to be drained for diagnostic or therapeutic reasons. Fluid samples collected by thoracentesis can be useful to identify a bacterial pathogen and its antibiotic sensitivities; however, after 48–72 hours of oral or IV antibiotic treatment, the yield of culture drops dramatically.

Diagnostic drainage is indicated if the clinical history is not compatible with a community-acquired pneumonia.

Features of sampled pleural fluid that may alter decision-making include the following:

- *Microbiology*: Bacterial culture and sensitivity, acid-fast bacilli
- *Cytology*: Presence of neutrophils, lymphocytes, malignant cells, and erythrocytes
- *Low pleural glucose and pH* (<7.2) help to predict those effusions that may benefit from aggressive drainage procedures.

Antibiotic treatment

Empyemas in children are most often caused by common pathogens of community-acquired pneumonia: *Streptococcus pneumoniae*, *Staphylococcus aureus*, and group A streptococcus. Antibiotics should be administered intravenously to cover these pathogens and their local antibiotic sensitivities (e.g., ceftriaxone or cefuroxime, plus clindamycin or vancomycin if *Staph. aureus* is suspected).

IV antibiotics are administered until children are afebrile for 24–48 hours. Oral antibiotics are generally continued, for variable durations, after discharge to prevent recurrence; this practice has not been studied.

Pleural fluid drainage

- *Repeated needle thoracentesis*: If early in the clinical course with thin, free-flowing pleural fluid
- *Large-bore chest tube drainage*: Effective early in the course when pleural fluid is rapidly accumulating and mass effect is large (e.g., mediastinal shift). This is not effective when the pleural effusion is loculated or organized.
- *Small-bore (pigtail) catheter with fibrinolytic therapy*: Small-bore catheters have the advantage of less pain at the insertion site than that with large-bore tubes; however, without fibrinolytics they are rarely effective due to clotting. Fibrinolytic agents are not universally available in all countries. Choices may include urokinase, streptokinase, or tissue plasminogen activator (t-PA). Use of fibrinolytic therapy, usually for 3–4 days, requires
  - Intrapleural instillation of fibrinolytic via the chest tube twice a day
  - Clamping of the tube with a dwell time of 2–4 hours
  - Withdrawal of liquefied pleural contents via closed drainage system under continuous suction (–20 to –30 cm H_2O)

Video-assisted thoracoscopic surgery (VATS)

VATS involves manual evacuation of simple or organized pleural fluid and air under direct thoracoscopic visualization under general anesthesia with subsequent chest tube placement for ongoing drainage. Postoperative morbidity is less with this procedure than with a thoracotomy.

Thoracotomy and decortication

This procedure is done infrequently with the advent of VATS, but is an option in advanced or severe cases.

Decisions to intervene with a drainage procedure depend on the presentation of the child. For children in overt respiratory failure due to pleural mass effect, drainage should be immediate and may be life saving. For children who are not improving on antibiotics alone over 48 hours, the choice of drainage techniques depends on local experience and surgical expertise.

Hospital care and discharge

- *Fever*: Monitoring and treatment with antipyretics. Children will often improve clinically before the fever resolves.
- *Hypoxemia*: Supplemental oxygen to keep saturations 92%–95%
- *Pain*: Often debilitating early in the course and may require narcotic analgesics
- *Nutrition*: Pain and nausea may limit oral intake, but adequate hydration and nutrition are critical for healing
- *Discharge criteria*: Afebrile for 24–48 hours and pain resolved. Tachypnea and unilateral reduction in breath sounds may persist after discharge and improve gradually. Radiographic abnormalities in extensive disease may persist for 3–6 months.

Pulmonary tuberculosis

Worldwide, tuberculosis of the lung is a major health problem. Tuberculosis (TB) should always be considered in children from endemic areas, as well as those at risk of immunodeficiency or taking immunosuppressive agents.

Mycobacterium tuberculosis is spread from person to person by droplet infection. Once inhaled, some bacilli remain at the site of entry and the rest are carried to regional lymph nodes; the bacilli multiply at both sites and can then spread via the blood and lymphatics. After inhaling *M. tuberculosis*, most children do not develop disease but rather latent infection (e.g., positive skin test but no clinical or radiographic findings).

The risk of developing clinical disease depends on host–organism interactions and is highly variable by age: from up to 50% in infants <1 year, to <10% in children 5–10 years. Pulmonary disease accounts for the majority of children affected, except for infants in whom meningitis and disseminated disease are common.

Clinical findings

Pulmonary TB causes a pathologic triad called the primary complex:
1. Localized parenchymal pneumonia (Gohn focus)
2. Associated infection of draining lymphatics (lymphangitis)
3. Infection of regional lymph nodes

Seventy percent of primary complexes are subpleural and 25% are multi-focal. In those who have disease progression, the pathological sequence is as follows:

0–4 weeks
- Asymptomatic incubation period

4–8 weeks
- Febrile illness
- Erythema nodosum

2–6 months
- Tuberculous meningitis
- Disseminated tuberculosis
- Formation of the primary complex of pulmonary disease
- Chronic cough and weight loss

6–9 months
- Progression and complications of the primary complex
- Calcification of parenchyma—"coin lesion" on chest radiograph
- Pleural effusions and pneumothorax (parenchymal focus rupture into pleural space)
- Cavitation: Parenchymal focus rupture into bronchus and endobronchial spread of disease
- Regional lymph nodes calcify and may compress or erode into bronchi.

>9 months
- Extrapulmonary disease: Osteomyelitis, renal disease, etc.

Chest radiograph

Pulmonary tuberculosis can manifest with many radiographic changes:

- *Regional lymphadenopathy*: Hilar, mediastinal, and subcarinal
- *Miliary tuberculosis*: Diffuse granular opacification of bilateral lung fields, the result of multiple infectious tubercles
- *Collapse-consolidation*: Atelectasis + parenchymal opacification is frequently seen in the right upper, right middle, and left upper lobes.
- Caseating consolidation, calcification and cavitatory lesions
- Pleural effusion, pneumothorax, or pyopneumothorax
- Bronchiectasis

Diagnosis

Tuberculin skin test (TST)

Infection with *M. tuberculosis* produces a delayed-type hypersensitivity reaction identifiable by skin test. Up to 10% of immunocompetent children will have false-negative tests, and false-positive tests occur if bacille Calmette–Guérin (BCG) vaccine was received.

Interferon-γ release assays (IGRAs)

The IGRA is a serum test for *M. tuberculosis*–specific interferon-γ release by circulating T cells and monocytes. IGRA is less sensitive than TST, but more specific (fewer false positives with BCG administration and non-*Tuberculous mycobacterium* infection). It is currently recommended as an adjunct to TST in diagnosis.

Gastric aspirates

This test requires serial samples of gastric fluid obtained in the morning before eating. *M. tuberculosis* recovery by cultures is ~40% in children with radiographic pulmonary disease and ~70% in infants, but fewer than 10% will be positive on acid-fast stain alone.

Sputum

α-Fetoprotein (AFB) smear and culture are less reliable in children because of their inability to expectorate sputum from lower airways. Culture positivity ranges from 5% to 20%.

Bronchoalveolar lavage

Sampling from the lower airways under direct visualization with a bronchoscope produces variable results, with cultures positive in 15%–60% of children.

Drug management (see also p.738)

Latent infection

- 9 months: Isoniazid

Pulmonary tuberculosis

- 2 months: Isoniazid, rifampicin, and pyrazinamide (add ethambutol if drug-resistant organisms are suspected)
- Then 4 months: Isoniazid and rifampicin

Miliary tuberculosis

- 3 months: Isoniazid, rifampicin, and pyrazinamide
- Then 12–18 months: Isoniazid and rifampicin

Once diagnosed, TB is a notifiable disease to public health agencies and contact tracing is required so that those exposed to the patient can undergo tuberculin testing and chest X-ray screening.

BCG vaccination

This vaccine is commonly given to newborns in most countries where *M. tuberculosis* remains endemic. BCG does not prevent pulmonary tuberculosis, but is protective against miliary disease and meningitis, with efficacy ranging from 0 to 80%.

Gastroesophageal reflux disease (GERD) and aspiration syndromes

Gastroesophageal reflux disease (see p. 382)

Gastroesophageal reflux disease (GERD) can produce pulmonary problems in addition to gastrointestinal complaints. GERD can be primary, due to abnormal esophageal sphincter tone, or secondary, worsened by increased inspiratory and expiratory respiratory effort (e.g., labored breathing or coughing). GERD is a common complication of chronic obstructive and restrictive lung disease, such as asthma, cystic fibrosis, and chronic lung disease of prematurity.

Pulmonary manifestations of GERD include the following:
• Apnea
• Hoarseness, stridor, laryngeal edema
• Bronchitis (mucus secretion)
• Aggravation of asthma (probably does not cause asthma) and recurrent wheezing in infants
• Recurrent pneumonia and atelectasis

Diagnostic assessment

Diagnosis of GERD is often based on objective measures including clinical emesis, and improvement of signs and symptoms with GERD-specific interventions (e.g., antacid medication trials). Standard diagnostic tools to identify GERD include the following:
• *Esophageal pH monitoring*: Calculation of total time with pH <4 at the upper and lower esophagus in 24 hours
• *Impedance monitoring* of the esophagus
• *Contrast radiography* of the upper GI tract is also used to rule out structural abnormalities of the stomach and esophagus that explain GERD.
• *Nuclear medicine scans* are used to detect stomach contents moving retrograde and to evaluate gastric emptying.

Treatment

Therapy for GERD:
• *Supportive measures*: Decreased caffeine intake, sleeping on an incline, thickened feedings in infants
• *Antiacids* (proton-pump inhibitors [PPI] or H₂-blockers) and *prokinetic agents* when delayed gastric emptying is present. Nighttime symptoms, apnea, and pain behavior improve within days if GERD is playing a role, but lower respiratory tract disease (wheezing and atelectasis) may take weeks to months. These therapies do not account for non-acid gastric constituents that may contribute to pulmonary disease (e.g., pepsin).
• *Fundoplication*: For severe disease, particularly in the presence of aspiration, surgical fundoplication may be indicated.

Aspiration syndromes

Children can aspirate particulate matter and liquids, leading to lower airway and parenchymal lung disease.

Acute aspiration of fluid or solids (foreign bodies) into the lungs may present as paroxysmal choking and coughing, with asymmetric air movement on auscultation.

Chronic aspiration may present with recurrent pneumonia, wheezing, and bronchitis. Aspiration is associated with GERD but can exist in the absence of GERD (and vice versa). Children often merit diagnosis of both conditions so that rational therapies can be devised.

Aspiration is more likely to occur when airway protection mechanisms are less active (e.g., fatigue, altered consciousness).

The following conditions predispose to pulmonary aspiration:

- Neurological disease (seizures, encephalopathy)
- Neuromuscular disease involving the upper airway muscles of swallowing
- Acute and chronic pulmonary diseases that produce tachypnea and increased work of breathing (fatigue-related aspiration)
- Structural abnormalities of the upper and central airways (e.g., vocal cord paralysis, laryngeal cleft)

Diagnostic assessments

Diagnosis is made by observations of coughing or choking on liquids or solids or by radiographic evaluations of swallow (video-fluoroscopic swallowing studies, or "milk scans") to evaluate dysphagia and descending aspiration with various liquid consistencies. Children more likely aspirate thin liquids than thick liquids. Children can aspirate after several minutes due to fatigue while drinking. Diagnosis is confirmed only after intervention to prevent aspiration is beneficial.

Treatment

Therapy can be temporary during episodes of increased respiratory work (e.g., bronchiolitis) or permanent when present with underlying chronic lung disease.

Interventions include the following:

- Thickening of liquid with gelatins or rice cereal. Bottle propping and supine positions for drinking should be avoided.
- Temporary bypass of the oropharynx with a nasogastric or nasoduodenal feeding tube
- Permanent gastrostomy tube (with fundoplication if GERD is also present)
- Long-term goals should include feeding therapy to improve motor deficits of swallowing and prevent feeding aversion.

Gastroenterology and clinical nutrition

Healthy eating for children

Infants

See also p. 124.
- Breast milk is the ideal feed for almost all infants.
- Solids are not recommended until age 6 months (↓ food allergies)
- Initial solids should be based on baby rice, fruit, and vegetables.
- Gluten is acceptable from age 6 months.
- Following introduction of solids, infants should experience and progress through a wide variety of tastes and appropriate textures.
- Finger foods should be introduced from age 7 months.
- Continue complimentary breast/formula feeds until age 1 year. Normal cow's milk can then be introduced thereafter.
- Do not add salt and sugar to food.
- Low-fat products are not suitable for infants.
- Vitamins A, C, and D are recommended until age 5 years.

Age 1–5 years

A well-balanced diet in early childhood is important for a lifetime pattern of healthy eating. The key recommendations for healthy eating to be achieved by age 5 years are listed below:
- Decrease fat to 35% energy intake by avoiding excess high-fat foods.
- Include whole-grain cereals and five portions per day of fruits and vegetables to increase fiber intake.
- Avoid obesity.
- Moderate salt intake, e.g., not adding salt to cooking or at the table
- Avoiding iron deficiency anemia by restricting milk intake to 1 pint per day and including foods rich in iron (red meat, cereals, beans, pulses, egg yolk, dark green vegetables, and dried fruit). Add vitamin C as fruit juice at a meal to increase iron absorption. Drinking tea with meals decreases iron absorption.
- Excessive consumption of fruit juices and squashes can contribute to toddler diarrhea and plays a role in food refusal.

Older children

Schoolchildren should eat a diet based on a wide variety of foods. Nutritional guidelines relating to school meals have been set out by nutritional authorities. A healthy diet should include the following:
- At least one starchy food at each meal time, e.g., whole-grain bread, potatoes, pasta, and rice
- Five portions per day of fruit and vegetables
- Two servings of meat or alternatives each day
- 2–3 portions a day of 2% milk, low-fat yogurt, fromage frais, or cheese (a portion = 1 yogurt, 1/3 pint milk, 30 g cheese)
- Only small and occasional amounts of sugar and fats

Nausea and vomiting

Three clinical scenarios are recognized (see Box 10.1):
- *Acute*: Discrete episode of moderate to high intensity. Most commonly associated with an acute illness
- *Chronic*: Low-grade daily pattern, frequently with mild illness
- *Cyclic*: Severe, discrete episodes associated with pallor, lethargy ± abdominal pain. The child is well in between episodes. Often there is a family history of migraine or vomiting.

Causes
- *Acute*: Gastrointestinal (GI) infection, non-GI infection (e.g., urinary tract infection [UTI]), GI obstruction (congenital or acquired), adverse food reaction, poisoning, ↑intracranial pressure, endocrine/metabolic disease (e.g., diabetic ketoacidosis)
- *Chronic* (usually GI): Peptic ulcer disease, GI obstruction (e.g., pyloric stenosis), gastroesophageal reflux (GERD), chronic infection, gastritis, gastroparesis, food allergy, psychogenic, bulimia, pregnancy
- *Cyclic* (usually non-GI cause): Idiopathic, CNS disease, abdominal migraine, endocrine (e.g., Addison's disease), metabolic (e.g., acute intermittent porphyria), intermittent GI obstruction, fabricated illness

Management
- *Full history*, e.g., early morning vomiting with CNS tumor, or family members with similar illness
- *Full examination*, including ear, nose, and throat (ENT), and growth parameters. Assess for dehydration.

Treatment
- *Supportive* treatment, e.g., oral or intravenous fluids
- *Treat cause*, e.g., pyloromyotomy for hypertrophic pyloric stenosis
- *Pharmacological*: Antihistamines; proton pump inhibitors (PPI); phenothiazines (side effects: extrapyramidal reactions); 5-HT3 antagonists, e.g., ondansetron, especially for treating postoperative or chemotherapy-induced vomiting

---

Box 10.1 Investigations for nausea and vomiting

Acute (if severe)
- Electrolytes
- BUN/creatinine, lipase
- Stool culture, *Clostridium difficile*, ova and parasite exam (O&P), virology
- Abdominal X-ray: three-way
- Surgical consultation if obstruction or acute abdomen is possible
- Exclude systemic disease

Chronic (tests to be considered)
- CBC
- ESR/CRP
- Urinalysis (UA)
- Liver function tests (LFTs), lipase
- *H. Pylori* stool antigen or urea breath test
- Abdominal and renal ultrasound
- Contrast upper GI
- Sinus X-rays
- Test feed (pyloric stenosis)
- Brain imaging (for CNS tumor)
- Consider urine pregnancy testing in teenage girls
- Upper GI endoscopy

Cyclic
As for chronic condition, plus:
- Glucose, lactate, pyruvate
- Ammonia
- Serum amino acids, urine organic acids

Complications

These include dehydration, electrolyte disturbance (e.g., $\downarrow K+$, $\downarrow Cl-$, $\downarrow pH$ with pyloric stenosis), acute or chronic GI bleeding (e.g., Mallory–Weiss tear), esophageal inflammation, stricture or Barrett's metaplasia with persistent vomiting or GERD, bronchopulmonary aspiration uncommonly, except in those unable to protect the airway, FTT, and anemia.

Psychogenic vomiting

- *Causes*: Anxiety, manipulative behavior, disordered family dynamics. A family history of vomiting is common.
- *Management*: Exclude organic disease and refer to a child psychologist.

Diarrhea

Diarrhea is the passage of an increased number of stools of less than normal form and consistency. Acute diarrhea has an onset of symptoms less than 14–30 days. Chronic diarrhea has an onset of symptoms greater than a month. Most acute diarrhea has an infectious etiology and is self-limiting.

There are three main types of diarrhea: osmotic, secretory, and inflammatory (see Box 10.2). Often there is overlap in clinical presentation.

Osmotic diarrhea

Excessive stool water is from ingestion of poorly absorbed substances, e.g., lactose intolerance or laxative abuse.
• *Presentation*: Watery stools with/without abdominal pain and distension that abates when made NPO or when offending agent is removed
• Individuals with steatorrhea or fat malabsorption have a subtype of osmotic diarrhea (cystic fibrosis or pancreatic insufficiency). These patients usually present with fatty or oily diarrhea.

Secretory diarrhea

Excessive stool water results from the presence of excessive stool electrolytes secondary to reduced electrolyte absorption or increase electrolyte secretion, e.g., cholera.
• *Presentation*: Voluminous water stools that continue despite being made NPO

Inflammatory diarrhea

Increased stools result from an inflammatory process within the intestines, e.g., inflammatory bowel disease (IBD), invasive bacterial infection.
• *Presentation*: Bloody stools with or without mucous

Investigations

Initial screening tests

Blood work

Complete blood count (CBC; anemia, leukocytosis); creatinine; albumin; total protein; Ca^{2+}; PO_4^{3-}; LFT; tissue transglutaminase and endomysial antibodies (celiac antibodies); sedimentation rate and C-reactive protein (CRP) (inflammatory markers)

Stool studies

pH and reducing substances (carbohydrate malabsorption); fecal fat staining (fat malabsorption); stool electrolytes (can help differentiate between osmotic and secretory diarrhea); hemoccult (inflammatory diarrhea); stool Gram stain (white blood cells in stool indicate inflammatory diarrhea)

Specific infectious stool studies

Stool for O&P (may need to specify for cryptosporidium), culture (usually evaluates for *E. coli*, *Klebsiella*, *Yersinia*, *Campylobacter*, *Shigella*, and *Salmonella*), *Clostridium dificile* toxin; stool for rotavirus; serology for *E. histolytica*

If diagnosis is still unclear, consider the following:
- 72-hour fecal fat stool measurement for fat malabsorption
- Stool elastase for pancreatic insufficiency
- Fecal α_1-antitrypsin for protein-losing enteropathy, e.g., IBD
- Sweat test for cystic fibrosis
- Breath hydrogen test for evaluation of carbohydrate malabsorption and bacterial overgrowth
- Serum iron, folate, vitamin B_{12}
- Abdominal imaging, e.g., upper GI with small-bowel follow-through (SBFT)/CT scan/MRI
- Upper endoscopy and/or colonoscopy with biopsy
- Capsule endoscopy

Box 10.2 Causes of diarrhea

Osmotic diarrhea
- Carbohydrate intolerance (lactose and fructose intolerance, see p. 253)
- Laxative abuse
- Malabsorptive syndromes, e.g., short bowel syndrome and celiac

Secretory diarrhea
- Congenital chloridorrhea
- Viral gastroenteritis, e.g., rotavirus
- Bacterial gastroenteritis, e.g., cholera
- Bacterial toxin or food poisoning
- Endocrine diarrhea e.g., carcinoid, VIPoma, hyperthyroidism

Inflammatory diarrhea
- Inflammatory bowel disease (Crohn's and ulcerative colitis)
- Infectious diseases e.g., *E. coli*, *Yersinia*, CMV, amebiasis
- Ischemic colitis
- Radiation colitis

Treatment

Most acute diarrheal illnesses are usually self-limiting and do not require any specific treatment except for maintaining good hydration. It is important to avoid antibiotic treatment unless the organism is known and there is specific indication. Indiscriminate use of antibiotics leads to resistant organisms and serious complications such as worsening of hemolytic–uremic syndrome (HUS) with *E. coli*.

Antidiarrheal medications such as loperamide should be also avoided because of potential complications, unless there are specific indications.

Treatment is disease specific. Some diarrheal processes require removal of the offending agent, such as lactose intolerance or celiac or allergic gastroenteritis. Others require treatment with antibiotics such as *Giardia* or *Entamoeba histolytica*. Still others, such as IBD or autoimmune enteritis, require anti-inflammatory or immunosuppressive medications.

Always monitor hydration status. In individuals with chronic diarrhea, monitor nutritional status.

Constipation

Constipation is infrequent or inefficient passage of stool associated with pain, difficulty, or delay in defecation. It may progress to encopresis.
- 95% of infants pass ≥1 stool/day
- 95% of school children pass ≥3 stools/week
- Approximately 5% of school children suffer from constipation.
- An organic cause is more likely if there is delayed passage of meconium beyond 48 hours, onset in early infancy, severe symptoms, FTT, or abnormal physical findings.

Causes
Idiopathic
This form is most often due to a combination of the following:
- Withholding
- Low-fiber diet, relative dehydration
- Lack of mobility and exercise
- Decreased colonic motility (common positive family history)

Gastrointestinal
- Anal disease (stenosis, ectopic, fissure, hypertonic sphincter)
- Hirschsprung's disease
- Food hypersensitivity
- Celiac disease
- Colonic obstruction (mass, inflammation)

Nongastrointestinal
- Hypothyroidism
- Hypercalcemia
- Hypokalemia
- Neurological disease (e.g., spinal disease)
- Sexual abuse
- Chronic dehydration (e.g., diabetes insipidus)
- Drugs (e.g., opiates and anticholinergics)

Presentation
- Straining and/or infrequent stools
- Anal pain on defecation
- Fresh rectal bleeding (anal fissure)
- Abdominal pain (diffuse, upper or lower; nocturnal or post-prandial)
- Anorexia, early satiety
- Involuntary soiling or spurious diarrhea (liquid feces passes around solid impaction, "overflow" diarrhea)
- Flatulence
- ↓ growth
- Abdominal distension
- Palpable abdominal or rectal fecal masses, usually indentible
- Anal fissure
- Abnormal anal tone

A rectal exam is needed to confirm diagnosis, check for rectal masses or tumors, and assess tone.

Management (see Box 10.3)

Investigations are usually not necessary. If an organic cause is suspected, consider a thyroid function test (TFT), serum Ca^{2+}, radioallergosorbent test (RAST), CBC, CRP, albumin, rectal biopsy (Hirschsprung's disease), and anal manometry. Spinal imaging is used for a neurological cause. Use of abdominal X-rays is controversial as they may miss pelvic masses.

Box 10.3 Treat constipation in a stepwise manner

- Treat any underlying organic cause.
- Treat anal fissure with topical anesthetic (2% lignocaine ointment) to reduce pain and remove voluntary inhibition to defecate.
- Dietary: ↑ oral fluid and fiber intake, natural laxatives, e.g., fruit juice.
- Behavioral measures: Regular 5-minute toilet time after meals. Interrupt withholding behavior. Use toilet footrests. Encourage parents to not show concern; use star charts and rewards.

Medications

- Emphasize the need for consistency, treat for at least 3 months.
- Poor adherence and failure to evacuate fecal masses preclude improvement.
- Regular oral fecal softeners, e.g., lactulose or polyethylene glycol electrolyte solution, sodium docusate
- Avoid oral stimulant laxatives (e.g., senna) for prolonged periods and avoid phosphate products.
- Magnesium citrate, magnesium phosphate or large-volume polyethylene glycol (PEG) electrolyte solution cleanout (may need nasogastric administration for rapid infusion)
- Enemas (e.g., bisacodyl, mineral oil) for persistent rectal fecal mass after intensive oral therapy (document normal anal tone, rule out masses prior)
- Hospital admission for either manual evacuation under sedation or general anesthesia (GA) if appropriate or oral PEG

Prognosis

Most children will improve with complete evacuation of any stool masses, maintaining soft stools and defecation training. This requires patience, consistency, and understanding of the mechanism by the child, family, and provider. Many children need long-term therapy. Don't underestimate the misery that constipation and encopresis can inflict on both the child and family.

Encopresis

Encopresis is voluntary defecation in unacceptable places, e.g., the child's pants. It has no organic abnormality and is a symptom of emotional disorder, more common in boys. Once organic disease or spurious diarrhea is excluded, refer patient to a child psychiatrist.

Failure to thrive (FTT)

Failure to thrive (FTT) is when growth "falls away" from standardized weight or height centile. Weight is the most sensitive indicator in infants and young children, while height is more likely factor in older children. Under stress, head circumference growth is preserved more than linear growth, and more than weight gain.

In infancy, birth weight is a poor guide to correct "genetic potential." Growth in the first few months of life reflects influences from the intrauterine environment, and the infant may fall to find his or her own "level" thereafter. In a well, happy child, consider constitutional small stature (characterized by normal growth velocity in a healthy child of small-stature parents).

Causes

Aside from genetic influence, FTT commonly is due to inadequate food offering or intake (socioeconomic difficulties, emotional deprivation, unskilled feeding, particular belief system regarding appropriate nutrition). Organic causes often overlap:

- Decreased appetite, e.g., psychological or secondary to chronic illness
- Inability to ingest, e.g., GI structural or neurological problems
- Excessive food loss, e.g., severe emesis (dysmotility, pyloric stenosis, achalasia), diabetes mellitus (urine)
- Malabsorption (see p. 371)
- Increased energy requirements, e.g., congenital heart disease, cystic fibrosis, malignancy, sepsis
- Renal tubular acidosis
- Impaired utilization, e.g., various syndromes, endocrinopathies

Management

- Detailed history, including age of onset of FTT, and timing of weaning. Consider detailed dietary history evaluation by pediatric dietitian.
- Full examination, including accurate measurement of growth (use percentile, weight–length, and BMI charts)
- If organic disease is possible, conduct *basic investigations*:
  - CBC with differential, ESR/CRP (CRP requires smaller sample), liver and kidney function tests, total protein and albumin, Ca^{2+}, PO_4^{3-}
  - Celiac antibodies
  - Urinalysis including microscopy, culture, and sensitivity (M, C & S)
  - Fecal occult blood
  - *Advanced investigations* include metabolic screen, karyotype, serum lead (pica), serum immunoglobulins, sweat test, upper endoscopy and small intestinal biopsy, chest X-ray, bone age, skeletal survey (non-accidental injury [NAI]), abdominal ultrasound, head CT/MRI, ECG, fecal fat, fecal elastase and α_1-antitrypsin, endocrine workup.

- If nonorganic disease is likely, get dietary advice, preferably from a pediatric dietitian. If FTT resolves in the next few weeks, give positive reinforcement and supervise subsequent growth as an outpatient. If FTT persists, admit the child to the hospital for basic investigations and observe their response to supervised adequate dietary input. Adequate growth in the hospital confirms a nonorganic cause, so explore and support the family dynamics. Should FTT occur again at home, refer the child to Social Services. If FTT continues in the hospital despite adequate dietary input, occult organic disease is most likely and requires extensive investigation.
- Dietetic input, whatever the cause, to support nutritional correction and education
- Identify and correct associated morbidities, e.g., developmental delay

Prognosis

The prognosis depends on the severity of FTT. It is good if the condition is mild, familial. Severe FTT, whatever the cause, may be associated with later developmental and behavioral impairment.

Recurrent abdominal pain

Recurrent abdominal pain is defined as more than two discrete episodes in a 3-month period that interfere with school and/or usual activities. Its incidence is 10%–15% among school-age children.

Causes

No organic cause is found in 90% of cases. Causes include constipation, dietary indiscretion, food intolerance (lactose or fructose), irritable bowel syndrome, psychogenic pain, peptic ulcer disease (*H. pylori*), celiac disease, abdominal migraine (cyclic vomiting syndrome), IBD, gallbladder disease, renal colic, dysmenorrhea, mittlelschmerz, urinary tract infection, and physical or sexual abuse. Abdominal pain is not consistently associated with pathologic esophageal acid reflux.

Presentation

Nonorganic disease
This form occurs in a thriving, generally well child, with short episodes of periumbilical pain, good appetite, no other GI symptoms, no family history of IBD or celiac disease, and a normal examination.

Organic cause
If presentation is different from that for nonorganic disease or the child is <6 years of age, the cause is likely organic.

Management

- *History*: Relationship to eating, stooling, precipitating events (e.g., cow's milk introduction in milk protein enteropathy), atopy, social history (e.g., start of school, parental separation), dietary history, weight loss, constitutional symptoms, family history (celiac disease, IBD).
- *Full examination*, including rectal exam.

Investigation

- If *nonorganic disease* is likely, no or very little investigation is needed (e.g., CBC, ESR/CRP [CRP needs less volume to sample], urinalysis, C&S; a plain abdominal X-ray is not very helpful for chronic pain).
- If *organic disease* is likely, investigate the same factors as for nonorganic disease, plus consider LFT, creatinine, *H. pylori* stool antigen, hydrogen breath test (lactose intolerance), fecal culture and microscopy (if diarrhea), ultrasound, CT imaging, GI endoscopy, colonoscopy, or other GI imaging modalities.

Treatment

Nonorganic disease
- Reassure confidence
- Education that condition is common and pain is genuine (just like headaches)
- Personal support
- Avoidance of associated stressful events (e.g., bullying)
- Acknowledgment of pain, while also playing it down

- Minimize secondary gains from abdominal pain, e.g., school avoidance
- Increased dietary fiber intake may be beneficial
- Formal psychotherapy in complex and resistant cases.

Organic disease
- Treat underlying cause.

Prognosis

Some 25% of children with functional abdominal pain continue to have pain or headaches into adulthood.

Abdominal migraine

Abdominal pain is associated with pallor, headaches, anorexia, and nausea ± vomiting. Abdominal migraine overlaps with periodic syndrome and cyclic vomiting syndrome. Usually there is a strong family history of migraine.

Treatment is dietary: avoid citrus fruits, chocolate, caffeine-containing drinks (e.g., cola), solid cheeses; and pharmacological: cyproheptadine, amitriptyline, beta-blockers, gabapentin, or sumatriptan may be helpful.

Gastrointestinal hemorrhage

This condition is relatively rare. Upper GI tract bleeding may present as hematemesis (vomiting of frank blood or "coffee grounds") or melena (black, tarry, foul-smelling stools). Hematochezia (bright or dark red blood per rectum) indicates lower GI tract bleeding (see Box 10.4).

Beware of spurious hemorrhage (e.g., black stools after bismuth/iron ingestion, red vomit after beetroot, urate crystals in diapers, or normal pseudomenstruation in newborns). Use Gastrocult or a Guaiac test to confirm blood if you are unsure.

Causes

Neonates
- Swallowed maternal blood
- Necrotizing enterocolitis (NEC)
- Dietary protein intolerance
- Infectious colitis (including pseudomembranous)
- Coagulopathy
- Stress ulcers
- Gastritis, vascular
- Malformations
- Duplication cyst

Infants
In addition to above:
- Esophagitis
- Swallowed blood from upper airway (e.g., epistaxis)
- Anal fissure
- Intussusception
- Meckel's diverticulum (often presents as a massive, painless bleed)

Older children
Most of the above causes, plus:
- Peptic ulcer disease
- Mallory–Weiss tear
- Esophageal varices
- Nonsteroidal anti-inflammatory drugs (NSAIDs)
- Intestinal or colonic polyps
- IBD
- GI infection (e.g., dysentery)
- Henoch–Schönlein purpura (HSP)
- Hemolytic uremic syndrome (HUS)

Box 10.4 Investigations for GI hemorrhage

Guided by findings, these may include the following:

- CBC
- Coagulation studies
- LFT
- Albumin
- Protein
- Electrolytes
- ESR/CRP
- Apt's test (confirms swallowed maternal blood by distinguishing adult from fetal Hb)
- Stool M, C & S
- Stool *Clostridium difficile* toxin assay
- Formal ENT examination
- Abdominal ultrasound (e.g., intussusception or portal hypertension)
- Nuclear medicine Meckel's scan (premedicate with histamine antagonist if possible)
- Tagged-RBC scan (occult bleeding)
- Chest X-ray (if hemoptysis is true cause)
- Endoscopy if melana or hematemesis, flexible sigmoidoscopy or colonoscopy if hematochezia

Management

- *Detailed history*, e.g., is there associated abdominal pain?
- *Examination*: Specifically, vital signs, skin (pallor, abnormal blood vessels), hepatic stigmata, ENT examination (e.g., epistaxis), organomegaly, abdominal tenderness, anal inspection (e.g., fissure or fistula), rectal examination. Examine vomit or stool to confirm nature of bleed, and place nasogastric tube to determine location and quantity of bleeding.
- *Supportive treatment*: Fluids, blood product transfusion, nasogastric tube, airway protection with ETT, as necessary
- *Drug treatment*: Octreotide reduces splanchnic blood flow and, thereby, upper GI bleeding.
- *Therapeutic endoscopy* in severe bleeds, e.g., balloon tamponade, electrocautery, bleeding-vessel ligation, variceal banding/injection
- *Treat underlying cause*, e.g., surgical removal of Meckel's diverticulum

Jaundice

Jaundice occurs when serum bilirubin >1.5 mg/dL. It is rare outside the neonatal period. First determine the serum total bilirubin level (SBR) and conjugated (direct) fraction. Unconjugated jaundice is rarely due to liver disease. Conjugated jaundice (>1.2 mg/dL) is due to liver disease and requires investigation (see also p. 144).

Unconjugated jaundice

This form is due to excess bilirubin production, impaired liver uptake, or conjugation.

Causes

- Hemolysis (e.g., spherocytosis, G6PD deficiency, sickle cell anemia, thalassemia, hemolytic uremic syndrome)
- Defective bilirubin conjugation (Gilbert syndrome, Crigler–Najjar syndrome)

Intrahepatic cholestasis

Here jaundice is due to hepatocyte damage ± cholestasis. There is unconjugated ± conjugated hyperbilirubinemia.

Causes

Infectious
- Viral hepatitis
- Bacterial hepatitis (e.g., leptospirosis or Weil's disease, septicemia, *Mycoplasma*, liver abscess)
- *Toxoplasma gondii*

Toxic
- Drugs or poisons (e.g., acetaminophen overdose, sodium valproate, anti-TB drugs, cytotoxic drugs)
- Fungi (*Amanita phalloides*)

Metabolic
- Galactosemia, hereditary fructose intolerance
- Tyrosinemia type 1
- Wilson disease
- α_1-antitrypsin deficiency
- Peroxisomal disorders (e.g., Zellweger syndrome)
- Hypothyroidism
- Dubin–Johnson syndrome; Rotor syndrome

Biliary hypoplasia
- Nonsyndromic
- Syndromic (e.g., Alagille syndrome)

Cardiovascular
- Budd–Chiari syndrome
- Right heart failure

Autoimmune
- Autoimmune hepatitis

Cholestatic (obstructive) jaundice

Conjugated hyperbilirubinemia is due to bile tract obstruction.

Causes

- Biliary atresia
- Choledochal cyst
- Caroli's disease
- Primary sclerosing cholangitis (commonly associated with IBD)
- Cholelithiasis (may be secondary to chronic hemolysis)
- Cholecystitis
- Cystic fibrosis
- Obstructive tumors or cysts

Management

- *Full history*, e.g., medications, family history, overseas travel, past blood transfusions, jaundice contacts, pale stools or dark urine (cholestasis)
- *Examination*: Vital signs; conscious level (hepatic coma); hepatic stigmata (= chronic liver disease); pallor (hemolysis); hepatomegaly; splenomegaly; ascites; peripheral edema

Investigations

Depending on the pattern, these may include the following:

- CBC, blood smear, reticulocyte count
- Coagulation
- Electrolytes; BUN and creatinine; bilirubin (total and conjugated); LFT; albumin; total protein; thyroid function tests
- Viral serology (hepatitis A, B, and C, EBV, CMV); blood culture; leptospira and toxoplasma antibody titers
- Inborn errors of metabolism (IEM) screen; ammonia; ceruloplasmin; 24-hour urinary copper excretion; blood glucose and lactate; α_1-antitrypsin phenotype; galactose-1-uridyl-phosphatase level; urinary succinylacetone
- Immunoglobulins, anti-nuclear antibody (ANA), smooth muscle (SMA) and liver/kidney microsomal (LKM) antibodies (autoimmune hepatitis)
- Abdominal ultrasound, abdominal CT/MRI, biliary scintigraphy (e.g., hepatoiminodiacetic acid [HIDA] scan)
- Liver biopsy

Treatment

- Remove or treat underlying cause.
- Correct blood glucose if it is low.
- Correct clotting abnormalities.
- Phototherapy may be helpful only if jaundice has a significant unconjugated component, e.g., Crigler–Najjar syndrome.
- Treat any associated anemia if it is due to hemolysis.
- Treat liver failure as appropriate.

Adverse reactions to food

Food allergy

Food allergy is defined as an abnormal immunological response to food (incidence of 6%–8% in children aged <3 years).

- Immediate allergic reactions involve production of food-specific IgE antibodies.
- Reactions may be delayed and cause by non-IgE mechanisms.
- 70% of cases have a family history of atopy.
- Allergy becomes less common as age increases.
- The most common food allergens are cow's milk proteins, eggs, peanuts, wheat, soy, fish, shellfish, and tree nuts.
- Children with primary eosinophilic gastroenteritis or eosinophilic esophagitis may react to one or multiple foods, or have inflammation independent of any food trigger.

Presentation

- Diarrhea ± blood or mucous
- Vomiting
- Dysphagia, possibly heartburn (acid reflux symptoms)
- Abdominal pain
- FTT
- Eczema
- Urticaria
- Erythematous rash, particularly perioral
- Asthma symptoms
- Anaphylaxis

Food intolerance

Intolerance involves adverse reactions to food that are mediated by nonimmunological responses. This condition is more common than food allergy. Its presentation is similar to that of food allergies. Fructose intolerance is very common due to the usage of high-fructose corn syrup in prepared foods and beverages. Other food intolerances may be due to

- Enzyme deficiency, e.g., lactose intolerance (see p. 362), congenital sucrase–isomaltase deficiency
- Pharmacological reactions to agents contained in food, e.g., caffeine, histamine, tyramine, tartrazine, acetylsalicylic acid
- Reactions to food toxins or microbes, e.g., hemagglutinins in soy or mycotoxin present in mold-contaminated cereals

Management of suspected food allergy or intolerance

- *Dietary treatment*: Exclusion of offending food(s) from diet, e.g., egg-free diet. Involve a pediatric dietitian in the diagnosis and management.
- *Drug treatment*: Regular therapy may have a role (e.g., oral sodium cromoglycate, corticosteroids, antihistamines), or IM adrenaline (e.g., Epipen) for emergency treatment by the child or parent for anaphylactic reactions.

- After at least 6–12 months of being symptom-free on an exclusion diet, consider food challenge if there is a food allergy. If the previous reaction was severe, this should only be done in the hospital with full resuscitation facilities.
- Prophylaxis: Data are not clear; in newborns with a first-degree relative with confirmed food allergy, temporary avoidance may lower risk of allergy.

Take a history, including diet history and examination. A food diary may be helpful.
- Investigations may include a radioallergosorbent test (RAST) or ELISA test to detect specific food IgE antibodies; serum ↑ total IgE or eosinophils; favorable response to dietary elimination of specific suspected food protein and recurrence after challenge; and allergen prick or patch skin testing. If the diagnosis is still in doubt, a double-blind, controlled food antigen challenge or small bowel endoscopy and biopsy (nonspecific inflammatory infiltrate) may be helpful.
- In severe cases when allergen(s) cannot be identified, start a full-elimination diet in which only a few hypoallergenic foods, e.g., lamb, rice, water, pears, or amino acid–based formula are given for 1–2 weeks, followed by gradual reintroduction of increasingly allergenic foods until a food reaction(s) is detected.

Prognosis
The prognosis depends on the cause. Most infantile food allergic reactions resolve by 2 years. Allergies that develop in older children may be chronic.

Lactose intolerance
- This is most commonly due to postviral gastroenteritis lactase deficiency; most cases are transient and short lasting (<4–6 weeks).
- In older healthy children and adults (especially Asian, African American), lactase levels commonly decline with subsequent variable degrees of intolerance.
- Rarely due to congenital genetic lactase deficiency (primary). Present with severe diarrhea with lactose exposure
- *Presentation*: Diarrhea, excessive flatus, colic, diaper rash, stool pH <5. Symptoms may be delayed post-ingestion.
- *Treatment*: Lactose-free milk. Use in acute gastroenteritis is controversial. Lactase supplementation can be helpful.

Cow's milk protein allergy

- Most common food allergy in infancy
- Symptoms depend on where the allergic inflammation is.
  - Upper GI tract: Vomiting, feeding aversion, pain
  - Small intestine: Diarrhea, cramping, protein-losing enteropathy, FTT
  - Large intestine: Blood in stools, diarrhea, pain
- Limited use for RAST or skin testing in infants
- May well occur in breast-fed infants (commonly allergic colitis—usually healthy-appearing, happy infant)
- First treat by limiting cow's milk protein intake (and commonly soy protein) in infant's or nursing mother's diet.
- Hydrolyzed formulas (shorter peptides), e.g., Alimentum, Nutramigen, pregestimil. If symptoms are severe or patient is unresponsive, an elemental (amino acid) formula may be required, e.g., Neocate, Elecare.
- Very rare need for anti-inflammatory medications
- Avoid using goat's or sheep's milk, as 25% of patients will also develop allergy to these milks (cross-reactivity). Rice milk is not a nutritionally adequate substitute.
- After starting solids, introduce cow's milk protein-free diet (supplement with oral calcium).
- Consider cow's milk protein challenge after 6–12 months.

Nutritional disorders

Malnutrition is a common cause of morbidity and mortality in pediatrics. There is a wide spectrum of nutritional disorders varying from protein-energy malnutrition to micronutrient nutritional deficiencies to morbid obesity. In nonindustrialized nations, protein-energy malnutrition in association with infection is a leading cause of death in pediatrics, while in industrialized nations, obesity in childhood is associated with morbidity such as atherosclerosis, asthma, depression, and increased adult mortality (see Table 10.1).

Assessment of nutritional status

- Accurately plot serial height and weight for age
  - Weight loss ≥10% over 3 months is a flag for nutritional concerns.
  - Falling across 2 percentile lines or below the third percentile is a flag for nutritional concerns.
- Percent (%) weight for height (proportionality) – (Expected weight for height percentile ÷ Actual weight) × 100
  - <10% or >90% may indicate under-nutrition or obesity, respectively
- Body mass index (BMI) – Weight (kg)/Height (m^2)
  - Widely accepted measure for obesity
- Triceps skin fold monitors changes in total body fat.
- A *food diary* is a detailed dietary assessment of food and drink over 3–7 days.
- Laboratory studies are only useful when used in conjunction with clinical history and physical (see below for specifics).

Protein-energy malnutrition

There are three main types: Kwashiorkor, Marasmus, and Kwashiorkor–Marasmus.

Kwashiorkor

This type is due to severe deficiency of protein and inadequate essential amino acids.

- *Clinical features*: Growth retardation; diarrhea; apathy and irritability; anorexia; edema; skin or hair depigmentation; abdominal distension with fatty liver
- *Weight* is a poor indication for nutritional status in these children, secondary to edema.
- *Labs*: Hypoalbuminemia, normo- and microcytic anemia, ↓Ca^{2+}, ↓Mg^{2+}, ↓PO_4^{3-}, and ↓glucose
- This type is often associated with concomitant gastrointestinal infection: you should check for culture, O&P, or viral infection.

Marasmus

The Marasmus type is due to severe deficiency in caloric intake.

- *Clinical features*: Height is relatively preserved compared to weight; "living skeleton," wasted appearance; muscle atrophy; listless; often constipated
- *Labs*: Low–normal albumin and normo- or microcytic anemia

Kwashiorkor–Marasmus

Most undernourished infants have clinical characteristics of both Marasmus and Kwashiokor.

Treatment

- Correct dehydration and electrolyte imbalance (IV if required).
- Treat underlying infection and/or parasitic infections.
- Treat concurrent or causative disease.
- Treat specific nutritional deficiencies.
- Orally refeed slowly—evaluate for refeeding syndrome.

Table 10.1 Specific nutritional deficiencies

Vitamin/Mineral Deficiency	Causes	Presentation
Vitamin A	Fat malabsorption states, e.g. cystic fibrosis; deficient indigenous diet.	↑morbidity and mortality from infections, follicular hyperkeratosis, xerophthalmia, night blindness. Plasma retinol <0.7 mmol/l.
Vitamin D	Dietary deficiency; low UV light; fat malabsorption, hepatic or renal failure.	Rickets (limb x-rays: distal bony cupping and fraying), ↑serum Ca^{2+} and PO_4^{3-}, ↑ alkaline phosphatase, plasma 25-hydroxy cholecalciferol <25nmol/l.
Vitamin K	Congenital, fat malabsorption states, small bowel bacterial overgrowth.	Bleeding, including hemorrhagic disease of the newborn (p. 194). ↑ protime ↑INR
Vitamin B_1 (Thiamine)	Dietary deficiency (particularly when polished rice staple diet).	Beri-beri (muscle weakness, edema, heart failure), Wernicke's encephalopathy. Red cell thiamine pyrophosphate <150 nmol/l.
Niacin	Dietary especially in countries where corn (maize) is the basic food source.	Classic triad: dermatitis, diarrhea and dementia
Vitamin B_6 (pyridoxine)	Malabsorptive diseases such as celiac and Vitamin B_6 dependent syndromes such as xanthurenic aciduria. Drug interactions, such as INH and penicillamine.	Convulsions in infants, peripheral neuritis, dermatitis and anemia
Vitamin B_{12}	Vegan diets, distal small bowel disease (e.g. Crohn's disease), pernicious anemia.	Macrocytic megaloblastic anemia, peripheral neuropathy, motor weakness. Vitamin B_{12} level <75pmol/l, Schilling test of B_{12} absorption.

Table 10.1 (Contd.)

Vitamin/Mineral Deficiency	Causes	Presentation
Vitamin C	Lack of fresh fruit and vegetables.	Scurvy: petechiae, ecchymosis, bleeding gums, painful sub-periosteal bleeding of legs, motor weakness. Plasma vitamin C level <6–11 µmol/l.
Vitamin E	Prematurity, fat malabsorption.	Hemolytic anemia. Serum vitamin E level <5 mg/l.
Folic acid	Small bowel disease, malignancy, drugs (anticonvulsants, cytotoxics).	Macrocytic megaloblastic anemia, irritability, failure to thrive, thrombocytopenia. Red cell folate <160 ng/ml.
Iron	Low dietary intake, chronic blood loss (e.g. intestinal parasites or malaria), prematurity.	Common. Microcytic hypochromic anemia, developmental delay, angular stomatitis, koilonychia, serum ferritin <7 mg/l, serum iron <5 nmol/l, total iron binding capacity >90 mmol/l.
Zinc	Prematurity, dietary insufficiency, intestinal disease or chronic diarrhea, acrodermatitis enteropathica (inborn error of zinc absorption).	Peri-orificial and anal dermatitis, diarrhea, alopecia, failure to thrive, neurological dysfunction. Serum zinc <11 µmol/l.
Iodine	Dietary deficiency. Endemic in some regions.	Hypothyroidism and retarded development. Low urine iodine: creatinine ratio.

Nutritional support

Nutritional support can be either enteral or parenteral. Enteral nutrition, when possible, is preferred over parenteral nutrition (PN). It is cheaper, technically less demanding, more physiological, and associated with fewer complications.

Involve a pediatric dietitian to assess nutritional status, requirements, and support. Be aware of refeeding syndrome (potentially fatal cardiac failure induced by electrolyte disturbance following nutritional therapy in severe malnutrition). Frequently reevaluate nutritional status and adjust therapy as needed.

Indications
- Severely ill patients, e.g., ill preterm infants
- Nutrition supplementation is required, e.g., in FTT or chronic illness such as CF
- Feeding difficulties, e.g., oropharyngeal aspiration
- Metabolic diseases, e.g., phenylketonuria
- Gastrointestinal diseases, e.g., malabsorption, short bowel syndrome
- Other primary disease states, e.g., chronic renal failure

Gastric tube feedings
- Can be orogastric, nasogastric, or via gastrostomy
- Liquid feeds are given as boluses or continuously (e.g., overnight)
- Feeds are standard polymeric diets (e.g., ready-to-feed nutritionally complete, whole-protein products); elemental diets and semi-elemental diets requiring little or no digestion; or disease-specific or metabolic formulations.
- Gastrostomy reduces orofacial complications and discomfort, although complications include gastric leakage, localized skin infection or inflammation, GI perforation, trauma, or hemorrhage.
- Complete or partial nutrition may be administered via a gastric tube.
  - Trophic feeding (synonym: minimal enteral feeding)

Indications for complete or partial nutritional support are during PN and for newborn infants, particularly if preterm. The rationale for their use is that prolongation of enteral starvation leads to loss of normal GI structure and function despite a PN-induced anabolic body state.

Small milk volumes appear to prevent this, as well as promote GI development in newborn infants. Typically, in newborn infants, 0.5–1 mL/kg/hr milk is fed within 2–3 days of birth. Evidence of beneficial effects (in newborns) includes fewer episodes of sepsis, fewer days of PN, improved growth, improved gut function, and a decrease in PN-associated cholestasis.

Duodenal and jejunal tube feedings
- These can be given with a nasoduodenal/jejunal, gastrojejunal, or primary duodenal tube (avoid primary jejunal tubes, as they have a high complication rate).
- Liquid feeds are given as continuously only. You may NOT use a bolus within the small intestines.
- Feeds are standard polymeric diets (e.g., ready-to-feed nutritionally complete, whole-protein products); elemental diets and semi-elemental diets requiring little or no digestion; or disease-specific or metabolic formulations.
- Used in settings of severe GERD or anatomic or physiologic problems with feeding into the stomach

Parenteral nutrition (PN)
- Intravenously administered nutrition
- Contains fluids, amino acid, dextrose, fats, and vitamins and minerals
- Can provide complete or partial nutrition
- ONLY use when unable to feed enterally
- Can be administered peripherally (PPN) or centrally (TPN). Strict nutritional criteria must be used when ordering PPN/TPN.

Parenteral nutrition (PN)

Intravenous parenteral nutrition may be supplemental or provide total (TPN). Parents can be trained to give prolonged PN at home to children.

Indications
- Postoperative (e.g., abdominal or cardiothoracic)
- Treatment of IBD
- After severe trauma or burns
- Acute pancreatitis
- Oral feeds are contraindicated (e.g., NEC)
- GI failure (e.g., short bowel syndrome)
- Protracted vomiting or diarrhea
- Chronic intestinal pseudo-obstruction
- Very preterm infants
- Oncology patients (e.g., severe mucositis, graft-versus-host disease [GVHD])

Administration
A multidisciplinary team of clinician, pharmacist, and pediatric dietitian should be involved in supervising PN. Follow unit or hospital dietetic and pharmacy guidelines for individual needs. Allowance should be made for body weight (you may need to estimate a working weight, e.g., if patient is edematous or has gross ascites), recent weight trends, clinical condition, fluid and nutritional requirements, and additional infused fluids.

Method
Once requirements are calculated, sterile pharmacy-prepared solutions are given via central (preferable) or peripheral venous lines. Rapid commencement of PN may risk refeeding syndrome in chronically undernourished patients. When significant malnutrition exists, measure and correct electrolyte abnormalities before commencing PN and introduce slowly.

PN is usually supplied and administered as two components:
- *Lipid component*. Contains fat (triglyceride emulsion, e.g., Intralipid 20%) and fat-soluble vitamins
- *Aqueous component*. Contains carbohydrate (glucose solution), protein (crystalline L-amino acid solution), electrolytes, water-soluble vitamins, minerals, and trace elements (zinc, copper, manganese, selenium, ± iron) (see Table 10.2)

Monitoring
Serious, unexpected biochemical disturbances occur rarely as a result of PN. An appropriate monitoring regimen is suggested in Table 10.2.

Weaning
PN should be weaned slowly so that hypoglycemia is prevented. This also allows GI mucosal recovery as enteral feeding is increased. When weaning is protracted, a pediatric dietitian should assess the contribution of both enteral and parenteral feeds to ensure nutritional adequacy.

Complications and problems

- Sepsis: Gram-positive and gram-negative bacteria, fungal
- Central-line occlusion, breakage, displacement
- Thrombophlebitis, thrombobosis, thromboembolism
- Extravasation injuries. Cardiac tamponade
- Electrolyte or metabolic disturbances—hypo- and hyperglycemia
- PN-associated liver disease; steatosis, cholestasis, cirrhosis, portal hypertension
- Metabolic bone disease (insufficient Ca^{2+} and PO_4^{3-})

Table 10.2 Guidelines for monitoring stable patients during short-term PN

Measurements	Pre- PN	1st week	2nd week	3rd and sub-sequent weeks
Creatinine BUN, Na, K	✓	x 2	x 2	x 2
Calcium	✓	x 1	x 1	x 2
Magnesium	✓	x 1	x 1	Monthly
Phosphate	✓	x 2	x 1	x 2
Alk phos, ALT, bilirubin, albumin	✓	x 1	x 1	x 2
Glucose	✓	Daily blood glucose	Urine dipstick daily	Urine dipstick daily
Cu, Zn, Se	—	—	—	Monthly
CBC	—	—	x 1	x 1
Triglycerides	✓	x 1	x 1	x 1
Weight	✓	Daily	Daily	Daily

Esophageal disorders

See also p. 986.

Gastroesophageal reflux disease (GERD)

Other causes in infancy and in older children include lower esophageal sphincter (LES) dysfunction (e.g., hiatus hernia); ↑gastric pressure (e.g., delayed gastric emptying); external gastric pressure; gastric hypersecretion (e.g., acid); and CNS disorders (e.g., cerebral palsy).

Gastroesophageal reflux occurs when there is inappropriate effortless passage of gastric contents into the esophagus. GERD exists when reflux is repeated and is severe enough to cause harm. Reflux is very common in infancy and is associated with slow gastric emptying, liquid diet (milk), horizontal posture, and low resting LES pressure.

Presentation of GERD

- *Gastrointestinal*: Regurgitation, nonspecific irritability, rumination, esophagitis (heartburn, difficult feeding with crying, painful swallowing, hematemesis), FTT (calorie deficiency due to profuse reflux)
- *Respiratory*: Apnea, hoarseness, cough, stridor, lower respiratory disease (aspiration pneumonia, asthma)
- *Neurobehavioral symptoms*, e.g., Sandifer's syndrome (bizarre extension and lateral turning of head, dystonic postures)
- *Complications*
  - Esophageal stricture (dysphagia)
  - Barrett's esophagus (intestinal metaplasia)
  - FTT
  - Anemia (chronic blood loss)
  - Lower respiratory disease

Management of GERD

- *History*, e.g., effortless regurgitation, relationship to feeds
- *Examination*, including growth, possible anemia, respiratory issues
- *Investigations* (appropriate when diagnosis is uncertain, there is poor response to treatment, or complications occur) may include upper GI endoscopy, esophageal biopsy, 24-hour esophageal pH probe, barium swallow with fluoroscopy, radioisotope "milk" scan (aspiration), esophageal manometry (esophageal dysmotility), and chest X-ray (associated respiratory disease).

Treatment

Treatment is carried out in a in stepwise fashion:
- *Positioning*: Nurse infants on head-up slope of 30° ± prone.
- *Dietary*: Thickened milk feeds (infants); small, frequent meals; avoid food before sleep; avoid fatty foods, citrus juices, caffeine, carbonated drinks, alcohol and smoking
- *Drugs*: Gastric acid–reducing drugs, e.g., ranitidine or omeprazole (if esophagitis); Gaviscon (contains antacids and an alginate that forms a viscous surface layer to reduce reflux); prokinetic drugs; mucosal protectors, e.g., sucralfate; corticosteroids

- *Surgery*. Usually Nissen fundoplication is done when medical treatment has failed. Indications for surgery are failed intense medical treatment; esophageal stricture, Barrett's esophagus, or severe esophagitis; recurrent apnea; lower respiratory disease; or FTT. Complications of surgery include "gas bloating" syndrome, dysphagia, profuse retching, and "dumping" syndrome.

Prognosis
Most infants outgrow symptoms by 1 year of age. In older children, 50% develop a chronic, relapsing course.

Esophageal foreign body
This condition usually occurs in toddlers or older children with neurologic or psychiatric conditions. If the object reaches the stomach, 90% will pass spontaneously. Confirm position with AP and lateral chest X-ray. Remove endoscopically if
- Dysphagia or drooling persists
- Object is still in esophagus for >12 hours
- Sharp object (perforation risk)
- Hazardous, e.g., mercuric oxide disc batteries, material is ingested

Upper esophageal dysfunction
This disorder is usually due to diffuse CNS dysfunction.
- *Presentation*: Choking, cough, drooling, dysphagia, nasal regurgitation
- *Diagnosis*: Barium swallow with video fluoroscopy or esophageal manometry
- *Treatment*: Treat primary underlying disorder. Rarely, cricopharyngeal myotomy is helpful.

Achalasia
This rare, idiopathic, condition of obstruction is due to failure of lower esophageal sphincter relaxation.
- *Presentation*: Vomiting, dysphagia with solids or liquids, FTT, aspiration
- *Diagnosis*: Barium swallow (dilated tapering lower esophagus) or esophageal manometry
- *Treatment*: Nifedipine (short term), endoscopic balloon dilatation, Heller's cardiomyotomy

Benign esophageal stricture
Causes include severe GERD, caustic ingestion, and radiation therapy.

Treatment
Treat the underlying cause, e.g., reduce gastric acid production in GERD; perform balloon endoscopic dilatation.

Pancreatitis

Acute pancreatitis

This disorder consists of acute pancreatic inflammation with variable involvement of local tissues and remote organ systems; it is rare.

Causes
- Blunt abdominal trauma
- Viral infection (e.g., mumps, hepatitis A, Coxsackie B)
- Multisystem disease (e.g., SLE, Kawasaki disease, hemolytic uremic syndrome, IBD, hyperlipidemia)
- Drugs and toxins (e.g., depakote, cytotoxic drugs)
- Pancreatic duct obstruction (e.g., CF, choledochal cyst, tumors)

Presentation
Abdominal pain involves upper central abdominal pain, radiating to the back, chest, or lower abdomen. There is also vomiting, fever, and abdominal tenderness.

Severe cases also exhibit the following:
- Hypotension
- Abdominal distension
- Cullen's or Grey–Turner's sign (bruising of periumbilical and flanks, respectively)
- Ascites
- Pleural effusion
- Jaundice
- Multi-organ failure

Investigations
- *Blood*: Amylase (↑↑), lipase (↑), Ca^{2+} (↓), abnormal LFT
- *Radiology*: Abdominal ultrasound or CT; after magnetic resonance retrograde cholangiopancreatography (MRCP) to diagnose ductal obstruction, endoscopic retrograde cholangiopancreatography (ERCP) to treat ductal obstruction

Treatment
Mild
- Supportive only, e.g., nasogastric tube, analgesia
- Start short period of NPO to "rest" pancreas

Severe
Treat as for the mild form, plus:
- Admit to intensive care unit
- Correct hypotension
- Treat multi-organ failure
- Surgery for significant pancreatic necrosis, major ductal rupture (trauma), gallstones (cholecystectomy), or presence of pseudocyst. ERCP may be therapeutic for a structural obstructive cause.

Prognosis
- Complete recovery is likely if there is minimal organ dysfunction.
- 20% mortality if there is severe disease or organ failure present, or if local complications develop (e.g., pancreatic pseudocyst)
- Most children have only a single acute episode.

Chronic pancreatitis

Chronic pancreatitis follows acute pancreatitis with continuing inflammation, destruction of pancreatic tissue, and fibrosis, leading to permanent exocrine or endocrine pancreatic failure. It is very rare, and usually caused by cystic fibrosis, congenital ductal anomalies, sclerosing cholangitis (IBD), hyperlipidemia, or hypercalcemia.

Presentation
- Repeated episodes of acute pancreatitis are separated by good health.
- Eventually, features of pancreatic exocrine failure or diabetes mellitus become apparent.

Investigations
- Abdominal ultrasound or CT scan confirms chronic pancreatitis.
- Pancreatic function tests may be useful, e.g., stool chymotrypsin (↑), pancreozymin-secretin test, 72-hour fecal fat measurement (↑)

Treatment
- Treat acute episodes as for acute pancreatitis, plus give pancreatic enzyme replacement and nutritional supplementation (well-balanced diet with moderated fat intake and fat-soluble vitamins).
- Relieve ductal obstruction by ERCP or surgery.

Prognosis
Recovery or long-term pancreatic exocrine or endocrine failure is dependent on cause.

Intestinal disorders

Gastritis and peptic ulcer disease
This disease is rare in children. It most commonly affects the duodenum.

Causes
- *H. pylori* infection (strong familial link, associated with increased risk of adult gastric cancer)
- Stress ulcers, (e.g., post-trauma)
- Drug related, (e.g., NSAIDs); ↑acid secretion (Zollinger–Ellison syndrome, multiple endocrine neoplasia type I, hyperparathyroidism)
- Crohn's disease
- Eosinophilic gastroenteritis
- Hypertrophic gastritis
- Autoimmune gastritis

Presentation
Often this condition is asymptomatic while the following occurs:
- Chronic abdominal and epigastric pain
- Nausea ± vomiting
- GI hemorrhage
- FTT ± anorexia
- Iron deficiency anemia
- Perforation (very rare)
- Obstruction

Investigation
- C^{14} urea breath test (*H. pylori*)
- Upper GI endoscopy and biopsy (*H. pylori* histology and culture)
- *H. pylori* stool antigen

Treatment
- Treat cause (e.g., eradicate *H. pylori* with 7–10 days oral clarithromycin, bismuth, metronidazole ± omeprazole [quadruple therapy])
- ↓gastric acid production, e.g., proton pump inhibitors (PPI), H_2 antagonists; sucralfate (cytoprotective)
- Antacids, e.g., aluminum hydroxide

Protein-losing enteropathy
This disorder is characterized by chronic intestinal protein loss.

Causes
- GI infection, e.g., giardiasis
- Severe food hypersensitivity
- Celiac disease or IBD
- Severe cardiac failure
- SLE; graft versus host disease
- Lymphatic obstruction

Presentation
There is hypoalbuminemia ± diarrhea or abdominal pain. ↑fecal α_1-antitrypsin confirms condition.

Treatment
Treat underlying disease; give albumin infusions as required.

Short bowel syndrome
Malabsorption, fluid and electrolyte loss, and malnutrition follow massive small bowel loss or resection.

Presentation
• Diarrhea, steatorrhea
• FTT
• Dehydration, electrolyte loss (Na, K, Mg, Ca)
• Cholestasis (bile salt loss)
• Peptic ulcer disease ($\uparrow$ gastrin)
• Specific (e.g., vitamin B_{12}) ± generalized malnutritional disorders
• Renal stones (oxalate)

Treatment
• Correct fluid and electrolyte disturbance
• Specific nutritional supplements; elemental diets
• PN
• PPI or H_2 antagonists
• Antidiarrheal drugs, e.g., loperamide
• Cholestyramine (chelates bile salts)
• Parenteral somatostatin
• Oral antibiotics ($\downarrow$ bacterial overgrowth)
• Surgery to $\downarrow$ GI motility or small bowel transplant

Prognosis
Prognosis is improving, with 90% 5-year survival. Retention of ileocecal valve significantly improves prognosis.

Intestinal polyps
Most juvenile polyps are hamartomas, single and located in the distal colon. Polyposis (multiple polyps) syndromes include the following:
• Peutz–Jegher's syndrome (mucocutaneous pigmentation)
• Familial polyposis coli
• Gardner's syndrome (osteomas and soft tissues tumors)

Presentation
• Often asymptomatic
• Hematochezia
• Rectal polyp prolapse
• Protein-losing enteropathy
• Intussusception

Investigation
• Colonoscopy or barium enema

Treatment
• Endoscopic or surgical removal
• Periodic colonoscopy surveillance is required in polyposis syndrome because of significant risk of neoplasm.

Inflammatory bowel disease

The incidence of IBD is ~5–15/100,000 per year. Crohn's disease (CD) is more common than ulcerative colitis (UC) in children. The cause is unknown, although there is a recognized genetic predisposition in Crohn's. A family history of IBD confers a high risk for developing IBD.

Ulcerative colitis

- Involves the colon only
- Rectal (proctitis) is most common or may extend continuously to involve entire colon (pancolitis)
- Terminal ileum may be affected by "backwash ileitis."

Crohn's disease

- May affect any part of the GI tract, but terminal ileum and proximal colon are the most common
- Unlike UC, bowel involvement is noncontinuous ("skip" lesions).
- Characteristic noncaseating granuloma is present on biopsy samples.

Presentation

Symptoms
- Anorexia; weight loss; lethargy
- Abdominal cramps
- Diarrhea ± blood/mucous; urgency and tenesmus (proctitis); rarely constipation
- Fever
- Anemia

GI signs
- Aphthous oral ulcers
- Abdominal tenderness
- Abdominal distension; RLQ mass (CD)
- Perianal disease (CD), i.e. abscess, sinus, fistula, skin tags, fissure, stricture

Non-GI signs and associations
- Fever
- Finger clubbing
- Anemia
- Erythema nodosum
- Pyoderma gangrenosum
- Arthritis; ankylosing spondylitis
- Iritis; conjunctivitis; episcleritis
- Poor growth
- Delayed puberty; hepatic disease
- Sclerosing cholangitis
- Renal stones
- Nutritional deficiencies (e.g., vitamin B_{12})

Complications
- "Toxic" colon dilatation (UC > CD)
- GI perforation or strictures, pseudopolyps
- Massive GI hemorrhage
- Colon carcinoma (higher risk with prolonged, severe disease)
- Fistula involving bowel only or bowel and skin, vagina, or bladder (CD)
- Abdominal and pelvic abscesses (CD)
- Hypercoagulability
- Depression, anxiety

Investigations
- Stool culture, P&P, *C. difficile* if at risk (infectious disease can mimic CD and UC)

Blood
- CBC; ESR/CRP (↑); albumin (↓); blood culture; iron indices (↓); vitamin B_{12} and folate (↓)

Serum serological markers
These are NOT indicated in the primary-care setting.

Endoscopy
- Esophagogastroduodenoscopy (EGD) and colonoscopy are used to determine the extent and pattern of abnormal mucosa and intestinal biopsy. UC histology shows crypt abscesses, mucosal and lamina propria inflammation only, and goblet cell depletion. CD histology shows granulomas and transmural inflammation.

Intestinal imaging
- Imaging is needed if stricture is suspected, there are disease complications (e.g., abscess) and to evaluate small intestinal involvement. Different options include barium study, CT scan, MR enterography, and capsule endoscopy.

Treatment

Supportive treatment

Provide supportive treatment if disease is severe, e.g., bowel rest, IV hydration, TPN.

Drug treatment

- *Mild–moderate disease*: 5-aminosalicylic acid (ASA) compounds (mesalamine, sulfazalazine) may be useful to induce and maintain colonic disease remission in UC. These are also available in enema form for treating rectal disease. Dietary therapy (exclusive liquid formula) is effective but has a high relapse rate.
- *Moderate–severe disease*
  - *Induce remission* with oral prednisone or IV methylprednislone, 1–2 mg/kg/day until condition is improved (<2 weeks), then wean over 6–8 weeks. Long-term steroid treatment must be avoided. Give infliximab infusion (approved in children). Cyclosporin is less commonly used. Surgery is indicated for severe, unresponsive disease and with perforation.
  - *Maintenance*: Azathioprine/6-mercaptopurine, which may need 3–6 months for results, close lab monitoring. Methotrexate weekly (add folic acid). Infliximab. Rarely tacrolimus, cyclosporine.
- Probiotics, antibiotics, e.g., ciprofloxacin or metronidazole may be helpful but have an unestablished role.
- Dietary support: Provide ample protein and calorie intake, vitamins, iron, and trace elements.
- Non-adherence is a major cause of treatment failure.

Surgery

- *UC*: Total colectomy and ileostomy, pouch creation and anal anastomosis (cures UC). Result in 10%–20% pouch complications (e.g., pouchitis), infertility
- *CD*: Ileocecal resection is considered in severe isolated CD inflammation of the terminal ileum; inflammation recurrence is universal. Surgery is needed for symptomatic strictures, internal fistula, and persistent abscesses.

Prognosis

UC and CD are marked by relapse and remission. Patients can have a very good quality of life with current therapy.

Celiac disease

Celiac disease is enteropathy due to intolerance of gluten protein (present in wheat, barley, and rye). Prevalence is ~1 in 2500. It is associated with
- Type I diabetes
- Down syndrome

Presentation

The condition may present at any age after starting gluten in the diet. The classic features include the following:
- Diarrhea
- Paleness
- Bulky, floating stools
- Anorexia
- FTT
- Irritability

Later, there is
- Apathy
- Gross motor developmental delay
- Ascites
- Peripheral edema
- Anemia
- Delayed puberty
- Arthralgia; hypotonia
- Muscle wasting
- Specific nutritional disorders

Celiac crises

Life-threatening dehydration is due to diarrhea accompanying malabsorption. This condition is rare, except in the less-developed world.

Investigations

Serum
- Anti-endomysial IgA antibody
- Tissue transglutaminase IgA antibody

Fecal
- Fat studies
- *Small bowel biopsy*: Endoscopy with biopsy of proximal small intestine shows diffuse, subtotal villus atrophy, increased intraepithelial lymphocytes, and crypt hyperplasia. Villi return to near normal on a gluten-free diet

Most clinicians consider positive mucosal histology and full clinical recovery on gluten-free diet ± positive IgA antibodies sufficient to make a diagnosis. Avoid gluten challenge (>10 g oral gluten per day for 3–4 months) and re-biopsy unless the diagnosis is in doubt (e.g., biopsy is inadequate or not typical, or alternative diagnosis is possible—transient gluten intolerance may occur after gastroenteritis, giardiasis, and cow's milk protein intolerance).

Treatment
- Gluten-free diet under supervision of pediatric dietitian
- Gluten avoidance should be life-long if celiac disease is confirmed.
- Nutritional supplements may be required.

Prognosis
Prognosis is excellent if patient is compliant with strict, lifelong gluten-free diet. There is a possible increased risk of intestinal lymphoma if gluten is ingested, even in asymptomatic celiac disease.

Gastrointestinal infections

These infections are the second-most common cause of primary care consultation after the common cold. It is a major cause of pediatric morbidity and mortality worldwide (see also p. 160).

Viral gastroenteritis

Transmission is by fecal–oral route, including contaminated water. Epidemics are frequent (usually in winter). Breastfeeding is protective. Severity is increased in malnourished children.

Causes
- Rotavirus (most common)
- Norwalk agent
- Enteric adenovirus
- Astrovirus
- CMV (in immunocompromised patients)

Presentation
- Watery diarrhea
- Vomiting
- Cramping abdominal pain
- Fever
- Dehydration
- Electrolyte disturbance
- Vomiting predominate with Norwalk virus

Investigation
Investigation is rarely necessary. See diarrhea (p. 358).

Treatment
Give supportive rehydration orally or with nasogastric (NG) tube or IV with glucose/electrolyte solution. Hospitalization is rarely needed (e.g., in patients with ≥10% dehydration or who are unable to tolerate oral fluids).

Prognosis
Symptoms generally last <7 days, except in enteric adenovirus, in which diarrhea frequently goes on beyond 14 days. The patient may develop transient secondary lactose intolerance.

Prevention
Rotavirus vaccine is now available and effective.

Bacterial gastroenteritis

Bacterial gastroenteritis causes secretory and inflammatory diarrhea It is more common under 2 years of age. Causative organisms include the following:

- *Salmonella* species
- *Campylobacter jejuni*
- *Shigella* species
- *Yersinia enterocolitica*
- *E. coli*
- *Clostridium difficile*
- *Vibrio cholerae*

Sources

These include contaminated water, poor food hygiene (meat, fresh produce, chicken, eggs, previously cooked rice), and fecal–oral route.

Presentation

The wide range of symptoms include

- Watery diarrhea
- Dysentery (bloody and mucus-like diarrhea)
- Malaise
- Abdominal pain may mimic appendicitis or IBD
- Fever
- Tenesmus

Complications

- Bacteremia
- Secondary infections (particularly *Salmonella*, *Campylobacter*), e.g., pneumonia
- Osteomyelitis, meningitis
- Reiter's syndrome (*Shigella*, *Campylobacter*)
- Hemolytic uremic syndrome (*E. coli* 0157, *Shigella*)
- Guillain–Barré syndrome (*Campylobacter*)
- Reactive arthropathy (*Yersinia*)
- Hemorrhagic colitis

Investigation (see Diarrhea p. 358)

- Stool ± blood culture (some organisms need specific culture medium)
- Stool *Clostridium difficile* toxin
- Sigmoidoscopy (colitis)

Treatment

- Rehydration as for viral gastroenteritis
- Antibiotics are not indicated, as the duration of symptoms is not altered and may increase chronic carrier status, unless there is a high risk of disseminated disease, presence of artificial implants (e.g., V-P shunt), severe colitis, severe systemic illness, age <6 months, enteric fever (see p. 802), cholera, or *E. coli* 0157. Most organisms are sensitive to ampicillin, cotrimoxazole, or third-generation cephalosporins. Consider
    - Erythromycin if campylobacter
    - Oral vancomycin or metronidazole if there is *Clostridium difficile*

Parasitic gastroenteritis

Infection is usually via the fecal–oral route. Pets and livestock can be hosts. Parasitic infection conditions can mimic IBD, hepatitis, sclerosing cholangitis, peptic ulcer disease, and celiac disease.

Presentation

- Abdominal pain
- Diarrhea; dysentery; flatulence
- FTT and malabsorption
- Abdominal distension
- Intestinal obstruction
- Biliary obstruction; liver disease
- Pancreatitis
- Fever

Investigations (see Diarrhea, p. 358)

Protozoa

Giardia lamblia

These are very common. Swallowed cysts develop into trophozoites that attach to the small intestinal, causing malabsorption.

Presentation

- Diarrhea, flatulence, abdominal discomfort

Treatment

- Metronidazole or nitazoxanide

Entamoeba histolytica

Symptoms are usually mild but may cause the following:
- Fulminating colitis (amoebic dysentery can mimic ulcerative colitis)
- Intestinal obstruction due to a chronic localized lesion (an "amoeboma")
- Amoebic hepatitis
- Liver abscess (right upper quadrant pain, fever, hepatomegaly)

Treatment

- Metronidazole

Cryptosporidium

This is a mild self-limiting illness, except in immunocompromised patients, in whom it can cause
- Severe chronic watery diarrhea
- Flatulence
- Malaise
- Abdominal pain
- Weight loss

Treatment

- Nitazoxanide, also erythromycin, metronidazole, or spiramycin

Nematodes

Ascaris lumbricoides

These look like earthworms and can cause Loeffler's syndrome (eosinophilic pneumonitis, which mimics asthma).

Treatment
- Mebendazole, albendazole, pyrantel pamoate

Trichuris trichiura (whip worm)

These nematodes live in the colon and causes diarrhea, abdominal pain, and weight loss.

Treatment
- Mebendazole or albendazole

Hookworms (Necator americanus, Ancylostoma duodenale)

Hookworms enter via the skin (e.g., bare feet) and live in the intestine, sucking blood. This leads to anemia and hypoproteinemia.

Treatment
- Mebendazole

Strongyloides stercoralis

- This species penetrates the skin and migrates to the lungs. They are then coughed up and ingested into the gut.
- This condition causes bloating, heartburn, and malabsorption.

Treatment
- Mebendazole, albendazole, or thiabendazole

Enterobius vermicularis (thread or pinworm)

This condition is very common and causes anal pruritus as females emerge and lay eggs in the perianal region. Diagnosis is confirmed by direct visualization of worms on the perianal area or in the stool, or via microscopy of clear tape applied to the anus.

Treatment
- Mebendazole

Cestodes (tapeworms)

Infection is by ingesting undercooked contaminated pork (*Taenia solium*), beef (*Taenia saginata*), or fish (*Diphyllobothrium latum*). Diagnosis is by microscopy of eggs or proglottides in the stool.

Treatment
- Praziquantel

Acute hepatitis

Viral causes

- *Hepatitis A (HAV)*: Incubation 2–6 weeks, fecal–oral transmission
- *Hepatitis B (HBV)*: Incubation 6 weeks to 6 months. Endemic in the Far East and Africa. Transmission is from
  - Blood products
  - IV drug abuse
  - Sexual intercourse
  - Close direct contact (e.g., intrafamilial)
  - Vertical transmission (may cause fulminant hepatitis)
- *Hepatitis C (HCV)*: Incubation 2 weeks to 6 months. Transmission is as for HBV. Usually asymptomatic. HCV rarely causes acute hepatitis.
- *Hepatitis E*: Fecal–oral transmission, endemic in India
- *Hepatitis D*: Requires previous HBV infection
- *Hepatitis G*: Parenteral transmission

Other organisms can cause hepatitis as part of systemic infection: Epstein–Barr virus (EBV; common in adolescents, 40% have hepatitis); TORCH organisms (neonatal hepatitis), HIV, CMV (immunocompromised), *Listeria*.

Other causes

- *Poisons and drugs*, e.g., acetaminophen, isoniazid, halothane
- *Metabolic disease*, e.g., Wilson's disease, tyrosinemia type I
- *Autoimmune hepatitis*. May present with acute hepatitis

Reye's syndrome

Acute encephalopathic illness is associated with aspirin therapy and microvesicular fatty infiltration of the liver. Reye's syndrome is rare. Prodrome (nausea, vomiting, hypoglycemia, abdominal pain) occurs 2–3 days before onset of jaundice or abnormal LFT.

Presentation

Acute hepatic failure (encephalopathy and coagulopathy) may rarely occur. Many infections are asymptomatic, particularly HAV and HCV. There are many presentations:

- Fever
- Fatigue
- Malaise
- Anorexia
- Nausea
- Arthralgia
- Right upper quadrant abdominal pain
- Jaundice ± hepatomegaly
- Splenomegaly
- Adenopathy
- Urticaria

Investigations

- LFT: ↑bilirubin >2 mg/dL; ↑AST/ALT (2x ULN)
- ↓blood glucose (especially in Reye' syndrome)
- Viral serology (IgM antibodies), viral PCR (HCV), EBV heterophil antibodies (Monospot). Get blood culture if appropriate
- Acetaminophen level or halothane antibodies, if relevant
- Serum immunoglobulin, complement (C3, C4), positive autoimmune antibodies (anti-smooth muscle, anti-nuclear or anti-liver kidney microsomal) in autoimmune hepatitis
- Serum copper/ceruloplasmin, 24-hour urinary copper (Wilson's disease)
- Urinary succinylacetone (tyrosinemia type I)

Management

Usually none is required, except support and rest.
- Alcohol avoidance in teenagers
- There is no place for antivirals unless the patient is immunocompromised.
- Fulminant hepatitis requires referral to a liver transplantation center.
- Reye's syndrome: Maintain blood glucose >60 mg/dL; prevent sepsis; provide intensive care support.

Prognosis

- Acute hepatitis is usually self-limiting.
- Mortality after fulminant hepatitis is ~30% if both cerebral edema and renal failure are absent, ~70% if both are present without liver transplant.

There is a long-term risk of
- Chronic hepatitis (HAV 0%, HBV 5%–90%, HCV ~85%)
- Cirrhosis
- Hepatocellular carcinoma (HBV and HCV)
- Glomerulonephritis (circulating immunocomplexes)

Prevention

Active immunization exists for both HAV and HBV. Following infectious contact, infection may be prevented by giving within 24 hours pooled serum immunoglobulin for HAV and CMV, or specific HBV serum immunoglobulin for HBV.

Chronic liver failure

Causes
- Chronic hepatitis (after viral hepatitis B or C)
- Biliary tree disease, e.g., biliary atresia
- Toxin induced, e.g., alcohol
- α_1-antitrypsin deficiency
- Autoimmune hepatitis
- Wilson's disease (age >3 years)
- Cystic fibrosis
- Alagille syndrome, or nonsyndromic paucity of the bile ducts
- Tyrosinemia
- Primary sclerosing cholangitis (PSC)
- TPN induced
- Budd–Chiari syndrome

Presentation
- Jaundice (not always)
- GI hemorrhage (portal hypertension and variceal bleeding)
- Pruritis
- FTT
- Anemia
- Enlarged hard liver (though liver is often small in cirrhosis)
- Non-tender splenomegaly
- Hepatic stigmata, e.g., spider nevi
- Peripheral edema and/or ascites
- Nutritional disorders, e.g., rickets
- Developmental delay or deterioration in school performance
- Chronic encephalopathy

Investigations
Blood tests
- LFT ($\uparrow$or $\leftrightarrow$bilirubin, $\uparrow$AST/ALT (2–10 x ULN), albumin <3.5 g/dL)
- CBC ($\downarrow$Hb if GI bleeding); $\downarrow$WBC and platelets (hypersplenism)
- Coagulation (prothrombin time [PT] $\uparrow$)
-    Blood glucose
- Electrolytes ($\downarrow Na^+$, or $\downarrow Ca^{2+}$, $\uparrow PO_4^{3-}$, $\uparrow$alkaline phosphatase if biochemical rickets)
- Viral serology or PCR for hepatitis B and C
- $\uparrow$IgG, $\downarrow$complement (C3, C4), autoimmune antibodies (see p. 398)

Metabolic studies
- Sweat test (CF); α_1-antitrypsin level and phenotype
- $\downarrow$serum copper and ceruloplasmin
- $\uparrow$24-hour urinary copper (Wilson's disease)

Abdominal ultrasound
- Hepatomegaly
- Echogenic liver
- Splenomegaly
- Ascites

Upper GI endoscopy
- Esophageal or gastric varices
- Portal gastritis

EEG
- To confirm chronic encephalopathy if suspected

Liver biopsy
- Histology; enzymes; electron microscopy (EM)

Management

Treat underlying cause and give nutritional support:
- Lower protein, increased kcal, carbohydrate diet
- Vitamin supplementation, particularly fat-soluble vitamins A, D, E, and K. Involve dietitian

Drug therapy
- Prednisone ± azathioprine for autoimmune hepatitis
- Interferon-γ ± ribavirin for chronic viral hepatitis
- Penicillamine and B_6 vit/trientine for Wilson's disease
- Cholestyramine may be useful to control severe pruritis.
- Vitamin K_1 and FFP (10 mL/kg) if there is significant coagulopathy or bleeding

Esophageal varices
- Endoscopy, i.e., sclerotherapy, or surgery

Ascites
- Na+ restriction (1 mmol/kg/day)
- Spironolactone (1–2 mg/kg 12 hourly) and furosemide
- Consider IV 25% albumin if ascites serum level <2.5 mg/dL

Encephalopathy
- ↓GI ammonia absorption: Use oral/rectal lactulose

Liver transplantation

Prognosis

There is up to 50% 5-year mortality without liver transplantation. Poor prognostic factors are as follows:
- Bilirubin >5 mg/dL
- Albumin <3 g/dL
- PT INR >2
- Poorly controlled ascites
- Encephalopathy
- Malnutrition

α_1-Antitrypsin deficiency

α_1-Antitrypsin is a serum protease inhibitor.
- It is the most common genetic cause of liver disease in children, with autosomal recessive inheritance.
- Prevalence is 1:2000 to 1:7000.
- Genetic variants are identified by enzyme electrophoretic mobility as medium (M), slow (S), or very slow (Z). S is associated with ~60% α_1-antitrypsin level of normal, Z ~15%. Normal genotype is PiMM. Only PiZZ individuals are at risk of liver disease.

Presentation
- Cholestasis in infancy, may progress to liver failure
- Cirrhosis in late childhood to adult. Chronic liver disease affects 25% of patients in late adulthood.
- Pulmonary emphysema is the most common presentation in adulthood.

Diagnosis
- α_1-antitrypsin phenotype or genotype

Treatment
- Supportive treatment of liver complications
- Advise against smoking
- Liver transplant for end-stage liver failure

Wilson's disease

This rare autosomal recessive disorder leads to toxic accumulation of copper in the liver and, subsequently, other tissues, especially the brain (see also p. 1012).

Presentation
- Kayser–Fleischer rings (copper deposition in the eye, Descemet's membrane) may be present (~45% with hepatic presentations and 90% with neurological) but may require slit-lamp examination for visualization.
- Hepatic presentations usually occur in childhood and adolescence (hepatitis, cirrhosis, fulminant hepatic failure)
- Adults (and older adolescents) usually present with neurological disease.

Investigations
- Ceruloplasmin is low (but a normal level does not exclude diagnosis).
- Serum copper may be low, normal, or elevated. Calculated free (non-ceruloplasmin bound) copper is usually elevated >25 µg/dL
- 24-hour urinary copper excretion >100 µg/day (normal <40 g/day)
- Liver copper >250 µg/g dry weight
- Wilson's disease gene (*ATP7B*) mutation analysis

Treatment
- Chelation therapy (penicilamine or trientine)
- Zinc
- Liver transplantation if there is end-stage hepatic failure

Liver transplantation

Indications for liver transplantation

- Fulminant hepatic failure (e.g., viral, toxic, Wilson disease)
- Acute liver failure post-liver transplant—primary non-function, hepatic artery thrombosis
- Chronic end-stage liver disease
- Chronic liver disease with unacceptable quality of life correctable by transplantation (e.g., severe pruritus, hepatopulmonary syndrome)
- Unresectable tumor confined to the liver (e.g., hepatoblastoma)
- Liver-based metabolic disease causing injury to other tissues (e.g., oxalosis, urea cycle disorder, Crigler–Najjar syndrome)

Clinical features of chronic liver disease requiring consideration for transplantation

- Portal hypertension with bleeding varices
- Growth failure or developmental delay
- Resistant ascites
- Encephalopathy and fatigue
- Intractable pruritus
- Coagulopathy (INR >2× normal)
- Hepatorenal syndrome
- Hepatopulmonary syndrome

Preparation for transplant

Multidisciplinary evaluation includes the following:
- Meet with transplant physician, surgeon, and nurse coordinator for education and counseling
- Social work support
- Nutritional support
- Developmental and psychological assessment
- Ensure that immunizations are current (e.g., MMR, varicella, hepatitis A and B)
- Cardiac evaluation (ECG, echocardiogram)
- Insurance and financial counseling

Post- transplant complications

- Primary non-function of the liver (<5%)
- Hepatic artery thrombosis (10%)
- Biliary leaks and strictures (20%)
- Acute rejection (40%)
- Chronic rejection (5%)
- Sepsis (main cause of death)

Prognosis

Long-term studies indicate psychosocial development and quality of life in survivors improve after transplantation. Patients require lifelong immuno-suppression drug therapy, e.g., tacrolimus.
- 1-year survival: 90%
- 5-year survival: 85%

Nephrology

Hematuria

Hematuria is the presence of red blood cells in the urine. The presence of 10 or more RBCs per high-power field is abnormal. Hematuria may be visible to the naked eye or it may be microscopic and detected only by dipstick testing or by microscopy. Urinary dipsticks are very sensitive and can be positive at <5 RBCs per high-power field. In one study, 3%–4% of unselected school-age children between 6 and 15 years of age had a positive dipstick for blood in a single urine sample.

It is important to distinguish hematuria into a proper category since evaluation and follow-up will vary. The categories are

- Asymptomatic isolated microscopic hematuria
- Asymptomatic microscopic hematuria with proteinuira
- Symptomatic hematuria and gross hematuria

In gross hematuria, glomerular bleeding often results in brown urine, while lower urinary tract bleeding often results in pink or red urine accompanied by blood clots.

Presentation

- Episode of macroscopic hematuria (causes alarm to child and family)
- Incidental finding of microscopic hematuria when being investigated for other urinary tract symptoms
- Family screening and routine urinalysis

Other causes of "red urine"

The following causes can usually be distinguished from hematuria by taking a careful history and with urine dipstick testing and microscopy:

- Hemoglobinuria, myoglobinuria
- Foods with coloring (e.g., beetroot)
- Drugs (e.g., rifampin, phenazopyridine)
- Urate crystals (in young infants usually "pink" diapers)
- External source (e.g., menstrual blood losses)
- Metabolites associated with other clinical conditions (e.g., porphyria)
- Fictitious—consider if no cause is found

Causes of hematuria

- Urinary tract infections
  - Bacterial
  - Viral (e.g., adenovirus)
  - Schistosomiasis (history of foreign travel)
  - Tuberculosis
- Glomerular
  - Postinfectious glomerulonephritis
  - IgA nephropathy, Henoch–Schönlein Purpura (HSP), focal segmented glomerulosclerosis (FSGS), SLE
  - Hereditary: Thin basement membrane, Alport syndrome
- Urinary tract stones—hypercalciuria
- Trauma
- Uretheral injury

- Other renal tract pathology
  - Renal tract tumor
  - Polycystic kidney disease
- Vascular
  - Renal vein thrombosis
  - Arteritis
- Hematological: Coagulopathy, sickle cell disease
- Drugs: cyclophosphamide
- Exercise-induced

History

- Urinary tract infection (UTI): Fever, frequency, dysuria
- Renal stones: Colicky abdominal pain, radiation
- Glomerular: Sore throat or rashes, brown urine
- Coagulopathy: Easy bruising
- Trauma
- Uretheral injury: Terminal hematuria
- Exercise induced
- Family history: Hematuria, deafness (Alport syndrome)

Examination

- Vitals: Weight and BP
- Abdomen: Palpable masses
- Skin: Rashes
- Extremities: Edema, pain and swelling at joints

Investigations and treatment

Asymptomatic isolated microscopic hematuria:
- Urinalysis (UA) with culture. If negative, repeat BP and UA in 1–2 weeks with no prior exercise
  - If patient remains asymptomatic, repeat physical exam, BP, and UA in 3–6 months
  - If isolated hematuria persists for 1 year, get urine calcium/creatinine ratio, test parents and siblings

Asymptomatic microscopic hematuria with proteinuria:
- Check renal function panel, spot U protein/creatinine ratio on first morning sample or 24-hour urine collection
  - If protein excretion is within an acceptable range, reevaluate in 2–3 weeks
  - If there is above-normal proteinuria, abnormal renal function, or persistent proteinuria, refer patient to pediatric nephrology and check CBC, C3, C4, albumin, microscopic examination of urine, and renal ultrasound.
- Consider Antistreptolysin O (ASO) titer, streptozyme, antinuclear antigen (ANA), and anti-neutrophil cytoplasmic antibodies (ANCA)

Symptomatic hematuria (may be nonspecific such as fever, malaise, and weight loss; extrarenal such as rash, purpura, and arthritis; or kidney related such as edema, hypertension, dysuria, and oliguria) and/or gross hematuria:

- UA with microscopic examination (look for RBC casts and dysmorphic RBCs) and a culture
- Check urine calcium/creatinine ratio and renal ultrasound.
- Tailor evaluation based on history and physical findings.
  - Recent trauma: CT scan of abdomen and pelvis
  - Suspect nephrolithiasis: Renal ultrasound and/or spiral CT scan
  - Suspect perineal/meatal irritation: Supportive care and reassurance
  - History of recent pharyngitis, impetigo, or upper respiratory infection: Glomerulonephritis evaluation
  - Suspect glomerular disease (proteinuira, RBC casts or dysmorphic RBC on urine microscopic examination, edema, hypertension): Serum electrolytes, renal function, CBC, C3, C4, albumin, and a referral to pediatric nephrology. Consider ASO titer, streptozyme, ANA, and ANCA
  - History of predisposing clinical conditions: Sickle cell disease or trait, a coagulopathy, or deafness
  - Recent vigorous exercise: Exercise-induced hematuria is a diagnosis of exclusion, including rhabdomyolysis
  - Cystoscopy is rarely indicated in children.

Refer patient to pediatric nephrology if there is a complex diagnosis (impaired renal function, proteinuria, or family history) or change in any parameters.

Proteinuria

Proteinuria is defined as excessive urinary protein excretion and is a well-established marker for renal disease. The challenge is to differentiate patients with transient or other benign forms of proteinuria from those with renal disease. Urinary protein excretion in a normal child is <100 mg/m^2/day or up to total of 150 mg/day. In neonates, the normal urinary excretion rate is higher, up to 300 mg/m^2/day.

Detection of proteinuria

Urinalysis
Performed by dipstick testing (see Box 11.1), urinalysis is a cheap, practicable, sensitive method that primarily detects albumin in the urine. It is less sensitive for other forms of proteinuria.

Box 11.1 Urinalysis by dipstick testing	
Test result	**Equivalent protein estimate**
Trace	15–30 mg/dL
+	20–100 mg/dL
++	100–300 mg/dL
+++	300–1000 mg/dL
++++	>1000 mg/dL

Protein/creatinine ratio (UP:UCr)
Collection of an early-morning urine specimen for measurement of the urinary protein to creatinine ratio is especially useful in young children, from whom it may be difficult to obtain timed urine. The ratio provides a gross estimate of 24-hour urinary protein excretion by multiplying the ratio by 1000 (e.g., ratio of 0.6 mg/mg creatinine approximately translates to 600 mg/24 hr of urinary protein excretion).

> Normal: <0.2 mg protein/mg creatinine (children >2 years old)
> <0.5 mg protein/mg creatinine (children 6–24 months)

24-hour urinary protein excretion
This is the gold-standard test and requires a 24-hour collection of urine to estimate urinary protein excretion. The patient should discard the first morning urine into the toilet, then collect every void thereafter into the collection container. The last void in the container will be the first morning void the next day to complete a 24-hour cycle.

> Normal   <100 mg/m^2/day or 4 mg/m^2/hr
>
> Nephrotic range   >1000 mg/m^2/day or 40 mg/m^2/hr

Causes
Proteinuria may be due to benign or pathological causes.

Nonpathological proteinuria

Transient
- Fever
- Exercise
- Urinary tract infection
- Seizures
- Hypovolemia

Orthostatic proteinuria (postural proteinuria)
This is a common cause of referral in older children, particularly girls. There is usually no history of significance, and a normal examination. Investigations reveal a normal UP/UCr ratio in early-morning urine, with an elevated level in the afternoon specimen. This is regarded as a benign finding and requires no treatment.

Pathological (persistent) proteinuria
This may be seen in a number of renal disorders:
- Nephrotic syndrome
- Glomerulonephritis
- Chronic kidney disease
- Tubulointerstitial nephritis
- Diabetes mellitus (DM)

Investigations
Asymptomatic patients
- UP/UCr on the first morning urine (if normal, confirm orthostatic proteinuria by dipstick proteinuria on the second upright specimen)
- UA and a culture (treat if +UTI). Microscopic examination looking for signs of glomerular disease (RBC casts, dysmorphic RBCs)

If there is persistent proteinuria, check BP, serum electrolytes, renal function, cholesterol, and albumin, and refer patient to pediatric nephrology. Consider adding renal ultrasound, C3, C4, ANA, ASO titer, streptozyme, hepatitis B and C serology, and HIV testing.

If there is a history of febrile UTI or abnormal renal ultrasound, consider a voiding cystourethrogram (VCUG). A referral to pediatric nephrology and renal biopsy are indicated if there is abnormal BP, persistently elevated proteinuria (>500 mg/m^2/day), or abnormal renal function.

Symptomatic patients can have nonspecific, nonurinary, or renal-related symptoms.
- If there is heavy proteinuria or edema, promptly evaluate for nephrotic syndrome (see Nephrotic syndrome, p. 488) and refer patient to pediatric nephrology.
- In non-nephrotic range proteinuria with hypertension, abnormal urinalysis, or abnormal renal function, refer patient to pediatric nephrology.
- If there is a history of febrile UTI or abnormal renal ultrasound, consider VCUG.

Urinary tract infection (UTI)

Up to 3% of girls and 1% of boys suffer from UTI during childhood. A UTI may be defined in terms of the presence of symptoms (dysuria, frequency, loin pain) plus the detection of an organism from a urine culture.

Note: Bacteriuria in the absence of symptoms does not necessarily need treatment but needs to be considered in the clinical context (e.g., previous UTI, predisposing urinary tract abnormalities).

Clinical features

Presentation varies; symptoms in infants may be nonspecific:
- Fever (can be the sole manifestation <2 years old. The presence of another source does not rule out UTI.)
- Vomiting and diarrhea
- Poor feeding or failure to thrive
- Prolonged neonatal conjugated hyperbilirubinemia
- Hematuria
- Dysuria, urgency, frequency, incontinence in older children

History and examination

- Chronic symptoms, constipation, vesicoureteral reflux (VUR), previous undiagnosed febrile illnesses, family history of GU abnormalities, antenatally diagnosed renal abnormality, hypertension, use of barrier contraception with spermicidal agents in sexually active girls
- Height and weight—plot on growth chart
- Blood pressure
- Examination for abdominal masses, suprapubic and costovertebral tenderness
- Examine genitalia and spine for congenital abnormalities.
- Examine lower limbs for evidence of neuropathic bladder.

Diagnosis

Try to distinguish between the more serious upper (fever, vomiting, loin pain) and lower urinary tract symptoms (dysuria, frequency, mild abdominal pain, enuresis). Differentiation is often not possible in a younger child.
- UTI is a major cause of sepsis in a young infant. A lumbar puncture should be obtained for infants <1 month of age.
- Dipstick test in the urine. "Leukocytes" and "nitrites" strongly suggest UTI. Urine should be sent for microscopy, culture, and antibiotic sensitivity.
- >10^5 organisms/mL in pure growth from a carefully collected urine sample (catheterized, clean-catch urine). Two consecutive growths of the same organism with identical sensitivities are ideal but not always practical.
- Any growth on culture of suprapubic aspirate

Acute treatment

Antibiotics should be started after urine collection.

If the symptoms are mild, treat empirically with oral antibiotic until sensitivities are available, then narrow coverage for 7–14 days (AAP clinical practice guideline):

- Amoxicillin   20–40 mg/kg/day divided tid
- TMP-SMX   6–12 (TMP) mg/kg/day divided bid
- Cephalosporins

There may be increased resistance to amoxicillin-clavulanate, TMP-SMX, and first-generation cephalosporins, so consider use of third-generation cephalosporin if resistant organisms are suspected. Give antibiotics for shorter duration in children >2 years old and with good response.

For children <2 months old, ill, or toxic (high fever, vomiting), give IV antibiotics:

- Third- and fourth-generation IV cephalosporin or
- IV gentamicin 2.5 mg/kg/dose q8h alone or with ampicillin 25 mg/kg/dose q6h

Treatment should continue for at least 48 hours without a fever. Thereafter, a 7- to 10-day course can be completed orally (see above). Re-evaluate and include repeat urine culture if no expected clinical response occurs in 2 days.

Follow-up and investigations

Children presenting with UTI should be investigated to identify any renal scarring and any predisposing urinary tract abnormalities. Oral antibiotic prophylaxis should be started and continued until investigation is complete. Imaging studies can occur as soon as symptoms are resolved. Although imaging modality is controversial, current recommendations are as follows for renal ultrasound and VCUG:

- Girls under 3 years of age with first UTI
- Boys at any age with first UTI
- Children at any age with first febrile UTI
- Children with recurrent UTI with no previous imaging
- Children at any age with UTI with family history of kidney disease, hypertension, or abnormal urinary history

Consult with pediatric nephrology and urology on abnormal studies.

Prediction of which patients with UTI will develop long-term sequelae is very difficult.

UTI prevention

Provide patient and family education to reduce predisposing factors to recurrent UTIs:

- Treat and prevent constipation
- Hygiene—clean perineum front to back
- Avoid nylon underwear and bubble baths
- Encourage fluid intake and regular toileting with double micturition

Use of oral antibiotic prophylaxis (TMP-SMX 2 mg/kg at night or nitrofurantoin 1 mg/kg at night) is controversial in patients with VUR and/or frequent infections, given increased resistance in organisms in subsequent UTI and no association with lower frequency of recurrent UTI. Current evidence challenges routine prophylaxis.

Hypertension: definition

- Defined as average systolic blood pressure (SBP) and/or diastolic blood pressure (DBP) ≥95th percentile for sex, age, and height on three or more occasions (see Table 11.1a and Table 11.1b)
- SBP and DBP between 90th and 95th percentile defined as prehypertension
- Adolescents with BP ≥120/80 mmHg are prehypertensive
- Stage I hypertension: 95th to 99th percentile plus 5 mmHg
- Stage II hypertension: 99th percentile plus 5 mmHg
- White coat hypertension is defined as a patient with BP greater than 95th percentile in physician's office but normotensive outside of the clinical setting. This often requires 24-hour ambulatory blood pressure monitoring for diagnosis.

Blood pressure measurement should be part of routine examination.

Measurement technique

- Cuff size
  - Bladder width 40% mid-arm circumference
  - Bladder length completely encircle arm

Note: Small cuff area is a common cause of false positive high BP.

- After 5 minutes rest (ideally!)
- Sitting position with right arm at level of heart (children)
- Supine position for infants
- On ausculation, the first and fifth (disappearance) Korotkoff sounds are used for systolic and diastolic values, respectively.

Measurement devices

- Manual auscultation sphygmomanometer (mercury is now withdrawn)
- Doppler, for infants (for systolic pressure)
- Automatic oscillometry—not all devices are suitable
- 24-hour ambulatory blood pressure monitoring
- Intra-arterial (in ICU setting)

BP centile figures

Table 11.1a BP Levels for Boys by Age and Height Percentile

Age, y	BP Percentile	SBP, mm Hg/DBP, mm Hg						
		Percentile of Height						
		5th	10th	25th	50th	75th	90th	95th
1	50th	80/34	81/35	83/36	85/37	87/38	88/39	89/39
	90th	94/49	95/50	97/51	99/52	100/53	102/53	103/54
	95th	98/54	99/54	101/55	103/56	104/57	106/58	106/58
	99th	105/61	106/62	108/63	110/64	112/65	113/66	114/66
2	50th	84/39	85/40	87/41	88/42	90/43	92/44	92/44
	90th	84/39	99/55	100/56	102/57	104/58	105/58	106/59
	95th	97/54	102/59	104/60	106/61	108/62	109/63	110/63
	99th	101/59	110/67	111/68	113/69	115/70	117/71	117/71
3	50th	109/66	87/44	89/45	91/46	93/47	94/48	95/48
	90th	86/44	101/59	103/60	105/61	107/62	108/63	109/63
	95th	100/59	105/63	107/64	109/65	110/66	112/67	113/67
	99th	104/63	112/71	114/72	116/73	118/74	119/75	120/75
4	50th	111/71	89/48	91/49	93/50	95/51	96/51	97/52
	90th	88/47	103/63	105/64	107/65	109/66	110/66	111/67

Table 11.1a (Contd.)

Age, y	BP Percentile	SBP, mm Hg/DBP, mm Hg						
		Percentile of Height						
		5th	10th	25th	50th	75th	90th	95th
	95th	106/66	107/67	109/68	111/69	112/70	114/71	115/71
	99th	113/74	114/75	116/76	118/77	120/78	121/78	122/79
5	50th	90/50	91/51	93/52	95/53	96/54	98/55	98/55
	90th	104/65	105/66	106/67	108/68	110/69	111/69	112/70
	95th	108/69	109/70	110/71	112/72	114/73	115/74	116/74
	99th	115/77	116/78	118/79	120/80	121/81	123/81	123/82
6	50th	91/53	92/53	94/54	96/55	98/56	99/57	100/57
	90th	105/68	106/68	108/69	110/70	111/71	113/72	113/72
	95th	109/72	110/72	112/73	114/74	115/75	117/76	117/76
	99th	116/80	117/80	119/81	121/82	123/83	124/84	125/84
7	50th	92/55	94/55	95/56	97/57	99/58	100/59	101/59
	90th	106/70	107/70	109/71	111/72	113/73	114/74	115/74
	95th	110/74	111/74	113/75	115/76	117/77	118/78	119/78
	99th	117/82	118/82	120/83	122/84	124/85	125/86	126/86

		94/56	95/57	97/58	99/59	100/60	102/60	102/61
8	50th	94/56	95/57	97/58	99/59	100/60	102/60	102/61
	90th	107/71	109/72	110/72	112/73	114/74	115/75	116/76
	95th	111/75	112/76	114/77	116/78	118/79	119/79	120/80
	99th	119/83	120/84	122/85	123/86	125/87	127/87	127/88
9	50th	95/57	96/58	98/59	100/60	102/61	103/61	104/62
	90th	109/72	110/73	112/74	114/75	115/76	117/76	118/77
	95th	113/76	114/77	116/78	118/79	119/80	121/81	121/81
	99th	120/84	121/85	123/86	125/87	127/88	128/88	129/89
10	50th	97/58	98/59	100/60	102/61	103/61	105/62	106/63
	90th	111/73	112/73	114/74	115/75	117/76	119/77	119/78
	95th	115/77	116/78	117/79	119/80	121/81	122/81	123/82
	99th	122/85	123/86	125/86	127/88	128/88	130/89	130/90
11	50th	99/59	100/59	102/60	104/61	105/62	107/63	107/63
	90th	113/74	114/74	115/75	117/76	119/77	120/78	121/78
	95th	117/78	118/78	119/79	121/80	123/81	124/82	125/82
	99th	124/86	125/86	127/87	129/88	130/89	132/90	132/90

Table 11.1a (Contd.)

Age, y	BP Percentile	SBP, mm Hg/DBP, mm Hg						
		Percentile of Height						
		5th	10th	25th	50th	75th	90th	95th
12	50th	101/59	102/60	104/61	106/62	108/63	109/63	110/64
	90th	115/74	116/75	118/75	120/76	121/77	123/78	123/79
	95th	119/78	120/79	122/80	123/81	125/82	127/82	127/83
	99th	126/86	127/87	129/88	131/89	133/90	134/90	135/91
13	50th	104/60	105/60	106/61	108/62	110/63	111/64	112/64
	90th	117/75	118/75	120/76	122/77	124/78	125/79	126/79
	95th	121/79	122/79	124/80	126/81	128/82	129/83	130/83
	99th	128/87	130/87	131/88	133/89	135/90	136/91	137/91
14	50th	106/60	107/61	109/62	111/63	113/64	114/65	115/65
	90th	120/75	121/76	123/77	125/78	126/79	128/79	128/80
	95th	124/80	125/80	127/81	128/82	130/83	132/84	132/84
	99th	131/87	132/88	134/89	136/90	138/91	139/92	140/92

15	50th	109/61	110/62	112/63	113/64	115/65	117/66	117/66
	90th	122/76	124/77	125/78	127/79	129/80	130/80	131/81
	95th	126/81	127/81	129/82	131/83	133/84	134/85	135/85
	99th	134/88	135/89	136/90	138/91	140/92	142/93	142/93
16	50th	111/63	112/63	114/64	116/65	118/66	119/67	120/67
	90th	125/78	126/78	128/79	130/80	131/81	133/82	134/82
	95th	129/82	130/83	132/83	134/84	135/85	137/86	137/87
	99th	136/90	137/90	139/91	141/92	143/93	144/94	145/94
17	50th	114/65	115/66	116/66	118/67	120/68	121/69	122/70
	90th	127/80	128/80	130/81	132/82	134/83	135/84	136/84
	95th	131/84	132/85	134/86	136/87	138/87	139/88	140/89
	99th	139/92	140/93	141/93	143/94	145/95	146/96	147/97

* The 90th percentile is 1.28 SD, the 95th percentile is 1.645 SD, and the 99th percentile is 2.326 SD over the mean.

Reprinted with permission from The Fourth Report on the Diagnosis, Evaluation, and Treatment of High blood Pressure in children and Adolescents Pediatrics. August 2004; **114** supplement: 557–558.

Table 11.1b BP Levels for Girls by Age and Height Percentile

| Age, y | BP Percentile | SBP, mm Hg/DBP, mm Hg Percentile of Height | | | | | | |
		5th	10th	25th	50th	75th	90th	95th
1	50th	83/38	84/39	85/39	86/40	88/41	89/41	90/42
	90th	97/52	97/53	98/53	100/54	101/55	102/55	103/56
	95th	100/56	101/57	102/57	104/58	105/59	106/59	107/60
	99th	108/64	108/64	109/65	111/65	112/66	113/67	114/67
2	50th	85/43	85/44	87/44	88/45	89/46	91/46	91/47
	90th	98/57	99/58	100/58	101/59	103/60	104/61	105/61
	95th	102/61	103/62	104/62	105/63	107/64	108/65	109/65
	99th	109/69	110/69	111/70	112/70	114/71	115/72	116/72
3	50th	86/47	87/48	88/48	89/49	91/50	92/50	93/51
	90th	100/61	100/62	102/62	103/63	104/64	106/64	106/65
	95th	104/65	104/66	105/66	107/67	108/68	109/68	110/69
	99th	111/73	111/73	113/74	114/74	115/75	116/76	117/76
4	50th	88/50	88/50	90/51	91/52	92/52	94/53	94/54
	90th	101/64	102/64	103/65	104/66	106/67	107/67	108/68

	95th		105/68	106/68	107/69	108/70	110/71	111/71	112/72
	99th	112/76	113/76	114/76	115/77	117/78	118/79	119/79
5	50th	89/52	90/53	91/53	93/54	94/55	95/55	96/56
	90th	103/66	103/67	105/67	106/68	107/69	109/69	109/70
	95th	107/70	107/71	108/71	110/72	111/73	112/73	113/74
	99th	114/78	114/78	116/79	117/79	118/80	120/81	120/81
6	50th	91/54	92/54	93/55	94/56	96/56	97/57	98/58
	90th	104/68	105/68	106/69	108/70	109/70	110/71	111/72
	95th	108/72	109/72	110/73	111/74	113/74	114/75	115/76
	99th	115/80	116/80	117/80	119/81	120/82	121/83	122/83
7	50th	93/55	93/56	95/56	96/57	97/58	99/58	99/59
	90th	106/69	107/70	108/70	109/71	111/72	112/72	113/73
	95th	110/73	111/74	112/74	113/75	115/76	116/76	116/77
	99th	117/81	118/81	119/82	120/82	122/83	123/84	124/84
8	50th	95/57	95/57	96/57	98/58	99/59	100/60	101/60
	90th	108/71	109/71	110/71	111/72	113/73	114/74	114/74
	95th	112/75	112/75	114/75	115/76	116/77	118/78	118/78
	99th	119/82	120/82	121/83	122/83	123/84	125/85	125/86

Table 11.1b (Contd.)

Age, y	BP Percentile	SBP, mm Hg/DBP, mm Hg						
		Percentile of Height						
		5th	10th	25th	50th	75th	90th	95th
9	50th	96/58	97/58	98/58	100/59	101/60	102/61	103/61
	90th	110/72	110/72	112/72	113/73	114/74	116/75	116/75
	95th	114/76	114/76	115/76	117/77	118/78	119/79	120/79
	99th	121/83	121/83	123/84	124/84	125/85	127/86	127/87
10	50th	98/59	99/59	100/59	102/60	103/61	104/62	105/62
	90th	112/73	112/73	114/73	115/74	116/75	118/76	118/76
	95th	116/77	116/77	117/77	119/78	120/79	121/80	122/80
	99th	123/84	123/84	125/85	126/86	127/86	129/87	129/88
11	50th	100/60	101/60	102/60	103/61	105/62	106/63	107/63
	90th	114/74	114/74	116/74	117/75	118/76	119/77	120/77
	95th	118/78	118/78	119/78	121/79	122/80	123/81	124/81
	99th	125/85	125/85	126/86	128/87	129/87	130/88	131/89

12	50th	102/61	103/61	104/61	105/62	107/63	108/64	109/64
	90th	116/75	116/75	117/75	119/76	120/77	121/78	122/78
	95th	119/79	120/79	121/79	123/80	124/81	125/82	126/82
	99th	127/86	127/86	128/87	130/88	131/88	132/89	133/90
13	50th	104/62	105/62	106/62	107/63	109/64	110/65	110/65
	90th	117/76	118/76	119/76	121/77	122/78	123/79	124/79
	95th	121/80	122/80	123/80	124/81	126/82	127/83	128/83
	99th	128/87	129/87	130/88	132/89	133/89	134/90	135/91
14	50th	106/63	106/63	107/63	109/64	110/65	111/66	112/66
	90th	119/77	120/77	121/77	122/78	124/79	125/80	125/80
	95th	123/81	123/81	125/81	126/82	127/83	129/84	129/84
	99th	130/88	131/88	132/89	133/90	135/90	136/91	136/92
15	50th	107/64	108/64	109/64	110/65	111/66	113/67	113/67
	90th	120/78	121/78	122/78	123/79	125/80	126/81	127/81
	95th	124/82	125/82	126/82	127/83	129/84	130/85	131/85
	99th	131/89	132/89	133/90	134/91	136/91	137/92	138/93

Table 11.1b (Contd.)

		SBP, mm Hg/DBP, mm Hg						
		Percentile of Height						
Age, y	BP Percentile	5th	10th	25th	50th	75th	90th	95th
16	50th	125/82	122/78	108/64	132/90	125/82	121/78	108/64
	90th	126/83	122/79	109/65	133/90	126/82	122/78	108/64
	95th	127/83	123/79	110/65	134/90	127/83	123/79	110/65
	99th	129/84	125/80	111/66	135/91	128/84	124/80	111/66
17	50th	130/85	126/81	113/67	137/92	130/85	126/81	112/66
	90th	131/85	127/81	114/67	138/93	131/85	127/81	114/67
	95th	132/86	128/82	115/68	139/93	132/86	128/82	114/68
	99th	125/82	122/78	108/64	132/90	125/82	121/78	108/64

* The 90th percentile is 1.28 SD, the 95th percentile is 1.645 SD, and the 99th percentile is 2.326 SD over the mean.

Reprinted with permission from The Fourth Report on the Diagnosis, Evaluation, and Treatment of High blood Pressure in children and Adolescents *Pediatrics.* August 2004; 114 supplement: 557–558.

Hypertension: causes and features

Box 11.2 Causes and features of hypertension (HTN)

Primary (essential) hypertension
This is a diagnosis of exclusion. High body mass index (BMI), excessive salt intake, lack of exercise, and family history may be underlying predisposing factors.

Secondary hypertension
- Renal (most common cause in hospital referral practice)
  - Chronic renal parenchymal disease (reflux/scarring)
  - Polycystic kidney disease
  - Obstructive uropathy
  - Acute nephritis
  - Chronic renal failure
- Vascular
  - Umbilical arterial/venous catheters
  - Renal artery stenosis
  - Renal vein thrombosis
  - Coarctation of aorta
  - Vasculitis
- Endocrine
  - Congenital adrenal hyperplasia
  - Hyperthyroidism
  - Increased steroids (iatrogenic or endogenous)
  - Pheochromocytoma (HTN is not always intermittent)
  - Hyperaldosteronism
- Trauma
- Neurological
  - Secondary to pain
  - Raised intracranial hypertension
- Tumors
  - Neuroblastoma
  - Wilms' tumor
- Medication
  - Steroids
  - Aminophylline/caffeine
  - Oral contraceptive pill
  - Erythropoietin
  - Calcineurin inhibitors
  - Decongestants
  - Amphetamines; cocaine
- Others
  - Bronchopulmonary dysplasia
  - Extracorporeal membrane oxygenation (ECMO)
  - White-coat hypertension

Clinical features

Most features are asymptomatic.

Infants
- Vomiting
- Failure to thrive (rare)
- Congestive cardiac failure or respiratory distress (in newborns)

Children
- Headache, nausea and vomiting
- Visual symptoms
- Irritable, tiredness
- Bell's palsy
- Epistaxis
- Growth failure
- Altered consciousness

Examination
- Check optic fundi.
- Feel abdomen for abdominal masses.
- Listen for renal bruits in abdomen and back.
- Feel femoral pulses and compare to radial/brachial pulses (to exclude coarctation) and check blood pressure in all four limbs.
- Examination of the heart

Investigations

A secondary cause is more likely with severe hypertension. Treatment and investigations may need to proceed together. Consult pediatric nephrology for investigation and treatment recommendations.

- Urine
  - Urinalysis, microscopy and culture
  - Pregnancy test for adolescent females
- Blood tests
  - Full blood count
  - Electrolytes, BUN, Cr, calcium, phosphorus, albumin
  - Consider plasma renin and aldosterone
- Chest X-ray
- Echocardiogram—left ventricular hypertrophy suggests long-standing HTN
- Ultrasound of urinary tract
  - + Doppler if renal artery stenosis is suspected
- Further imaging will depend on suspected cause and ultrasound findings, e.g., DMSA, CT scan, arteriogram
- Specialized tests, e.g., for pheochromocytoma: plasma metanephrines

Hypertension: management

Hypertensive urgency and emergency

Acute, severe hypertension may require careful monitoring in a pediatric intensive care unit (ICU) and treatment with drugs shown below.

- Hypertensive urgency: Elevated BP without the presence of acute target-organ damage
- Hypertensive emergency: Elevated BP accompanied by acute target-organ damage. In children, encephalopathy is most common.

Treatment of severe hypertension

The aim is to reduce systolic and diastolic blood pressure to <95th centile for age and sex, but if the patient is severely hypertensive, only aim to decrease BP by <25% over the first 8 hours, then aim for controlled reduction in blood pressure over 26–48 hours (see Table 11.2). A quick decrease in BP may cause end-organ ischemia due to the autoregulatory mechanism of a chronically hypertensive patient.

Maintenance antihypertensive therapy

The exact dosing schedules of many antihypertensive drugs have not been evaluated in depth in children. The most often used classes of medications are calcium channel blockers, ACE inhibitors, and beta-blockers. ACE inhibitors should be avoided if renal artery stenosis is suspected but are useful for renin-mediated hypertension. Phenoxybezamine is used if catecholamine-induced hypertension is suspected (e.g., pheochromocytoma). See Table 11.3.

Encourage lifestyle changes (diet and physical activity modification) for stage I primary hypertension before treating with medication. Refer patient to pediatric nephrology if antihypertensive medication is indicated.

Table 11.2 Antihypertensive Drugs for Management of Severe Hypertension in Children 1–17 years

Useful for severely hypertensive patients with life-threatening symptoms

Drug	Class	Dose*	Route	Comments
Esmolol	β-adrenergic blocker	100–500 mcg/kg/min	IV infusion	Very short-acting—constant infusion preferred. May cause profound bradycardia.
Hydralazine	Direct vasodilator	0.2–0.6 mg/kg/dose	IV, IM	Should be given every 4 hr when given IV bolus.
Labetalol	α- and β-adrenergic blocker	bolus: 0.20–1.0 mg/kg/dose, up to 40 mg/dose infusion: 0.25–3.0 mg/kg/hr	IV bolus or infusion	Asthma and overt heart failure are relative contraindications.
Nicardipine	Calcium channel blocker	bolus: 30mcg/kg up to 2 mg/dose infusion: 0.5–4 mcg/kg/min	IV bolus or infusion	May cause reflex tachycardia.
Sodium Nitroprusside	Direct vasodilator	0.5–10 mcg/kg/min	IV infusion	Monitor cyanide levels with prolonged (>72 hr) use or in renal failure; or co-administer with sodium thiosulfate.

Table 11.2 (Contd.)

Useful for severely hypertensive patients with less significant symptoms

Drug	Class	Dose*	Route	Comments
Clonidine	Central α-agonist	0.05–0.1 mg/dose, may be repeated up to 0.8 mg total dose	PO	Side effects include dry mouth and drowsiness.
Enalaprilat	ACE inhibitor	0.05–0.10 mg/kg/dose up to 1.25 mg/dose	IV bolus	May cause prolonged hypotension and acute renal failure, especially in neonates.
Fenoldopam	Dopamine receptor agonist	0.2–0.8 mcg/kg/min	IV infusion	Produced modest reductions in BP in a pediatric clinical trial in patients up to 12 years.
Hydralazine	Direct vasodilator	0.25 mg/kg/dose up to 25 mg/dose	PO	Extemporaneous suspension stable for only 1 week
Isradipine	Calcium channel blocker	0.05–0.1 mg/kg/dose up to 5 mg/dose	PO	Stable suspension can be compounded.
Minoxidil	Direct vasodilator	0.1–0.2 mg/kg/dose up to 10 mg/dose	PO	Most potent oral vasodilator; long-acting.

FDA indicates Food and Drug Administration; IM, intramuscular; IV, intravenous; PO, oral.

* All dosing recommendations are based on expert opinion or case series data except as otherwise noted.

Courtesy of Joseph T. Flynn, MD, MS, Professor of Pediatrics, University of Washington School of Medicine, and Seattle Children's Hospital.

Table 11.3 Recommended doses for selected antihypertensive agents for use in hypertensive children and adolescents

Class	Drug	Starting dose	Interval	Maximum dose*	Comments
Aldosterone receptor antagonists	Eplerenone	25 mg/day	QD-BID	100 mg/day	1. Electrolytes should be monitored shortly after initiating therapy and periodically thereafter.
	Sprionolactone[††]	1 mg/kg/day	QD-BID	3.3 mg/kg/day up to 100 mg/day	2. Best use is probably in combination with other classes of antihypertensives.
Angiotensin-converting enzyme (ACE) inhibitors	Benazepril[††]	0.2 mg/kg/day up to 10 mg/day	QD	0.6 mg/kg/day up to 40 mg/day	1. Monitor serum chemistries shortly after initiating therapy and periodically thereafter.
	Captopril[††]	0.3–0.5 mg/kg/dose	BID–TID	6 mg/kg/day up to 450 mg/day	2. Contraindicated in patients with bilateral RAS or RAS in single kidney, and in pregnancy
	Enalapril[††]	0.08 mg/kg/day	QD	0.6 mg/kg/day up to 40 mg/day	3. May cause cough and angioedema
	Fosinopril	0.1 mg/kg/day up to 10 mg/day	QD	0.6 mg/kg/d up to 40 mg/day	4. Many ACEI are available in combination preparations containing a diuretic
	Lisinopril[††]	0.07 mg/kg/day up to 5 mg/day	QD	0.6 mg/kg/d up to 40 mg/day	
	Quinapril	5–10 mg/day	QD	80 mg/day	

Table 11.3 (Contd.)

Class	Drug	Starting dose	Interval	Maximum dose*	Comments
Angiotensin-receptor blockers	Candesartan	4 mg/day	QD	32 mg/day	1. Monitor serum chemistries shortly after initiating therapy and periodically thereafter.
	Irbesartan	75–150 mg/day	QD	300 mg/day	2. Contraindicated in patients with bilateral RAS or RAS in single kidney, and in pregnancy
	Losartan††	0.75 mg/kg/day up to 50 mg/day	QD	1.4 mg/kg/day up to 100 mg/day	3. Many ARB are available in combination preparations containing a diuretic
	Olmesartan	2.5 mg/day	QD	40 mg/day	
	Valsartan††	1.3 mg/kg/day up to 40 mg/day <6 years: 5-10 mg/d	QD	2.7 mg/kg/day up to 160 mg/day <6 years: 80 mg/day	

α- and β-adrenergic antagonists	Labetalol††	2–3 mg/kg/day	BID	10–12 mg/kg/day up to 1.2 g/day	1. Contraindicated in asthma, heart failure (labetalol only) and diabetes
	Carvedilol	0.1 mg/kg/dose up to 12.5 mg BID	BID	0.5 mg/kg/dose up to 25 mg BID	2. Heart rate is dose-limiting. 3. May impair athletic performance. 4. Carvedilol beneficial in heart failure
β-adrenergic antagonists	Atenolol††	0.5–1 mg/kg/day	QD–BID	2 mg/kg/day up to 100 mg/day	1. Propranolol contraindicated in asthma, CHF.
	Bisoprolol/HCTZ	0.04 mg/kg/day up to 2.5/6.25 mg/day	QD	10/6.25 mg/day	2. Atenolol accumulates in patients with GFR<35 ml/min/1.73m2
	Metoprolol	1–2 mg/kg/day	BID	6 mg/kg/day up to 200 mg/day	3. Heart rate is dose-limiting. 4. Should not be used in insulin-dependent diabetics.
	Propranolol	1 mg/kg/day	BID–TID	16 mg/kg/day up to 640 mg/day	5. Sustained-release formulations of propranolol and metoprolol are available that are dosed once-daily; suspension of propranolol available.

Table 11.3 (Contd.)

Class	Drug	Starting dose	Interval	Maximum dose*	Comments
Calcium channel blockers	Amlodipine[††]	0.06 mg/kg/day	QD	0.3 mg/kg/day up to 10 mg/day	1. Felodipine and extended-release nifedipine tablets must be swallowed whole.
	Felodipine	2.5 mg/day	QD	10 mg/day	2. May cause mild tachycardia, flushing and headache.
	Isradipine[††]	0.05–0.15 mg/kg/dose	TID–QID	0.8 mg/kg/day up to 20 mg/day	3. Gingival hyperplasia may occur with prolonged use, especially in combination with calcineurin inhibitors.
	Extended-release nifedipine	0.25–0.5 mg/kg/day	QD–BID	3 mg/kg/day up to 120 mg/day	
Central α-agonists	Clonidine[††]	5–10 mcg/kg/day	BID–TID	25 mcg/kg/day up to 0.9 mg/day	1. May cause dry mouth and sedation. 2. Clonidine also available in a transdermal preparation.
	Methyldopa[††]	5 mg/kg/day	BID–QID	40 mg/kg/day up to 3 g/day	3. Sudden withdrawal of clonidine may cause severe rebound hypertension.

Diuretics				
Amiloride	5–10 mg/day	QD	20 mg/day	1. Electrolytes should be monitored shortly after initiating therapy and periodically thereafter.
Chlorothiazide	10 mg/kg/day	BID	20 mg/kg/day up to 1.0 gram/day	2. All diuretics are best used as add-on therapy in combination with other classes of antihypertensives.
Chlorthalidone	0.3 mg/kg/day	QD	2 mg/kg/day up to 50 mg/day	3. Chlorothiazide and furosemide are commercially available as suspensions
Furosemide	0.5–2.0 mg/kg/dose	QD-BID	6 mg/kg/day	
HCTZ	0.5–1 mg/kg/day	QD	3 mg/kg/day up to 50 mg/day	
Triamterene	1–2 mg/kg/day	BID	3–4 mg/kg/day up to 300 mg/day	

Table 11.3 (Contd.)

Class	Drug	Starting dose	Interval	Maximum dose*	Comments
Peripheral α-antagonists	Doxazosin	1 mg/day	QD	4 mg/day	1. All may cause first-dose hypotension
	Prazosin	0.05–0.1 mg/kg/day	TID	0.5 mg/kg/day	
	Terazosin	1 mg/day	QD	20 mg/day	
Vasodilators	Hydralazine	0.25 mg/kg/dose	TID–QID	7.5 mg/kg/day up to 200 mg/day	1. Tachycardia and fluid retention are common side effects.
					2. Hydralazine can cause a lupus-like syndrome in slow acetylators.
	Minoxidil	0.1–0.2 mg/kg/day	BID–TID	1 mg/kg/day up to 50 mg/day	3. Prolonged use of minoxidil causes hypertrichosis.

* The maximum recommended adult dose should never be exceeded.

†† Information on preparation of a stable extemporaneous suspension is available for these agents.

Abbreviations used in table: ACEI, angiotensin converting enzyme inhibitor; ARB, angiotensin receptor blocker; BID, twice-daily; HCTZ, hydrochlorothiazide; QD, once-daily; QID, four times daily; RAS, renal artery stenosis; TID, three times daily.

Courtesy of Joseph T. Flynn, MD, MS, Professor of Pediatrics, University of Washington School of Medicine, and Seattle Children's Hospital.

Nephrotic syndrome

This is defined as a combination of
- Heavy proteinuria (urinary protein excretion > 1000 mg/m^2/day)
- Hypoalbuminemia (serum albumin <3 g/dL)
- Edema
- Hyperlipidemia

Epidemiology
- Incidence is approximately 2–7 per 100,000 children.
- It is more common in boys than in girls.
- Peak age of onset is less than 6 years old.
- Hispanic and black patients are more likely to have steroid-unresponsive disease than whites.
- Age of presentation is important in disease frequency:
  - First year of life: Genetic disorder and congenital infection are most common.
  - 70% of minimal-change disease (MCD) below age of 5 years
  - Increase in incidence of focal segmental glomerulosclerosis (FSGS) at older ages: median age of presentation is 6 years old

Causes
Nephrotic syndrome can be either primary or secondary.

Congenital and infantile
- Primary: Most cases have a genetic basis and poor outcome.
- Secondary: Usually infection

Primary nephrotic syndrome is in absence of an identifiable systemic disease.
- MCD is most common.
- Incidence of FSGS is on the rise.
- Membranoproliferative glomerulonephritis (MPGN)
- Proliferative disease
- Membranous nephropathy

Secondary nephrotic syndrome is in presence of an identifiable systemic disease.
- Infection: HIV, malaria
- Systemic disease: DM, SLE, HSP
- Drugs and toxins: NSAIDs, penicillin, ACE inhibitors
- Mechanical factors: Renal vein thrombosis
- Tumors: Hodgkin disease

Classification
Nephrotic syndrome can be clinically classified as being either steroid sensitive (SS) or steroid resistant (SR). Responsiveness to steroid also has prognostic implications (see Prognosis, p. 441).
- MCD (SS) = 90%
- FSGS (SS) = 20%
- MPGN (SS) = 55%

Clinical features

Most children present with an insidious onset of edema, which is initially periorbital but becomes generalized with pitting edema. Periorbital edema is often most noticeable in the morning. Ascites and pleural effusions may subsequently develop.

Examination

This should establish the extent of edema (e.g., facial, ankle, scrotal, etc). Assessment should also include the following:

- Height and weight (compare with previous or recent measurements)
- Blood pressure
- Peripheral perfusion
- Respiratory status
- Abdominal exam: Evaluate for peritoneal signs

Investigations
Urine

- Urinalysis: protein +++
- Microscopy: Hematuria/casts suggest causes other than MCD
- Culture
- Protein/creatinine ratio

Blood

- Serum albumin (reduced <3 g/dL)
- CBC; electrolytes, BUN, Cr
- C3/C4 (if decreased, this suggests not MCD)
- Total cholesterol, triglycerides, and total lipids
- Consider ANA
- Varicella zoster immunity status: Most of the time, the patient will be started on prednisone and therefore are at a higher risk of developing more severe complications of varicella.

Management

Patients should be admitted if there are any signs of complications or decreased glomerular filtration rate (GFR), or if they are ill appearing. Management is initially aimed at fluid restriction and prevention of hypovolemia. A trial of oral steroid therapy to induce remission is started after testing PPD negative.

Treatment

- Treat hypovolemia if present, but albumin infusion is NOT routine
- Salt restriction and fluid restriction to 800–1000 mL per 24 hours
- Steroid therapy
  - Oral prednisone 60 mg/m^2/day (max 80 mg/day) for 6 weeks followed by 40 mg/m^2/alternate days for 6 weeks then stop, or consider slow wean over next 4 months. Observe for side effects of corticosteroids.

Other measures

- Diet (no added salt, and healthy eating—<u>not</u> high protein)
- Immunize with pneumococcal vaccine

Nephrotic syndrome: complications and follow-up

Complications

Complications are secondary to the relative hypovolemia, to impaired immunity, and to the hypercoagulable state.

Respiratory distress

This is secondary to pulmonary effusions.

Infection

Predisposition to infection is secondary to decreased IgG levels from urinary losses and to impaired opsonization due to steroids immunosuppression. Bacterial peritonitis (especially *Strep. pneumoniae*) is an important complication and should be considered in any child with nephrotic syndrome who complains of abdominal pain or unexplained fever. Urgent assessment, cultures, and IV antibiotic therapy are required.

Thrombosis

Nephrotic syndrome produces a hypercoagulable state and predisposition to both arterial and venous thrombosis.

Hypovolemia

Hypovolemia is suggested by development of oliguria and/or presence of low BP caused by massive fluid shift into the extravascular compartment. Patients may also complain of abdominal pain. Treatment considerations include IV fluid (giving saline may worsen edema due to salt load) and 25% albumin 1 g/kg given over 4 hours. Consider furosemide (0.5–1 mg/kg/dose) IV following albumin if there is concern for too-rapid fluid shift back into the intravascular compartment and respiratory distress. Fluid balance is very delicate (furosemide may worsen hypovolemia and cause prerenal renal failure and acute tubular necrosis [ATN]), so consult an experienced clinician and/or pediatric nephrologist.

Acute renal failure

This is usually prerenal secondary to hypovolemia.

Indications for renal biopsy

Most patients will have MCD and will respond to steroids. Biopsy is therefore reserved for those with atypical features:

- Age <12 months or >12 years (unresponsive to prednisone)
- Increased BP
- Macroscopic hematuria
- Impaired renal function
- Decreased C3/C4
- Failure to respond after 6–8 weeks of daily prednisone

Follow-up

Prognosis

Response to initial therapy (first 8 weeks) is prognostic of both progression of end-stage renal disease (ESRD) and frequency of relapses.

- 30% with no relapse
- 10%–20% with occasional relapse (<4) while off steroids before permanent remission
- 30%–40% steroid dependent: ≥4 relapse per year or relapse while on steroid

Relapse

Many patients with steroid-sensitive nephrotic syndrome will relapse. A relapse is defined as detection of urine dipstick + 2 proteinuria for greater than 3 days or presence of edema.

Frequent relapse is defined as greater than two relapses within 6 months of initial response or four or more relapses in any 12 months.

Management of relapses

Each relapse is treated with high-dose oral steroids. Alternative strategies for frequent-relapsing patients include a trial of therapy with other agents:

- Cyclophosphamide
- Cyclosporin A/tacrolimus
- Levamisole

Other immunosuppressive agents such as mycophenolate mofetil also may be considered.

Glomerulonephritis

Glomerulonephritis (GN) consists of a combination of hematuria, oliguria, edema, and hypertension with variable proteinuria. Presentation can vary from asymptomatic incidental findings of hematuria and/or proteinuria to rapidly progressive glomerulonephritis (RPGN) in need of dialysis. Most cases are postinfectious, usually with a history of antecedent URI and/or sore throat 1–2 weeks before renal symptoms. Use the following guidelines to direct the evaluation.

- Acute vs. chronic process (see Box 11.3)? Chronic GN may be suggested by the presence of anemia, elevated parathyroid hormone, small echogenic kidneys on ultrasound, or left ventricular hypertrophy from long-standing HTN.
- Isolated kidney disease vs. involvement of extrarenal organ systems? Common multisystem diseases with GN: HSP, SLE, systemic vasculitis, hemolytic–uremic syndrome (HUS), and Goodpasture syndrome
- Depressed complement levels (C3, C4)? If so, this is most likely postinfectious GN, SLE, MPGN, or chronic infection (bacterial endocarditis, shunt nephritis)
- History of recurrent gross hematuria? If so, this is likely IgA nephropathy or, rarely, Alport syndrome
- Age of the patient? Many etiologies have characteristic age of presentation.
- Evidence of RPGN? Prompt referral, diagnosis, and initiation of therapy are crucial.
- Nephrotic syndrome? Combination of nephrotic syndrome and low C3 are suggestive of MPGN or SLE. Post-strep GN rarely presents with nephrotic syndrome.

Box 11.3 Causes of acute glomerulonephritis

Postinfectious
- Bacterial: Streptococcal (most common), *Staph. aureus*, *Mycoplasma pneumoniae*, *Salmonella*
- Viral: Herpes viruses (EBV, varicella, CMV), chronic hepatitis, HIV
- Fungi: *Candida*, *Aspergillus*
- Parasites: *Toxoplasma*, malaria, *Schistosomiasis*

Others (less common)
- MPGN
- IgA nephropathy/HSP
- Systemic lupus erythematosis (SLE)
- Subacute bacterial endocarditis
- Shunt nephritis
- Crescentic GN including anti-glomerular basement membrane disease
- Vasculitis (e.g., ANCA disease)

Investigations

- Urine
  - Urinalysis by dipstick: Hematuria ± proteinuria
  - Microscopy: Dysmorphic RBCs, RBC casts
- Blood
  - CBC
  - Electrolytes, BUN, creatinine, calcium, phosphate and albumin
  - ASO titer, streptozyme, anti-DNAse B
  - C3, C4
  - ANA, ANCA, and other antibodies, depending on clinical suspicion
- Renal ultrasound
- Chest X-ray (if fluid overload is suspected)
- Dental evaluation if chronic tooth carries is suspected

Management

Many patients require admission because of fluid imbalance, worsening renal function, or hypertension. Treat life-threatening complications first:
- Hyperkalemia
- Hypertension
- Acidosis
- Seizures
- Hypocalcemia

Otherwise, give supportive treatment:
- Fluid balance
  - Daily weights
  - No added/restricted salt diet
  - If patient is oliguric, fluid restrict to insensible losses (400 mL/m^2/day) + urine output
- Hypertension
  - Treat fluid overload
  - Calcium channel blocker is usually the first choice. Beta-blockers are also commonly used. If there is normal renal function and patient is euvolemic, consider diuretics like furosemide for hypertension in patients with postinfectious GN.
  - **NOTE**: Do not use ACE inhibitors in acute setting (this may worsen renal function)

When to refer to pediatric nephrology

- Patients with life-threatening complications
- Those with atypical features, including the following:
  - Worsening renal function
  - Nephrotic state
  - Evidence of systemic vasculitis (e.g., rash)
  - Normal complement levels
  - + ANA
  - Persisting proteinuria at 6 weeks
  - Persisting low C3 at 3 months

Prognosis
- 95% of patients with postinfectious GN show complete recovery. Microscopic hematuria may persist for 1–2 years. Discharge from follow-up once UA, blood pressure, and creatinine are normal.
- Prognosis is much worse for non-postinfectious GN (e.g., MPGN, SLE, crescentic GN, and ANCA disease). Refer patient to pediatric nephrology for further management.

Nephrolithiasis

The incidence of nephrolithiasis varies according to geography and socio-economic conditions around the world. In the United States, nephrolithiasis is most common in the Southeast, and more common in Caucasian children and rare in African-American children.

Stone composition

- Calcium oxalate: 45%–65% of cases
- Calcium phosphate: 14%–30%
- Struvite 13%
- Cystine 5%
- Uric acid 4%

Etiology

This is usually determined in 75% to 85% of affected children.

Metabolic

- Hypercalciuria is most common. It is defined as >4 mg/kg/day. Spot UCa/UCr is most often used (see Investigations for normal ranges).
  - Idiopathic: Most cases are likely from a combination of genetic and environmental factors.
  - Dehydration
  - Prolonged immobilization
  - Medication: loop diuretics
  - Excess amounts of vitamin D
  - Primary hyperparathyrodism
- Hyperoxaluria and oxalosis
  - Idiopathic hyperoxaluria often occurs with hypercalciuria.
  - Primary hyperoxaluria type I and II
  - Fat malabsorption
- Hypocitraturia
  - Citrate is an inhibitor to calcium oxalate and calcium phosphate crystallization.
  - Chronic metabolic acidosis causes enhanced citrate reabsorption leading to stones.
- Hyperuricosuria
  - Uric acid excretion is highest in infants.
  - Idiopathic hyperuricosuria occurs often in conjunction with hypercalciuria.
  - Tumor lysis syndrome, lymphoproliferative and myeloproliferative disorders
  - Lesch–Nyhan syndrome, glycogen storage disease
- Cystinuria is an autosomal recessive condition.
  - Disorder of renal tubular transport
- Ketogenic diet
- Cystic fibrosis

Infective

- Struvite stones: *Proteus*, *Providencia*, *Klebsiella*, *Pseudomonas*, and enterococci

Associated with urinary stasis
- Congenital malformations
  - Medullary sponge kidney, autosomal dominant polycystic kidney disease (ADPKD)
  - Ureteropelvic junction obstruction, horseshoe kidney, bladder exstrophy, megaureter
  - Bladder augmentation
  - Neurogenic bladder

Clinical features

Most children will present with either gross or microscopic hematuria. They may be otherwise asymptomatic. The classic symptoms of renal colic are less common than in adults (e.g., intense pain located in the abdomen or in the loins and back). Symptoms and signs of a urinary tract infection may also be present. Some children may describe a sensation of "having passed gravel."

Investigations

Urine
- UA with microscopy (pH, cells, crystals) and culture
- Spot U calcium/U creatinine ratio. Normal range:
  - <0.8 mg/mg Cr for <6 months of age
  - <0.6 mg/mg Cr for 6–12 months of age
  - <0.2 mg/mg Cr for >2 years old
- Consider U oxalate/U creatinine ratio. Normal range:
  - <0.3 mg/mg Cr for < 6 months of age
  - <0.15 mg/mg Cr for 6 months to 4 years old
  - <0.1 mg/mg Cr for >4 years old
- Urine uric acid when appropriate. Adjust for GFR by

  (U uric acid $\times$ P creatinine)/U creatinine

- Normal <0.56 mg/dL for age 3 years and older

Serum
- Electrolytes, including Ca and Phos, BUN, Cr
- Parathyroid hormone (PTH)
- Uric acid

Renal tract ultrasound
This is used to evaluate location of stones, signs of obstruction, and anatomical abnormality, and is a good first-line imaging tool. If images are inconclusive or show obstruction, consider a spiral CT scan.

Other investigations
- Spiral CT scan is the gold standard.
- Abdominal X-ray
  - Radio-opaque stones: Calcium, cysteine, infective
  - Radiolucent stones: Uric acid, xanthine
- Urine composition study for stone formation risk
- Renal stone analysis for composition

Treatment

The acute treatment of renal colic secondary to renal stones is based on the provision of adequate analgesia and hydration. Treat any underlying urinary tract infection with antibiotics. If severe renal impairment and urinary tract obstruction are evident, refer patient to the pediatric urology team for consideration of extracorporeal shock-wave lithotripsy. Surgery (e.g., percutaneous nephrolithotomy or open surgery) is now seldom indicated. Long-term management is aimed at preventing further obstruction and bouts of renal colic. The simplest and most effective measures to achieve this are to ensure adequate hydration and diuresis maintain a good urinary flow and dilute urine. Treatment of any underlying urinary tract infection and metabolic disorder is also required.

Primary hyperoxaluria type 1

This is an autosomal recessive condition. Three forms are recognized:
- Infantile form
  - Early nephrocalcinosis and progression to ESRD
- Child and adolescent form
  - Recurrent urolithiasis and progression to ESRD
- Adult form
  - Urolithiasis only

Combined liver–kidney transplantation is the treatment of choice for patients with ESRD. The liver provides the missing enzyme.

Polyuria and frequency

This is often subjective and difficult to assess, particularly in small children. Frequency can be considered the inappropriate and frequent passage of small amounts of urine. Polyuria can be quantitatively defined as the passage of >2000 mL/1.73 m^2/24 hour.

Assessment of polyuria and frequency requires a detailed history of urinary frequency habit.

Causes of polyuria

- Renal disorders
  - Chronic renal failure
  - Postobstructive uropathy
  - Nephrogenic diabetes insipidus
  - Fanconi syndrome
- Metabolic and endocrine disorders
  - Diabetes mellitus
  - Central diabetes insipidus
  - Hypoadrenalism
- Excess and inappropriate water intake
  - Psychogenic polydipsia

Causes of urinary frequency

- Urinary tract infection
- Bladder irritability and instability
- All causes of polyuria
- Small bladder capacity

Investigations

Baseline screening investigations should include the following:

- Urine
  - Urinalysis by urine dipstick testing and measurement of specific gravity
  - Urine culture
  - Urine osmolality
  - Urine glucose
- Blood
  - Electrolytes, BUN, Cr
  - Plasma osmolality
  - Blood glucose (random or fasting)

Enuresis

Enuresis is the involuntary emptying of the bladder. Although children may "wet" themselves by day or night, the term *enuresis* is applied to nocturnal enuresis. When it occurs during the day, while awake, it is known as *diurnal enuresis*. Nocturnal enuresis is the more common disorder.

In order to learn bladder control, the young child needs to overcome the infant pattern of automatic voiding. For the young child, conscious awareness of fullness and the ability to postpone voiding by suppressing the urge to void is not perfect. This response is first learned for daytime control. Eventually, bladder control becomes automatic and does not require a conscious act. Nighttime bladder control requires that the brain, during sleep, suppress the automatic emptying reflex. Learning bladder control at night occurs gradually and in some children and families takes much longer than average.

Girls achieve bladder control earlier than boys. *Enuresis* is defined as the continued wetting in girls beyond the age of 5 years, and in boys beyond the age of 6 years.

Enuresis may be primary, with children not having established an appropriate period of adequate bladder control in early childhood, or secondary, occurring after a period of established bladder control.

Primary enuresis
- A strong family history
- Boys more commonly than girls (2:1)
- 15% of 5-year-olds, 5% of 10-year-olds, and 1% of 16-year-olds have not established total bladder control and will wet the bed once a week or more.
- Most cases have no underlying organic cause and are thought to be due to delayed maturation.

Secondary enuresis
This condition needs careful history and investigations because of a probable organic cause.

- Renal tract
  - Urinary tract infection
- Neurological
  - Spina bifida
- Endocrine
  - Diabetes mellitus, diabetes insipidus
- Behavioral problems
- Abuse

Daytime wetting is usually caused by bladder detrusor instability.

Assess pattern and types of drink
- Often limited fluid in the day
- Drink after school and evening

Voiding habits
- Infrequent (<4 daily)
- Frequent (>7 daily)
- Dysfunctional or inappropriate place of voiding

Urine testing
- Culture
- Urinalysis

Ultrasound of the renal tract
- Assess pre- and post-micturition bladder urine residual volume
- Underlying anatomical abnormalities

Treatment
Primary (nocturnal) enuresis
- Encourage regular drinks (water) but restrict in last hour before bed
- Give drinking and voiding chart

If primary nocturnal enuresis is associated with arousal from sleep or disturbance, then an enuresis alarm should be considered. This requires careful discussion with families. Compliance is often an issue and the family and child need to be motivated. If enuresis is associated with a small bladder, "bladder training" exercises are the first-line approach. Also consider using bladder-stabilizing drugs (i.e., oxybutynin). If nocturnal enuresis and urine output exceed bladder capacity, consider using Desmopressin (antidiuretic hormone) and limit fluid intake 1 hour before until 8 hours after administration.

If the problem is resistant to the above treatments, other pathologies need to be considered:
- Urinary outflow obstruction in boys
- Chronic constipation
- Neurodevelopmental problems
- Psychological problems

Abdominal and renal masses

These masses are a rare presentation of urinary tract problems and need to be differentiated from other causes of abdominal mass and swelling.

Causes
Intrarenal
- Wilms' tumor (young child with rapidly growing mass)
- Renal vein thrombosis (newborn with hematuria)
- Mesoblastic nephroma (rare neonatal problem, rarely malignant)
- Horseshoe kidney
- Pyelonephritis (renal abscess)

Cystic
Hydronephrosis associated with
- Ureteropelvic junction (UPJ) obstruction
- Ureterovesicular junction (UVJ) obstruction
- Large bladder: bladder outlet obstruction, e.g.:
  - Posterior urethral valves (PUV)
  - Prune belly
  - Neurogenic bladder
- Urinoma: An encapsulated extrapelvocalyceal collection of urine that forms from urine leakage through a tear in the collecting system or the proximal ureter
- Single cyst (benign renal cyst)
- Multicystic dysplastic kidney—usually newborn
- Polycystic disease
  - Autosomal recessive
  - Autosomal dominant—can present as infants and children
- Hematoma (trauma)

Extrarenal
- Adrenal mass (neuroblastoma)

History
- Palpable abdominal or flank mass discovered by caretakers and providers
- Incidental finding during an evaluation for another reason. e.g., abdominal CT after a trauma

Investigation
Ultrasound will distinguish between most of the above. Further investigation depends on likely causes and discussion with the radiologist and urologist, and can include CT/MRI.

Acute kidney injury (AKI)

AKI is a sudden reduction in glomerular filtration rate, resulting in an impaired excretion of nitrogenous waste product and disturbed fluid, electrolyte, and acid–base homeostasis.

Classification

The causes of AKI can be broadly divided into prerenal, renal, and postrenal (see Box 11.4). Overlap exists, and a patient may have more than one cause for their renal injury.

> ### Box 11.4 Causes of acute kidney injury
>
> *Prerenal*
> - Hypovolemia, e.g., GI loss, hemorrhage, nephrotic syndrome
> - Peripheral vasodilatation, e.g., sepsis
> - Impaired cardiac output, e.g., congestive heart failure
> - Drugs, e.g., ACE inhibitors
>
> *Renal*
> - Acute tubular necrosis (usually following prerenal cause)
> - Interstitial nephritis (usually drug induced)
> - Glomerulonephritis
> - Hemolytic–uremic syndrome (HUS)
> - Malignant hypertension
> - Cortical necrosis
> - Myoglobinuria, hemoglobinuria
> - Nephrotoxic drugs, e.g., aminoglycoside, IV contrast, NSAIDs
> - Tumor lysis syndrome
> - Renal artery/vein thrombosis
> - Bilateral pyelonephritis
>
> *Postrenal*
> - Obstruction
>   - Posterior urethral valves (PUV)
>   - Neurogenic bladder
>   - Calculi
>   - Tumor (rhabdomyosarcoma in infancy)

History

It is important to include the following points:
- History of vomiting or diarrhea, hemorrhage, sepsis
- History of sore throat or rash (e.g., strep. glomerulonephritis)
- History of bloody diarrhea
- Urinary symptoms of
  - Hematuria, frequency, dysuria (e.g., pyelonephritis)
  - Poor stream (e.g., PUV)
- Significant antenatal history
- Drugs

Examination

It is important to assess and document the following:
- Height and weight (compare with any recent or past measurements)
- Fever
- Hydration status–any evidence of edema or dehydration
- Hemodynamic status including BP
- Presence of any rashes or arthritis
- Abdomen–tenderness or masses
- Neurology–exclude possible neuropathic bladder

Investigations

Urine
- Urinalysis with microscopy of fresh urine, e.g., evidence of casts
- Culture, e.g., pyelonephritis
- Osmolality, Na, creatinine; calculate fractional excretion of sodium (FENa)
- Protein/creatinine ratio if dipstick is positive for protein
- Myoglobin if there is evidence of rhabdomyolysis
- Urine calcium/oxalate to creatinine ratios if renal calculi are suspected

Blood investigations
- Electrolytes, BUN, creatinine, Ca^{2+}, PO_4, albumin, glucose
- Plasma osmolality
- CBC
- Blood culture if patient is clinically septic
- C3, C4, ASO titer, streptozyme, anti-DNAse B, ANA, ANCA in suspected nephritis
- Uric acid if tumor lysis is suspected
- Creatine kinase if possible myoglobinuria
- Coagulation studies if patient is septic or there is a potential need for biopsy or dialysis access
- Drug levels if relevant (e.g., gentamicin)

Cultures
- Stool culture, specifically for *E. coli* O157:H7 if HUS is suspected

Radiology
- Ultrasound (± Doppler) of kidneys and bladder
- Chest X-ray if there is evidence of fluid overload

AKI: diagnosis and treatment

Diagnosis

First urinary indices may be helpful if no diuretics are given (Table 11.4).

Table 11.4 First urinary indices indicating AKI

Test	Prerenal	Renal	Postrenal
Urine osmolality	>400–500	<350	Variable
Urine Na (mEq/L)	<10	>30–40	Variable
FENa	<1%	>2%	Variable

To accurately interpret FENa, patients should not have recently received diuretics. FENa is greater than 1% (and usually greater than 3%) with acute tubular necrosis and severe obstruction of the urinary drainage.

$$FENa = \frac{U_{Na} \times P_{Cr}}{P_{Na} \times U_{Cr}} \times 100$$

Treatment

Communicate with pediatric nephrology **early** and treat the following:
- Hyperkalemia (K^+ >6.5 mmol/L)
- Metabolic acidosis
- Hypertension
- Shock
- Fluid overload
- Hyperphosphatemia
- Hypocalcemia
- Hypo- or hypernatremia

Specific treatment depends on the underlying cause; however, the following general management principles apply:
- *Observations*: Daily weight, BP, strict fluid input and output monitoring
- *Fluids management*: Prerenal: fluid bolus (20 mL/kg of normal saline); otherwise, restrict to insensible losses (400 mL/m^2/day) + urine output. Consider adding diuretic therapy.
- *Electrolytes*: Monitor at least 12 hourly until stable
  - K^+ and PO_4 restricted diet. Consider adding PO_4- binder
- *Blood pressure*: Treat hypertension
- *Medications*: Adjust drug doses according to estimated GFR

The patient requires transfer to a pediatric nephrology center if dialysis looks likely or there is uncertainty about the diagnosis.

Indications for dialysis

The following are indications for urgent dialysis in AKI:
- Severe hyperkalemia
- Symptomatic uremia with vomiting or encephalopathy
- Azotemia
- Symptomatic fluid overload, especially cardiac failure or pericardial effusion
- Uncontrollable hypertension
- Severe electrolyte abnormalities and acidosis refractory to supportive medical therapy
- Prolonged oliguria: Conservative regimen controls AKI but causes nutritional failure
- Removal of exogenous toxins or endogenous metabolite (inborn error)

Note: Patients with hemolytic uremic syndrome should be referred as soon as the child becomes oliguric or if urea is raised, as early dialysis may reduce neurological complications and allow transfusion.

Acute dialysis methods
- Peritoneal dialysis (abdominal catheter)
- Hemodialysis (femoral or jugular access)
- Continuous renal replacement therapy (CRRT) is better tolerated by hemodynamically unstable patients.

Hemolytic–uremic syndrome

Hemolytic–uremic syndrome (HUS) is one of the most common causes of acute kidney injury in the United States. It typically has a seasonal variation with peaks in the summer and autumn months. It presents with a triad of
- Microangiopathic hemolytic anemia
- Thrombocytopenia
- Acute renal failure

Two forms of HUS are recognized:
- Diarrhea associated (D+ HUS): 90% of HUS cases
  - Commonly associated with *Shiga* toxin producing *E. coli* 0157:H7, although other pathogens have also been implicated (e.g., *Shigella*). Frequently there is bloody diarrhea.
- Atypical (D- HUS)
  - Not diarrhea associated
  - Some cases are familial while others are infectious
  - More insidious onset
  - Relapsing progressive course with worse outcomes
  - More often with permanent renal sequelae

E. coli are common bacteria, normally found in the gut of warm-blooded animals. There are many types of *E. coli*, many of which are harmless.

However, the enterohemorrhagic *E. coli* (EHEC) produce toxins, which can cause gastroenteritis with blood in the stool. The toxins are called *Shiga* toxins or verotoxins, hence EHEC is also called STEC or VTEC. EHEC is found in the gut of cattle and can also be found in the gut of humans without causing illness. The bacteria can be passed on to humans by
- Eating improperly cooked beef, in particular, ground or minced beef
- Drinking unpasteurized milk
- Close contact with a person who has the bacteria in their feces
- Drinking contaminated water
- Swimming or playing in contaminated water
- Contact with farm animals

Clinical features
Acute kidney injury
Gut
- Prodrome of diarrhea, often bloody
- Rectal prolapse
- Hemorrhagic colitis
- Bowel wall necrosis and perforation

Pancreas (occurs in <10%)
- Glucose intolerance or insulin-dependent diabetes mellitus
- Pancreatitis

Liver
- Jaundice
Neurological
- Irritability to frank encephalopathy

Cardiac
- Myocarditis (rare)

Manifestations can vary from mild diarrhea with no other organ involvement to multi-organ failure.

Investigations
- CBC with differential and smear
- Lactate dehydrogenase (LDH)
- Blood cultures
- Electrolytes, BUN, Cr, Phos
- Transaminases
- Lipase/amylase
- Stools: microscopy and culture—specify to culture for *E. coli* O157:H7

Treatment
Early referral to pediatric nephrology is required, as early dialysis may be needed. Management is mainly supportive and directed at treating the clinical features of HUS. Antibiotics for underlying *E. coli* infection are NOT indicated.
- Monitor electrolyte balance
- Monitor fluid balance
- Monitor neurological status
- Nutrition: TPN/IL is often required
- Blood transfusion (note risks and concerns regarding fluid overload and hyperkalemia)
- Treat hypertension
- Dialysis if needed
- Consider plasmapheresis for D- HUS

Outcome
- Generally good (for D+ HUS)
- Mortality <5%
- Long-term: Up to 30% of patients may develop mild impairment of GFR.

D- HUS has a worse prognosis, with relapsing and a progressive course, and permanent renal sequelae such as hypertension and chronic kidney disease.

Chronic kidney disease (CKD)

Most children with CKD are asymptomatic until significant progression of the disease (see Table 11.5). CKD should be considered with the following:
- Failure to thrive
- Polyuria and polydipsia
- Lethargy, lack of energy, poor school concentration
- Anemia
- Other abnormalities such as rickets

Table 11.5 Stages of CKD

Stage	Description	GFR (mL/min/1.73m^2)
1	Kidney damage with or without increased GFR	>90
2	Kidney damage with mild decrease in GFR	60–89
3	Moderate decrease in GFR	30–59
4	Severe decrease in GFR	15–29
5	End stage	<15 (or dialysis)

CKD: common misconceptions
- A normal serum creatinine may not mean a normal GFR. The relationship between GFR and serum creatinine is not linear.
- Urine flow rate may not mean a good GFR, as many children with renal dysplasia have polyuria and nocturia.
- Minor urinary abnormalities such as proteinuria and glycosuria can be an indicator of tubular dysfunction.

The focus is on GFR and not plasma creatinine
- GFR can be formally measured by iothalamate clearance, ^{51}Cr EDTA method, and inulin clearance, among a number of methods
- In ordinary clinical practice, GFR (mL/min/1.73 m^2) may be estimated by the Schwartz equation

$$= (k*height (cm))/serum creatinine$$

Where k = 0.33 in premature infants, 0.45 in term infants to 1 year old, 0.55 in all children and postpubertal females, and 0.7 in postpubertal males

Box 11.5 Causes of chronic kidney disease

Congenital: most common
- Renal hypoplasia/dysplasia
- Obstructive uropathies
- Vesicouretral reflux nephropathy

Glomerulopathies
- Focal segmental glomerulosclerosis
- Chronic glomerulonephritis

Hereditary nephropathies
- Polycystic kidney disease
- Alport/hereditary nephritis
- Nephronophthisis
- Cystinosis
- Oxalosis

Multisystem disorders
- Systemic lupus erythematous (SLE)
- Henoch–Schönlein purpura
- Hemolytic–uremic syndrome

Others
- Wilms' tumor from kidney loss or nephrectomy
- Renal vascular disease
- Unknown

Investigations
- Urinalysis
- Blood
  - CBC + iron studies if anemic
  - Electrolytes, Ca, PO_4, albumin
  - pH/bicarbonate
  - Parathyroid hormone (PTH)
- Renal tract ultrasound
- VCUG if there is a history of multiple UTIs or you suspect reflux nephropathy
- Left hand and wrist X-ray for bone age
- Echocardiography for signs of left ventricular hypertrophy if patient is hypertensive

CKD treatment

Treatment

There should be a referral to a pediatric nephrology center.

Urgent life-threatening abnormalities

- High/low K^+
- Low Na^+
- Acidosis
- Low Ca^{2+}
- High PO_4
- High/low BP

Nutrition

Early involvement of the pediatric renal dietician is needed.

- Patients often require supplemental nutrition.
  - Nasogastric or gastrostomy feeds
- Vitamins supplements (but not vitamin A)

Fluid and electrolyte balance

- Avoid high K^+-containing foods (e.g., banana, chocolate)
- Many causes of CKD cause polyuria and Na^+ wasting, therefore the patient may need Na^+ supplements
- If fluid overloaded: Na^+ restriction and diuretics

Acid–base balance

- Sodium bicarbonate supplements

Renal osteodystrophy

- Control of plasma PO_4: Restrict dietary intake and PO_4 binders
- 1, 25-dihydroxycholciferol (vitamin D) and/or other vitamin D analogues
- Monitor PTH
- Annual X-ray to assess bone age

Anemia

- Assess iron status, oral iron supplements
- Subcutaneous erythropoietin

Hypertension (see Hypertension, p. 414)

Preservation of renal function

- Control hypertension
- Reduce proteinuria–e.g., ACE inhibitor or angiotensin receptor blocker therapy

Growth

- Optimize nutrition, acid–base balance, electrolyte balance
- If there is failing height velocity (HV ≤ −2 SDS) or short stature (Ht ≤ −2 SDS) treatment with recombinant human growth hormone is indicated.

Education and preparation for dialysis or transplantation
- Information provision
- Meet team
- Meet other families

Peritoneal dialysis (PD)
- The preferred choice is automated peritoneal dialysis (APD) performed in the patient's home (with mobile machines) so there is minimal disruption.
- The main risks are peritonitis and catheter blockage.
- The patient needs family and social support.

Hemodialysis (HD)
- Extracorporeal circuit
- The preferred long-term vascular access is an AV fistula (upper extremities). Therefore, avoid venopuncture and IVs.
- The most common form of vascular access is a right internal jugular venous catheter. This is more convenient than an AV fistula to place and can be used immediately. There is a higher risk of infection and line dysfunction.
- Frequency and time per dialysis session is dependent on patient's size and dialysis needs (metabolic balance and fluid removal requirement).
- Home HD is possible, but few families are suitable.

Renal transplantation
This is the ultimate goal in ESRD.
- Minimum is 10 kg, although not a rigid requirement
- Deceased donor vs. living donor source
- Preemptive transplantation before dialysis is suitable for certain patients and families.
- Living donor by a laparoscopic donor nephrectomy is now standard.
- 3-year graft survival is 88% for living-related graft, 76% for deceased donor (North American Pediatric Renal Transplant Cooperative Study [NAPRTCS], 2007)
- Lifelong immunosuppression is required.

Psychosocial support
- Continuous patient and family support is a MUST. Patients and families with CKD face multiple challenges lifelong.
- Focus on prevention of cardiovascular disease, which is a major cause of mortality and morbidity in adult life.

Congenital urinary tract anomalies

- Increasingly, urinary tract anomalies are being detected earlier by the use of routine antenatal ultrasound scans.
- Accounts for 20%–30% of all anomalies detected in the prenatal period
- Close communication between obstetricians, pediatricians, and surgeons with regard to counseling the parents and follow-up is vital

Amniotic fluid volume

- Oligohydramnios—low urine production or obstruction of urine excretion that may lead to pulmonary hypoplasia
- Polyhydramnios—polyuria or swallowing problems

Renal size

- Enlarged: Cystic kidneys (any cause), hydronephrosis
- Small: Dysplasia

Hydronephrosis

- Unilateral: Ureteropelvic junction (UPJ) or ureterovesical junction obstruction (UVJ), vesicoureteral reflux (VUR)
- Bilateral: Bladder outlet obstruction (e.g., PUV, VUR, prune belly syndrome)

Renal cysts

- Multicystic dysplastic kidneys (MCDK)
- Cystic dysplasia

Abnormal renal parenchyma

- Echogenic
- Cystic kidneys (any cause)
- Congenital nephrotic syndrome (may have polyhydramnios, large placenta)
- Bilateral or unilateral agenesis, dysgenesis
- Ectopic kidney

Investigations

- If bilateral involvement or a solitary affected kidney is suspected, and/or history of oligohydramnios, then a renal ultrasound should be performed immediately after stabilization of the neonate (within the first 24 hours of life). Otherwise conduct a postnatal investigation with ultrasound (at 2–4 weeks) followed by VCUG and/or radionuclide scan, if indicated.
- Serum creatinine of newborns will reflect maternal creatinine. In term infants, it will take about a week to normalize and 2–3 weeks for preterm infants.

Clinical management

In the postnatal period, ensure that boys have voided with a good urinary stream. The initial postnatal ultrasound finding guides further management:

- If ultrasound shows obstruction, consult pediatric urology for drainage with Foley catheter or nephrostomy.
- VCUG only if there is strong suspicion of VUR (e.g., dilated ureters or intermittent dilatation of pelvis). The patient will need antibiotics for the procedure.
- Give antibiotic prophylaxis (amoxicillin 20 mg/kg daily) to all babies with suspicion of VUR until VCUG performed
- Radionuclide scan depends on the lesion
  - DMSA if focal renal parenchymal abnormality is suspected or if helpful to know the differential function of each kidney
  - MAG3 renogram if obstruction is suspected (e.g., UPJ, UVJ)

Most infants with nonobstructive hydronephrosis can be conservatively observed until it resolves. Refer patient to pediatric nephrology and/or urology if persistent.

Vesicoureteral reflux (VUR)

This is the retrograde flow of urine from the bladder into the upper urinary tract. VUR is usually congenital in origin but may be acquired (e.g., post-surgery). The incidence of VUR is approximately 1% in newborn infants. It is observed in 30%–45% of young children presenting with febrile UTI.

Traditionally, VUR combined with infected urine was believed to lead to progressive renal scarring (reflux nephropathy) and progress to CKD/ESRD. However, there is new evidence suggesting that CKD may be a result of renal maldevelopment (hypoplasia and dysplasia) associated with VUR, instead of continuous damage from infection and/or urinary back-pressure into the upper urinary tract.

There is often a strong family history of reflux:

- VUR is seen in two-thirds of children whose parents had VUR.
- There is a 35% incidence rate among siblings of affected children.

Grade of VUR

The extent of retrograde reflux from the bladder can be graded according to the International Reflux Study grading system:

- I   Into ureter only, without dilation
- II   Into ureter and collecting system, without dilation
- III Fills and mildly dilates the ureter and the collecting system with mild blunting of the calyces
- IV   Fills and grossly dilates the ureter and the collecting system. One-half of the calyces are blunted.
- V   Massive reflux grossly dilates the collecting system. All the calyces are blunted with a loss of papillary impression and intrarenal reflux may be present. There is significant ureteral dilation and tortuosity.

Presentation

- *Prenatal*: VUR is suggested by hydronephrosis on antenatal ultrasound.
- *Postnatal*: most often after UTI, less often from screening siblings of a VUR patient

Diagnosis

The diagnosis of VUR is established by radiological techniques.

Voiding cystourethrogram (VCUG)

This is the first choice of technique. It involves urinary catheterization and administration of radiocontrast medium into the bladder. Reflux is detected on voiding.

- Advantages: Grade of reflux seen, more sensitive
- Disadvantages: Requires bladder catheterization, radiation dose

Radionuclide cystogram

This procedure involves introduction of radionuclide tracer by a urinary catheter.

- Advantages: Lower radiation dose
- Disadvantages: Lower sensitivity, especially for other anatomical anomalies

Evaluation

- Prenatal presentation
  - Ultrasound after delivery. If there is moderate or greater hydro-nephrosis or a dilated ureter, proceed to VCUG. If VCUG is normal, proceed to a dynamic functional study such as MAG3 renal scan to rule out obstruction.
  - If postnatal ultrasound is normal or shows mild hydronephrosis, then repeat ultrasound in 3 months
  - If there is a strong family history of VUR, proceed to VCUG.
- Postnatal presentation: VCUG for
  - Any males with first UTI
  - Girls younger than 3 years old with first UTI
  - Any child under 5 years old with febrile UTI
  - Children with recurrent UTI
  - Children with other renal or urinary tract anomaly

Follow-up and treatment

Current management recommendations are based on a premise that CKD results from VUR and infection, thus the aim is to prevent renal scarring. This approach may change in the future (see previous page for controversy of the mechanism leading to CKD).

- Medical therapy
  - Antibiotic prophylaxis therapy (TMP-SMX or nitrofurantoin) has been recommended until reflux has resolved. Current evidence challenges routine prophylaxis.
- Surgical management is considered, depending on the patient's age, severity of reflux, presence of renal scarring, failed medical therapy, poor compliance, and family preference. Discuss this with the pediatric urologist and/or nephrologist.
  - The "STING" procedure (subureteric transurethral injection) is an outpatient procedure involving endoscopic injection of a copolymer substance beneath the mucosa of the UVJ. Success rates are higher with lower grades of VUR. Recurrence is possible but high success rates accompany the second attempt.
  - Open surgery involves reimplantation of ureters. This has a higher success rate than that of the STING procedure, but is more invasive and requires hospitalization.
- Follow-up
  - Mandatory urine culture with UTI symptoms or unexplained fever
  - Periodic VCUG or radionuclide cystogram while on medical ther-apy or follow-up study after surgery

Prognosis

- Spontaneous resolution of VUR often occurs, especially with lower grade of reflux.
- Bilateral reflux (grades IV and V) and reflux into duplex systems is associated with a lower probability of resolution.

Inherited renal disease

Many renal abnormalities are inherited. Recognition of these is important, not only in terms of diagnosis and treatment of the patient, but also for screening and genetic counseling for the whole family.

- New therapies may become available.
- Ethical considerations are very important in this group in terms of family screening and counseling.
- Databases such as Online Mendelian Inheritance in Man (OMIN) provide comprehensive lists. A few of the more common conditions follow.

Autosomal dominant inheritance

Polycystic kidney disease (ADPKD)

ADPKD is the most common inherited renal disease (1:400 to 1:1000 live births), which can present anytime over a lifetime with progression to ESRD mostly during adulthood. It may have multiorgan involvement (intracranial aneurysms, liver and pancreatic cysts, mitral valve prolapse). It may present with hypertension, abdominal mass, hematuria, or pain (a rare presentation in neonatal period with abdominal masses and/or high or low blood pressure, renal impairment). Genetic tests for PKD1 and PKD2 are available.

Tuberous sclerosis

PKD1 and TSC2 are adjacent to each other on chromosome 16 and are often associated with each other.

- An inherited neurocutaneous disorder involving multiple organs, including benign neoplasm of the brain, kidney, and skin. Diagnosis is made using specific criteria based on clinical features.
- Renal involvement: Cysts, angiomyolipomas, high or low blood pressure, renal impairment. Angiomyolipoma may enlarge and hemorrhage.

Autosomal recessive inheritance

Polycystic kidney disease (ARPKD)

- Incidence is 1:10,000 to 1:40,000
- It typically presents in infancy with oligohydramnios and large echogenic kidneys.
- Microcysts are usually less than 3 mm in diameter.
- Fusiform dilatation of collecting tubules
- There is always hepatic involvement with cysts, fibrosis, and portal hypertension.
- Neonatal prognosis depends on the degree of pulmonary involvement.
- It usually presents at an earlier age than for ADPKD and progresses to renal failure in a shorter time.

Cystinosis
- Accumulation of cystine is due to defective transport system out of lysozomes.
- Multi-organ involvement: Cornea, liver, thyroid, brain, growth failure
- Renal: Tubulopathy eventually progresses to end stage (Fanconi syndrome).
- Cysteamine will slow renal progression and improve growth.

Nephronophthisis
- A group of chronic tubulointerstitial nephritis disorders with varying rates to progression to end stage and extrarenal involvement

Primary hyperoxaluria
See Nephrolithiasis (p. 446).

Cystinuria
- A defect in proximal tubule cystine reabsorption leads to cystine stone formation (it sounds similar to cystinosis but is a completely different disease).

Bartter syndrome
See Bartter syndrome (p. 473).

Gitleman syndrome
See Gitleman syndrome (p. 474)

X-linked

Alports syndrome
- Sensorineural deafness with progressive nephritis

Nephrogenic diabetes insipidus

Fabry disease
- Deficiency of α-galactosidase A with eventual progression to end stage.

Sporadic

VATER association
- **V**ertebral, **A**nal, **T**racheo**E**sophageal, **R**adial/**R**enal renal problems include agenesis, ectopy or obstruction

CHARGE association
- **C**oloboma, **H**eart defects, choanal **A**tresia, **R**etarded growth, **G**enital anomalies, **E**ar abnormalities (renal anomalies include dysplasia, agenesis, and ectopy)

Turner (XO) syndrome
- Horseshoe or duplex kidneys, abnormal vascular supply, hypertension

William syndrome
- Renovascular hypertension, nephrocalcinosis from hypercalcemia

Renal tubular disorders

The renal tubules are responsible for the regulation of fluid, acid–base, and electrolyte balance. Abnormalities of renal function may occur at any point along the length of the renal tubule system and may lead to a disturbance in the equilibrium of any of the substances handled by it. It is essential to consider these disorders with any of the following:

- Glycosuria, amino-aciduria, or impaired ability to concentrate or acidify urine shown on urinalysis
- Stones or nephrocalcinosis
  - Distal tubular acidosis and hyperoxaluria are major causes.
- Polyhydramnios and failure to thrive in a newborn
  - E.g., Bartter syndrome associated with hypokalemic alkalosis
- Failure to thrive with rickets
  - Cystinosis is the most common inherited cause of Fanconi syndrome in children
- Major rickets with low plasma phosphate levels
  - Familial hypophosphatemic rickets
- Failure to thrive with low urine osmolality
  - Nephrogenic diabetes insipidus

Renal tubular acidosis

Renal tubular acidosis (RTA) is a state of systemic hyperchloremia resulting from impaired urinary acidification—either the net retention of hydrogen chloride or its equivalent or the net loss of sodium bicarbonate or its equivalent. All forms of RTA result in normal anion gap metabolic acidosis. Three types of RTA exist (see Box 11.6):

- Type 1, or distal RTA
- Type 2, or proximal RTA
- Type 4, or hypoaldosteronism RTA

Box 11.6 Causes of renal tubular acidosis

Distal (type 1)
- Isolated
  - Sporadic or inherited
- Secondary
  - Tubulointerstitial diseases
  - Obstructive nephropathy
  - Inherited
  - Ehlers–Danlos syndrome
  - Hereditary hypercalciuria
  - Sickle cell anemia
  - Hypercalciuria
  - Acquired
  - Sjögren syndrome
  - Chronic active hepatitis
  - Systemic lupus erythematosus (SLE)
  - Toxins
  - Amphotericin B
  - Lithium

Proximal (type 2)
- Isolated
  - Sporadic or inherited
- Fanconi syndrome
  - Primary
  - Secondary
  - Inherited
- Cystinosis
- Galactosemia
- Glycogen storage disease
- Wilson disease
- Lowes syndrome
- Dent disease
  - Acquired
- Vitamin D–deficient rickets
- Sjögren syndrome
  - Hyperparathyroidism
  - Toxins
- Ifosfamide
- Aminoglycosides
- Heavy metals

Distal RTA (type 1)

This type is due to impaired capacity for hydrogen-ion (ammonium) secretion in the collecting tubules, resulting in abnormally high urine pH even during systemic acidosis (urine pH >5.5). This presents with hyperchloremic hypokalemic acidosis with an inappropriately high urine pH, often associated with hypercalciuria, sometimes resulting in nephrolithiasis and nephrocalcinosis. Distal RTA may be isolated or secondary.

Proximal RTA (type 2)

This type of RTA results from reduced proximal tubular reabsorption of bicarbonate.
- Fall in plasma bicarbonate concentration is self-limited (~15–18 meq/L) as acid–base balance is reached when all the filtered bicarbonate can be reabsorbed.
- Urine pH can vary.

Proximal RTA less often occurs as an isolated disorder. This form may be transient and is occasionally inherited. It usually occurs as a more generalized defect of proximal tubular transport (Fanconi syndrome; see Box 11.6) characterized by
- RTA
- One or more of following: glucosuria, phosphaturia, uricosuria, aminoaciduria, and tubular proteinuria

Clinical features of type 1 and 2 RTA

Children with isolated forms of proximal and distal RTA usually present with failure to thrive in infancy. Those with the secondary forms of RTA may present in a similar way.

Diagnosis

Other causes of systemic acidosis (e.g., chronic diarrhea, lactic acidosis, diabetic ketoacidosis) should be excluded. Investigation to establish a diagnosis of RTA should include the following:

- Blood: pH; bicarbonate (low); potassium (low); chloride (high)
- Urine: Early-morning sample
  - pH ≥5.5 suggests distal RTA
  - Proximal RTA can have variable pH

If proximal RTA is detected, then blood tests and urinalysis to establish other tubular defects should be undertaken.

Treatment

The main aims are correction of acidosis and maintenance of normal bicarbonate and potassium. This can be achieved by alkali (citrate or bicarbonate) or potassium-containing solutions.

Hypoaldosteronism (type 4)

This is due to either aldosterone deficiency or tubular resistance to the action of aldosterone. Patients usually present with mild metabolic acidosis, hyperkalemia, and low urinary pH (<5.3). Most patients are managed with dietary restriction of potassium and, if necessary, with diuretics.

Bartter syndrome

This is a relatively rare autosomal recessive form of renal tubular dysfunction. The condition is best described as a defect in sodium chloride reabsorption in the ascending loop of Henle, resulting in
- Excessive potassium excretion
- Increased prostaglandin synthesis
- Stimulation of the renin–angiotensin–aldosterone system
- Polyuria due to sodium and water losses

Clinical features

The syndrome usually presents in infancy or early childhood with the following traits:
- Poor growth
- Muscle weakness
- Constipation
- Polyuria and polydipsia due to excessive salt and water loss
- History of polyhydramnios and prematurity are common.
- May be associated with mental retardation

Diagnosis

Diagnosis is largely one of exclusion: rule out vomiting and diuretic use. Typically, characteristic findings include
- Hyopkalemia
- Metabolic alkalosis
- Hypochloremia
- Some cases with hypomagnesemia (much less frequent than in Gitelman syndrome)
- Impaired urine concentration capacity
- Hyperreninemia and hyperaldosteronemia
- Low/normal blood pressure
- Increased urinary calcium excretion

Treatment

The goals are to maintain serum potassium levels in the normal range and adequate nutrition. Therapy includes a combination of oral potassium supplement together with a potassium-sparing diuretic (e.g., spironolactone) and indomethacin (prostaglandin inhibitor). ACE inhibitors may also be used if they do not cause hypotension.

Gitelman syndrome

This is another rare autosomal recessive form of renal tubular dysfunction, resulting from mutation in the gene coding for thiazide-sensitive Na-Cl co-transporter in the distal tubule. It is usually more benign than Bartter syndrome.

Clinical features

Unlike Bartter syndrome, Gitelman syndrome typically presents late in childhood or early adulthood. Features are comparable to patients taking thiazide diuretic:
- Cramps
- Fatigue
- Nocturia and polyuria
- Salt craving

Diagnosis

Diagnosis is similar to that of Bartter syndrome, with overlapping features (see Table 11.6 for comparison):
- Hyopkalemia
- Metabolic alkalosis
- Hypochloremia
- **ALWAYS** with hypomagnesemia
- Hyperreninemia and hyperaldosteronemia
- Normal to below normal blood pressure
- Low urine calcium excretion: UCa/UCr <0.1

Table 11.6 Comparison of Bartter and Gitelman syndromes

	Bartter syndrome	Gitelman syndrome
Location of defect	Currently, 5 different channel defects described in the ascending loop of Henle	Thiazide-sensitive Na-Cl channel in the distal tubule
Typical age and presenting features	Infancy or early childhood with poor growth	Late childhood or early childhood with cramps, tetany, and/or fatigue
Biochemical differences	High urinary calcium excretion, impaired urinary concentration capacity	Hypomagnesemia invariably, low urine calcium excretion

Treatment

Give potassium and magnesium supplements to replace urinary losses.

Endocrinology and diabetes

Obesity

Obesity has become an important public health problem that has achieved epidemic levels in the developed world. In the United States approximately 33% of children and adolescents are either overweight or obese.[1] Obesity in childhood strongly predicts obesity in adulthood. Obesity is an important risk factor for the development of life-threatening disease in later life, including type 2 diabetes mellitus (DM), hypertension, cardiovascular disease, and cancer.

Definition and diagnosis

Obesity implies increased central (abdominal) fat mass, and can be quantified using a number of clinical surrogate markers. Body mass index (BMI) is the most convenient indicator of body fat mass (see Fig. 12.1).

BMI = weight (kg) / height (m)^2
- Overweight   BMI = > 85th centile – < 95th centile
                                      > +1.0 SDS – < +1.6 SDS
- Obese   BMI = > 95th centile
                                        > +1.6 SDS

(SDS = standard deviation score)

Other measures of obesity include
- Waist circumference
- Waist–hip ratio

Epidemiology

The worldwide increase in incidence in obesity has been observed mainly in Western countries and in other developed societies. Risk factors for the development of obesity include the following:
- Parental or family history of obesity
- African-American, Asian, Hispanic, or Native American ethnic origins
- Catch-up growth (weight) in early childhood (0–2 years): Infants born small for gestational age who demonstrate significant weight catch-up (>2 SDS) in the first 2 years of life.

Causes

So-called idiopathic (or "simple") obesity is by far the most common cause of obesity, accounting for up to 95% of cases. It is multifactorial in origin and represents an imbalance in normal nutritional–environmental– gene interaction, whereby daily calorie (energy) intake exceeds the amount of calories (energy) expended:
- Genetic predisposition (energy conservation)
- Increasing sedentary lifestyle (energy expenditure)
- Increasing consumption and availability of high-energy foods
Obesity may be associated with other identifiable underlying pathological conditions.

1. Ogden CL, Carroll MD, Curtin LR, et al. (2006). Prevalence of overweight and obesity in the United States 1999–2004. *JAMA* **295**:1549–1555.

Endocrine (rare)
- Hypothyroidism (see p. 502)
- Cushing's'syndrome/disease (see p. 516)
- Growth hormone deficiency (see p. 552)
- Pseudohypoparathyroidism (see p. 522)
- Polycystic ovarian syndrome
- Acquired hypothalamic injury (see p. 502) i.e., CNS tumors and/or surgery resulting in disruption to the neuroendocrine pathways regulating appetite and satiety

Genetic
Obesity is a recognized feature characterizing the phenotype of a number of genetic syndromes:
- Prader–Willi syndrome (see p. 1075)
- Bardet–Biedl syndrome (see p. 1075)
- Monogenic causes: Leptin deficiency (rare), melanocortin-4 receptor gene (5%–6% of all causes)

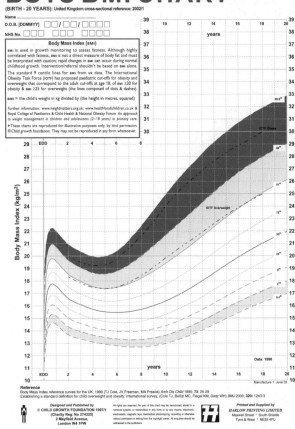

Figure 12.1a Body mass index (BMI) centile charts. Copyright Child Growth Foundation.

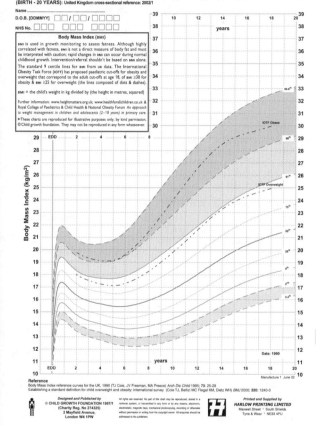

Figure 12.1b Body mass index (BMI) centile charts. Copyright Child Growth Foundation.

Obesity: management

Evaluation and investigations

This includes taking a detailed clinical and family history:

- Birth weight (*note*: small for gestational age)
- Feeding habits and behavior, particularly infancy and early childhood.
- Hyperphagia may suggest a genetic cause.
- Weight gain and growth pattern (check previous health records)
- Physical activity
- Neurodevelopment and school performance
- Screen for comorbid factors (see below)
- Family history: Obesity; type 2 DM; cardiovascular disease

Laboratory investigations are directed at excluding secondary causes of obesity:

- Blood biochemistry: Thyroid function test, serum cortisol (midnight, or late in day) or 24-hour urine free cortisol, liver function test, fasting lipid profile
- Genetic studies (e.g., Prader–Willi syndrome)
- Oral glucose test (see Obesity and OGTT)

Complications and co morbid conditions

Obesity is associated the following comorbid conditions, which should be screened for at the time of assessment:

- *Psychological*: Low self-esteem, depression.
- *ENT and respiratory*: Obstructive sleep apnea, obesity–hypoventilation syndrome, pulmonary hypertension
- *Orthopedic*: Bowing of legs, slipped femoral epiphysis, osteoarthritis
- *Metabolic*: Impaired glucose tolerance or type 2 diabetes, hypertension, dyslipidemia, polycystic ovarian syndrome
- *Hepatic*: Nonalcoholic steatohepatitis
- *Other*: Hypertension

Obesity and oral glucose tolerance testing (OGTT)

In children and adolescents with obesity the prevalence of impaired glucose tolerance (IGT) and type 2 diabetes mellitus (T2DM) has been estimated to be in the region of 20%–25% and 4%, respectively.

An oral glucose tolerance test (see Box 12.1) should be considered when one or more of the following risk factors are present:

- Severe obesity: BMI SDS >1.6
- Acanthosis nigricans
- Positive family history of T2DM
- Ethnic origin: African-American, Asian, Hispanic, or Native American
- Polycystic ovarian syndrome
- Hypertension

Box 12.1 Oral glucose tolerance testing (OGTT)

- *Conditions*: Performed in the morning after 8–10 hours fast
- *Dose:* Glucose 1.75 g/kg, to a maximum of 75 g, drunk within 5–10 minutes
- *Sampling:* Blood glucose at 0 minutes and at 30-minute intervals thereafter for 120 minutes

Interpretation of OGTT:

	Blood glucose 0 minutes	Blood glucose 120 minutes
Normal	<100 mg/dL	<140 mg/dL
IGT	>100 to <126 mg/dL	>140 to <200 mg/dL
T2DM	>126 mg/dL	>200 mg/dL

Management

There is currently no consensus on the best approach to treating childhood obesity. Treatment requires a multidisciplinary approach:

- Nutrition and lifestyle education and counseling are important.
- Decrease calorie intake and increase exercise
- Behavior modification and family therapy strategies
- Drug therapies (currently limited, not licensed for children)
- Obesity (bariatric) surgery (rarely)

Community or population-based intervention and prevention strategies may be more effective than approaches targeted at the obese individual. Parental commitment is essential to success when treating the obese child.

Type 1 diabetes mellitus (T1DM)

This the most common form of diabetes mellitus in children and adolescents (90% of cases). It is an autoimmune disorder characterized by T-cell-mediated destruction and progressive loss of pancreatic β cells leading to eventual insulin deficiency and hyperglycemia.

Epidemiology

The incidence of T1DM has been increasing shows marked geographical variation. The incidence of T1DM in the United States is approximately 25/100,000/year.[1,2] There are data to show, as in Europe, an annual increase in incidence of approximately 3%.

During childhood there are two peaks in presentation—one between ages 5 and 7 years and the other, larger peak, just before or at the onset of puberty. Seasonal variation in presentation of T1DM is also observed, with a peak seen in the winter months.

Etiology

The cause of T1DM involves both genetic and environmental factors. Over 20 different T1DM susceptibility genes have been identified. The IDDM1 gene locus, which represents the HLA DR/DQ locus on the major histocompatibility complex, accounts for the greatest susceptibility.

The role of various environmental interactions and triggers is controversial.

Pathophysiology

T1DM is a chronic autoimmune condition:
- Immune tolerance is broken and antibodies against specific β-cell autoantigens are generated (e.g., anti-islet cell; anti-insulin; anti-GAD65; anti-IA2 antibodies).
- T-cell activation leads to β-cell inflammation ("insulitis") and to subsequent cell loss through apoptosis.
- The rate of β-cell loss varies (months–years) and the timing and presentation of symptomatic diabetes may depend on factors that increase insulin requirements (e.g., puberty).

Clinical presentation

The onset of symptoms generally evolves over a period of weeks. Symptoms are a reflection of insulin deficiency resulting in increased catabolism and hyperglycemia. In most patients, first presentation is usually made in the early symptomatic phase with the following:
- Weight loss
- Polyuria, polydipsia
- Nocturia, nocturnal enuresis

Other less common symptoms include
- Candida infection (e.g., oral thrush, balanitis, vulvovaginitis)
- Skin infections

Failure to recognize these symptoms will result in delayed or late diagnosis of T1DM and possible presentation with diabetic ketoacidosis (DKA) (see p. 106). The risk of first presentation of T1DM with DKA is increased when nonspecific symptoms of diabetes go unrecognized:

• Intercurrent or febrile illness
• Infants and preschool-age child

Assessment of new patient

Emphasis should be made on the following:

• History: Duration of symptoms
• Family history of diabetes or other autoimmune disease
• Examination: Weight, BMI; signs of DKA (see p. 106)

Diagnosis and investigations

The diagnosis is readily established in a symptomatic child with a random blood glucose level >200 mg/dL. Other investigations:

• Blood urea nitrogen (BUN) and electrolytes
• Blood pH (to exclude DKA)
• Diabetes-related autoantibodies: Islet cell antibody (ICA), anti-insulin antibody (IAA), anti-GAD65 antibody (GAD), anti IA-2
• Other autoimmune disease screening: Thyroid function test, thyroid antibodies; celiac disease antibody screen (anti-tissue transglutaminase IgA or anti-endomysial antibodies)

1. The Writing Group for the SEARCH for Diabetes in Youth Study Group (2007). Incidence of Diabetes in Youth in the United States. *JAMA* **297**:2716–2724.
2. Vehik K, Hamman RF, Lezotte D, et al. (2007). Trends in the incidence of type 1 diabetes mellitus in 0–17 year-old Colorado youth (1978–2004). *Diabetes Care* **30**:503–509.

T1DM: management

The initial care and subsequent long-term management of patients with T1DM should be delivered by a specialist pediatric diabetes team. All newly diagnosed patients must start insulin therapy as soon as possible. An intensive program of education and support is needed for the child and parents (see Box 12.2).

> **Box 12.2 Aims of management of T1DM**
>
> - Education of the child and family about diabetes
> - Insulin therapy
> - Nutritional management
> - Monitoring of glycemic control
> - Avoidance and management of hypoglycemia
> - Management of acute illness and avoidance of DKA
> - Screening for development of associated illness
> - Screening for diabetes-related microvascular complications
> - Prevention and treatment of microvascular complications

Education, counseling, and support

An intensive program of education and counseling is needed in the first few days and weeks to cover the fundamental principles about T1DM and its management:
- Basic pathophyisology of T1DM
- Insulin therapy
  - Actions of insulin
  - Subcutaneous (SC) injection techniques
  - Dose adjustment principles
- Home and self blood-glucose monitoring
- Acute complications
  - Avoidance, symptom recognition, and treatment
  - Hypoglycemia
  - Diabetic ketoacidosis
  - "Sick-day rules" during illness to prevent DKA
- Diet
  - Healthy, low fat
  - High complex carbohydrate
- Long-term complications
  - Risk factors and avoidance
- Psychological issues

A considerable amount of time and need for repetition are required to deliver this information. The process of education and support is a continual one, along with regular review and updates of knowledge.

Nutritional management

Diet and insulin regimen need to be matched to optimize glycemic control. A healthy diet is recommended with a high complex-carbohydrate and relatively low-fat content (see Box 12.3).

Box 12.3 Daily dietary balance in T1DM

- Healthy diet
- 50%–60% carbohydrate–complex and high fiber
- <30% fat (<10% in form of saturated fat)
- 15%–20% protein
- Refined sugars limited to <25 g/day

Blood glucose monitoring

Regular daily blood-glucose monitoring and testing when blood levels are suspected to be low or high are recommended. Home blood-glucose monitoring is carried out using a portable glucose meter and lancet device.

Regular testing is required to assist with decisions on insulin dose adjustment and to learn and predict how changes in lifestyle, food, and exercise affect glycemic control.

Minimal testing frequency is before meals and bedtime, 3 to 4 times per day. However, this will vary and depend on the patient's and family's motivation and desire for intensive glycemic control, balanced against the negative aspects of testing (finger-pricks).

T1DM: insulin therapy

Insulin and insulin analog preparations (created by minor amino acid substitutions to the "native" human insulin molecule) are described in Table 12.1.

Table 12.1 Characteristics of various insulin preparations

Type	Example	Onset	Peak	Duration
Short acting	Regular/soluble	30–60 min	1.5–3 hr	4–6 hr
Rapid (analog)	Insulin lispro	10–15 min	30–90 min	3–5 hr
	Insulin aspart	10–20 min	1–3 hr	3–5 hr
	Insulin glulisine	15–20min	45–75 min	3–5 hr
Intermediate acting	NPH	1–4 hr	5–10 hr	10–16 hr
Long acting (analog)	Insulin Detemir	2–4 hr	None	12–20 hr
	Insulin glargine	1–2 hr	None	20–24 hr

Data taken from Tanner JM (1962). *Growth at Adolescence*. Oxford: Blackwell Scientific Publications.

The daily requirement for insulin varies with age:

units/kg per day

- At diagnosis: 0.5–1
- Childhood or prepubertal: 0.5–1
- Puberty: 1.2–2
- Post-puberty: 0.7–1.2

Insulin is administered subcutaneously, usually as a bolus injection. A number of patients receive insulin in the form of a continuous subcutaneous insulin infusion (CSII) delivered by a pump device. Insulin injection sites include the subcutaneous tissues of the upper arm, the anterior and lateral thigh, the abdomen, and buttocks.

There are a variety of different daily insulin-injection therapy regimens. The choice of regime is a compromise between achieving optimal therapy and minimizing psychosocial development. The patient and family must have input into the choice.

Insulin regimens

Basal bolus regimen

This regimen attempts to mimic physiological secretion. Low-level, background, basal insulin provides for fasting and between-meal insulin requirements, and larger acute doses of fast-acting insulin are given to provide for prandial requirements:

- *Basal insulin*: Once-a-day intermediate or long-acting insulin (traditionally at bedtime, although often administered in the morning or divided into morning and bedtime for younger children).
- *Fast-acting insulin*: At meal times (i.e., 3 × per day) and with between-meal snacks.

Advantages

- Increase flexibility with meal times and exercise planning
- Insulin dose adjustment with carbohydrate (CHO) counting

Disadvantages

- Need for more injections
- Need more frequent blood glucose monitoring

Continuous subcutaneous insulin infusion (CSII)

Current insulin infusion pumps are reliable and portable. CSII therapy can be used in children of all ages. Short or rapid-acting insulin is administered as a continuous insulin infusion. Mealtime boluses and "blood glucose correction" boluses are administered when required.

Advantages

- No bolus injections and reduced injection frequency
- Increased flexibility of meal times and exercise planning
- Insulin dose adjustment with CHO counting
- Reduced frequency of hypoglycemia

Disadvantages

- No long-acting insulin. Infusion interruption introduces risk of rapid DKA
- Need more frequent blood glucose monitoring
- Greater management expertise required

Two-dose regimen

This is the simplest regimen, with two injections per day. Each injection is a mix of short and rapid-acting insulin PLUS an intermediate-acting insulin. Traditionally, two-thirds of the total daily dose is given at breakfast and one-third is given before or at the evening meal.

Disadvantages

- Need to mix insulins
- Peak action of insulin does not correspond with timing of main meals of day
- Increased frequency of between-meal and nocturnal hypoglycemia. Between-meal snacks are required to minimize hypoglycemia.

Note: There is less hypoglycemia with rapid analog insulin use than with regular insulin.

Three-dose regimen

This regimen is an improvement and intensification of the two-dose regimen.

- 1. At breakfast: Mix of short or rapid-acting insulin PLUS an intermediate-acting insulin
- 2. Before or at evening meal: Short or rapid-acting insulin only
- 3. At bedtime: Intermediate-acting insulin only

Advantages

Delayed evening intermediate-acting insulin results in reduced frequency of nocturnal hypoglycemia.

Insulin requirements and dose adjustment

Insulin doses are adjusted on the basis of home blood-glucose monitoring. Generally it is best not to alter the basic insulin regimen every time the blood glucose levels are outside the target range (e.g., 80–180 mg/dL). Rather, recorded blood glucose levels should be reviewed and insulin adjustments made to correct recurrent profiles that are either too low or too high. Insulin doses are adjusted by 5% to 10% at a time.

Carbohydrate counting: insulin dose adjustment system

This system applies the principle that the amount of fasting and rapid-acting insulin given at mealtimes is adjusted and matched according to the amount of carbohydrates consumed.

Acute complications of T1DM

Hypoglycemia

Almost all children with T1DM will experience an episode of hypoglycemia; early detection will hopefully allow the child to avoid severe hypoglycemia. Symptoms develop when blood glucose <60 mg/dL, or with rapid falls in blood glucose levels. The frequency of hypoglycemia is higher with more intensive insulin regimens and in young children. Symptoms and signs include the following:

- Hunger feeling
- Sweatiness
- Feeling faint or dizzy
- "Wobbly" feeling
- Irritability, confusion, misbehavior
- Pallor

Hypoglycemia unawareness

Occasionally, sudden onset of hypoglycemia may result in unconsciousness and seizures. Children experiencing frequent episodes of hypoglycemia may fail to develop the typical (i.e., counterregulatory, adrenergic) symptoms of hypoglycemia. Avoidance of hypoglycemia usually results in restoration of warning symptoms.

Nocturnal hypoglycemia

The frequency of nocturnal hypoglycemia is thought to be high in T1DM (up to 50%). Nocturnal hypoglycemia should be considered when fasting early-morning blood sugars are repeatedly high, despite seemingly adequate overnight insulin cover (secondary to hypoglycemia counterregulation).

Detection and confirmation of nocturnal hypoglycemia can be achieved by using a subcutaneous continuous glucose monitoring system (CGMS) device or through frequent monitoring of nighttime and early-morning blood glucose.

Hypoglycemia: management

Acute episodes of mild to moderate symptomatic hypoglycemia can be managed with oral glucose (glucose tablets or a sugar-containing drink such as juice). Oral glucose gels (e.g., Insta-glucose) applied to the buccal mucosa can be used in the child who is unwilling or unable to cooperate to eat. Severe hypoglycemia can be managed in the home with Glucagon (0.3–1 mg). This is available as a specific injection kit.

Sick-day management

During illness and other physiological stresses (e.g., following injury), insulin requirements may dramatically increase in response to the body's increased catabolic state.

Blood glucose should be monitored more frequently than usual and insulin doses may need to be increased. Insulin must be continued at all times, even although oral intake of food and fluids may be decreased. Urine or plasma ketones must be monitored and, if elevated, are a sign of increased insulin needs and possible impending DKA.

- In the presence of moderate to high ketone levels, doses of rapid-acting insulin must be increased (by 25%–100%) and supplemental doses may need to be given. Supplemental doses can be calculated as 5%–10% of total daily insulin dose for small–moderate ketones, 10%–20% of total daily dose when marked ketones are present.
- Carbohydrate and fluid intake should be maintained as much possible to avoid hypoglycemia and dehydration.

If the child is unable to maintain hydration (e.g., due to excessive vomiting) or cannot take in adequate carbohydrate to avoid hypoglycemia, the child should be evaluated by the diabetes or other medical team and treatment with IV fluids and insulin infusions should be considered (see DKA).

Diabetic ketoacidosis (DKA) (see also p. 106)

DKA is caused by a decrease in effective circulating insulin associated with elevations in counterregulatory hormones (glucagon, catecholamines, cortisol, growth hormone [GH]). This leads to increased glucose production by the liver and kidney and impaired peripheral glucose utilization with resultant hyperglycemia and hyperosmolality. Increased lipolysis, with ketone-body (β-hydroxybutyrate, acetoacetate) production causes ketonemia and metabolic acidosis.

Hyperglycemia and acidosis result in osmotic diuresis, dehydration, and obligate loss of electrolytes. Ketoacid accumulation also induces an ileus, resulting in nausea and vomiting and an exacerbation of the dehydration.

DKA: frequency

The frequency of DKA occurring at T1DM onset, or diagnosis, is 10 per 100,000 children and is more common in children <4 years of age. In established T1DM the frequency of DKA is approximately 1%–10% per patient per year.

The risk of DKA is increased in children with poor metabolic control; previous episodes of DKA; peripubertal and adolescent girls; and children with psychiatric disorders, including those with eating disorders and those with difficult family circumstances.

DKA: mortality and morbidity

Mortality rates for DKA are 0.15%–0.31%. Cerebral edema (CE) accounts for 57%–87% of all DKA-related deaths. The incidence of DKA-associated CE is 0.46%–0.87%. Reported mortality from CE is high (21%–25%) and significant morbidity is evident in 10%–26% of all CE survivors.

T1DM: long-term complications

The risk of developing microvascular or macrovascular complications (see Box 12.4) is related to the duration of diabetes and to the degree of glycemic control achieved over time. Patients who achieve and maintain good glycemic control (i.e., HbA1c 7.0% or less) have a lower risk. Genetic factors may also influence the risk of complications.

> **Box 12.4 Long-term complications of T1DM**
>
> *Microvascular complications*
> • Renal: Microalbuminuria, diabetic nephropathy
> • Eyes: Retinopathy
> • Nervous: Peripheral neuropathy, autonomic neuropathy
>
> *Macrovascular complications*
> • Hypertension
> • Coronary heart disease

Macrovascular complications are almost never seen in children and adolescents.

Microvascular complications may be seen during the childhood and adolescent years of T1DM. The incidence and frequency is low before puberty. Risk factors for the development of early microvascular disease are duration of diabetes, glycemic control (long-term), and the onset of puberty.

Microalbuminuria (MA)

MA is rare before puberty, and may be intermittent and transient. It may be associated with increased blood pressure, and require treatment with angiotensin-converting enzyme (ACE) inhibitor or angiotensin receptor blocker if MA persists (± hypertension).

Retinopathy

Significant changes are rare before the onset of puberty. Background retinopathy (microaneurysms, retinal hemorrhages, soft and hard exudates) may be seen. Preproliferative and proliferative retinopathy are rare.

T1DM: associated illnesses

Patients with T1DM are at increased risk for a number of other autoimmune disorders. The most important of these are the following:
- Autoimmune thyroiditis
  - Up to 5% of patients develop hypothyroidism
- Celiac disease
  - Prevalence rate is 5%–10%
  - Usually atypical symptoms or asymptomatic
- Adrenal insufficiency
  - Uncommon

Testing for thyroid autoantibodies, thyroid function tests (thyroid-stimulating hormone [TSH] and free T4), together with a celiac disease antibody screen (transglutaminase or endomysial antibodies) should be carried out on an annual basis for the early detection and treatment of these disorders.

Screening and long-term monitoring
Glycemic control
- Glycated hemoglobin index (HbA1c) measured every 3–4 months

Growth and development
- Height, weight, BMI (regular at clinic)
- Puberty stage (annual)

Microvascular complications
- Blood pressure monitoring (regular at clinic)
- Microalbuminuria screening
- 3 x early morning urinary albumin/creatinine ratio (annual)
- Retinopathy screening
- Retinal photography (annual, from age 12 years or after 5 years T1DM)
- Neuropathy (rare)

Type 2 diabetes mellitus (T2DM)

Type 2 diabetes mellitus (T2DM) is a multifactorial and heterogeneous condition in which the balance between insulin sensitivity and insulin secretion is impaired. The condition is characterized by relative insulin insufficiency to overcome underlying concomitant tissue insulin resistance.

Epidemiology

T2DM in children is emerging as a significant health problem, with increasing incidence in most developing countries. The increasing frequency of T2DM parallels the upward trend in childhood obesity in these populations. In the United States, T2DM now accounts for up to 45% of the new cases of diabetes diagnosed in childhood.

Etiology

T2DM is not an autoimmune disease. There is no association with HLA-linked genes, however, there is a strong genetic basis, which is thought to be polygenic (see Box 12.5).

> **Box 12.5 Known risk factors for the development of T2DM**
>
> - Obesity
> - Family history of T2DM
> - Polycystic ovarian syndrome
> - Small for gestational age
> - Ethnic origin
>   - Asian or Pacific Islander
>   - African-American
>   - Hispanic
>   - Native American

Clinical features

Clinical presentation ranges from mild incidental hyperglycemia to the typical manifestations of insulin deficiency. Presentation with DKA may be occasionally seen. Frequent clinical findings include evidence of obesity and acanthosis nigricans.

Diagnosis

> *Current diagnostic prerequisites for T2DM*
> - Presence of T2DM risk factors (as above)
> - Lack of absolute or persistent insulin deficiency
> - Absence of pancreatic autoantibodies

Not infrequently, the distinction between T1DM and T2DM at initial presentation may be difficult.

Management

All patients with T2DM require the same type and degree of educational support and clinical follow-up as for patients with T1DM. Long-term management goals are the same as T1DM (see p. 492).

Specific treatment goals should in addition include the following:
- Aim to improve insulin sensitivity and insulin secretion.
- Manage obesity and its comorbidities via lifestyle changes.
- Screening and management of T2DM comorbidities such as hyperlipidemia and hypertension

Depending on the degree of hyperglycemia, T2DM may initially be managed with lifestyle interventions aimed at lowering caloric intake (low-fat, reduced-CHO diet) and increasing physical activity. When these interventions fail, pharmacological therapy is added. In children, the oral insulin-sensitizing agent Metformin is added as a first step; however, if glycemic targets remain difficult to achieve, insulin therapy should be included.

Children or adolescents with T2DM may present with severe hyperglycemia, such as DKA or hyperosmolar hyperglycemic nonketotic coma (HHNK). Such presentations require intensive treatment including insulin infusion. Insulin therapy may be required only transiently.

Other forms of diabetes mellitus

Maturity onset diabets of young (MODY)

MODY is a clinical heterogeneous group of disorders characterized by an autosomal dominant mode of inheritance; onset is usually before age 25 years and nonketotic diabetes is at presentation. The condition is due a primary defect in B-cell function and insulin secretion. Six different types have been identified due to mutations in six different genes (Box 12.6).

Neonatal diabetes mellitus

Neonatal DM is rare (1 in 400,000–500,000 live births). It is defined as hyperglycemia requiring insulin therapy occurring in the first few weeks of life; transient (50%–60%) and permanent forms are recognized.

Transient neonatal diabetes mellitus (TNDM)

TNDM is a disorder of developmental insulin production that resolves spontaneously in the postnatal period. Intrauterine growth restriction (IUGR) is evident at birth, and failure to thrive and hyperglycemia occur in the first few days. Most patients will achieve remission and insulin independence within 1 year; however, in many patients persistent diabetes recurs in late childhood or adulthood. TNDM is usually sporadic. Chromosome 6 abnormalities are observed in many patients (paternal duplications; paternal isodisomy; methylation defects).

Permanent neonatal diabetes mellitus (PNDM)

PNDM is rare. It may be caused by a defect in KCJN11 or SUR1, defects in two subunits of the potassium channel that plays a key role in insulin release. This defect results in defective insulin secretion.[1] Mutations in the insulin gene are a recently discovered cause of PNDM. PNDM may also be associated with a number of clinical syndromes (IPEX syndrome— diffuse autoimmunity; severe pancreatic hypoplasia associated with IPF-1 mutation; Walcott–Rallison syndrome).

Cystic fibrosis–related diabetes (CFRD)

The prevalence of CFRD increases with age (~9% between ages 5 and 9 years; 26% between ages 10 and 19 years). It is primarily due to a defect in pancreatic insulin secretion, although modest insulin resistance is also recognized. Insulin is recommended for all patients with CFRD.

Severe insulin resistance syndromes

This is a rare, heterogeneous, group of disorders. Genetic mutations resulting in insulin receptor and post-receptor signaling defects underlie the mechanism of severe insulin resistance. Hyperinsulinemia is present. Common clinical features include acanthosis nigricans, and evidence of ovarian hyperandrogenism in females. Syndromes associated with severe insulin resistance include the following:

- Type A insulin resistance
- Donohue's syndrome
- Rabson–Mendenhal syndrome
- Partial lipodystrophy

Box 12.6 Types of MODY

MODY 1
- 5% of MODY cases
- Mutation in HNF4α gene (20q)
- Presents or has onset at adolescence, <25 years age
- Severe hyperglycemia
- Oral agents, insulin therapy often required
- Microvascular complications are frequent and high risk.

MODY 2
- 10%–63% of MODY cases
- Heterozygous for mutation in glucokinase gene (7p)
- Altered glucose sensing by pancreatic β cell
- Presents incidentally, with onset in early childhood
- Mild hyperglycemia
- Diet therapy alone
- Complications are rare.

MODY 3
- 20%–70% of MODY cases
- Mutation in HNF1α gene (12q24)
- Presents or has onset at adolescence, <25 years of age
- Severe hyperglycemia
- Oral agents, insulin therapy often required
- Microvascular complications are frequent and high risk.

MODY 4
- Rare
- Heterozygous for mutation in IPF-1gene (13q)
- Onset is postpubertal
- Moderately severe diabetes
- Microvascular complications are rare.

MODY 5
- Rare
- Mutation HNF-1β/TCF2 gene (17cen-q21.3)
- Onset is postpubertal
- Severe diabetes
- Associated renal insufficiency
- Microvascular complications are unknown.

MODY 6
- Rare
- Mutation NeuroD1/β2 gene (2q32)
- Onset is postpubertal.
- ? Severe diabetes
- Microvascular complications are unknown.

1. Stoy J, Edghill EL, Flanagan SE, et al (2007). Insulin gene mutations as a cause of permanent neonatal diabetes. *Proc Natl Acad Sci USA* **104**:15040–15044.

Goiter

A *goiter* is an enlargement of the thyroid gland. It may be congenital or acquired. Thyroid function may be normal (euthyroid), underactive (hypothyroid), or overactive (hyperthyroidism). Enlargement is usually secondary to increased pituitary secretion of TSH but may, in certain cases, be due to an infiltrative process that is either inflammatory or neoplastic.

Congenital goiter

The most common causes of congenital goiter in the United States relate to the transplacental transmission of factors from the mother to the fetus that interfere with fetal thyroid function:
- Maternal anti-thyroid drugs
- Maternal iodine exposure
- Maternal hyperthyroidism (Graves' disease)

Other rare causes include
- Thyroid teratoma
- Endemic iodine deficiency
- Thyroid hormone biosynthetic defects (e.g., Pendred syndrome)

Acquired goiter
- Simple (colloid) goiter
- Multinodular goiter
- Acute thyroiditis (see p. 510)
- Graves' disease
- Anti-thyroid chemical exposure: Iodine intoxication
- Anti-thyroid drugs: Lithium, amiodarone

Simple (colloid) goiter

This is a euthyroid, nontoxic goiter of unknown cause. It is not associated with disturbance of thyroid function and is not associated with either inflammation or neoplasia. Thyroid function tests and radioisotope scans are normal. It is most common in girls during or around the peripubertal years. Treatment is not needed, although follow-up is recommended.

Multinodular goiter

This form is rare, constituting a firm goiter with single or multiple palpable nodules. Thyroid function studies are usually normal, although TSH and anti-thyroid antibody titers may be elevated. Abnormalities on thyroid ultrasound and areas of reduced uptake on radioisotope scanning may be seen.

Solitary thyroid nodule

Solitary nodules of the thyroid are uncommon. Approximately 15% may be associated with underlying thyroid cancer. Careful evaluation is required. Potential causes of a solitary thyroid nodule include the following:

- Benign adenoma
- Thyroglossal cyst
- Ectopic, normal thyroid tissue
- Single median thyroid gland
- Thyroid cyst or abscess
- Thyroid carcinoma

Investigation should include a radioisotope (^{99m}Tc) scan. Cold nodules or nodules that feel hard on palpation or are rapidly growing should raise suspicion of thyroid cancer. Biopsy and surgical excision are indicated.

Thyroid carcinoma

Thyroid cancer is rare in childhood. In the past, many carcinomas of the thyroid were associated with previous direct irradiation to the head and neck tissues for other conditions.

Carcinomas of the thyroid are histologically classified as being either papillary, follicular, or mixed. They are usually slow growing. Girls are affected twice as often as boys.

Presentation is usually with a painless thyroid nodule. Cervical lymph node involvement is often evident at time of diagnosis. Metastases to the lung may be observed radiologically but are usually asymptomatic.

Diagnosis is established by biopsy. Radioisotope scanning (^{123}I or ^{99m}Tc) demonstrates reduced uptake. Thyroid function tests are usually normal.

Treatment and prognosis

Thyroidectomy (subtotal or complete) is indicated. Radioiodine therapy after surgery is often given. Postablative oral thyroid hormone replacement therapy is needed, with a goal of near suppression of TSH.

Prognosis is usually very good, even with presence of cervical node and or metastases at diagnosis.

See also Medullary thyroid cancer (p. 779).

Congenital hypothyroidism

Hypothyroidism may be due to a number of conditions that result in insufficient secretion of thyroid hormones. Congenital hypothyroidism is a relatively common condition occurring in approximately in 1 in 4000 births. It is twice as common in girls than in boys.

Etiology

The cause of congenital hypothyroidism includes the following:
- Thyroid dysgenesis (85%): Usually sporadic; resulting in thyroid aplasia or hypoplasia; ectopic thyroid (lingual/sublingual)
- Thyroid hormone biosynthetic defect (15%) is hereditary (e.g., Pendred's syndrome).
- Iodine deficiency (rare in the United States but common worldwide)
- Congenital TSH deficiency (rare) is associated with other pituitary hormone deficiencies.

Clinical features

These are usually nonspecific and difficult to detect in first month of life. They include the following:
- Umbilical hernia
- Prolonged jaundice
- Constipation
- Hypotonia
- Hoarse cry
- Poor feeding
- Excessive sleepiness
- Dry skin
- Coarse facies
- Delayed neurodevelopment

Diagnosis

In all U.S. states, as well as in most developed countries, there are national neonatal biochemical screening programs:
- Test in the first week of life, usually at 48 hours, often followed by a second test at 1–2 weeks of life.
- Blood spot with filter paper collection (e.g., "Guthrie card")
- TSH (high) and/or fT4 (low) estimation

Thyroid imaging is also recommended to determine whether the cause is due to thyroid dysgenesis or hormone biosynthetic disorder:
- Thyroid ultrasound
- Radionucleotide scanning (^{99}Tc or ^{131}I)

Treatment

Without early hormone replacement therapy, a number of adverse sequelae may occur:
- Neurodevelopmental delay and mental retardation
- Poor motor coordination
- Hypotonia
- Ataxia
- Poor growth and short stature

The earlier the treatment with oral thyroid hormone replacement therapy is initiated, the better the prognosis:
- *L*-thyroxine (initial dose 10–15 µg/kg/day)

Monitoring therapy

Monitor serum TSH and T4 levels
- Every 1–2 months the first year; every 2–3 months at age 1–2 years; every 4–6 months over age 2 years
- Maintain T4 level in upper half of normal range; TSH in lower end of normal range

Transient hyperthyrotropinemia

This is uncommon and is usually detected at the time of neonatal thyroid screening. It is characterized by a slightly elevated serum TSH level in the presence of otherwise normal serum T4 levels. It is probably due to the transplacental transmission of maternal thyroid antibodies to the child in utero.

Presumed cases do not need treatment, but must be monitored. TSH levels that remain persistently elevated after a few weeks or if associated with low T4 levels should be treated with oral *L*-thyroxine.

Acquired hypothyroidism

This is a relatively common condition with an estimated prevalence of 0.1% to 0.2% in the population. The incidence in girls is 5–10 times greater than in boys.

Etiology

Acquired hypothyroidism may be due to a primary thyroid problem or indirectly to a central disorder of hypothalamic–pituitary function.

Primary hypothyroidism (raised TSH; low T4/T3)

- Autoimmune (Hashimoto's or chronic lymphocytic thyroiditis)
- Iodine deficiency
  - Most common cause worldwide
- Subacute thyroiditis
- Drugs (e.g., amiodarone, lithium)
- Postirradiation thyroid (e.g., bone marrow transplant, total body irradiation)
- Postablative (radioiodine therapy or surgery)

Central hypothyroidism (low serum TSH and low T4)

Hypothyroidism due to either pituitary or hypothalamic dysfunction:
- Intracranial tumors or masses
- Post cranial radiotherapy or surgery
- Developmental pituitary defects (genetic, e.g., *PROP-1; Pit-1* genes):
- Isolated TSH deficiency; multiple pituitary hormone deficiencies

Clinical features

The symptoms and signs of acquired hypothyroidism are usually insidious and can be extremely difficult to diagnose clinically. A high index of suspicion is needed.
- Goiter: Primary hypothyroidism
- Increased weight gain or obesity
- Decreased growth velocity or delayed puberty
- Delayed skeletal maturation (bone age)
- Fatigue; mental slowness; deteriorating school performance
- Constipation; cold intolerance; bradycardia
- Dry skin; coarse hair
- Pseudopuberty
  - Girls: Isolated breast development
  - Boys: Isolated testicular enlargement
- Slipped upper (capital) femoral epiphysis: hip pain or limp

Diagnosis

Diagnosis is dependent on biochemical confirmation of hypothyroid state.
- Thyroid function tests: High TSH, low T4, low T3
- Thyroid antibody screen: Raised antibody titers:
  - Anti-thyroid peroxidase
  - Anti-thyroglobulin
  - TSH receptor (blocking type)

Treatment
- Oral *L*-thyroxine (25–200 µg/day; typically 100 µg/m^2/day)
- Monitor thyroid function test every 4–6 months during childhood
- Monitor growth and neurodevelopment

Thyrotoxicosis

Thyrotoxicosis refers to the clinical, physiological, and biochemical findings that result when the tissues are exposed to excess thyroid hormones (see Box 12.7). *Hyperthyroidism* denotes those conditions resulting in hyperfunction of the thyroid gland leading to a state of thyrotoxicosis.

Box 12.7 Causes of thyrotoxicosis

Hyperthyroidism
- Excessive thyroid stimulation
  - Graves disease (p. 508)
  - Hashimoto's disease (Hashitoxicosis) (p. 506)
  - Neonatal (transient) thyrotoxicosis (p. 502)
  - Pituitary thyroid hormone resistance (excess TSH)
  - McCune–Albright syndrome
  - HCG-secreting tumors
- Thyroid nodules (autonomous)
  - Toxic nodule or multinodular goiter (p. 498)
  - Thyroid adenoma or carcinoma (p. 500)

Not hyperthyroidism
- Thyroiditis
  - Subacute
  - Drug induced
- Exogenous thyroid hormones

Clinical features (all causes)
Thyrotoxicosis may be associated with the following symptoms:
- Hyperactivity, irritability
- Poor concentration; altered mood; insomnia
- Heat intolerance, fatigue, muscle weakness, wasting
- Weight loss despite increased appetite
- Altered bowel habit; diarrhea
- Menstrual irregularity
- Sinus tachycardia; increased pulse pressure
- Hyperreflexia; fine tremor
- Pruritis

Investigations
- Thyroid function tests (serum): Raised T4 and T3; suppressed TSH
- Thyroid antibodies: Anti-thyroid peroxidase; anti-thyroglobulin; TSH receptor antibody (stimulatory type; also known as thyroid-stimulating immunoglobulin [TSIG])
- Radionucleotide thyroid scan: Increased uptake (Graves' disease)
- Decreased uptake (thyroiditis)

Graves' disease

Graves' disease

Graves' disease is a complex autoimmune disorder with both genetic and environmental factors contributing to susceptibility. Several HLA-DR gene loci (DR3; DQA1*0501) have been identified as susceptibility loci and there is often a strong positive family history of autoimmune thyroid disease (occurring more often in girls than in boys). Graves' disease occurs from a predominance of stimulating type autoantibodies to the TSH receptor.

Clinical features

In addition to features of hyperthyroidism (see p. 506), Graves' disease is characterized by specific features:
• Diffuse goiter (most cases)
• Graves' ophthalmopathy: Exophthalmos, proptosis; eyelid lag or retraction; periorbital edema, chemosis; ophthalmoplegia or extraocular muscle dysfunction

Diagnosis

Clinical suspicion of Graves' disease requires confirmatory blood test:
• Thyroid function tests: High T4, high T3, low TSH
• Thyroid antibody screen: Anti-thyroid peroxidase; anti-thyroglobulin positive; TSH receptor antibody (stimulatory type) positive; radionucleotide thyroid scan shows increased uptake

Treatment

Treatment options include medical therapy, radioactive ablation, and surgery, although surgery is rarely used. The aims of medical therapy are to induce remission of Graves' disease with anti-thyroid drugs (methimazole or propylthiouracil) and, if necessary, bring the symptoms of thyrotoxicosis (anxiety, tremor, tachycardia) under control with a beta-blocking agent (propranolol). Two alternative regimens are practiced.

Dose titration regimen

Anti-thyroid treatment is titrated to achieve normal thyroid function.

Block and replace regimen

Anti-thyroid treatment is maintained at the lowest dose necessary to induce complete thyroid suppression and therapeutic hypothyroidism. In this situation, replacement thyroxine therapy is also necessary to achieve euthyroidism.

Anti-thyroid therapy is usually given for 12–24 months in children before considering a trial of treatment. Thyroid function (serum free T4; TSH levels) should be monitored at regular intervals (1–3 months). Methimazole and PTU can cause neutropenia and hepatitis, so blood counts and hepatic transaminases should be monitored.

Radioactive iodine

While not recommended in young children because of the risk of thyroid cancer, this may be given as definitive treatment in older children once diagnosis is established or after a patient is stabilized on medical therapy.

Prognosis

Following completion of treatment, 40%–75% of children will relapse over the next 2 years. Relapses may be treated with a further course of anti-thyroid drugs, although definitive therapy with radioiodine is being offered as first-line treatment. Thyroid surgery is another approach for management of relapses, although it is rarely employed in otherwise healthy children.

Following definitive treatment (either radioiodine or surgery), lifelong thyroxine replacement therapy will be required.

Neonatal thyrotoxicosis

This condition is rare and due to the passive transfer of maternal thyroid antibodies from a thyrotoxic mother to the fetus. Affected neonates are irritable, flushed, and tachycardic. Weight gain is poor and cardiac failure may be present.

The condition is self-limiting. Supportive treatment (e.g., beta-blocker therapy, digoxin) and transient blockade of thyroid hormone production (e.g., with iodine-containing preparations such as SSKI) may be required.

Thyroiditis

Thyroiditis is inflammation of the thyroid gland, which may result in goiters. Initial thyrotoxicosis is usually followed by hypothyroidism. Recognized causes include
• Autoimmune thyroiditis (Hashimoto's)
• Acute suppurative (pyogenic) thyroiditis
• Subacute (de Quervain) thyroiditis

Autoimmune thyroiditis (Hashimoto's)

This is the most common cause of thyroid disease in childhood and adolescence and is the most common cause of hypothyroidism in developed countries.
• Characterized by lymphocytic infiltration of the thyroid gland and early thyroid follicular hyperplasia, which gives way to eventual atrophy and fibrosis
• Associated with a positive family history of thyroid disease, and there is an increased risk of other autoimmune disorders (e.g., type 1 diabetes)
• 4 to 7 times more common in females than in males
• Children with Down or Turner syndrome are at increased risk.
• Peak incidence is in adolescence, although it may occur at any age.

Presentation

The clinical presentation is usually insidious with a diffusely enlarged, non-tender, firm goiter. Most children are asymptomatic and biochemically euthyroid. Some children may present with hypothyroidism. A few children may have symptoms suggestive of hyperthyroidism (i.e., Hashitoxicosis).

The clinical course is variable. Goiters may become smaller and disappear or may persist. Many children who are initially euthyroid eventually develop hypothyroidism within a few months or years of presentation. Periodic follow-up is therefore necessary.

Investigations

• Thyroid biochemistry may be normal or abnormal.
• Antimicrosomal thyroid antibody titers are usually raised, whereas anti-thyroglobulin titers are increased in only approximately 50%.
• Diagnosis can be established by thyroid biopsy (but not indicated).

Treatment

Treatment is only required for the management of either hypothyroidism (see p. 504) or hyperthyroidism, if present (see p. 508).

Acute suppurative thyroiditis

This is uncommon. It is often preceded by respiratory tract infection. Organisms include *Staph. auerus*, streptococci, and *E. coli* (rarely fungal infection). Abscess formation may occur.

- Presentation is with painful, tender swelling of the thyroid.
- Thyroid function is usually normal, however, hyperthyroidism may occur.
- Markers of inflammation are positive (e.g., C-reactive protein).
- Recurrent infection should raise suspicion of the presence of a thyroglossal tract remnant.
- Treatment requires administration of antibiotics and surgical drainage of abscess if present

Subacute thyroiditis (de Quervain's)

- A self-limiting condition of viral origin, associated with tenderness and pain overlying the thyroid gland
- Symptoms of thyrotoxicosis may be present initially, although hypothyroidism may develop later.
- Treatment includes nonsteroidal inflammatory agents and, in severe cases, corticosteroids (prednisolone). Beta-blocker therapy (e.g., propranolol) may help to control thyrotoxic symptoms.

Adrenal insufficiency

Primary adrenal failure results in both reduced glucocorticoid (cortisol) and mineralocorticoid (aldosterone) production. Adrenocorticotrophin (ACTH) levels are elevated due to reduced cortisol negative feedback.

Secondary adrenal failure is due to either reduced corticotrophin-releasing hormone (CRH) or reduced ACTH production (or both) and results in reduced cortisol production only. Mineralocorticoid activity remains normal, as this is mainly regulated by the angiotensin–renin system.

Causes of adrenal insufficiency

Primary

Acquired

- Autoimmune adrenalitis (Addison's disease)
- Adrenal infection (e.g., tuberculosis)
- Adrenal hemorrhage, infarction
- Iatrogenic: Adrenolectomy; drugs (e.g., ketoconazole)

Congenital

- Congenital adrenal hyperplasia
- Congenital adrenal hypoplasia
- Adrenoleukodystrophy
- Familial glucocorticoid deficiency

Secondary

- Defects of hypothalamus or pituitary structures
  - Congenital—pituitary hypoplasia
  - Intracranial masses: Tumors (e.g., glioma, germinoma); craniopharyngioma
  - Intracranial inflammation: Langerhan's histiocytosis
  - Intracranial infections
  - Cranial radiotherapy, irradiation
  - Neurosurgery
  - Traumatic brain injury
- Suppression of hypothalamic–pituitary–adrenal axis
  - Glucocorticoid therapy
  - Cushing's disease (after pituitary tumor removal)

Clinical features

The age of onset and manifestations will depend on the underlying cause. Clinical features may be *subtle and a high index of suspicion is often required*. Typically, clinical features are gradual in onset, with partial insufficiency leading to complete adrenal insufficiency with impaired cortisol responses to stress and illness (adrenal crisis):

- Anorexia and weight loss
- Fatigue, tiredness, and generalized weakness
- Dizziness (hypotension)
- Salt craving (primary adrenal insufficiency)
- Hyperpigmentation (primary adrenal insufficiency)
- Reduced pubic and axillary hair (primary adrenal insufficiency)
- Hypoglycemia (neonates, infants, young children)

Diagnosis

Basal serum cortisol and ACTH

Note: Random basal cortisol levels are often within the normal range and cannot be relied on. Inappropriately low basal cortisol during "stress" suggests adrenal insufficiency. A basal cortisol level of >20 μg/dL (550 nmol/L) usually excludes this diagnosis.

An elevated early-morning (9 AM) ACTH level for the level of cortisol is suggestive of primary adrenal insufficiency.

Adrenal stimulation tests

These tests are usually required to establish a diagnosis of adrenal insufficiency and are used to demonstrate inappropriately low serum cortisol responses to physiological or pharmacological stimulation of the adrenal glands.

Insulin tolerance test

This is considered the gold standard test. Insulin-induced mild hypoglycemia is used to assess the integrity of the entire hypothalamic–pituitary–adrenal axis. Serum cortisol response to hypoglycemia (>550 nmol/L) is normal.

ACTH stimulation (cosyntropin) test

Serum cortisol is measured at baseline and at +30 and +60 minutes after IV/IM of synthetic ACTH (short cosyntropin test). Serum cortisol response >20 μg/dL at 60 minutes is considered normal. Standard (250 μg) and low-dose (1 μg) tests have been used. Recent-onset secondary adrenal insufficiency may produce a normal response, especially standard dose.

Other investigations

- Serum electrolytes and glucose: Serum sodium (low); serum potassium (high); serum glucose (low)
- Adrenal antibodies titers (Addison's disease)
- Adrenal imaging: Ultrasound, CT scan
- Adrenal androgens profile: Serum, urine
- Molecular genetic studies
- Pituitary imaging: MRI scan

Adrenal insufficiency: treatment

Primary adrenal insufficiency requires both glucocorticoid and mineralo-corticoid replacement therapy. Secondary adrenal insufficiency requires glucocorticoid therapy only.

Glucocorticoid therapy

- Hydrocortisone: Oral, 10–15 mg/m^2/day in 2 to 3 divided doses per day. Usually about two-thirds of the dose is given in the morning, in an attempt to mimic normal diurnal variation in cortisol secretion.
- During times of illness and stress (e.g., infection, trauma, surgery) patients are advised to increase their normal daily maintenance dose of hydrocortisone by 2 to 3 times. Parenteral preparations are provided to families in the event that an illness or trauma is such that oral glucocorticoids are not tolerated.

Mineracorticoid therapy

- Fludrocortisone: Oral, 50–150 μm/day. Monitor electrolytes, blood pressure, and plasma renin levels.

Adrenal crises

An adrenal (or Addisonian) crisis is an acute exacerbation of an underlying adrenal insufficiency brought on by "stresses" that necessitate increased production and secretion of cortisol from the adrenal gland. This is a life-threatening emergency and should be treated if there is a strong clinical suspicion, rather than waiting for confirmatory test results. Typical causes include infection, trauma, and surgery. Symptoms include the following:

- Nausea and vomiting
- Abdominal pain
- Lethargy and somnolence
- Hypotension

Treatment

- Immediate IV bolus of hydrocortisone followed by 6-hourly repeat injections, or hydrocortisone continuous infusion
- IVI fluids, glucose

Adrenal excess

This is a state of glucocorticoid (cortisol) excess. The most common cause of hypercortisolemia is iatrogenic, due to exogenous steroids. Hyperfunction of the adrenal cortex resulting in excess cortisol secretion may have primary (adrenal or ACTH-independent) or secondary (ACTH-dependent) causes. The term *Cushing's disease* applies to an ACTH-secreting pituitary tumor. All other causes of glucocorticoid excess are often referred to as Cushing's syndrome.

Causes of adrenal (cortisol) excess

- Iatrogenic
- Primary adrenal hyperfunction (ACTH independent)
  - Adrenal tumor (carcinoma, adenoma)
  - Nodular adrenal hyperplasia
  - McCune–Albright syndrome
- Secondary adrenal hyperfunction (ACTH dependent)
  - Cushing's disease: Pituitary adenoma, hyperplasia
  - Ectopic ACTH secretion (tumor)

In young children (<5 years), adrenal disorders are the most common, noniatrogenic, cause of hypercorticolism; in neonates and infants, McCune–Albright syndrome should be considered. In older children and adolescents, Cushing's disease is most common.

Clinical features

All causes of hypercortisolemia are characterized by the following pattern of clinical signs and symptoms:
- Obesity: Central adiposity—face, trunk, abdomen
- "Moon" facies
- Buffalo hump: Prominent, enlarged posterior cervical or supraclavicular fat pads
- Muscle wasting
- Proximal muscle weakness
- Skin abnormalities: Thinning (rare in children); easy bruising; striae (abdomen and thighs)
- Hypertension
- Growth impairment: Reduced growth velocity, short stature
- Pubertal delay, amenorrhea
- Osteoporosis

Note: Other signs may be present depending on the underlying cause. Children with adrenal tumors may have signs of abnormal virilization and masculinization (early pubic hair, hirsuitism, acne, clitormegaly) due to excess adrenal androgen secretion.

Investigations

These are directed at establishing a diagnosis of hypercortisolism and, thereafter, at differentiating between ACTH-dependent and ACTH-independent causes (see Box 12.8).

Box 12.8

Is hypercortisolism present or not?
- Cortisol circadian rhythm
  - Midnight serum cortisol. *Note:* Patients must be asleep at the time of sampling for test to be valid.
  - Loss of normal diurnal variation—raised midnight value observed
  - Salivary cortisol can also be measured in some commercial laboratories.
- Urinary free cortisol excretion
  - 24-hour collection
- Dexamethasone suppression test
  - Overnight test (1 mg dexamethasone at midnight)
  - Low dose test (0.5 mg every 6 hours for 48 hours)
  - High dose test (2 mg every 6 hours for 48 hours)
  - Failure of suppression of plasma cortisol levels is observed.

Other investigations
- Plasma ACTH
  - High in ACTH-dependent causes
- Dexamethasone suppression test
  - High-dose test (2 mg every 6 hours for 48 hours)
  - In Cushing's disease, serum cortisol levels decrease by approximately 50%. Ectoptic ACTH secretion indicates no suppression.
- Corticotropin-releasing hormone (CRH) test
- CT scan of adrenal glands
- MRI scan of brain
- Bilateral inferior petrosal sinus sampling (in conjunction with CRH administration)

Management
Cushing's disease
- Preoperative treatment to normalize blood cortisol levels
  - Ketaconazole
- Pituitary surgery
  - Transsphenoidal surgery
- Pituitary radiotherapy

Adrenal disease or tumor
- Surgery, i.e., adrenalectomy

Congenital adrenal hyperplasia

Congenital adrenal hyperplasia (CAH) is a family of disorders characterized by enzyme defects in the steroidogenic pathways that lead to the biosynthesis of cortisol, aldosterone, and androgens. The relative decrease in cortisol production, acting via the classic negative feedback loop, results in increased secretion of ACTH from the anterior pituitary gland and to subsequent hyperplasia of the adrenals. All forms of CAH are inherited in an autosomal recessive manner, and their clinical manifestation is determined by the effects produced by the particular hormones that are deficient and by the excess production of steroids unaffected by the enzymatic block.

The causes of CAH include deficiencies in the following steroidogenic pathway enzymes:
- 21α-hydroxylase (CYP21)
- 11β-hydroxylase (CYP11)
- 3β-hydroxysteroid dehydrogenase
- 17α- hydroxylase/17–20 lyase (CYP17)
- Side-chain cleavage (SCC/StAR)

Deficiency of the 21α-hydroxylase enzyme is the most common form of CAH, accounting for over 90% of cases.

21α-hydroxylase deficiency

CAH due to deficiency of the 21α-hydroxylase enzyme arises as a result of deletions or deleterious mutations in the active gene (*CYP21*) located on chromosome 6p. Many different mutations of the *CYP21* gene have been identified that cause varying degrees of impairment of 21α-hydroxylase activity, resulting in a spectrum of disease expression.

CAH can be classified according to symptoms and signs and to age of presentation:
- *Classic CAH* includes a severe "salt-wasting" form that usually presents with acute adrenal crisis in early infancy (usually males at 7–10 days of life), and a "simple virilizing" form in which patients demonstrate masculinization of the external genitalia (females at birth) or signs of virilization in early life in males.
- *Nonclassic (late-onset) CAH* presents in females with signs and symptoms of mild androgen excess at or around the time of puberty.

The incidence of CAH due to 21α-hydroxylase deficiency has been reported to be in the region of 1 in 10,000 to 17,000 in Western Europe and the United States, with an overall worldwide figure of approximately 1 in 14,000 births.

Diagnosis

"Classic" CAH is diagnosed by demonstrating characteristic biochemical abnormalities, which are present regardless of severity, age, and sex of the infant:
- Elevated plasma 17-hydroxyprogesterone levels
- Elevated plasma 21-deoxycortisol levels
- Increased urinary adrenocorticosteroid metabolites

Note: It may be difficult to distinguish elevated androgen levels from the physiological hormonal surge that occurs in the first 2 days of life. These tests should be postponed or repeated after 48 hours of age. Newborn screening is offered for CAH in many U.S. states.

In the salt-wasting form, the aldosterone deficiency results in hyponatremia, hyperkalemia, and metabolic acidosis. However, these are not specific findings and can cause diagnostic confusion when children present with more common causes of renal tubular dysfunction, such as acute pyelonephritis.

Treatment

Glucocorticoid replacement therapy

This therapy is required in all patients. In addition to treating cortisol deficiency, it also suppresses the ACTH-dependent excess adrenal androgen production. Standard therapy usually consists of

- Hydrocortisone: oral 15 mg/m^2/day in three divided doses

As in other disorders associated with cortisol insufficiency, during periods of stress and illness increased amounts (e.g., triple dose) of glucocorticoid therapy are required (see p. 514).

Mineralocorticoid therapy

This is for the salt-wasting form of CAH only.

- Fludrocortisone: Oral 50–300 μg/day

Sodium chloride therapy

Resistance to mineralocorticoid therapy is usually seen in infancy. Sodium chloride supplements are often required during this period of life to maintain normal electrolyte balance. Once a normal solid diet is established, salt supplements may be discontinued.

- Sodium chloride solution: Oral, added to feed, 2–10 mmol/kg/day in divided doses

Urogenital surgery

Reconstructive surgery (clitoral reduction and vaginoplasty) is usually performed in infancy in females with significant virilization of the external genitalia.

Long-term management and monitoring

Regular monitoring of patients by a specialist team is required to ensure the child's optimal growth and development.

Mineralocorticoid excess

The principal mineralocorticoid secreted by the *adrenal gland* is aldosterone. Increased production may result from a primary defect of the adrenal gland (primary hyperaldosteronism) or from factors that activate the renin–angiotensin system (secondary hyperaldosteronism). Hypokalemia and hypertension are typical features.

Primary hyperaldosteronism

This is characterized by hypokalemia and hypertension. There is suppression of the renin–angiotensin system with low plasma renin levels. Children may have no symptoms, the diagnosis being established after the incidental finding of hypertension. Chronic hypokalemia may result in muscle weakness, fatigue, and poor growth.

> *Causes of primary hyperaldosteronism*
> - Bilateral adrenal hyperplasia (see p. 578)
> - Adrenal tumors (see p. 516)
> - Glucocorticoid-remediable hyperaldosteronism

Secondary hyperaldosteronism

This occurs when excess aldosterone production is secondary to elevated renin levels. Hypertension may or may not be present.

> *Causes of secondary hyperaldosteronism*
> *Associated with hypertension*
> - Renovascular malformations, stenosis
> - Primary hyperreninemia
> - Juxtaglomerular tumor
> - Wilms' tumor
> - Postrenal transplantation
> - Urinary tract obstruction
> - Pheochromocytoma
>
> *Associated without hypertension*
> - Hepatic cirrhosis (see p. 400)
> - Congestive cardiac failure (see p. 263)
> - Nephrotic syndrome (see p. 440)
> - Bartter syndrome (see p. 473)
> - Anorexia nervosa (see p. 596)
> - Syndrome of apparent mineralocorticoid excess: Type 1 and type 2 variants

Mineralocorticoid deficiency

Reduced aldosterone production or activity is rare and may be due to congenital or acquired causes:

- Aldosterone synthase deficiency
  - Type 1
  - Type 2
- Pseudohypoaldosteronism
  - Type 1
  - Type 2
- Hyporeninemic hypoaldosteronism
- Hyperreninemic hypoaldosteronism
- Transient hypoaldosteronism in infancy
- Congenital adrenal hyperplasia
  - 17α-hydroxylase (CYP17) deficiency
  - 11β-hydroxylase (CYP11) deficiency
- Congenital adrenal hypoplasia
- Primary adrenocortical insufficiency
- Iatrogenic hypoaldosteronism

Inherited endocrine syndromes

Multiple endocrine neoplasia

This is a family of endocrine neoplasia syndromes that are inherited in an autosomal dominant manner:

- Multiple endocrine neoplasia (MEN) type 1
- Multiple endocrine neoplasia (MEN) type 2
- von Hippel–Lindau (VHL) syndrome

The molecular genetic defects for these syndromes have been identified and genetic screening is available. Patients with these conditions require close surveillance and screening (biochemistry, radiology, etc).

Multiple endocrine neoplasia (MEN) type 1

MEN type 1 is characterized by the following clinical features:

- Hyperparathyroidism (90%), due to parathyroid hyperplasia. Usually present in second decade of life
- Pancreatic endocrine tumors (75%), typically multifocal, pancreatic islet cell tumors. Include insulinoma (60%); gastrinoma (30%); VIPoma (rare); glucagonoma (rare). Usually occur in adulthood
- Pituitary adenomas (10%–65%): Prolactinoma (60%); GH secreting (30%)
- Other features: Thyroid adenoma; thymic or bronchial carcinoid tumors; lipomas

Multiple endocrine neoplasia (MEN) type 2

MEN type 2 belongs to a family of three syndromes (MEN type 2A, MEN type 2B, familial medullary thyroid cancer) characterized by activating mutations in the *RET* protooncogene. Medullary thyroid cancer is a common feature in all the syndromes.

MEN type 2A

- Medullary thyroid cancer (90%)
- Pheochromocytoma (50%)
- Parathyroid ademona (25%)

MEN type 2B

- Medullary thyroid cancer (90%)
- Pheochromocytoma
- Mucosal or intestinal ganglioneuromas
- Marfanoid body habitus
- Hirschprung's disease

Familial medullary thyroid cancer

- Isolated medullary thyroid cancer

von Hippel–Lindau syndrome (VHL)

This condition is due to a mutation in the *VHL* gene, a tumor repressor gene located on chromosome 3. The condition is characterized by the following features:

- Retinal hemangioblastomas (40%)
  - Uncommon before age 10 years
  - Bleeding and retinal detachment
- CNS hemangioblastomas: 75% occur in cerebellum
- Pheochromocytomas (20%): Bilateral in 40%
  - Renal cysts and carcinomas
  - Late feature from fourth decade
  - Occur in 70% by age 60 years
- Pancreatic neuroendocrine tumors are uncommon
  - 50% are malignant. Most are nonfunctioning tumors but they may be secreting (insulin, glucagons, VIP).
- Simple adenomas and cysts are uncommon
  - Pancreas, liver, epididymis, lung
  - Meningioma

McCune–Albright syndrome (MAS)

This syndrome is characterized by the following triad of clinical features:

- Skin has hyperpigmented (café au lait) macules
  - Classically there is an irregular edge ("coast of Maine" appearance")
  - Do not cross midline
- Polyostic fibrous dysplasia
  - Slowly progressive bone lesion
  - Any bones, although facial and base of skull bones are most commonly affected
- Autonomous endocrine gland hyperfunction
  - Ovary is most commonly affected
  - Precocious puberty (gonadotrophin independent)
  - Thyroid (hyperthyroidism)
  - Adrenal (Cushing's syndrome)
  - Pituitary (adenoma, gigantism)
  - Parathyroid (hyperparathyroidism)

Neurofibromatosis (see also p. 616)

Two types of neurofibromatosis (NF) are recognized (see section 25). NF type 1 (also known as von Recklinghausen's disease) is an autosomal dominant condition due to a mutation of the *NF1* gene (Ch17).

NF1 may be associated with endocrine abnormalities:

- Hypothalamic and pituitary tumors
  - Optic glioma (15%)
- Growth hormone deficiency
- Precocious puberty
- Delayed puberty

Calcium disorders: hypocalcemia

Most causes of low calcium (hypocalcemia) can be explained by abnormalities of vitamin D, or parathyroid hormone (PTH) metabolism, or by disordered kidney function. The principal manifestations of hypocalcemia are related to neuromuscular irritability and include tetany and parasthesias.

- Hypocalcemic seizures (grand-mal type) or laryngeal spasm may occur acutely.
- Cardiac conduction abnormalities (prolonged QT interval QRS and ST changes and ventricular arrhythmias) may be seen.

Chronic hypocalcemia may be asymptomatic. The child's age is helpful in determining the differential diagnosis of hypocalcemia (see Box 12.9)

Box 12.9 Causes of hypocalcemia

Early neonatal causes
- Prematurity
- Maternal diabetes
- Maternal preeclampsia
- Respiratory distress syndrome

Late neonatal causes
- Cow's milk hyperphosphatemia
- Maternal hypercalcemia
- Congenital hypoparathyroidism

Infancy causes
- Nutritional rickets
- Pseudohypoparathyroidism type 1a

Childhood causes
- Pseudohypoparathyroidism type 1b
- Hypoparathyroidism

Iatrogenic causes
- Chemotherapy agents, e.g., cisplatin
- Anticonvulsant agents, e.g., phenytoin

Investigations
- Plasma calcium
- Plasma phosphate
- Serum PTH: *Note:* Low or even normal PTH concentrations imply failure of PTH secretion.
- Plasma Vitamin D
- Plasma magnesium
- X-ray of skull. Chronic hypocalcemia: basal ganglia calcification may be seen.

Treatment

See p. 102 for acute treatment.

Chronic treatment
- Should be directed at the underlying cause
- Oral calcium supplements, together with oral vitamin D therapy in the form of Calcitriol (1-α calcidiol), are often required to maintain plasma calcium levels within the normal range.

Hypoparathyroidsm

Low serum parathyroid hormone levels in childhood may be due to the following factors.

Failure in parathyroid development (agenesis/dysgenesis)
- Isolated defect
  - X-linked recessive
- Associated with other abnormalities
  - DiGeorge syndrome
  - Kearnes–Sayre syndrome

Destruction of parathyroid glands
- Autoimmune
  - Type 1 autoimmune polyendocrinopathy (see p. 522)
- Surgery (post-thyroidectomy)
- Radiotherapy

Failure in PTH secretion
- Magnesium deficiency

Failure in PTH action
- Pseudohypoparathyrodism (PHP)

Investigations
- Plasma calcium–low
- Plasma phosphate–high
- Serum PTH–low
- Serum magnesium–low

Pseudohypoparathyrodism

This disorder is characterized by end-organ resistance to the actions of PTH. It is a genetic disorder due to a defect in the $G_s\alpha$-adenylate cyclase signaling system common to the PTH receptor and other endocrine receptors belonging to the G-protein receptor family (e.g., thyroid-stimulating hormone [TSH], luteinizing hormone [LH], follicle-stimulating hormone [FSH]) (see Table 12.2).

Table 12.2 Classification of pseudohypoparathyroidism (PHP)

Classification	Pathophysiology	AHO	Other hormone resistance	Urinary cAMP response to PTH
PHP la	GNAS1 mutation	Yes	Yes	Decreased
Pseudo PHP	GNAS1 mutation	Yes	No	Normal
PHP lb	$G_s\alpha$-related protein	No	No	Decreased
PHP lc	? Receptor signal transduction	Yes	Yes	Decreased
PHP II	cAMP-dependent protein	No	No	Normal

Rickets

Rickets is a disorder of the growing skeleton due to inadequate mineralization of bone as it is laid down at the epiphyseal growth plates. There is characteristic widening of the ends of long bones and characteristic radiology. *Osteomalacia* occurs when there is inadequate mineralization of mature bone. Rickets and osteomalacia may be present at the same time.

Causes

Malnutrition and calcium deficiency are common causes worldwide. Vitamin D deficiency is rare in developed countries, although inadequate exposure to sunlight and exclusive breast-feeding of 6–12 months during infancy is a well-recognized cause.

- Calcium deficiency: Dietary, malabsorption
- Vitamin D deficiency: Dietary; malabsorption; lack of sunlight; Iatrogenic (drug induced e.g., phenytoin therapy)
- Defective vitamin D metabolism: Vitamin D–dependent rickets type I (1α-hydroxylase deficiency); liver disease; renal disease
- Defect in Vitamin D action: Vitamin D–dependent rickets type II
- Phosphate deficiency
  - Renal tubular phosphate loss,
  - Non-genetic hypophosphatemic rickets
    —X-linked (see p. 470)
    —Autosomal recessive
    —Autosomal dominant
  - Acquired hypophosphatemic rickets
    —Fanconi syndrome (see p. 470)
    —Renal tubular acidosis
    —Nephrotoxic drugs
  - Reduced phosphate intake

Clinical features

- Growth delay or arrest
- Bone pain and fracture
- Muscle weakness
- Skeletal deformities
  - Swelling of wrists
  - Swelling of costochondral junctions ("rickety rosary")
  - Bowing of the long bones
  - Frontal cranial bossing
  - Craniotabes (softening of skull)

Diagnosis

Laboratory (see Table 12.3)
- Plasma calcium, phosphate, alkaline phosphatase, PTH
- Vitamin D metabolites (25-hydroxyvitamin-D3 (25OHD), 1,25-dihydroxyvitamin-D3 (1,25 OHD)

Radiological
- X-ray of wrists (generalized osteopenia, widening, cupping and fraying of metaphyses)

There are three characteristic stages in disease progression:
- Stage 1: Low plasma calcium, normal plasma phosphate
- Stage 2: Normal plasma calcium (restored due to compensatory hyperparathyroidism)
- Stage 3: Low plasma calcium and phosphate. Advanced bone disease

Stages 1 and 2 are biochemically evident only; stage 3 has clinical features.

Table 12.3 Laboratory findings in different types of rickets

	Plasma Ca	Plasma PO₄	Alk Phos	25, OHD	1, 25 OHD	PTH
Vitamin D deficiency	↑	↑	↑	↑	↑	↑
VDDR type I	↑	↑	↑	N	↑	↑
VDDR type II	↑	↑	↑	N	↑	↑
X-linked hypophosphatemic	N	↑	↑	N	N	N or ↑
Renal tubular acidosis	↑ or N	↑	↑	N	N or ↑	N

N, normal; ↑, increase; ↓, decrease.

Vitamin D–dependent rickets (VDDR) type I

VDDR type I is an autosomal recessive condition due to a deficiency in renal 1α-hydroxylase, the enzyme responsible for the conversion of 25-hydroxyvitamin-D3 to 1,25 dihydroxyvitamin-D3. The condition results from mutations in the 1α-hydroxylase gene P450c1α.

Patients usually present with evidence of severe clinical rickets within the first 24 months of life. Treatment requires a replacement dose of 1,25 dihydroxyvitamin-D3 (calcitriol).

Vitamin D–dependent rickets (VDDR) type II

Type II is an autosomal recessive condition due to mutations in the vitamin D receptor gene, leading to end-organ resistance to vitamin D. The condition is also referred to as vitamin D–resistant rickets.

Clinical, laboratory, and radiological features are similar to those seen in vitamin D deficiency and VDDR type I. However, a striking feature observed in most patients with VDDR type II is sparse body hair development or total alopecia. This finding is usually present at birth or develops during the first year of life.

Treatment with supraphysiological doses of 1,25 dihydroxyvitamin-D3 (e.g., up to 60 μg/day of calcitriol) is often successful, although responses are highly variable.

Hypercalcemia

There are a number of different causes of high plasma calcium levels:
- William's syndrome
- Idiopathic infantile hypercalcemia
- Hyperparathyroidism
- Hypercalcemia of malignancy
- Vitamin D intoxication
- Familial hypocalciuric hypercalcemia
- Other uncommon causes: Sarcoidosis and other granulomatous disease; chronic immobilization; renal failure; hyperthyroidism; Addison's disease; iatrogenic, e.g., thiazide diuretics

Clinical features

Symptoms and signs of hypercalcemia are nonspecific:
- Gastrointestinal: Anorexia; nausea and vomiting; failure to thrive; constipation; abdominal pain
- Renal: Polyuria and polydipsia
- CNS: Apathy; drowsiness; depression

Investigations

Laboratory
- Plasma calcium (total and corrected for albumin)
- Serum PTH
- Vitamin D metabolites
- Urea and electrolytes, liver function tests
- Thyroid function test
- Urinary calcium excretion (UCa:UCr ratio; 24-hour UCa)

Radiological
- Renal ultrasound scan (screen for nephrocalcinosis)

Treatment

For treatment of acute cases see p. 690. Treatment of chronic conditions is directed at the underlying cause.

Hyperparathyroidism

Uncommon in children, excessive production of PTH may result from a primary defect of the parathyroid glands or may be secondary and compensatory to either hypocalcemia or hyperphosphatemic states.
- Primary hyperparathyroidism
  - Parathyroid adenoma
  - Parathyroid hyperplasia: MEN type 1 (see p. 522); MEN type 2 (see p. 522); neonatal severe form
- Secondary
  - Hypocalcemic states: Rickets (see p. 528)
  - Hyperphosphatemia: Chronic renal failure (see p. 462)
- Transient neonatal hyperparathyroidism
  - Maternal hypoparathyroidism

Primary hyperparathyroidism

This is rare in children. In the neonatal period it usually associated with generalized parathyroid hyperplasia. In older children it is usually due to a parathyroid adenoma and most often associated with MEN type 1.

Transient neonatal hyperparathyroidism

This condition is observed in neonates born to mothers with previously undetected and/or untreated hypoparathyroidism or pseudohypoparathyroidism. Chronic intrauterine hypocalcemia results in hyperplasia of the fetal parathyroid glands.

Neonatal severe hyperparathyroidism

See Familial hypocalciuric hypercalcemia, below.

Hypercalcemia of malignancy

Rarely, in children with endocrine tumors (e.g., pheochromocytoma) or other tumors (e.g., lymphoma), production of humoral factors such as PTH-related peptide (PTHrP) results in hypercalcemia.

Treatment requires resection and removal of the tumor to reverse the hypercalcemic state. Interim control can be achieved with a single intravenous infusion of a bisphosphonate agent (e.g., pamidronate). The latter enhances calcium bone resorption. Calcitonin may be used as a very short-term agent.

Familial hypocalciuric hypercalcemia

This autosomal dominant disorder is caused by a mutation of the calcium-sensing receptor (CaSR) gene. This is a benign, mostly asymptomatic disorder, which is often an incidental finding during routine biochemistry analysis. Plasma calcium levels are raised (but usually <3 mmol/L), and urinary calcium excretion is low. PTH levels are inappropriately normal for the degree of hypercalcemia.

Note: Those homozygous for the mutation have severe, life-threatening primary hyperparathyroidism at birth. This form of neonatal severe hyperparathyroidism requires immediate parathyroid surgery.

Disorders of the pituitary gland

Hypopituitarism

This refers to either partial or complete deficiency of the anterior and/or posterior pituitary function. Hypopituitarism may be congenital or acquired, with pituitary function. Clinical features depend on the type of hormone deficiency, its severity, and rate of development.

Congenital hypopituitarism

Mutations in pituitary transcription factor genes can result in isolated or multiple anterior pituitary hormone deficiencies. A number of specific inherited genetic defects have been characterized. Abnormalities in the hypothalamic–pituitary structures and other midline brain structures (e.g., septo-optic dysplasia, optic nerve hypoplasia, absent corpus collosum) are often detected on imaging.

Acquired hypopituitarism

Potential causes of pituitary hormone deficiency include the following:
- Intracranial (sellar/suprasellar) tumors
- Cranial irradiation or radiotherapy: The GH axis is the most sensitive to radiation damage; the thyroid and adrenal axes are more often affected at higher doses of radiation. Precocious puberty may occur, or gonadotropin at higher doses of radiation.
- Traumatic brain injury
- Inflammatory or infiltrative disease: Langerhans cell histiocytosis, sarcoidosis
- Pituitary infarction (apoplexy)
- Intracranial infection

Investigations

- Basal hormone levels, e.g., LH, FSH; TSH; fT4; prolactin; cortisol (8–9 AM); IGF-I
- Dynamic endocrine testing: Specific tests to assess secretory capacity of the anterior pituitary gland
- MRI scan of the brain

Treatment

Treatment involves adequate and appropriate hormone replacement therapy and, where applicable, management of the underlying cause.

Posterior pituitary

The posterior pituitary gland secretes two hormones: arginine vasopressin (AVP) and oxytocin.

Diabetes insipidus (DI)

This is defined as the inappropriate passage of large volumes of dilute urine (<300 mOsml/L). DI is due to either deficiency in AVP production (central DI) or resistance to its actions at the kidney (nephrogenic DI).

The most common cause of DI is primary deficiency of AVP production (i.e., central DI), acquired or inherited in origin (see Box 12.10).

Box 12.10 Classification of diabetes insipidus

Central DI

Inherited/familial
- Autosomal dominant
- Autosomal recessive
- X-linked recessive (Xq28)
- Wolfram syndrome (4p WFS1)

Congenital
- Midline craniofacial defects
- Holoprosencephaly

Acquired
- Intracranial tumors
  - Craniopharyngioma
  - Germinoma
- Traumatic brain injury
- Infiltrative or inflammation
  - Langerhans cell histiocytosis
- CNS infection

Primary polydipsia
- Psychogenic
- Dipsogenic (abnormal thirst)

Nephrogenic

Inherited/familial
Autosomal dominant
  - (Aquaporin-2 gene)
- Autosomal recessive
  - (Aquaporin-2 gene)
- X-linked recessive
  - (ADH receptor-2 gene)

Acquired
- Idiopathic
- Drugs (lithium, cisplatin)
- Metabolic (hypercalcemia)

Children present with polydipsia, polyuria, and nocturia, which must be distinguished from more common causes. Infants may exhibit failure to thrive, fever, and constipation. Other symptoms may be related to the underlying cause, e.g., headache, visual acuity, or visual-field impairment

Diagnosis

When suspected, assessment of 24-hour urinary volume and osmolality under conditions of *ad libitum* fluid intake should be undertaken. Serum osmolality, urea and electrolytes (Na^+), and blood glucose should also be measured.

Blood hypertonicity (serum osmolality >300 mOsm) with inappropriate urine hypotonicity (urine osmolality <300 mOsm) should be demonstrated. Diabetes mellitus and renal failure should be excluded.

A water deprivation test (Box 12.11) together with assessment of responses to exogenously administered ADH is often required to diagnose the type of DI. Other tests to determine the underlying cause of DI will also be needed (e.g., cranial MRI imaging).

Box 12.11 Water deprivation test

The test should be carried out in conditions of strict monitoring and in centers with experience with this test.

1. Allow fluids overnight. If primary polydipsia is suspected, consider overnight fluid deprivation to avoid overhydration.
2. Commence fluid deprivation at 8 AM.
3. Serum osmolality, serum Na$^+$, urine volume recorded, and urine osmolality should be checked each time the urine sample is voided.
4. Duration of water deprivation is seldom longer than 8 hours in children and 6 hours in infants. In any case, the water deprivation is terminated if there is either
   • Urine osmolality concentrated at 800 mOsm/kg or greater
   • Thirst becomes intolerable or
   • 5% dehydration (5% weight loss) or
   • Serum osmolality 300 mOsmol/L or greater.
5. In those with inadequate urinary concentration, administer desmopressin (DDAVP) 0.1 mg/kg to maximum of 4 mg IM.
6. Interpret results.

Urine osmolality (mOsm/kg)

	After fluid deprivation	After DDAVP
Central DI (CDI)	<300	>800
Nephrogenic DI	<300	<300
Primary polydipsia	>800	>800
Partial CDI/polydipsia	300–800	<800

Treatment

Central DI

The synthetic analogue of ADH, desmopressin (DDAVP), which has a longer duration of action, can be given intranasally or orally. The dose required varies considerably and must be titrated for each patient. The dose and frequency of administration (once to three times a day) is adjusted to maintain 24-hour urine output volume to within the normal range.

Water retention should be avoided. It is essential to educate all patients and families about the hazards of excessive water intake. Patients with an intact thirst sensation mechanism should achieve this, but much closer monitoring may be needed for those without an intact thirst mechanism.

Nephrogenic DI

Correct underlying metabolic or iatrogenic causes, if possible. Maintenance of an adequate fluid input is essential. Thiazide diuretics (e.g., hydrochlorthiazide), amiloride, and prostaglandin synthase inhibitors (e.g., indomethacin) can be effective.

Primary polydipsia

Treatment is often difficult. Behavior modification strategies are usually required.

Posterior pituitary: syndrome of inappropriate ADH secretion (SIADH)

SIADH is a heterogeneous disorder characterized by hypotonic hyper-natremia and impaired urinary dilution that cannot be accounted for by a recognized stimulus to ADH secretion. Plasma ADH is elevated or inadequately suppressed. Several different types of pathogenic mechanisms are likely to be responsible for this. There are many causes of SIADH (see Box 12.12).

Box 12.12 Causes of SIADH

Congenital
- Agenesis of corpus collosum

Acquired
- CNS: Traumatic brain injury, cerebrovascular bleeding
- Tumors: Brain, lung, thymus
- Infection: Pneumonia, meningitis, encephalitis, TB
- Neurological: Guillain–Barré syndrome
- Respiratory: Asthma, pneumothorax
- Drugs: Vincristine, cyclophosphamide

Up to 15% of children presenting with brain trauma or infection develop SIADH. Clinical features include development of
- Confusion
- Headache
- Lethargy
- Seizures and coma

Symptoms do not necessarily depend on the concentration of serum sodium but on its rate of development. Slow, gradual development of hyponatremia may be asymptomatic (see Box 12.13).

Box 12.13 SIADH diagnostic criteria

- Hyponatremia (serum Na^+ <135 mmol/L)
- Hypotonic plasma (osmolality <270 mOsm/kg)
- Excessive renal sodium loss (>20 mmol/L)
- No hypovolemia or fluid overload
- Normal renal, adrenal cardiac, and thyroid function
- Increased plasma ADH

Management

Treatment of the underlying cause is necessary. Fluid restriction is the mainstay of therapy.

- Hypertonic (3%) saline solution may be used to correct severe hyponatremia, or hyponatremia resistant to fluid restriction.
- Slow correction of hyponatremia is essential to avoid rapid overcorrection, a possible complication of which is central pontine demyelination.
- Longer-term management and treatment with demeclocycline may be effective for fluid balance by inducing nephrogenic DI.

Growth and puberty

Normal growth

Normal human growth can be divided into two distinct phases: prenatal (fetal) and postnatal

Prenatal and fetal growth

This is the fastest period of growth, accounting for around 30% of eventual height. Factors that determine growth during this period include maternal size, maternal nutrition, and intrauterine environment. Hormonal factors such as insulin, insulin-like growth factor (IGF)-II, and human placental lactogen are important regulators of growth during this period.

Postnatal growth

This is classically divided into three overlapping periods.

Infantile period

This period, from birth to 18–24 months of age, is marked by a rapid but decelerating growth rate (growth velocity range: 22–8 cm/year). Growth is largely under nutritional regulation during this period. Some infants (15%–20%) may show significant catch-up or catch-down in length and weight. By age 2 years, height is more predictive of final adult height than at birth.

Childhood period

This period is from age 2 years until onset of puberty and is characterized by a slow, steady growth velocity (range 8–5 cm/year). Growth is primarily dependent on growth hormone (GH), provided there is adequate nutrition and health.

Puberty

Growth during this period is dependent on GH and the actions of sex steroid hormones (testosterone and estrogen). This combination induces the characteristic growth spurt of puberty. In both males and females, estrogen induces the maturation of the epiphyseal growth centers of the bones, eventually resulting in fusion of the growth plates, the cessation of linear growth, and the attainment of final height.

Sex differences in growth

The onset of the pubertal growth spurt is earlier in females than in males. Females are, therefore, on average taller than males between the ages of 10 and 13 years. In males the pubertal growth spurt is later in onset and greater in magnitude. As a result, males are on average 12–13 cm (5 inches) taller than females at final height.

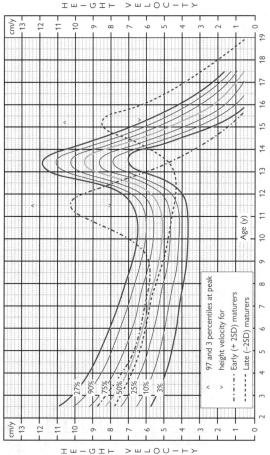

Figure 13.1a Growth velocity in males. Reprinted from Tanner JM (1985). Clinical longitudinal standards for height and height velocity for North American children. *J Pediatr* 107(3):317–329, with permission from Elsevier.

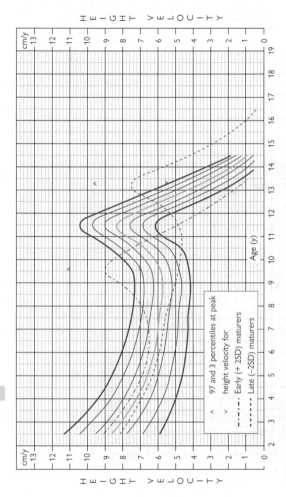

Figure 13.1b Growth velocity in females. Reprinted from Tanner JM (1985). Clinical longitudinal standards for height and height velocity for North American children. *J Pediatr* **107**(3):317–329, with permission from Elsevier.

Normal puberty

Puberty is a well-defined sequence of physical and physiological changes occurring during the adolescent years that culminates in attainment of full physical and sexual maturity.

- Nocturnal, pulsatile secretion of the hormone LHRH by the hypothalamus is the first step in the initiation of puberty. This results in the pulsatile secretion of the gonadotropin hormones LH and FSH by the anterior pituitary gland. LH stimulates sex hormone production from the gonads.
- The age of onset of puberty is earlier in females (mean [range] 10.4 [8.0–13.0] years) than in males (11.5 [9.0–14.0] years). In each sex, puberty progresses in an orderly or "consonant" manner through distinct stages (see Table 13.1).
- In females, the first sign of puberty is breast development, followed by pubic hair growth and growth acceleration. Menarche (the onset of menstruation) occurs, on average, 2.5 years after the start of puberty (median age 12.5 years in Caucasians, 12.06 years in African Americans, and 12.25 years in Mexican Americans).
- In males, the first sign of puberty is an enlargement of testicular size to ≥4 mL in volume. Pubic hair development and growth acceleration follow.

Pubertal growth spurt

In females, peak growth (height) velocity occurs relatively earlier in girls (Tanner stage 2–3) compared to boys (Tanner stage 3–4; testicular volumes 10–12 mL)

Note: The age of onset of puberty varies slightly between children of different races. In Afro-Caribbean and African-American children, average age of onset of puberty may be earlier than in Caucasian children, which is earlier than in Hispanic-American children.

Table 13.1 The normal stages of puberty ('Tanner stages')

Boys

Stage	Genitalia	Pubic hair	Other events
I	Prepubertal	Vellus not thicker than on abdomen	TV[a] <4mL
II	Enlargement of testes and scrotum	Sparse long pigmented strands at base of penis	TV 4–8 mL Voice starts to change
III	Lengthening of penis	Darker,curlier and spreads over pubes	TV 8–10 mL Axillary hair
IV	Increase in penis length and breadth	Adult type hair but covering a smaller area	TV 10–15mL Upper lip hair Peak height velocity
V	Adult shape and size	Spread to medial thighs (Stage 6: Spread up linea alba)	TV 15–25 mL. Facial hair spreads to cheeks Adult voice

Girls

Stage	Breast	Pubic hair	Other events
I	Elevation of papilla only	Vellus not thicker than on abdomen	
II	Breast bud stage:elevation of breast and papilla	Sparse long pigmented strands along labia	Peak height velocity
III	Further elevation of breast and areola together	Darker, curlier and spreads over pubes	
IV	Areola forms a second mound on top of breast	Adult type hair but covering a smaller area	Menarche
V	Mature stage: areola recedes and only papilla projects	Spread to medial thighs (Stage 6: spread up linea alba)	

[a] TV, testicular volume: measured by size-comparison with a Prader orchidometer. Adapted from Tanner JM (1962) *Growth at adolescence*, 2nd edn. Blackwell Scientific Publications, Oxford.

Assessment of growth

Growth must be measured accurately. The equipment used to measure weight and height must be regularly maintained, checked, and calibrated. Ideally, growth measurements should be carried out by someone with specific training and experience in measurement techniques. This will minimize measurement error.

Assessment of height

From birth to age 2 years, length is measured horizontally using a specifically designed measuring board (e.g., Harpenden neonatometer). Two people are required to ensure the child is lying straight with legs extended.

In children age 2 years or over, standing height is measured against a wall-mounted Harpenden stadiometer. A specific technique is required, with the person measuring applying moderate upward neck traction to the child's head with the child looking forward in the horizontal plane.

Measurement of sitting height using a modified stadiometer and calculation of the leg length (standing height *minus* sitting height) allows an estimate of upper and lower body segments and body proportion.

Growth data interpretation

Weight and height measurement data should be plotted as a simple dot on a sex-appropriate, standard growth centile chart (e.g., the Center for Disease Control and Prevention [CDC] 2000 growth charts). Height measurements should also be plotted on specific population growth charts where necessary or applicable (e.g., Turner syndrome; Down syndrome).

Single growth measurements should not be assessed in isolation of other previous measurements. Serial measurements are used to show a pattern of growth and determine growth rate. To minimize error in the assessment of growth rate, calculation of height velocity (cm/yr) should be taken from measurements a minimum of 3 to 6 months apart, ideally using the same equipment and by the same person.

Final height and target height

This is the height reached after the completion of puberty and is estimated to be achieved when growth velocity has slowed to <2.0 cm/year. This can be confirmed by finding epiphyseal fusion of the small bones of the hand and wrist on assessing the bone age X-ray.

Final height is largely genetically determined. A target height range can be estimated in each individual from their parents' heights.

Mid-parental height (MPH)

[(mother's height + father's height cm)/2] + 6.5 cm for boys
OR – 6.5 cm for girls

Target height range

MPH ±10 cm

Bone age

This is a measure of skeletal maturation, which can be assessed by the appearance of the epiphyseal centers of the long bones. Conventionally, this is quantified from X-rays of the left hand and wrist, either compared with standard radiograph images (e.g., Gruelich & Pyle method) or assessed using an individual bone scoring system (Tanner–Whitehouse methods). It is a very subjective assessment.

The difference between bone age (BA) score and chronological age at the time of assessment may be used as an estimation of the tempo of maturation. The BA may also be used as an indicator of the likely timing of puberty, which usually starts when BA is around 10.5 years in females and 11.5 years in boys. The relationship between BA and age of onset of menarche is more robust.

Girls usually reach skeletal maturity at a BA of 15.0 years and boys when BA is 17.0 years. The BA can therefore be used as an estimation of the remaining growth potential and can be used to predict final adult height. However, these predictions are not very accurate and can only be used in children who have normal growth velocities.

Assessment of puberty

Puberty stage can be rated using the Tanner staging system (Table 13.1). This involves identification of pubertal stage, particularly by assessment of stage of breast development in girls and testicular volume (by comparison with an orchidometer) in boys.

Short stature

This is defined as a height less than two standard deviations (2 SD) below the mean for the population. On a standard growth chart this represents a height below the second centile. However, note that abnormalities of growth may be present long before height falls below this level (see Box 13.1) and can be identified much earlier by monitoring growth velocity and observing a child's height crossing centile lines plotted.

Causes of short stature

These are summarized in Box 13.2. By far the most common cause is familial, in which case either one or both parents will also be short. Height correlates well with parental height and is probably of polygenic inheritance. However, it should be remembered that short parents may have dominantly inherited growth disorder.

Box 13.1 Assessment of short stature

Prenatal history
- Pregnancy illness, drugs, complications

Perinatal and infancy history
- Gestational age and complications
- Birth weight (length and head circumference)
- Feeding and weight gain

Past medical history
- Chronic illness

Drug history
- Glucocorticoids

Systematic enquiry
- Headaches, visual disturbance
- Gastrointestinal symptoms

Growth history
- Examine previous growth records if available

Neurodevelopmental history
- Developmental delay
- School performance

Family history
- Short stature, pubertal delay
- Endocrine disease

Examination

- Measure height, weight, and head circumference
- General systems examination
- Puberty (Tanner) staging
- Observe for goiter, dysmorphic features, malnutrition
- Assess growth velocity at 3- to 6-monthly intervals
- Measure parent's height and calculate MPH and family height target

Box 13.2 Causes of short stature

- Familial (genetic) short stature
- Constitutional delay in growth and puberty (p. 50)
- Intrauterine growth retardation (p. 154)
- Growth hormone deficiency (p. 552)
- IGF-1 deficiency
- Other endocrine disorders
  - Hypothyroidism (p. 504)
  - Cushing's syndrome (p. 516)
- Dysmorphic syndromes
  - Turner syndrome (pp. 551, 1074)
  - Noonan syndrome (p. 1067)
  - Down syndrome (p. 1064)
- Celiac disease (pp. 392)
- Chronic renal failure (p. 460)
- Chronic inflammatory disorders (p. 890)
  - Inflammatory bowel disease (p. 388)
  - Rheumatic disease (p. 888)
- Skeletal dysplasia (p. 886)
  - Achondroplasia, hypochondroplasia
- Metabolic bone disease
  - X-linked hypophosphatemic rickets (p. 470)
- Malnutrition

Investigations

The following baseline screening tests should be carried out:
- BUN, creatinine and electrolytes (renal function)
- Liver function tests
- Full blood count and CRP or ESR (chronic disease, inflammation)
- Calcium and phosphate (bone disorder)
- Karyotype (chromosomal abnormalities, especially Turner syndrome)
- Thyroid function tests
- Serum IGF-I (IGFBP-3) (GH or IGF-1 deficiency)
- Celiac disease antibody screen
- Urinalysis

Where clinically indicated:
- Bone age X-ray
- GH stimulation test

Management

This will depend on the underlying cause (see p. 556). Familial short stature does not necessarily require any specific treatment. Recombinant human growth hormone (hGH) therapy is FDA approved for idiopathic short stature if indicated.

Constitutional delay in growth and puberty

Relative short stature occurs because of a delay in the timing of onset of puberty. It is a variation in the timing of normal puberty rather than an abnormal condition. It usually presents in early adolescence, although it may be recognized in earlier childhood.

There is often a familial basis, often having occurred in one of the parents. It is more common in males, although this may reflect a bias in the level of concern.

Characteristic features include short stature and delayed pubertal development by >2 SD. Typically there is a mild degree of skeletal disproportion with evidence of a shorter back (sitting height percentile) relative to leg length. There is invariably delay in bone age (BA) maturation, which usually remains consistent over time. Height velocity is appropriate for BA.

Laboratory investigations are normal, including GH stimulation tests.

Management

Usually no treatment is required, as the onset of puberty and the accompanying growth spurt will occur spontaneously and an appropriate final adult or target height is achieved.

Treatment

Treatment is sometimes indicated in those adolescents who have difficulty coping with their short stature or with the delayed physical development. Administration of sex steroids for a period of 3–6 months can be used to induce pubertal changes and to accelerate growth rate (boys >14 years: depot testosterone enanthate or cypionate 50–100 mg IM every 4 weeks for 3–4 doses).

Intrauterine growth retardation (see p. 154)

Intrauterine growth retardation (IUGR) refers to reduction and restriction in expected fetal growth pattern. IUGR affects 3%–10% of pregnancies and 20% of stillborn infants are thought to have evidence of IUGR. Perinatal mortality rates are 4–8 times higher for growth-retarded infants, and morbidity is present in 50% of surviving infants.

Growth outcome

In placental causes of IUGR, "catch-up growth" occurs after birth in the majority of infants during the first 1 to 2 years of life, with infants regaining their genetically determined weight and height centiles. However, in approximately 15%–20% of infants with IUGR, catch-up growth does not occur and patients are at risk of short stature.

GH therapy has been FDA approved for the use in children with IUGR who fail to catch up in height. Recent studies implicate IUGR with adult onset of hypertension and coronary heart disease, and with early-onset obesity, polycystic ovarian disease, and type 2 diabetes. These studies suggest that IUGR has long-term affects on insulin sensitivity and endocrine function.

Turner syndrome (see also p. 1062)

This condition must always be considered in girls presenting with short stature, or height below parental target height range. Karyotype confirms the diagnosis.

The majority of girls with Turner syndrome will not have the classical phenotype of dysmorphic features and it may be difficult to identify, particularly when there is mosaicism in the karyotype.

- Short stature is frequent. Typically the growth rate begins to slow from age 3–5 years due to an underlying skeletal dysplasia.
- Ovarian dysgenesis and consequent gonadal failure result in loss of pubertal growth spurt.
- Mean final height is consistently 20 cm below the norm.

Treatment with daily subcutaneous injections of recombinant human growth hormone (rhGH 0.05 mg/kg/day) increases final height, although individual responses are variable. Oral estrogen (ethinyl estradiol or conjugated estrogen) is required to induce puberty between ages 12 and 14 years. Combination therapy, which also includes the anabolic steroid oxandrolone, may further improve final height.

Celiac disease (see p. 392)

Celiac disease may be asymptomatic or atypical in its presentation with few if any gastrointestinal symptoms or signs. Poor height velocity and evolving short stature may be presenting features.

Chronic inflammatory disorders

Poor growth and short stature are common features of long-term inflammatory conditions such as inflammatory bowel disease and rheumatic disorders. They may be presenting features in Crohn's disease when gastrointestinal symptoms are initially minimal.

Short stature is due to long-term use of immunosuppressive agents (e.g., glucocorticoids) and to the generation of inflammatory factors (e.g., IL-6). Both lead to GH/IGF-I resistance and suppression of bone growth.

Management should be aimed at minimizing inflammation and reducing immunosuppressive therapy. rhGH may have a place.

Skeletal dysplasias

This heterogeneous group of disorders includes achondroplasia and hypochondroplasia. Most disorders are characterized by severe short stature and often evidence of disproportion in body segment development. Skeletal survey may allow identification of the specific condition.

Growth hormone deficiency

Physiology: secretion

Growth hormone (GH) is secreted from the somatomammotropic cells of the anterior pituitary gland in a pulsatile pattern. Secretion is diurnal and largely nocturnal and is controlled by a rhythmically changing equilibrium between two hormones secreted by the hypothalamus: GH-releasing hormone (GHRH) and GH-inhibiting hormone (or somatostatin). GHRH induces GH synthesis and secretion whenever somatostatin is low.

Different factors act at the level of the hypothalamus to regulate GH hormone secretion. GH secretion is regulated by negative feedback by circulating IGF-I at the pituitary and hypothalamus, and by short loop-feedback by GH on the hypothalamus.

Causes of GH deficiency

These may be primary (or congenital) or secondary (acquired) in origin (see Box 13.3). In clinical practice, the most frequent cause of GH deficiency is secondary to cranial radiotherapy.

Box 13.3 Causes of GH deficiency

Primary or congenital causes
- Idiopathic, isolated
- Congenital hypopituitarism (see Chapter 12)
- Midline brain anomalies

Secondary or acquired causes
- Intracranial tumors
- Craniopharyngioma
- Cranial irradiation or radiotherapy
- Psychosocial deprivation
- Traumatic brain injury
- Inflammatory or infiltrative disease
- Langerhans cell histiocytosis
- Sarcoidosis
- Intracranial infection

Clinical features

Presentation depends on the age of onset of GH deficiency.

GH deficiency in infancy

This may present with hypoglycemia. Coexisting deficiencies in the adrenal, thyroid, and gonadal axes may cause prolonged jaundice and micropenis. Size at birth and growth during the first year of life may be normal, as growth during this period is not GH dependent.

GH deficiency in childhood

This typically presents with slow growth rate and short stature. Other characteristics include increased subcutaneous fat, truncal obesity, and decreased muscle mass.

Children with congenital GH deficiency develop relative hypoplasia of the mid-facial bones, frontal bone protrusion, and delayed dental eruption. Delayed closure of the anterior fontanel may also be observed.

Investigations

Laboratory

- Baseline, random serum IGF-I and IGFBP-3
  - GH dependent and may be low in GH deficiency. However, normal levels do not exclude GH deficiency.
- GH stimulation tests

All tests should be performed in the morning after an overnight fast and serial blood samples are collected (see Box 13.4). The insulin tolerance test (ITT) is considered the gold-standard test but is not routinely used in children secondary to the risk of hypoglycemia.

The GH stimulation test should only be performed in those centers with experience and with appropriate technical and laboratory support.

Box 13.4 GH deficiency assessment commonly used in children and adolescents

Pharmacological stimulation tests

- Insulin tolerance test (gold standard; children age 5 years or over), used rarely
- Glucagon stimulation tests
- Clonidine test
- Arginine test
- Levodopa test
- Propranolol test
- GHRH test

Physiological tests

- Random serum IGF-1 and/or IGFBP3 level
- Exercise is rarely done
- Overnight or 24-hour GH serum profiles—rarely done

Radiological investigation

- Bone age
- MRI scan of brain (hypothalamic, pituitary structures)

Box 13.5 Criteria for diagnosis of GH deficiency

Update of guidelines for the use of growth hormone in children is available from the Lawson Wilkins Pediatric Endocrine Society Drug and Therapeutics Committee (2003) (www.LWPES.org), and from Growth Hormone Research Society (2000). Consensus guidelines for the diagnosis and treatment of growth hormone (GH) deficiency in childhood and adolescence: summary statement of the Growth Hormone Research Society. *J Clin Endocrinol Metab* **85**:3990–3993.

- GH deficiency is primarily a clinical diagnosis supported by auxological, biochemical, and radiological findings.
- Confirmation of the diagnosis is usually by GH stimulation testing.
- Two such tests should be used in children with suspected isolated GH deficiency together with evaluation of other aspects of pituitary function.
- Definition of GH deficiency is a peak GH <10 µg/L after stimulation.

Growth hormone deficiency: management

GH deficiency is treated with rhGH, which is administered as a once-daily subcutaneous injection (25–50 µg/kg/day or 0.7–1.0 mg/m^2/day if patient is obese).

- Treatment should be undertaken in experienced centers.
- Responses to treatment (height velocity increase) and dose adjustments should be reviewed once every 3 to 6 months.
- Catch-up growth is optimal if GH therapy is stated as early as possible.

Transition to adulthood GH deficiency care

Treatment with rhGH is continued until final adult height is achieved. At this point, the GH deficiency should be reconfirmed, particularly in those with isolated or so-called idiopathic GH deficiency, for which the cause is unclear. Up to 50% of patients with the latter may have normal GH secretion when retested in early adulthood. Those patients with persisting GH deficiency should be offered the opportunity to continue rhGH therapy (0.2–0.5 mg/day).

Studies have demonstrated that rhGH replacement in adulthood may maintain lean body mass, muscle strength, and bone mineral density. In addition, improved quality of life has been reported with treatment.

Cranial irradiation and GH deficiency

Cranial radiotherapy used in the treatment of tumors (intracranial, face, and nasopharynx) may cause GH deficiency. The GH axis is the most sensitive to radiotherapy, followed by the gonadal and adrenal axes and, finally, the thyroid axis, which is least sensitive.

There is a good correlation between radiotherapy dose and the occurrence of hypothalamic–pituitary dysfunction (Table 13.2). Risk of dysfunction is also related to dose fractionation (single is more toxic than divided) and age (younger more sensitive).

Table 13.2 Correlation between radiotherapy and GH deficiency

Radiotherapy dose	% GH deficient*
18 Gy	None
24 Gy	55%
25–45 Gy	68%–76%
>45 Gy	100%

* Assessed 4 years after radiotherapy.

Psychosocial deprivation

Children subjected to physical or emotional abuse may exhibit growth failure. This may be due to a reversible inhibition of GH secretion, which improves within 3 to 4 weeks of being removed from the adverse environment. Catch-up growth is usually dramatic.

GH insensitivity syndrome

Moderate to severe short stature may be due to GH resistance. This may result from a defect in the GH receptor or a defect in post-receptor GH signaling.

Complete GH insensitivity syndrome (GHIS) results in severe short stature. It may be inherited as an autosomal recessive trait (Laron syndrome). Affected individuals have high GH levels and low circulating IGF-I levels. Exogenous rhGH administration fails to increase IGF-I levels further (IGF-I generation test).

GHIS and IGF-1 deficiency can be treated with recombinant human IGF-1, which is administered twice daily subcutaneously (80–240 µg/kg/day).

Tall stature

Referral for tall stature is much less common than for short stature. Socially it is more acceptable to be tall, particularly for boys. Nevertheless, tall stature, particularly when associated with inappropriately increased growth rates, may indicate an underlying growth disorder.

Causes of tall stature

In most cases tall stature is genetic in origin and inherited from tall parents. Other causes need to be considered, although rare.

- Familial
- Early (normal) puberty
- Obesity
- Endocrine disorders
  - Precocious puberty (see p. 564)
  - GH excess
  - Pituitary adenoma
  - Androgen excess
  - Congenital adrenal hyperplasia (p. 518)
  - Hyperthyroidism (p. 506)
  - Aromatase enzyme deficiency (very rare)
  - Estrogen receptor defects (very rare)
- Chromosomal abnormalities
  - Klinefelter syndrome (XXY), XYY, XYYY (p. 1062)
- Other syndromes
  - Marfan, homocystinuria, Soto's syndrome, Beckwith–Wiedemann

Assessment

History

A detailed history should be obtained.

Perinatal and infancy history

- Size at birth
- Birth weight (head circumference)
- Feeding and weight gain

Systematic enquiry

- Headaches, visual disturbance
- Growth history
- Examine previous growth records if available
- Recent growth acceleration
- Signs of puberty

Neurodevelopmental history

- Developmental delay
- School performance

Family history

- Tall stature
- Early puberty
- Endocrine disease

Examination

Measure
• Height
• Weight
• Head circumference

Puberty staging (Tanner)
• Observe dysmorphic features; goiter

Assess growth
• Velocity over a minimum 6-monthly interval

Family history
• Measure parents' height
• Calculate MPH
• Family height target

Investigations

The following baseline screening tests should be carried out:
• Karyotype (chromosomal abnormalities for Klinefelter syndrome)
• Thyroid function tests, serum IGF-I (and IGFBP-3)
• Sex hormone, LH and FSH levels
• Androgen levels (DHEAS, 17-OH progesterone)
• Bone age X-ray

Where clinically indicated:
• GH suppression test (i.e., modified oral glucose tolerance test; GH levels normally suppressed to low levels)

Management

In familial tall stature, reassurance and information about predicted final height are usually sufficient. Early induction of puberty using low-dose sex steroid to advance the pubertal growth spurt and cause earlier epiphyseal closure is occasionally considered. However, this produces variable results and there is a theoretical risk of complications (including thromboembolic disease and oncogenic risk).

Delayed puberty: assessment

This is defined as the lack of initiation and progress of pubertal development by greater than +2 SD later than the average age of onset of puberty for the population. In the United States, this equates to >13 years for females and >14 years for males.

The causes of delayed puberty are shown in Box 13.6.

History

A detailed history should screen for the many possible physical and functional causes of delayed puberty. Careful enquiry about the age of onset of puberty (including menarche in females) in other family members is required.

Examination

- Measure height, weight, head circumference
- Puberty (Tanner) staging
- Review previous growth records if available
- Measure parent's height and calculate MPH and family height target

Investigations

The following baseline screening tests should be carried out.

Blood

- LH and FSH levels
- Sex hormone: estrogen, testosterone
- Karyotype (chromosomal abnormalities)
- Thyroid function tests
- Routine biochemistry, and inflammatory markers (e.g., CRP or ESR)

Radiologic

- Bone age X-ray
- Pelvic ultrasound (ovarian morphology)
- Abdominal ultrasound (e.g., intra-abdominal testes)
- Brain MRI scan

Tests

- *Human chorionic gonadotrophin (hCG) stimulation test* (3- or 21-day test): measurement of testosterone pre- and post-hCG (as indicator of functional testicular tissue)
- *Gonadotrophin-releasing hormone agonist (GnRHa) test*: measurement of basal and post-GnRHa LH and FSH levels (an indicator of hypothalamic–pituitary function)

Note: It is difficult to distinguish between constitutional delay in growth and puberty (CDGP) from other causes of hypogonadotropic hypogonadism (HH) using current tests. In both conditions, basal and stimulated gonadotropin (LH/FSH) levels are low. Differentiation may only be possible after induction of puberty with sex steroid therapy and attainment of final height, when reassessment of the hypothalamic–pituitary–gonadal axis should be repeated after withdrawal of treatment.

Box 13.6 Causes of pubertal delay

Delay of growth and puberty
(Undetectable basal and stimulated gonadotropin levels)
- Congenital
  - Kallmann syndrome
  - Congenital hypopituitarism (e.g., *LHX-3; PROP-1*; see p. 534)
  - Isolated LH deficiency
  - Isolated FSH deficiency
  - Other causes of gonadotropin deficiency, e.g., congenital adrenal hypoplasia (*DAX-1* gene)
  - Syndromic associations e.g., Prader–Willi syndrome
- Acquired
  - Intracranial tumors (e.g., craniopharyngioma)
  - Cranial irradiation
  - Traumatic brain injury
  - Langerhans cell histiocytosis
  - Anorexia nervosa
  - Excess physical training
  - Chronic childhood disease, e.g., inflammatory bowel disease

Primary gonadal failure (hypergonadotropic hypogonadism)
(High basal and stimulated gonadotropin levels)
- Congenital
  - Chromosomal disorders, Turner syndrome, Klinefelter syndrome
  - Gonadal dysgenesis
  - LH resistance
  - Disorders of steroid biosynthesis, e.g., congenital adrenal hyperplasia—StAR, CYP17, 3βHSD; see p. 518)
- Acquired
  - Chemotherapy
  - Gonadal irradiation (local radiotherapy)
  - Gonadal infection (e.g., mumps orchitis)
  - Gonadal trauma, gonadal torsion
  - Cranial irradiation
  - Autoimmune (ovarian)

Delayed puberty: management

Children with CDGP may be treated with a short course of sex steroid therapy to promote physical development and growth.

Children with permanent gonadotropin deficiency or gonadal failure requiring complete induction of puberty and thus long-term treatment can have puberty induced with gradually increasing doses of sex steroids over a period of 2 to 3 years.

Boys

Give testosterone enanthate or cypionate by IM injection at incremental increases in dosage, starting from 50 mg every 4–6 weeks to 250 mg every 3–4 weeks.

Girls

Give ethinyl estradiol (EE) or conjugated estrogen, orally. Increase doses every 6 months, starting from 2 µg/day increasing to 4, 6, 10, and then 15–20 µg/day for EE or starting from 0.3 mg/day for conjugated estrogen. Medroxyprogesterone acetate, given on days 14–25 of the cycle, should only be added when the dose of EE is 10–15 µg/day or when vaginal bleeding or spotting is first observed.

The aims of long-term sex steroid therapy are maintenance of secondary sexual features, libido, and menstruation in females. There are also positive benefits in terms of bone mineralization and cardiovascular health.

Note. In males, testosterone therapy does not promote testicular growth, and testicular size remains prepubertal unless spontaneous puberty occurs.

Constitutional delay of growth and puberty (CDGP)

This is the most common cause of delayed puberty. Usually observed in boys, this condition reflects a delay in the timing mechanisms that regulate the onset of puberty. There is often a family history of delayed puberty in parents or siblings.

• Children presenting with CDGP are invariably healthy.
• Onset and progress through puberty will occur normally with time.
• Children achieve a final adult height in keeping with their predicted familial target range.

It is likely that most children with CDGP are not referred for medical attention, as they and their parents will not perceive that there is a problem. For many others, however, concerns about the lack of physical development and the lack of anticipated adolescent growth spurt can be a source of anxiety and psychological stress.

There is often evidence of delayed or slow growth in childhood, which is most pronounced in the peripubertal years due to lack of anticipated growth spurt. Children will also have evidence of delayed skeletal maturation on bone age assessment.

No specific therapy is required. For many children and families, explanation of the benign nature of the condition and reassurance that puberty will occur normally is sufficient. However, children who are experiencing significant social or psychological difficulties may request treatment. In this situation, low-dose sex steroids may be used (e.g., boys: depot testosterone enanthate or cypionate 50 mg IM monthly for 4–6 months).

This approach will:
- induce sexual development,
- promote an increase in growth rate, and
- stimulate activation of the hypothalamic–pituitary–gonadal axis so that puberty may continue once the administration of sex steroids has been stopped.

Any decision of whether or not therapy is required must include the views of the child and their parents.

Hypogonadtropic hypogonadism (HH)

HH indicates impaired gonadotropin release from the pituitary gland. Congenital and acquired causes are recognized (see Box 13.6). The condition is characterized by low or undetectable gonadotropin levels either under basal or stimulated (GnRHa test) conditions.

Congenital causes of HH may be characterized by micropenis and undescended testis at birth in boys, whereas in girls physical signs are absent.

Kallmann syndrome (KS)

KS is a genetic disorder characterized by the association of HH and anosmia (absent sense of smell). This arises from a defect in the co-migration of GnRH-releasing neurons and olfactory neurons that occurs during early fetal development.

X-linked, autosomal dominant, and recessive modes of inheritance are recognized. The X-linked form of KS results from a mutation in the *KAL* gene (encoding the glycoprotein anosmin-1). It is also characterized by a range of clinical features, including synkinesia (mirror-image movements), renal agenesis, visual problems, and craniofacial anomalies, although their expression is highly variable.

Precocious puberty

This is defined as the early onset and rapid progression of puberty. Age criteria vary. In Caucasian children, precocious puberty (PP) is defined as <8 in females and <9 years in males, whereas in African Americans PP is defined as <6.6 in females and <8 years in males.

Classification and causes

PP is either central or peripheral in origin. The various causes of PP are described below.

Central (true) PP (gonadotropin dependent)

- *Idiopathic* (familial/nonfamilial)
- *Intracranial tumors*: e.g., hypothalamic hamartoma; craniopharyngioma; astrocytoma, optic glioma
- *Other CNS lesions*: Hydrocephalus, arachnoid cysts, traumatic brain injury, cranial irradiation
- *Secondary CPP*: Early maturation of the hypothalamic–pituitary–gonadal axis due to long-term sex steroid exposure, e.g., congenital adrenal hyperplasia (CAH); McCune–Albright syndrome

Puberty occurs as a consequence of early physiological (true) activation of the hypothalamic–pituitary–gonadal axis (central). A normal sequence of pubertal development is observed.

CPP may also be idiopathic and familial. Girls with CPP are more likely to have idiopathic CPP, whereas in boys there is a much greater risk of intracranial tumors.

Peripheral PP (gonadotropin independent)

- *Gonadal*: McCune–Albright syndrome; ovarian tumors; e.g., benign cyst; granulosa cell tumor; testicular tumor; familial testitoxicosis (LH receptor is activating mutation)
- *Adrenal*: CAH; adrenal tumor (carcinoma; adenoma)
- *Human chorionic gonadotropin (hCG) secreting tumors* E.g., CNS—chorioepithelioma; germinoma
- *Iatrogenic* (exogenous sex steroid administration)

Puberty is due to mechanisms that do not involve physiologic gonadotropin secretion from the pituitary. The source of sex steroid may be endogenous (gonadal or extragonadal) or exogenous. Endogenous hormone production is independent of hypothalamic–pituitary–gonadal activity. An abnormal sequence of pubertal development is usually observed. Peripheral PP can lead to central PP, however, if the bone age has advanced sufficiently.

Assessment

History

A detailed history should be obtained:

- Age when first signs of pubertal development observed
- Which features of puberty are present and in what order did they appear?
- Evidence of growth acceleration
- Family history: careful enquiry about the age of onset of puberty (including age of menarche in females) within other family members

Examination

- Puberty (Tanner) staging
- Measure height, weight, head circumference
- Review previous growth records if available
- Measure parent's height and calculate MPH and family height target
- Skin lesions, e.g., café-au-lait marks (McCune–Albright syndrome; NF1)
- Abdominal or testicular masses
- Neurological examination of visual fields; fundoscopy

Investigations

Baseline screening tests should be considered:

- Third-generation or ultra-sensitive LH and FSH levels
- Sex hormone: Estrogen or testosterone
- Other serum androgen levels, e.g., 17-OH progesterone, DHEAS, androstenedione

In addition, undertake the following:

- Bone age X-ray
- Pelvic ultrasound (ovarian morphology; testicular masses)
- Abdominal ultrasound (e.g., adrenal glands)
- Brain MRI scan
- GnRHa test for measurement of basal and post-GnRHa LH and FSH levels as indicator of hypothalamic–pituitary function

Precocious puberty: management

Diagnosis

The diagnosis is based on demonstrating progressive pubertal development and increased growth rate, together with laboratory evidence of increased sex steroid production. Distinguishing between central and peripheral PP and from other normal variants of pubertal development may be difficult. In CPP there is usually a normal sequence of pubertal development that is in keeping with the normal physiological activation of puberty.

Management

The management of precocious puberty is aimed at the following:
• Detection and treatment of underlying pathological causes of PP.
This is especially important in males in whom early puberty is invariably due to organic disease.
• Reducing the rate of skeletal maturation, if necessary.

Accelerated skeletal maturation and growth rate occur and will result in the affected child being tall during childhood relative to peers. However, skeletal maturation exceeds height and thus growth potential is reduced. Growth is completed prematurely and final adult height is reduced and potentially below the predicted expected familial target height range.
• Reducing and halting, if necessary, the rate of physical pubertal development.
• Addressing potential behavioral and psychological difficulties.

Table 13.3 Characteristic findings of disorders of pubertal development

	Sequence of pubertal changes	Height velocity	Sex steroids	LH / FSH (basal/ stimulated)	Bone age
Central PP	Normal	++	++	++ LH predominant	++
Peripheral/ PP	May be atypical	++	++	Pre-pubertal Suppressed	++
Premature thelarche	Breast tissue only	N	N	Pre-pubertal/ FSH +	N
Thelarche 'variant'	Breast tissue only	+	N	Pre-pubertal/ FSH +	N/+
Premature adrenarche	Pubic hair Skin changes only	N	N/DHEAS +	Pre-pubertal Suppressed	N

+ slightly raised or advanced   ++ raised or advanced   N normal

- Sexual and reproductive characteristics advance inappropriately for age, leading to mature appearance. Early menstruation occurs in girls, and spermatogenesis and ejaculation in boys. Sexualized behavior may occur and, interactions with age-peers and adults may be based on assumed, but age-inappropriate, mental and social expectations.

Before therapy is considered, it is essential that an explanation of the physiology and physical consequences of precocious puberty be discussed with the parents and the child. The decision regarding therapy should be made jointly with the parents.

Treatment of precocious puberty
Central PP

- Suppression of the hypothalamic–pituitary–gonadal axis with a long-acting GnRH agonist is the only currently effective treatment for CPP. These agents work by providing continuous stimulation of the GnRH receptor on the pituitary gonadotropes, resulting in down-regulation of the receptor and, thus, decreased LH and FSH secretion.
- GnRH agonists are administered by IM injection, monthly (or 3-monthly in depot preparations), SC injection, or implantation.
- Treatment efficacy should be assessed by monitoring growth rate and pubertal stage. In addition, serum LH and FSH levels (basal and stimulated) should be measured to ensure hypothalamic–pituitary–gonadal axis suppression.

Variants of normal puberty

This includes premature thelarche and premature adrenarche. Neither condition is associated with pubertal activation of the hypothalamic–pituitary–gonadal axis.

Premature thelarche

- Isolated premature breast development occurring in the absence of any other signs of puberty
- Typically, females present in infancy and usually by 2 years of age.
- Breast development is due to the action of physiologic or mild increases in the amounts of circulating estrogen.

The clinical course is characterized by a waxing and waning of breast size, normal growth (height) rate, and the absence of any further sexual development. Breast development may be asymmetrical, and there is usually a resolution of any breast enlargement by age 4–5 years.

The cause is unknown, but small increases in basal and stimulated serum FSH levels are usually observed, whereas LH levels remain suppressed in the prepubertal range. Ovarian follicle development is often observed, but no changes in ovarian or uterine size are seen. Serum estradiol levels are increased when measured by sensitive assays, but typically within normal range by standard radioimmunoassay.

The condition is benign. Bone maturation, age of onset of menarche, and final adult height are not affected. Management is conservative with reevaluation of growth and puberty stage at 3- to 6-monthly intervals.

Thelarche variant

- An intermediate condition between premature thelarche and central precocious puberty
- It represents a nonprogressive form of early pubertal development.

Patients have evidence of breast development, increased growth rate, and advanced skeletal maturation on bone age assessment. There may also be evidence of ovarian enlargement and raised serum estradiol levels. For most patients the tempo of progression of pubertal development will be slow and they will have laboratory findings within normal range for age. Management is usually conservative with regular reevaluation of growth and pubertal status at 3- to 6-monthly intervals. Decisions to treat (as for CPP) are based on height velocity, final height predictions, and psychosocial concerns.

Premature adrenarche

Early onset of pubertal adrenal androgen secretion is a common variation of normal pubertal development. Premature adrenarche is the result of premature secretion of androgens from the zona reticualris of the adrenal gland.

- Children typically present with premature appearance of androgen-dependent secondary sexual hair development (axillary hair, pubic hair, or both), acne, and axillary (body) odor.
- Patients may have mild acceleration in height velocity and a slight increase in bone age.
- Laboratory investigations reveal an increase in serum DHEAS levels that are appropriate for pubic-hair stage rather than for age.
- Serum concentrations of testosterone and 17-OH progesterone are normal.

When evaluating patients for premature adrenarche, it is important to assess for clinical signs and symptoms that might indicate other causes of excess androgen production (e.g., adrenal tumor, congenital adrenal hyperplasia). The latter are characterized with signs of virilization, rapid growth rate, and significantly advanced bone age.

Premature adrenarche is a benign condition. The timing of onset of true puberty is normal and final adult height is unaffected. Management is conservative with reassurance after exclusion of other causes of adrenal androgen excess. Symptomatic treatment may be required if adrenarche is pronounced, particularly in females who may go on to develop features of ovarian hyperandrogenism and the polycystic ovarian syndrome.

Sexual differentiation

Terminology

- *Sexual determination* refers to the process that occurs from the time of conception until the fetal bipotential gonad has been fully determined as either an ovary or testis.
- *Sexual differentiation* refers to the process that occurs from the time gonadal sex is determined until secondary sexual characteristics are fully expressed and fertility achieved.

Disorders of sexual development (DSD)

The complex process of sexual determination and differentiation may be interrupted. Numerous disorders are recognized that can result in genital ambiguity and uncertainty about an infant's sex. Disorders of sexual development may be classified as genetic defects of gonadal determination (see Box 13.7), or defects in androgen biosynthesis, metabolism, and action (excess or deficiency).

Box 13.7 Genetic disorders of gonadal determination

- Gonadal dysgenesis
  - 45 X: Turner syndrome
  - 46 XY: Complete gonadal dysgenesis
  - 45 X/46 XY: Mixed gonadal dysgenesis
- Ovotesticular DSD (true hermaphroditism)
- 46 XX testicular DSD
- Camptomelic dysplasia (*SOX-9* mutation)
- *DAX-1* mutation
- Denys–Drash syndrome (*WT-1* mutation)

46 XX DSD (virilization of 46 XX infants [female pseudohermaphrodite])
- Excessive androgen production
- Congenital adrenal hyperplasia (CAH)
  - 21α-hydroxylase deficiency
  - 11β-hydroxylase deficiency
  - 3βHSD
- Defect in androgen exposure
  - Placental–fetal aromatase deficiency
- Maternal steroid exposure

46 XY DSD (undervirilization of 46 XY male [male pseudohermaphrodite])
- Defect in testosterone production
  - Leydig cell hypoplasia or agenesis
  - Defects of testicular and adrenal steroidogenesis
  —StAR
  —3βHSD
  —17α-hydroxylase/17,20 lyase deficiency
- Defect in testosterone metabolism
  - 5a-reductase deficiency
- Defects in testosterone action
- Androgen insensitivity syndrome: Complete or partial

Assessment

History

A detailed history should be obtained and should include the following:
- *Family history*: Ambiguous genitalia, disorders or problems of puberty, inguinal hernia
- *Prenatal history*: Maternal health, drugs taken during pregnancy, maternal virilization during pregnancy
- History of previous stillbirths or neonatal death?

Examination

General examination

- Dysmorphic features or midline defects; state of hydration; blood pressure

Genitalia

- Are the gonads palpable?
  - If "yes," they are likely to be testes or ovotestes
- Assess the degree of virilization.
  - Prader stage (Fig. 13.2)
  - External Masculinization Score
- Penis: Measure the length of the phallus.
  - Normal-term penis is about 3 cm (stretched length from pubic tubercle to tip of penis).
  - Micropenis has a length <2.0–2.5 cm.
- Penis—presence of chordee
- Vagina—locate opening?
- Appearance of labioscrotal folds
- Position of urethral opening
- Pigmentation of genital skin
  - Hyperpigmentation with excessive ACTH and opiomelanocortin in CAH
- In preterm girls, clitoris and labia minora are relatively prominent
- In boys, testes are undescended until 34 weeks

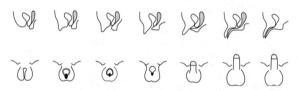

Figure 13.2 Prader staging: of virilization. From *Helvetica Paediatrica Acta* 1958;**13**:5–146. With kind permission of Springer Science and Business Media.

Sexual differentiation: management

Investigations

Laboratory

- Genetic sex determination: FISH for Y and X chromosomes, karyotype (takes 3–5 days)
- Serum electrolytes
- Blood sugar (hypoglycemia)
- Adrenal androgens: Plasma testosterone; 17-OH progesterone; LH and FSH
- Molecular genetic studies; blood for DNA

If a male/mosaic karyotype is confirmed, further investigations are directed at establishing whether testicular tissue is capable of producing androgens:
- hCG stimulation test
- Testosterone/DHT ratio
- Androgen receptor DNA testing

Imaging studies

- Ultrasound scan of pelvis for anatomy of urogenital sinus, vagina, and uterus
- Ultrasound scan abdomen for renal anomalies
- Urogenital sonogram
- MRI

Internal examination

- Examination under anesthesia (±cystography)
- Laparoscopy
- Gonadal biopsy

Management

This is professionally challenging and requires a multidisciplinary team including the following:
- Pediatric endocrinologist
- Neonatologist
- Pediatric urologist
- Gynecologist
- Geneticist
- Radiologist
- Psychologist
- Clinical biochemist

Most infants presenting with a disorder of sexual differentiation will have ambiguous genitalia at birth.
- Parents and their relatives will be anxious to know the sex of their newborn baby.
- Decisions about an infant's sex (sex assignment) must be delayed until the multidisciplinary team has carried out a thorough assessment.
- Birth registration must be delayed until this has been completed and an agreement on sex assignment has been made with the parents.

The general principles of making this assessment are presented in Box 13.8.

Box 13.8 General principles of sex assignment

Virilized females
- Should be brought up as female
- Clitromegaly: Perform clitoral recession (clitorplasty) in infancy or childhood if necessary; often there is "regression."
- Vaginoplasty is deferred until late childhood or early adolescence

Undervirilized male
The decision regarding sex assignment is more complex. This depends on the following:
- Degree of sexual ambiguity
- Underlying cause if known
- Potential for normal sexual function and fertility
- Phallic size
  - If >2.5 cm, reconstructive surgery is more likely to be successful.
  - A trial of IM testosterone may improve phallic size.

Gonadectomy is required
- If there is dysgenetic testis
- If complete AIS is present (controversial)
- If decision is to raise child as female

Hormone replacement therapy
- Testosterone therapy if decision is to raise child as male
- Estrogen therapy if decision is to raise child as female

Psychological support
- Experienced counseling is essential.
- Patient support groups are available.

Issues regarding assignment of gender, timing of reconstructive surgery, and hormone replacement therapy are complex. See Hughes IA, Houk C, Ahmed SF, et al. (2006). Consensus statement on management of intersex disorders. *Arch Dis Child* **91**:554–563.

Androgen insensitivity syndrome (AIS)

This condition is due to defects in the androgen receptor and results in a spectrum of undervirilized phenotypes in the 46 XY patient.

Complete AIS

Deletions of the gene and certain mutations can result in a complete female phenotype.

- External genitalia are unambiguously female, with normal clitoris, hypoplastic labia majora, and blind-ending vaginal pouch. Mullerian structures are absent.
- Testes may be located in the abdomen, inguinal canal, or labia.
- AIS should be strongly suspected and excluded in any female presenting with inguinal hernia.
- Patients with complete AIS often present in adolescence with primary amenorrhea.
- At puberty, serum levels of testosterone and LH are elevated. Conversion of testosterone to estradiol in the testis and in peripheral tissues results in normal breast development.
- Pubic and axillary hair development is absent or sparse.
- Diagnosis is confirmed by demonstrating 46XY karyotype and gene testing.

In view of the potential risk of malignant transformation, if retained, removal of the testis either soon after diagnosis or after the completion of puberty is often carried out. However, there is recent controversy over the actual risk of malignant transformation and thus the need for gonadectomy. After gonadal removal, estrogen replacement therapy is given.

Partial AIS

Certain mutations of the androgen receptor gene result in a partial form of AIS. There is a wide spectrum of phenotypic expression ranging from ambiguous genitalia to a normal male phenotype presenting with fertility difficulties. There is however, poor genotype–phenotype correlation and patients with the same mutation present with different phenotypes.

Management is much more challenging. Sex assignment depends on the degree of genital ambiguity.

Ovotesticular DSD (true hermaphroditism)

Individuals have both ovarian tissue with follicles and testicular tissue with seminiferous tubules either in the same gonad (ovotestis) or an ovary on one side and a testis on the other. The etiology of this condition is unclear. In 70% of cases the underlying karyotype is 46XX; 20% 46XX/46XY; 10% 46XY.

Ovotestes may be present bilaterally and be located in the inguinal canal. The external genitalia are most often ambiguous, although in 10% the phenotype may be female. The degree of feminization and virilization that occurs varies widely. Management is dictated by sex assignment. Dysgenetic testicular tissue should be removed because of the risk of malignant transformation.

Micropenis

Micropenis is often an incidental finding on newborn examination.

An intact hypothalamic–pituitary–gonadal axis is required for the formation of a normal-sized phallus and for descent of the testis. Both growth hormone and the gonadotropins are required for phallic growth.

The finding of micropenis warrants assessment of hypothalamic–pituitary function and exclusion of both growth hormone deficiency and hypogonadotropic–hypogonadism. Micropenis may also be part of a syndrome causing ambiguous genitalia.

Evaluation
Penile size
- Measured from pubic tubercle to tip of stretched penis in a term baby
- Normal size at birth is usually >3 cm.
- Micropenis <2.2–2.5 cm (varies with ethnicity)

General examination
- Dysmorphism
- Midline craniofacial defects

Ophthalmic examination
- Optic nerve hypoplasia, septo-optic dysplasia

Investigations
- Ultrasound of head for midline defects
- MRI of brain with emphasis on pituitary and hypothalamic region
- Anterior pituitary hormone levels (basal and stimulated)
  - ACTH and cortisol; GH [IGF-I, IGFBP3]; LH and FSH; TSH and fT4
- Karyotype

Management
Referral to a pediatric urologist is often required. If severe micropenis is present, a decision regarding sex assignment may be needed.

Treatment with a short course of intramuscular testosterone may stimulate penile growth and improve appearances.

Gynecomastia

This condition, which affects boys, involves hyperplasia of the glandular tissue of the breast, resulting in enlargement of one or both breasts. It is a common condition with three well-defined time periods of occurrence:

- Neonatal
- Puberty
- Older adult life

It is due to either an imbalance in the normal systemic or local estrogen/androgen ratio. An absolute or relative increase in estrogen levels, local breast tissue hypersensitivity to estrogens, or a decrease in the production or action of free androgen levels may induce gynecomastia.

A number of diverse causes are recognized (see Box 13.9). Gynecomastia must be differentiated from pseudogynecomastia, which is breast enlargement due to fat accumulation.

Box 13.9 Classification and causes of gynecomastia

- Pubertal gynecomastia
- Neonatal gynecomastia
- Impaired gonadal function
  - Hypogonadotropic hypogonadism
  - Hypergonadotropic hypogonadism
- Androgen insensitivity syndrome
- Adrenal tumors
- Testicular tumors
  - Leydig cell tumor
  - Sertoli cell tumor
  - Germ cell tumor
- Iatrogenic
  - Exogenous hormones, e.g., estrogen, anabolic steroids
  - Ketoconazole
  - Psychoactive drugs, e.g., diazepam, phenothiazines
- Alcohol excess
- Cannabis

Pubertal gynecomastia

This is most common form of gynecomastia in children and adolescents. The exact cause remains unclear. Proposed mechanisms include alterations in the rate of change in estrogen and androgen production during puberty and/or hypersensitivity of breast tissue to estrogen.

It may affect 40%–70% of boys to some degree, depending on ethnicity and nutritional status. The usual age of onset of development is early puberty (ages 10–12 years), peaking during puberty (age 13–14 years). In most children the gynecomastia usually involutes after 1–2 years and is generally resolved by the end of puberty (ages 16–17 years).

The diagnosis is established by excluding other possible causes of gynecomastia. A detailed clinical and family history and examination should be conducted, with the following investigations:
• Serum estrogen, testosterone, LH, FSH
• Serum prolactin
• Liver function test; thyroid function tests
• Karyotype

If testicular, adrenal, or hepatic tumor is suspected, the following investigation should be considered:
• Ultrasound of abdomen or testis
• MRI of abdomen or testis
• Serum βHCG levels

Management

Reassurance and explanation are usually sufficient for pubertal gynecomastia. In severe cases in which pubertal gynecomastia is causing significant psychological distress or gynecomastia persists beyond puberty, surgical resection of excess glandular breast tissue is warranted. The role of medical therapy with aromatase inhibitors or with selective estrogen receptor blocking agents (e.g., tamoxifen) is currently unclear.

Neurology

Examination: over 5 years

This is the most useful tool in assessing children with neurological disorders. Nevertheless, it is often thought to be difficult and therefore either neglected or performed incompletely.

Children over the mental age of 5 years who can walk

Older children can undergo a complete neurological examination by making it a game. Pay particular attention to their

- Affect
- Gait and spine
- Head size
- Skin, for neurocutaneous stigmata
- Abdomen, for organomegaly

Children between the time they walk and a mental age of 5 years

Such children can be examined by observing them playing and interacting with their parents and/or siblings in the examination room while you obtain a history.

Observe and note

- Gait
- Visual acuity, hearing, speech
- Behavior
- Movements

Play with the child and get the child to

- Walk in a straight line "on a tight rope" and turn quickly around (cerebellar function)
- Perform the Gowers' maneuver (assessing proximal muscle strength)

Examine

- Dorsiflexion by walking on heels
- Skin, abdomen, spine, fundi, and head circumference
- Coordination (taxis) and formation of movement (praxis) by playing simple games—e.g., "take this toy from my hand"; "pretend to open a door."

Cranial nerves (II, III, IV, VI)

- Look at the child's eyes. Do they fix and follow?
- Move an interesting toy and watch the child's eye movements. Get the child to look at you. Will they look left or right when the toy comes in from each side of their visual field?
- Get a parent to stand behind you and wiggle their nose. Ask the child to "see if you can count how many times daddy wiggles his nose."
- Quickly look at their fundi.

Other cranial nerves

- Watch the facial movements (VII).
- Say something with your hand covering your mouth and see if the child responds appropriately (VIII).
- Does the child dribble excessively? Ask a parent about this or watch the child swallow and listen to their articulation of speech (IX, X).
- Children love to shrug their shoulders and stick out their tongues (XI, XII).

Neuromuscular examination

Children who can walk, run, jump, and hop well are very unlikely to have an abnormality of the peripheral nervous system that will be identified on further examination. However, if there is an abnormality:

- Remove clothes as far as underwear if the child does not object.
- *Look at the gait:* Where does the foot strike? Heel or toe? Is it waddling or asymmetrical, is there abnormality of posture?
- *Observe the muscle bulk and joint positions* with particular reference to scoliosis, lordosis, hip flexion, and ankle inversion or eversion.
- *Assess the upper limbs* for joint ranges, tone, and power by playing with the child. Laugh and keep praising the patient during the examination. Use an adult reflex hammer and elicit the reflexes but place your thumb over the biceps and brachioradialis.
- Continue to play with the child as you assess the same in the lower limbs.
- Try to categorize the pattern into increased or decreased tone. Is it mainly unilateral, or bilateral but mainly in the legs, or in all four limbs, and possibly the bulbar muscles?

Sensation

- If indicated, assess sensation by asking the child to close their eyes and say "touch" every time the child feels your touch.

Examination: under 5 years and not walking

These children need a modified neurological examination incorporating primitive reflexes and development.

Observe and note
- Developmental stage: Can the child see, hear, or move?
- Characterize the child's vocalizations.
- Are there dysmorphic features?

Examination
Don't rush to get the clothes removed, as this may frighten the child and limit your physical assessment. Examine the following:
- Skin, for neurocutaneous stigmata
- Abdomen, for organomegaly
- Spine
- Fundi
- Head circumference (when the child likes you, or at the end of the examination if you haven't managed to break the ice)
- Check for dysmorphic features.

Cranial nerves (II, III, IV, VI)
- Check visual acuity: Will the patient fix on a small toy or large object (e.g., toy, face, bright light)?
- Will the child follow it?
- Are the eyes symmetrical with a full range of movement, when following small and large toys?
- Check pupil reaction to light.

Other cranial nerves
- Will the child respond to a quiet, moderate, or loud sound (VIII)?
- Elicit a smile, or wait to see if there is a spontaneous grimace (VII).
- Ask about or watch the child swallow (IX, X).

Neuromuscular examination
- Observe the child's *best motor function*: Antigravity movement, rolling over, lifting head up, sitting up, and pulling to stand
- Place your little fingers in the child's hands while they lie supine. Does the patient have a primitive grasp reflex? Then pull the child up off the bed, watching for head lag, which would imply low tone, reduced power, or both.
- If the patient has developed head control, see if the child can sit with or without support.
- Carefully pick the child up under their armpits: if the patient slips through your hands, this is a sign of hypotonia.
- Then assess their parachute and Moro reflexes (see Chapter 15, p. 632).

Children with age-appropriate motor development are very unlikely to have an abnormality of the peripheral nervous system that will be identified on further examination. If there is an abnormality:

- *Power:* Observe the movements and pattern of any paucity.
- *Tone:* Gently manipulate joints but take extreme care in infants to avoid trauma.
- *Reflexes:* Use an adult reflex hammer and elicit the reflexes but place your thumb over the tendons.
- *Coordination:* If age-appropriate, assess fine-motor ability by presenting an attractive target for the child to take or grasp with either a primitive or pincer grasp.

Sensation

- Check for symmetry of sensation by tickling or stroking the palms and soles and observing for changes in facial expression, vocalizations, and withdrawal of the stimulated extremity.

Nonepileptic paroxysmal episodes

Up to one-third of children diagnosed with "epilepsy" actually have nonepileptic events. Think carefully about other paroxysmal episodes before diagnosing a form of epilepsy and treating the child.

Etiology

It is best to consider the cause of paroxysmal episodes according to the age of the child.

Neonates and infants

- *Benign neonatal sleep myoclonus*: These are single or repetitive episodes of jerking of arms and legs (typically while falling asleep after a feed) and which resolve upon wakening.
- *Shuddering attacks*: These attacks resemble a chill, lasting a few seconds with preserved consciousness. They are benign events of unclear etiology. Affected patients have normal brain imaging and there are no EEG discharges during the events.

Older infants and toddlers

- *"Breath-holding attacks" and reflex anoxic seizures (RAS)*: A history of suddenly going limp (or syncope), which may be followed by clonic jerking (e.g., RAS). On closer questioning at least one episode has been triggered by a noxious stimulus (e.g., banging head). Typically there is a short cry and then the child goes limp, collapses to the floor, and has a brief seizure. Other episodes are characterized by "blue" breath-holding, when the child starts to cry for any reason, the crying builds up, and then the child collapses to the floor at the end of expiration.
- *Masturbation and other gratification phenomena*: When the child is bored he or she indulges in self-stimulation. In girls, the legs are held outstretched and the eyes are glazed. Sweatiness almost invariably raises the possibility of a tonic seizure, and these episodes are commonly mistreated as epilepsy.
- *Febrile myoclonus*: Short jerks associated with high fever
- *Benign paroxysmal vertigo of childhood*: Acute onset of fear, nausea, vertigo, and unsteadiness if forced to walk. Rarely, the child vomits and they may have nystagmus. This condition is considered to be a migraine-equivalent syndrome.
- *Benign paroxysmal torticollis*: Acute episodes of head tilt, at times with associated clinical features similar to those seen in children with benign paroxysmal vertigo
- *Parasomnias*: Night terrors. While in deep sleep, about 1–2 hours after going to bed, the child suddenly wakes up and is inconsolable. This lasts some 10–20 minutes and then child "wakes up" looks confused, rolls over, and sleeps again.

Childhood

Daydreaming

This episode can appear very similar to an absence seizure, but the latter will occur at home during activity as well as at school. Classical absences, as part of idiopathic generalized epilepsy (see p. 589), can be elicited on

EEG (taken during normal and sleep-deprived state) in over 95% of cases. They are short, associated with abrupt psychomotor arrest, and abrupt resumption of activity, speech, and thought. Absences as part of a partial-seizure disorder will only rarely occur without some other suggestive feature such as an automatism, abnormal movement, or postictal state.

Syncope
Also known as fainting, syncope occurs from age 9 months onward. There may well be a history of precipitating events (e.g., fright, head bang, sudden standing, hair brushing). Often the child has an aura of loss of vision, tingling, and auditory phenomena. Then loss of consciousness and posture change ensue; the child falls over if standing.

Not all syncopal events result in a loss of tone. In some cases the fall is accompanied by increased tone. Myoclonic jerks or even a generalized tonic–clonic seizure may follow.

Useful tools in diagnosis include a history of a precipitant, jerking less than a minute, and the movements not being rhythmic. If in doubt, assume that it is syncope until there is evidence to the contrary.

Caution. If there is a history of sudden death in the family, or a history of syncope induced by sudden physical stress such as exercise or fright, long QT syndrome should be investigated (see Chapter 8, p. 290).

Psychologically determined paroxysmal events (PDPE)
PDPE is a less pejorative term to describe episodes of psychological origin that used to be described as hysteria and more recently as pseudo-seizures or malingering, factitious, or conversion disorders. The episodes are a psychological phenomenon, although identifying or looking for the psychological causes at the time of diagnosis can be misleading or even counterproductive (see Box 14.1). There is no single event separating these events from epilepsy. Rarely, some children may even have both.

Box 14.1 Features suggestive but not diagnostic of psychologically determined paroxysmal events

- Events triggered by specific situations
- Events with convulsive movements that are not explained anatomically, e.g., left arm jerking, then lull followed by right leg
- Thrashing movements that wax and wane, and pelvic thrusting
- Eyes open during the episode
- Slumping to the floor in a dramatic manner, often via a person or object to break the fall and prevent injury
- Violence, rather than violent movements
- Gain
- Prolonged generalized movements with rapid return to normal

These features are not diagnostic; there is no *never* or *always*. In particular, young people can injure themselves and pass urine in PDPE. These events are often erroneously reported as diagnostic features of genuine seizures.

Nonepileptic paroxysmal episodes: general management

Assessment

History

Most paroxysmal episodes can be classified with a careful history. No episode can be safely classified, even after EEG and MRI, if an adequate history has not been taken. You will need details of the following:

- *First episode*: When, where, what happened and the child's responsiveness, how long, and recovery; talk to the witness
- *Subsequent episodes*: Situation, precipitants, duration, frequency
- Full medical history, family history, developmental and psychosocial history

Video

If you are unsure about the diagnosis, ask the parents to videotape the event. Do not treat the patient until the diagnosis is confirmed.

Caution. Even when the diagnosis is likely to be a nonepileptic disorder, until this is confirmed, the parents should be advised on how to manage a genuine seizure. The child should avoid specific dangers:
- Injury from fall
- Proximity to swimming water without an identified lifeguard
- Unprotected heat
- Moving objects and machinery

Management

Infantile disorders

- Reassure the caregivers.

Syncopal episodes and jerks

- Allay parents' concerns over the diagnosis.

Psychologically determined paroxysmal events

PDPE can be difficult to treat, but these patients do respond to well-organized management. The principal areas include the following:
- Unambivalent diagnosis explained to both the parent and the child or young person
- Stabilization phase when the family develops understanding
- Strengthen coping abilities and remove secondary gain from the behavior.
- Psychological support is essential. Some families will feel very threatened when the possibility is raised of looking at psychological issues that may have triggered these events in the child.

Seizures and childhood epilepsies

One percent of children will have had one seizure, not associated with fever, by the age of 14 years. Most of these seizures will be generalized tonic–clonic episodes.

Forms of epilepsy

The two main forms of seizures can be categorized as generalized or focal.

Generalized

Generalized seizures can have the following qualities:

- *Myoclonic*: Shock-like movement of one or several parts of the body, or generalized
- *Tonic*: Sustained contraction and stiffness
- *Clonic*: Rhythmic jerking of one limb, one side, or all of the body (contrast this with description of psychologically determined clinical events)
- *Tonic–clonic*: A combination of the above forms
- *Absence*: These are episodes of abrupt psychomotor arrest lasting 5–15 seconds in younger children, but can be longer in the older child. They can be associated with retropulsion of the head, upward deviation of eyes, and eyelid or perioral myoclonia. (Facial myoclonia can be asymmetrical and give the impression of a "partial" seizure.)

Focal

These seizures start in one area of the brain and then may spread and, ultimately, generalize. If the latter part of the event is witnessed, it may be described incorrectly as being primarily generalized. The semiology depends on the locality of the initial electrical activity. "Typical" seizure semiology includes the following:

- *Occipital*: Multicolored bright lights spreading from one area of homonymous visual fields
- *Centroparietal*: Sensorimotor phenomena spreading from one limb and marching up one side of the body
- *Temporal*: Feelings of gastric discomfort, strangeness, anxiety, memory disturbances (e.g., familiarity, déjà vu), automatisms (such as nose rubbing), and contralateral clonic or dystonic movements
- *Frontal*: Dystonic posturing, and strange guttural noises

Status epilepticus

Status epilepticus (SE) can be convulsive with tonic/clonic movements. Alternatively, it can be nonconvulsive with impairment of consciousness, and often subtle twitching.

Technically, SE is a seizure lasting for more than 30 minutes, or repeated seizures lasting more than 30 minutes without recovery of consciousness in between. Practically, though, the treatment algorithm can be used once a convulsive seizure has lasted longer than 5 minutes (see p. 95).

Seizures: management

First unprovoked seizure

- *History*: A full personal, social, and family history should be obtained.
- *Examination*: Perform a thorough examination, looking for markers of neurological diseases or insults.
- *Electroencephalography (EEG)*: There is debate over whether an EEG should be obtained. The current opinion is that, in most children, it is unlikely to influence drug management. In fact, few specialists would start therapy at this point, regardless of what the EEG showed. With expert neurophysiology a more accurate prognosis may be given, which in turn may influence therapy.
- *Imaging*: An MRI is not indicated after a single seizure alone. However, if there are some abnormalities found on physical examination, MRI is very important to obtain, to exclude a space-occupying lesion or congenital abnormality.

Febrile seizures

Febrile seizures can occur in infants or small children. Most last a minute or two, but can be just a few seconds. Others last for more than 15 minutes. Typically these patients have no prior neurological disease and no focal deficits on examination. Here are some key facts about febrile seizures (see also Box 14.2).

- They occur in up to 4% of all children, generally between the ages of 6 months and 6 years (although it is unusual to have one's first episode at >4 years).
- These children often have a temperature >39°C.
- The seizure tends to occur during the first day of fever.
- Children prone to febrile seizures are not considered to have epilepsy.
- Recurrence risk of febrile seizures is 35% during childhood, 25% during the next 12 months.
- The vast majority of febrile seizures are harmless.
- 95%–98% of children who have experienced febrile seizures do not go on to develop epilepsy.
- Children who have febrile seizures that are lengthy, affect only part of the body, or recur within 24 hours or who have neurological abnormalities have a higher incidence of subsequent epilepsy.

Classification

- *Simple febrile seizures* (typical): Generalized tonic–clonic activity lasting less than 15 minutes with associated fever
- *Complex febrile seizures* (atypical): These occur in up to 15% of cases and are characterized by focal seizure activity, a prolonged seizure longer than 15 minutes, or multiple seizures within a day.

Box 14.2 Management of febrile seizure

Safety
- Move any danger away from the child and consider their privacy.
- Place the child on a protected surface on their side.
- It is good practice to note the length of the seizure.

Assistance
- The family should call for help if unfamiliar with febrile seizures.
- Then call the ambulance.

Treatment
- If the seizure lasts longer than 10 minutes, the child should be treated for status epilepticus.
- Once the seizure has ended, the child should be assessed for the source of the fever and investigated and treated appropriately.
- Consider admission and observation, especially if this is the first episode.

Meningitis?
- Consider meningitis if the child shows symptoms of stiff neck, extreme lethargy more than 4 hours post-seizure, or abundant vomiting, or is under 12 months old.
- If there is concern, perform a lumbar puncture. If the child has a focal neurological deficit or prolonged postictal lethargy, a head CT scan should be obtained before performing the lumbar puncture.

Seizure prevention and home care
- There is poor evidence to support interventions to prevent febrile seizures.
- Parents should give standard antipyretics early in any febrile illness.
- Parents should get expert advice if a previous seizure lasted longer than 10 minutes.

Epilepsies: neonatal

Neonatal seizures are rarely part of a benign epilepsy syndrome (see also pp. 206). Rather:

- They are more commonly a symptom of underlying, severe cerebral dysfunction.
- Seizures are never generalized tonic–clonic seizures, because the brain has not matured enough to produce synchronous epileptic activity.

Management

- *History*: Is there a family history of similar convulsions with benign prognosis? Take a history for cerebral insults such as hypoxia–ischemia. Is there a relevant family history, including consanguinity?
- *Examination*: Look for neurocutaneous stigmata and dysmorphic features.
- *Blood investigations*: Full blood count; blood glucose; serum electrolytes, calcium, and phosphate
- *Lumbar puncture*: Cerebrospinal fluid (CSF) glucose, red blood cell (RBC) and white cell count (WCC); CSF microscopy and bacterial culture; CSF lactate and glycine; CSF polymerase chain reaction (PCR) for herpes simplex virus (HSV)
- *Electroencephalography (EEG)* to determine localization and pattern of epileptiform discharges, and to determine if subclinical electrographic seizures are present. Continuous EEG monitoring should be used if clinical seizures are not easily controlled with moderate doses of phenobarbital.

Epileptic encephalopathy: If no cause is evident, consider the investigations for epileptic encephalopathy (see Box 14.3). Follow advice of the neurologist and biochemical geneticist for further investigation or management of relevant results.

Drug treatment

- *Phenobarbital*: Treat by loading with 20 mg/kg IV. Continue on 6 mg/kg once daily for at least 2 weeks. If the infant does not respond to the initial loading dose, additional 5–10 mg/kg IV loading doses may be administered up to a maximum cumulative dose of 45 mg/kg. Follow serum phenobarbital levels (maximum 45 µm/ml).
- *Fosphenytoin*: If the infant is unresponsive to phenobarbital, continue treatment by loading with fosphenytoin 20 mg/kg (phenytoin equivalent) IV.
- *Pyridoxine*: If the infant is unresponsive to phenobarbital and fosphenytoin, treat with pyridoxine, 15–18 mg/kg/day. If possible, wait for 48 hours to assess the effect.
- *Continuous midazolam infusion*: If the pyridoxine has proved ineffective, treat by loading with 0.2–0.5 mg/kg midazolam IV, followed by a continuous infusion of IV midazolam at 1 µg/kg/min increasing as seizures continue up to a maximum of 4 µg/kg/min.

Box 14.3 Investigations for epileptic encephalopathy

Examinations
- *Wood's light*: Tuberous sclerosis
- *Ophthalmology*: Retinitis pigmentosa, phakomata, and other ophthalmological markers of neurological disorders
- *Magnetic resonance imaging*: Neuronal migration defects, structural abnormalities

Blood: routine
- *Urea and electrolytes, urate*: Renal and purine disorders
- *Liver function tests*: Liver dysfunction
- *Ammonia*: Urea cycle defects and liver failure
- *Lactate*: Mitochondrial disease
- *Thyroid function tests*: Thyroid disease
- *Chromosomes*: Major structural chromosomal abnormalities

Blood: special biochemistry
- *Plasma amino acid (including glycine and serine) and total homocysteine*: Amino acidemias and defects in homocysteine remethylation
- *Transferrin isoelectric focusing*: Congenital defects of glycosylation
- *Biotinidase*: Biotinidase deficiency
- *Acyl-carnitine profile*: Mitochondrial fatty acid β-oxidation defects
- *Pipecolic acid*: Pyridoxine-dependent seizures

Blood and cerebrospinal fluid (CSF)
- *Plasma glucose matched with CSF glucose*: Glucose carrier transport deficiency
- *CSF lactate*: Mitochondrial cytopathies
- *CSF glycine and serine*: Nonketotic hyperglycinemia and 3-phosphoglycerate dehydrogenase deficiency

Urine
- *Amino and organic acids*: Amino and organic acidurias, sulfite oxidase deficiency, and molybdenum cofactor deficiency
- *Purine and pyrimidine*: Disorders of purine and pyrimidine metabolism

Epilepsies: infantile

Infantile epilepsies are challenging and expert advice should be sought.

Benign myoclonic epilepsy of infancy

This form of epilepsy requires no further investigation or therapy provided that what is observed meets the following criteria:
- Myoclonic seizures
- No other seizure type
- Normal interictal EEG
- Normal development

West's syndrome

The diagnosis of this condition is based on a classic triad:
- Infantile spasms: Short tonic contraction of trunk with upward elevation of arms which may be confused with gastroesophageal reflux or colic
- Developmental delay or regression
- Hypsarrhythmia on the EEG

Often children have only some of these, or the EEG is reported as being chaotic, with high voltage sharp and slow waves, but not "classical hypsarrhythmia."

Investigations

Take a thorough history and examination and make sure that you have excluded tuberous sclerosis (TS). Then, use the series of investigations in Box 14.3 for epileptic encephalopathy.

Treatment

- Treatment for infantile spasms should be directed by a child neurologist. Treatment protocols vary by center and are dependent, in part, on the availability of therapeutic agents.
- Hormonal treatments include courses of either prednisolone or ACTH (synthetic or gel). Treatment may last from 1 to several weeks and include titration followed by tapering of the medication, depending on clinical response. Patients must be followed carefully for the development of corticosteroid adverse effects, including increased risk of infection, hypertension, hyperglycemia, and GI bleeding.
- Anticonvulsants treatments include zonisamide, topiramate, clonazepam, and vigabatrin (not currently FDA approved, but available in certain centers, particularly for treatment of infantile spasms secondary to tuberous sclerosis).

Severe myoclonic epilepsy of infancy

This is severe, progressive epilepsy that occurs from the first year onward and includes
- Prolonged (>1-hour) febrile and shorter afebrile seizures
- Focal seizures
- Atypical absences
- Segmental myoclonus

Investigations
- *EEG* may be normal initially, but may develop photosensitivity (i.e., within 12 months in 50% of cases) and generalized discharges once the different seizures are frequent.
- *Genetics*: 70% of patients have a mutation in the *SCN1a* gene. However, if this test is unavailable or the clinical picture is atypical, use the screening investigations for epileptic encephalopathy (p. 589)

Treatment
The treatment should follow a sequence, adding anticonvulsants if there is no response. Lamotrigine should be avoided in this form of epilepsy. The sequence is as follows:
- Start with divalproex sodium (but only after inborn errors of metabolism and mitochondrial disorders have been thoroughly investigated)
- Add levetiracetam
- Add clobazam (not FDA approved, but available in certain centers)
- Consider stiripentol if seizures are resistant to therapy (needs expert supervision; not FDA approved, but available in certain centers)

Myoclonic astatic epilepsy

This is a condition with
- Myoclonic astatic seizures
- Myoclonic jerks
- Generalized tonic–clonic seizures

The EEG demonstrates predominantly generalized discharges once seizures are established. Seek advice about further investigation and treat in the same manner as for idiopathic generalized epilepsy (p. 590). Seizures in this condition are likely to be unresponsive, so consider using the ketogenic diet early in refractory cases.

Lennox–Gastaut syndrome

This is a condition with
- Tonic seizures with trunk flexion (often evolving out of infantile spasms)
- Atonic seizures, myoclonic jerks, atypical absences

Invariably there is developmental delay once the seizures are established. This condition rarely responds to drugs. Seek advice about further investigation and treat in the same manner as for idiopathic generalized epilepsy (p. 590). Treat with sodium valproate, and add lamotrigine.

Epilepsies: mid to late childhood (1)

Idiopathic generalized epilepsies

The diagnosis of epilepsy rests on the history. The EEG helps with classi-fication. It should be remembered that generalized discharges on EEG (particular with photic stimulation) may occur in children without seizures. There is no need for MRI or blood tests after the first episode. Seizures include combinations of the following:

- Typical absences
- Myoclonus
- Tonic seizures and generalized tonic–clonic seizures
- Myoclonic jerks

In these patients more than 80% of standard EEG recordings and 95% of sleep-deprived EEG recordings will show generalized discharges.

Myoclonic absence epilepsy

- Typical absences with short, symmetrical jerks of mainly the upper limbs with abduction and elevation
- Early onset: <5 years
- EEG demonstrates generalized discharges of three cycles/second spike and wave—that is, not well formed—and may also have short bursts of polyspike discharges.
- This form has poor prognosis and can deteriorate into epileptic encepha-lopathy requiring treatment with the ketogenic diet.

Childhood absence epilepsy

- Previously known as *"petit mal"*
- Typical absences only
- Present during the first decade
- Patients rarely develop generalized tonic–clonic seizures.
- Absences can be associated with mild myoclonus.
- EEG demonstrates regular bursts of three cycles/second spike and wave.

Juvenile absence epilepsy

- Onset toward the start of the first and during the second decade
- All patients have absences.
- Up to 30% have myoclonic jerks.
- The majority develop generalized tonic–clonic seizures during the second decade if untreated.
- EEG: Discharges are more fragmented and irregular than in childhood absence epilepsy, with more bursts of polyspike.
- Prognosis is guarded, even after many years of being seizure-free as an adult; relapse is common.

Juvenile myoclonic epilepsy
- Onset is in the second decade.
- Invariable myoclonic jerks are classically within the first hour of wakening.
- There is a high risk of generalized tonic–clonic seizures. These are common and up to 86% of adolescent girls will have further generalized tonic–clonic seizures if they withdraw medication completely.
- EEG may have absences and photosensitivity; discharges are more fragmented and irregular than in juvenile absence epilepsy, with bursts of polyspike.

Treatment of idiopathic generalized epilepsies

The evidence is contradictory, but the general clinical consensus is as follows:

- *First-line*: For childhood absence epilepsy, ethosuximide is the first-line therapy. For other conditions, divalproex sodium is the first-line therapy except in girls over age 9 years, when lamotrigine should be used because of the endocrine profile and appetite stimulation of divalproex sodium.
- *Second-line*: Lamotrigine is the next choice, but it needs to be introduced more slowly when divalproex sodium is being used concurrently. In girls older than 9 years, divalproex sodium is used as the second-line drug after appropriate counseling.
- *Third-line*: There is no consensus. Some clinicians advocate using a benzodiazepine and suggest clonazepam as being the most effective. However, it is extremely difficult to withdraw if it is used in moderate to high dosage.

Epilepsies: mid to late childhood (2)

Idiopathic focal epilepsies

Benign childhood epilepsy with centrotemporal spikes

The classic presentation of this condition is as follows:

- Predominantly nocturnal sensorimotor seizures
- Onset in one side of the face or a hand, then spreading down one side and may generalize
- EEG may be relatively normal while patient is awake.
- EEG in slow-wave sleep or drowsiness will develop frequent centrotemporal spike-and-wave discharges with an easily recognizable shape and distribution.

Most children with this condition have infrequent, short seizures, and the decision of whether or not to treat it is made after discussion with the parents and child. Some clinicians feel strongly that therapy should be the same as for idiopathic generalized epilepsy, but others will consider using carbamazepine.

Benign childhood occipital seizure syndrome (Panayiotopoulos syndrome)

- Young children (age 1–7 years)
- Bizarre seizures: Prolonged (<30 minutes), stereotyped episodes of encephalopathy often associated with ictal vomiting, headache, and eye deviation
- Often misdiagnosed
- Heterogeneous EEG abnormalities
- Good prognosis
- Treatment is rarely indicated.

Landau–Kleffner syndrome (LKS) and electrical status in slow-wave sleep

This condition is considered an extreme variant of idiopathic focal epilepsy. These severe epilepsies are marked by

- Intellectual regression: these children have deteriorating cognition and behavior with relatively few seizures.
- LKS is marked by striking language impairment—an epileptic aphasia.
- EEG may show nonspecific abnormalities in the waking state, but once the patient is drowsy or in slow-wave sleep, the EEG develops electrical status.

This condition is difficult to treat and normally refractory to first-line drugs. Steroids are advocated and have been shown to be of temporary benefit; they may even improve long-term outcome. Children with LKS should be evaluated and managed through a pediatric epilepsy center.

Epilepsies: mid to late childhood (3)

Focal epilepsies

These epilepsies are symptomatic of a focal area of dysfunction, but the electrical discharges may generalize (i.e., secondary generalization).

- While the electrical discharges are focal, consciousness may be maintained. (Previously they were known as simple partial seizures.)
- When the discharges become more widespread, consciousness will be impaired or lost. (Previously these were known as complex partial seizures.)
- They all may develop into a secondarily generalized seizure. At that point it is not possible to classify them if the onset has not been witnessed.
- Their expression will depend on the principally affected area of the brain.

Frontal lobe epilepsies

These children tend to have short but frequent seizures, particularly arising out of sleep. Seizures are often associated with asymmetric dystonic posturing. Recovery can be quick, and they may be difficult to assess on the EEG.

Temporal lobe epilepsies

The seizures affect memory and emotion and have associated disturbances such as "déjà vu," fear, abdominal discomfort, and automatisms.

Occipital lobe epilepsies

These episodes are associated with the perception of simple, multicolored blobs of light in one side of a visual field. They often produce headache.

Management of focal epilepsies

Investigation

MRI is always indicated. While children rarely have malignant brain tumors, they can have dysplasias, gliosis, and benign tumors. The temporal lobe may show hippocampal sclerosis (mesial temporal sclerosis).

Treatment

- *First-line*: Carbamazepine is generally recommended.
- *Second-line*: Therapy is widely debated. There are few good studies comparing antiepileptic drugs against each other. However, divalproex sodium is a logical choice among the older anticonvulsants (but it should not be used in girls over 9 years of age). Of the newer anticonvulsants, lamotrigine, topiramate, and levetiracetam could be used, but licensing conditions should be noted.

Macrocephaly and microcephaly

Macrocephaly

Macrocephaly is defined as a head circumference above the 99.6th centile. Most of these children will have a benign and familial cause for this condition. However, hydrocephalus and degenerative disorders need to be considered.

History
- Take a full history, including developmental progression.
- Are there any features of autism or degenerative disorders?
- Are there signs of raised intracranial pressure?

Examination
- Perform a thorough examination.
- Plot occipitofrontal circumference (OFC) on a growth chart along with previous measurements.
- Look at the skin for signs of neurofibromatosis.

Findings and investigation
- *Abnormal*: If there are any abnormalities these will need further investigation.
- *Normal*: If the examination is normal, try and compare the child's head circumference with parental head circumferences. If they are all large, then the likely diagnosis is familial macrocephaly. If the parents' head circumferences are normal, then the child's condition is still probably benign, but it would be appropriate to follow measurements for the next 12 months. If there is further crossing of percentiles perform a CT scan.

Some children, boys more than girls, present with macrocephaly, mild developmental delay, and mild hypotonia. If there is nothing else in the history and examination, then manage as above. They will, however, need to be investigated for developmental delay (p. 644).

Microcephaly

Microcephaly is defined as a head circumference below the 0.4th centile. It is associated with a small brain. Most of these children will have developmental and neurological abnormalities (see also p. 644).

History
- Take a full history, including developmental progression and infection during pregnancy.
- Was newborn screening done? (phenylketonuria [PKU], hypothyroidism, etc.)

Examination
- Perform a thorough examination.
- Plot OFC on a growth chart along with previous measurements.
- Look for features of craniosynostosis.

Investigation
- Repeat newborn screening
- MRI scan
- Obtain results for karyotype, plasma lactate, and amino acids, and urine organic acids. Consider an evaluation for TORCH infections, including a full ophthalmologic assessment.

Management
- *Genetic advice*: An opinion is needed on whether you have the diagnosis. There may be a risk of up to 25% (autosomal recessive microcephaly) if no cause is found.

Hydrocephalus

Hydrocephalus may be present irrespective of whether there is obstruction to CSF flow (see also p. 198). The causes are as follows:
- *Obstructive (noncommunicating)*: Aqueductal stenosis, posterior fossa developmental anomalies, and tumors
- *Communicating*: Secondary to previous meningitis, subarachnoid hemorrhage, intraventricular hemorrhage

Clinical features
- *History*: Older children may present with a history of headache and vomiting; babies present usually because there is concern about head growth (i.e., crossing percentiles) and delay in development.
- *Examination*: Plot OFC on a growth chart along with previous measurements. Look for macrocephaly or bulging fontanelle in those with open sutures, "sunsetting" of the eyes, papilledema, hyperreflexia, spasticity, and poor head control.
- *Diagnosis*: Order cranial imaging, looking for enlarged ventricles. Imaging may also reveal associated congenital abnormalities such as Arnold–Chiari or Dandy–Walker malformations.

Treatment
- *Neurosurgical referral* for placement of ventricular shunt system or other surgery
- *Children with shunt systems* in place are at risk of shunt blockage, infection (e.g., ventriculitis), and subdural hematoma. Acute changes in behavior, new-onset headache, or persistent fever will need to be assessed with these problems in mind. Again, referral to the neurosurgical team for imaging and CSF sampling will need to be carried out.

Headache

Children with headache are commonly evaluated by general pediatricians and other primary-care providers.
- Over 90% of patients will have chronic childhood headache.
- Many will have migraine.
- Malignant brain tumors obstructing CSF flow, causing hydrocephalus and consequent headache, are less common. These are almost always associated with focal signs on examination or a suggestive history.

Chronic headache

This form of headache is
- Regular
- Often frontal
- Not associated with vomiting, paraesthesia, visual disturbance, or abnormality on examination (including BP)

History

The headache may be reported to be severe enough to take time off from school, but have few objective signs of pain. A full history is important, not only to exclude migraine and symptoms of raised ICP (see below), but also to elucidate stresses that may be causing the headache, or gains the child may have from the behavior.

Treatment

- Reassure the family that, with a thorough history and examination, migraine and tumors can be excluded.
- It is inappropriate to perform either a CT or MRI scan.

Sympathize with the family over the problem and suggest analgesia, although at best it is likely to make no difference. Therefore, dosage and number of drugs should be reduced to the minimum acceptable. Encourage the child or young person to continue doing all the normal activities for somebody of their age: "I can't take away the headache, but the more normal things you do and the fewer drugs you take, the less you will notice the pain". Regular aerobic exercise and appropriate sleep hygiene need to be emphasized.

Raised intracranial pressure

This is a potent cause of headache and will be associated with either or both of the following:
- *Abnormal examination*: In particular heel–toe walking, finger–nose co-ordination, eye movements and fundi (i.e., papilledema)
- *Severe short history*: Vomiting, morning headache, visual disturbance

Clinically, the main concern is a mass obstructing CSF flow, particularly a malignant posterior fossa tumor. However, the intracranial pressure can be raised without abnormality evident on a CT scan. In some of these children there may be thrombosis of a cerebral sinus. A subgroup has raised pressure of unknown cause, benign intracranial hypertension. There is no indication for further imaging unless there is an abnormal examination or severe short history as described above.

Benign intracranial hypertension (BIH)

BIH, or pseudotumor cerebri, may occur at any age in childhood, although typically it is associated with obesity, female gender, and adolescence. The causes are as follows:

- *Drugs*: Steroid withdrawal, vitamin A, thyroid replacement, oral contraceptive pills, phenothiazine
- *Systemic disease*: Iron deficiency, Guillain–Barré syndrome, systemic lupus erythematosus (SLE)
- *Endocrine changes*: Adrenal failure, hyperthyroidism, hypoparathyroidism, menarche, pregnancy, obesity
- Head injury

History

- *Infants*: Irritability and vomiting
- *Children*: Headache that worsens with coughing or bending over, blurred or double vision, tinnitus, vomiting

Examination and investigation

- *General*: Check blood pressure
- *Neurology*: There may be ataxia.
- *Eyes*: Papilledema, scotoma on visual-field testing
- *Imaging*: Normal
- *Lumbar puncture*: Raised intracranial pressure (>20 cm CSF) normal CSF cell count, protein, and glucose

Management

- Weight loss in the obese
- Try and remove the causal medication.
- Diuretics to reduce CSF formation (e.g., acetazolamide, frusemide)
- Steroids may be effective but can cause rebound problems when withdrawn.
- Serial lumbar punctures or surgical intervention
- Monitoring of eyes and visual fields is essential. Most patients without visual deficit do well, but some patients with eye problems may deteriorate.

Headache: migraine

Up to 10% of children may have migraine headache. These are debilitating episodes; the criteria are listed in Box 14.4. If they do not occur frequently (more than 4 times per month, for more than 3 months), the diagnosis is unlikely. If the headache occurs daily the term *chronic headache* should be used and managed as described in the Headache section.

Treatment

- *Exclude triggers* such as diet, dehydration, overtiredness, and stress.
- *Ibuprofen* should be tried initially, at the onset of symptoms, to treat the headache.
- *Sumatriptan*: When administered early in the course of the headache, sumatriptan (or other triptan agents) may reduce the severity and duration of migraine. Licensing conditions for these agents should be noted.
- *Prochlorperazine or metoclopramide* may be used for the emergency department treatment of severe nausea associated with migraine.
- *Prophylaxis*: If the migraine is frequent enough to disrupt schooling or social activity, consider prophylaxis. The evidence base for different therapies is poor. Initially, try a 3-month trial of propranolol. Antidepressants such as amitriptyline have also been used.

Box 14.4 Diagnostic criteria for pediatric migraine

Migraine without aura

A. At least five attacks fulfilling B–D
B. Headache attack lasting 4–72 hours
C. Headache has at least *two of the following*:
- Unilateral location
- Pulsating quality
- Moderate to severe intensity
- Aggravation by routine physical activity
D. During headache, at least *one of the following*:
- Nausea and/or vomiting
- Photophobia and/or phonophobia
E. Not attributed to another disorder

Migraine with aura

A. Idiopathic recurring disorder manifesting in attacks of reversible focal, neurological symptoms (the aura) that usually develop gradually and last for less than 60 minutes, then usually followed by headache with the features of migraine without aura
B. At least *two attacks fulfilling C and D*
C. At least two *of the following*:
- One or more fully reversible aura symptoms indicating focal cortical and/or brainstem dysfunction
- At least one aura developing gradually over more than 5 minutes, or two or more symptoms occurring in succession
- No aura lasting more than 60 minutes
D. Headache follows in less than 60 minutes
E. Not attributed to another disorder

Neuromuscular disorders

See also the floppy infant (p. 208). In children with neuromuscular problems, first think about the anatomical site that is affected:

- Brain (p. 602)
- Spine (p. 608)
- Anterior horn cell (p. 608)
- Peripheral nerve (p. 609)
- Neuromuscular junction (p. 611)
- Muscle (p. 612)

Cerebral insult

Any brain insult may make a child unreactive and move less. In these children there may be obvious signs of cerebral dysfunction, such as encephalopathy. Facial movement and peripheral power are good if the child is able to follow commands. However, they may have low tone in the trunk, with relatively better tone at limb extremities. Reflexes should be present.

Spinal cord lesions

Spinal tumors and transverse myelitis should produce a horizontal level, beneath which there will be upper motor neuron signs or a sensory level, or both.

Anterior horn cell disorders

A disorder here produces flaccid, areflexic limbs, normally sparing the face.

Polio

- Now rare, but may still be seen following vaccination or in immigrants
- Long term, the limb becomes flaccid and wasted

Spinal muscular atrophies (see also p. 624)

Confirmation of these conditions includes fibrillation on electromyography and genetic homozygous deletion of the survival motor neuron gene.

- *Type 0 (neonatal form)* is very severe, often with arthrogryposis.
- *Type 1 (Werdnig–Hoffman)* is severe with onset in the first months of life. Typically these infants have severe hypotonia, a "frog-like posture," areflexia, and weakness that is present more in the legs than in the arms, but with preserved cognition and interaction ("bright eyes," facial movements). This type is invariably fatal by 2 years of age.
- *Type 2* has onset in the first years of life, with low tone, peripheral weakness, absent reflexes, and scoliosis.
- *Type 3* has adolescent onset, with progressive weakness and gait disturbance, loss of reflexes, and low tone.

Peripheral neuropathies

Charcot–Marie–Tooth disease (hereditary motor and sensory neuropathies)

This refers to a group of disorders with mainly autosomal dominant inheritance.

- The hallmark is progressive distal weakness, initially presenting in the lower limbs, with peroneal muscle weakness and atrophy.
- There is also clumsiness and loss of fine-motor control.
- Later, these patients develop sensory disturbances with pins and needles in a glove-and-stocking distribution.

The most common types are as follows:

- *Type 1* demonstrates reduced conduction velocities on nerve conduction studies due to demyelination.
- *Type 2* shows near-normal nerve conduction velocities, but decreased amplitude of action potentials due to axonal degeneration.
- *Type 3* has an onset much earlier and is sometimes called Dejerine–Sottas syndrome. It is noted by very slow motor nerve conduction velocities.

The diagnosis of these conditions is based on the clinical picture, nerve conduction studies, and molecular analysis of the MPZ or PMP22 genes and, less commonly, the GJB1 gene (X chromosome), among many others. Treatment is symptomatic with physiotherapy and orthoses to encourage joint mobility and maintain range of movement.

Neuropathy

Neuropathy may also occur in the following conditions:

- Leukodystrophies
- Porphyria
- Diabetes
- Uremia
- Hypothyroidism
- Vitamin deficiencies (B_1, B_6, B_{12}, and E)
- Autoimmune disorders such as SLE
- Acutely, as part of the Guillain–Barré syndrome

Guillain–Barré syndrome (GBS)

GBS is an acute, potentially fatal, demyelinating polyneuropathy. It often follows an intercurrent infection. Initially, there are motor signs that progress up the body. That is, first there is gait disturbance, which then progresses to involvement of the arms, and then respiratory and bulbar involvement occurs in severe cases. Children may complain of muscle pain, which can mask the weakness. Sensory involvement, generally later in the course of the illness, may occur.

Etiology
- Epstein–Barr virus, cytomegalovirus (CMV)
- Measles, mumps
- Enterovirus
- *Mycoplasma pneumoniae*
- *Borrelia burgdorferi*
- *Campylobacter*

Diagnosis
The differential diagnosis includes myasthenia gravis, polio, spinal cord compression/myelitis, and botulism. The main diagnostic features of GBS are the following:
- *Clinical picture*: Muscle weakness, with loss of reflexes in an ascending fashion
- *Nerve conduction studies* demonstrate characteristic features.
- *Cerebrospinal fluid* shows elevated protein in the absence of pleocytosis, but this does not occur at onset.
- *Variants*: Miller–Fisher variant includes bulbar cranial nerve involvement, ophthalmoplegia, ataxia, and areflexia.

Course
- *Onset*: Starts 1–2 weeks after an antecedent illness
- *Ascending weakness*: This initial deterioration normally lasts less than 2 weeks.
- *Plateau phase*: Symptoms are static, normally lasting for 1–2 weeks.
- *Recovery* should begin within 2–4 weeks, in a descending manner, although full recovery sometimes takes a number of months. The reflexes are last to recover.

Management
- Immediate admission for monitoring of respiratory status (use FVC; see Chapter 5, p. 60) and autonomic involvement. Dysautonomia leads to tachycardia, fluctuating blood pressure, and gastrointestinal disturbance.
- Early introduction of physiotherapy and occupational therapy to avoid joint contracture
- Control of pain
- Immunoglobulin: IV treatment (total dose 2 g/kg over 3–5 days) is normally used initially, with plasmapheresis reserved for refractory cases.

Neuromuscular junction: autoimmune myasthenia gravis

The hallmark of this condition is fluctuating, fatigable weakness. At onset, 50% of patients have ptosis, with eventually more than 80% developing it. The condition is caused by autoantibodies against the nicotinic acetylcholine (ACh) receptor, which blocks transmission at the neuromuscular junction. Normally the condition is insidious, but sometimes an acute onset of fluctuating weakness of the extraocular, facial, oropharyngeal, respiratory, and limb muscles may occur.

Diagnosis

- *Clinical picture*: Fatigability of power/reflexes, particularly upward gaze with eyelids and elevation
- *Response to a trial of edrophonium (Tensilon)*: Video recording is essential, as the response may be brief.
- *ACh-receptor antibodies* are present in more than 50% of cases.

Management

- Immediate assessment of respiratory status using bedside measurement of forced vital capacity (FVC)
- Immediate assessment of bulbar function, looking at swallowing
- *First-line*: Cholinesterase inhibitors such as pyridostigmine
- *Refractory cases*: Acute, severe cases may respond to plasmapheresis. Subsequent immunosuppression with steroids, azathioprine, cyclosporin, methotrexate, and thymectomy. Needs to be monitored by an expert

Muscular disorders

Duchenne muscular dystrophy (DMD)

The muscular dystrophies are a group of genetic disorders characterized by dystrophic change on muscle biopsy. The best known of these conditions is DMD (see also p. 1070). This condition classically presents within the first 4 years with either delayed motor milestones or loss of motor function and may also be associated with mild speech and cognitive deficits. DMD is an X-linked recessive condition that lies at the severe end of this spectrum of disorders. It is due to a molecular abnormality of muscle fiber structural protein dystrophin.

Examination

- Waddling, lordotic gait
- Calf hypertrophy
- Weakness in limb girdles (lower more than upper): Gowers' sign
- Sparing of the facial, extraocular, and bulbar muscles

Investigation

- Markedly raised creatine kinase
- Genetic analysis: This frequently does not differentiate between the milder Becker and more severe Duchenne MD

Management

Symptomatic care within a neuromuscular clinic is needed. Glucocorticoid treatment has been shown to slow progression of weakness in boys with DMD. Patients must also be followed by a cardiologist for evaluation and management of associated cardiomyopathy. While DMD is an X-linked disorder, a large number of cases are due to a spontaneous mutation of the dystrophin gene. Genetic counseling is essential.

Myotonic dystrophy (see also p. 1070)

This is an autosomal dominant disorder with expanded CTG trinucleotide repeats in the DMPK gene on chromosome 19 (and anticipation when transmitted from the mother).

Congenital form

Severe cases may present in the neonatal period and are almost always of maternal inheritance. Infants present with hypotonia, feeding difficulty, tent-shaped mouth, respiratory impairment, and clubfoot. Treatment is supportive, but the symptoms become less disruptive as the child grows.

Later-onset form

Children and adolescents present with myopathic face, distal weakness, and myotonia. Later complications include diabetes mellitus, cataracts, and cardiac involvement. The diagnosis will initially be made from the characteristic clinical picture. Confirmation can be made on DNA analysis. Electromyography demonstrates the characteristic myotonic discharges, but it is not needed for diagnosis. Treatment is supportive and includes physiotherapy and occupational therapy, particularly for the foot drop. In addition, these children need cardiac and visual assessment. Genetic counseling is important, since there are likely to be other affected family members.

Caution
There is a risk of malignant hyperthermia during general anesthesia.

Congenital myopathies

This is a group of disorders characterized by
- Muscle weakness
- Hypotonia
- Variable involvement of the facial, bulbar, and extraocular muscles

The congenital myopathies tend to be autosomal recessive and can be associated with arthrogryposis. These are diagnosed by the clinical picture, electromyography, and nerve conduction studies (to exclude the myasthenias). Muscle biopsy is used when the more common disorders (myotonic dystrophy, DMD, and spinal muscular atrophy) have been excluded by DNA analysis.

Cerebral palsy

- *Definition*: Cerebral palsy (CP) is a chronic disorder of movement and/or posture that presents early (i.e., before the age of 2 years) and continues throughout life (see also p. 628).
- *Causation*: CP is caused by static injury to the developing brain.
- *Associations*: Children with CP are at increased risk of impairments relating to vision, hearing, speech, learning, epilepsy, nutrition, and psychiatric disorders.
- *Clinical forms*: Most children will have a mixed disorder, but some can have pure components of spasticity, choreoathetosis, or ataxia.

Spastic cerebral palsy

This is the most common label, and children can be hemiplegic, diplegic, or quadriplegic. Monoplegic cerebral palsy is extremely rare. Spasticity is a stretch-related response characterized by a velocity-dependent, increased resistance to passive stretch. It is caused by disruption to the spinal reflex arc by the upper motor neuron. It can affect all the skeletal muscles and causes the following symptoms:

- Increased tone and reflexes
- Clasp-knife phenomenon on rapidly stretching tendons, often described as a "catch"
- In the leg, ankle plantar flexion and either valgus or varus deformity of the foot
- In the hip, flexion, limited adduction, and often internal rotation
- Wrist is flexed and pronated
- Elbow is flexed
- Shoulder is adducted
- Bulbar muscles may be spastic, producing dysphagia and dribbling.

Choreoathetosis

This condition presents as a four-limb disorder with greatly increased tone while awake and less so during the early stages of sleep. These patients do not have the stretch-related response and increased reflexes of pure spastic CP. However, there may be combinations of these features in mixed CP. As the child matures, he or she will often develop fixed reduction in joint range of movement; the signs will then be more difficult to distinguish from spastic CP.

Ataxic cerebral palsy

This form of CP is extremely rare and poorly understood. It is also known as the dysequilibrium syndrome. Children have a congenital ataxia, giving them a striking loss of balance in the early years (i.e., dysequilibrium). They often have a mild diplegia and are thought to be etiologically distinct from the other types of CP, in which hypoxia and ischemia may be causal factors in certain cases.

Investigation
- *Cerebral palsy*: This is a descriptive term of disability and not the cause.
- All children need investigation.
- *History*: The cause may be evident from a good history, in particular for prematurity and periods of hypoxic ischemia or perinatal infection.
- *Imaging (MRI)*: Scan of the brain, with particular reference to the pyramidal tracts in children with spasticity and the basal ganglia in others.

If there is nothing evident in the history, examination, or MRI, then further investigations are unlikely to yield an etiology. Unfortunately, many children will not have an etiology identified. When the presentation is not typical for CP, children will need expert assessment.

Management
Complex multidisciplinary input
The primary therapists are the child's parents, as they will provide at least 90% of the therapy to the child. In the early years, experts in speech, physiotherapy, and occupational therapy will support this treatment.

Posture and movement
Optimize function by improving symmetry, joint ranges, muscle length, and power. Treatments and support include stretching exercises, orthoses (e.g., ankle foot orthosis), wheelchair for mobility, sleeping and standing systems, and botulinum toxin (Botox) to the gastrocnemius muscle. Surgery is used as a last resort.
- *Communication* with speech therapy and aids
- *Independence* with a tailored educational program, aids, and supervision from occupational therapy
- *Cognition and learning support* with a tailored educational program
- *General medical*: Watch for seizures, constipation, malnutrition, and behavioral or psychiatric disturbance.
- *NOTE*: DOPA-responsive dystonia will very rarely present with an unexplained diplegia and normal MRI. These children will need a trial of DOPA/carbidopa (e.g., Sinemet) with a gradually increasing dose of up to 10 mg/kg/day of the DOPA component over 3 months. If there is no significant improvement, the child is unlikely to be DOPA responsive.

Neurocutaneous disorders

Tuberous sclerosis complex (TSC)

- TSC is an autosomal dominant inherited disorder affecting brain, skin, heart, kidney, eye, and lung (see also p. 1073).
- The disorder is associated with hamartomata affecting the above organs, although other neoplasms also occur.
- Two genes have been identified: *TSC1* and *TSC2*.

Diagnosis

The diagnosis is made when a child has either two major or one major and two minor criteria (see Box 14.5).

Box 14.5 Criteria for diagnosis of TSC

Major criteria
- Facial angiofibromas
- Ungual fibroma
- Hypomelanotic macules (>3)
- Shagreen patch
- Cortical tubers
- Subependymal (SE) nodules
- SE giant cell astrocytoma
- Retinal nodular hamartoma
- Cardiac rhabdomyomata
- Lymphangiomyomata
- Renal angiomyolipoma

Minor criteria
- Pits in dental enamel
- Rectal polyps
- Bone cysts
- Cerebral white matter "migration tracts"
- Gingival fibromas
- Nonrenal hamartoma
- Retinal achromic patch
- Confetti skin lesions
- Multiple renal cysts

Management

Treatment is symptomatic depending on the organ-specific effects of the hamartoma and neoplasms. All cases require expert assessment of the following:

- Recurrence risk in family members (genetic counseling)
- Symptomatic epilepsies, particularly if West syndrome (infantile spasms) occurs
- Cardiac, renal, pulmonary and ophthalmological hamartomata
- Cystic kidneys

Neurofibromatosis

There are two distinct autosomal dominant disorders, characterized by multiple benign tumors of the peripheral nerve sheath (see also p. 1072).

NF1: chromosome 17

The diagnosis is based on having at least two of the following:
- >6 café-au-lait macules: >5 mm in diameter before puberty; >15 mm in diameter after puberty
- Skin fold or axillary freckling
- Two or more neurofibromas or one plexiform neurofibroma
- Two or more Lisch nodules in iris
- Optic glioma
- Skeletal dysplasia
- Affected first-degree relative

The management of this condition is symptomatic and depends on the local effects of the neurofibroma. However, all cases require expert assessment of the following:
- Recurrence risk in family members (genetic counseling) and need assessment annually
- Neoplasia and optic gliomata
- Renal artery stenosis
- Skeletal dysplasia
- Cognitive performance

NF2: chromosome 22

The diagnosis is based on having one major criterion or two minor criteria:
- *Major criteria*: Unilateral vestibular schwannoma and first-degree relative with NF2; bilateral vestibular schwannomas
- *Minor criteria*: Meningioma, schwannoma, ependymoma, glioma, cataract

The management of NF2 is complex, as in many cases the tumors themselves do not need to be removed when identified, although they may become symptomatic over time.

Sturge–Weber syndrome

- Leptomeningeal angiomatosis associated with a unilateral port-wine nevus in the distribution of the first branch of the trigeminal nerve
- Children can have severe focal epilepsies, learning disability, hemiplegia, glaucoma, and transient stroke-like episodes and severe headaches.

Bell's palsy

- Acute paralysis of the muscles of facial expression; the child may be unable to close the eye on the affected side
- Normally unilateral, but may be bilateral lower motor neuron lesion
- Secondary to edema of the facial nerve as it passes through the temporal bone

Etiology

- Idiopathic
- Varicella, herpes simplex and other viruses
- *Borrelia burgdorferi* (Lyme disease), particularly if bilateral

Management

Examination

- Check whether other branches of the facial nerve are affected, e.g., hyperacusis
- Full systemic examination, in particular look for signs of leukemia and vasculitides
- Full neurological examination: Look for other motor and sensory signs and exclude an idiopathic Bell's palsy

Investigation

- MRI if presentation is atypical or other neurological signs are present
- Thorough ENT examination for middle ear or temporal bone pathology if condition does not resolve

Treatment

- *Steroids*: Evidence for the use of steroids is limited, but the general opinion is to use 2 mg/kg (maximum 60 mg) prednisolone, once daily for 5 days, if the symptoms are no more than 7 days old.
- *Acyclovir*: Recent evidence indicates that oral acyclovir is not useful.

Prognosis

Most children will either recover fully or recover to a good degree. When this does not occur, referral for facial nerve grafting is appropriate.

Stroke in childhood

Cerebrovascular stroke is rare in childhood, but it does cause significant morbidity. The cause can be ischemic, hemorrhagic, or venous in origin. The majority of cases will have a likely cause identified on history and examination; the main causes are
- Sickle cell disease
- Thrombophilia
- Congenital cardiac defects
- Cerebral infection
- Trauma (arterial dissection)

Management

Children with stroke will need initial attention to ABC and treatment of acute conditions such as meningitis before early transfer to a specialist unit.

Investigation

Once stable, all children will require brain imaging—preferably magnetic resonance imaging and angiography, rather than CT scan, although this will show the distribution of injury. Even with a known cause such as trauma, all children require screening for underlying thrombophilia, as these conditions may coexist. If there is no obvious cause, the investigations in Box 14.6 should be considered.

Treatment

After stabilization, treatment should be undertaken in a tertiary referral center.

Box 14.6 Investigation for stroke

Blood: hematology
- Full blood count, ESR
- Thrombophilia screen

Blood: biochemistry
- Electrolytes, magnesium
- Liver function tests
- CRP for inflammation
- Plasma lactate and cerebrospinal fluid lactate: Mitochondrial disorders
- Fasting glucose for diabetes
- Fasting lipid screen for hyperlipidemias
- Thyroid function tests for Hashimoto thyroiditis and encephalopathy
- Ammonia for urea cycle disorders
- Homocysteine (free and total): Methyltetrahydrofolate reductase (MTHFR) deficiency can also be picked up by common mutation analysis on the thrombophilia screen or by plasma homocysteine analysis on a plasma sample.
- Serum iron, total iron binding capacity, ferritin, red cell folate, and vitamin B_{12}: Iron deficiency and other nutritional disorders
- Plasma amino acids for amino acidurias
- Carnitine (acyl, free, and total): β-oxidation defects

Urine: biochemistry
- Urine organic and amino acids: Homocystinuria, MTHFR deficiency

Blood immunology and infection screen
- IgG, IgM, IgA for immunodeficiency
- Titers for infection screen of *Mycoplasma, Chlamydia, Helicobacter, Borrelia, Brucella*; viruses (echo, Coxsackie, Epstein–Barr, varicella, hepatitis B)
- ASO, anti-DNAase B for streptococcal disease
- ANA, ANCA, anticardiolipin, and antiphospholipid antibody: SLE and autoimmune disease

Imaging studies
- MRI and angiography for vascular disease
- Doppler angiography for carotid stenoses
- Echocardiogram for endocarditis and other cardiac disease

Abnormal movements

Ataxia

An abnormality in gait that is wide-based, staggering, and unsteady may have a number of causes:

- Poisoning
- Posterior fossa tumour
- Brain stem encephalitis
- Postinfectious or autoimmune: Acute cerebellar ataxia, Guillain–Barré syndrome, multiple sclerosis
- Trauma
- Vascular disorders
- Congenital malformations: Dandy–Walker
- Neurological: Olivopontocerebellar degeneration, ataxia–telangiectasia (AT), adrenoleukodystrophy, Friedreich's ataxia (FA)
- Conversion disorder

Clinical review

- Speech: Increased separation of syllables and varied volume—scanning speech
- Neurology: Sensory disturbance in proprioception, positive Romberg, nystagmus with eye movement
- Systemic: Immunodeficiency in AT, hypertrophic cardiomyopathy and diabetes in FA

Investigation

- Brain imaging
- Cerebral spinal fluid examination for suspected infectious or post-infectious disorders
- Molecular analysis for suspected genetic etiologies

Chorea

Jerk-like movements may involve the face, arms, or legs. In childhood the causes include the following:

- *Drugs*: Anticonvulsants, psychotropics, benzodiazepine withdrawal after intensive care
- *Systemic illness*: Sydenham's chorea, SLE, hyperthyroidism
- *Genetic*: Huntington's chorea, glutaric aciduria, ataxia telangiectasia, pantothenate kinase–associated neurodegeneration (PKAN, Hallervorden–Spatz), benign familial chorea
- *Other*: Pregnancy

Streptococcal infection

Sydenham's chorea is often associated with streptococcal infection.

- About 20% of rheumatic fever cases include chorea.
- *Treatment*: High-dose penicillin V 40 mg/kg/day PO divided tid for 10 days, then daily prophylaxis
- Benzodiazepines, phenothiazine, haloperidol, may control the movement
- Improvement may occur over weeks to months.

PANDAS

PANDAS (**P**ediatric **A**utoimmune **N**europsychiatric **D**isorder **A**ssociated with **S**treptococcus) has specific diagnostic criteria and is accompanied by behavioral problems, e.g., obsessive-compulsive disease and tics.

Conversion disorders

A high percentage of children older than 5 years of age presenting with rapidly progressing and bizarre neurological symptoms are eventually diagnosed with a conversion disorder. These children are more likely to be teenage girls. However, it is important that this tendency not prejudice your clinical assessment—major oversights and mistakes can be made. These children tend to be well and have signs that cannot be explained anatomically, e.g., paralyses, sensory disturbances, and visual phenomena.

Management

The initial diagnosis should be that of a genuine physical disorder until all assessments (medical, psychological, and social) are complete.

Examination

- Must be thorough: You may reveal inconsistent signs such as an inability to lift the leg off the bed but able to walk across the room.

Investigation

- Imaging: Brain imaging (MRI, CT) is at the physician's discretion, but the family is likely to become very distressed if a psychological diagnosis is given while there are outstanding investigations.

Treatment

- Support and treatment is covered in Chapter 15 (p. 660), treatment of psychologically dependent paroxysmal episodes.

Degenerative disorders

There are many disorders that can present with developmental regression—that is, "loss of skills." Developmental regression is always alarming and it requires intensive investigation.

Assessment

History
- Full developmental history: Try and exclude autism.
- Family and social history with particular emphasis on consanguinity

Examination
- All systems: Storage disorders often involve other systems besides the brain.
- Neurological examination: This must be thorough; look particularly for evidence of ataxia, myoclonus, dementia, dystonia, and pyramidal signs.

Investigations (see also p. 1058)
- MRI: This imaging modality will give the largest yield. Look particularly at the white matter for leukodystrophies and at the cerebral and cerebellar cortices for evidence of atrophy.
- Other laboratory investigations are outlined in Box 14.7.

Box 14.7 Investigations for developmental regression

Blood biochemistry
- *Urea and electrolytes*: Renal failure
- *Liver function tests*: Liver disease
- *Plasma glucose and matching cerebrospinal (CSF) glucose*: Glucose carrier transport (GLUT1) deficiency
- *Plasma lactate and matching CSF lactate*: Mitochondrial cytopathy
- *Ammonia*: Urea cycle defects
- *Thyroid function tests*: Thyroid disease
- *Urate*: Lesch–Nyhan disease
- *Plasma amino acids*: Amino acidopathies
- *Very long-chain fatty acids*: Peroxisomal disorders
- *Copper level*: Menkes disease
- *Ceruloplasmin*: Wilson disease

Special blood investigations
- *Vacuolated lymphocytes*: neuronal ceroid lipofuscinosis (Batten's disease) and other storage disorders
- *White blood cell lysosomal enzymes*: Leukodystrophies, gangliosidoses and other lysosomal storage disorders

Urine
- *Amino and organic acids*: Organic acidurias, MTHFR deficiency, sulfite oxidase deficiency
- *Urate, creatinine, purine, and pyrimidine* excretion over 24 hours: Lesch–Nyhan, purine/nucleotide phosphorylase deficiency
- *Hydroxybutyric acid*: Succinate semialdehyde dehydrogenase deficiency
- *Mucopolysaccharides*: Mucopolysaccharidoses

Tissue biopsies
- *Liver*: Alpers' disease
- *Skin* (sphingomyelin degradation): Niemann–Pick type C
- *Muscle*: Mitochondrial disease
- *Rectal*: Batten's disease

Eyes
- *Ophthalmology review*: Retinitis pigmentosa and ophthalmological markers of neurological disorders

Electrophysiology
- *Visual-evoked responses*: Batten's disease
- *Electroencephalography*: Specific electrographic patterns for Batten's disease, SSPE, and other degenerative disorders

Genetic testing
- Confirmatory genetic testing via DNA analysis is available for many of these conditions. Specific testing, if available, may be done in place of tissue biopsies or other studies. Consultation with a child neurologist or geneticist should be obtained early in the course of the child's evaluation.

Child and adolescent development and behavior

Definitions

Neither development nor behavior can be considered in isolation, as each one shapes the other and is influenced by environmental and psychosocial factors.
- *Development*: Manifestations of maturation of the nervous system
- *Behavior*: Manifestations of individual and interpersonal conduct

A *CSHCN* (**C**hild or youth with a **S**pecial **H**ealth **C**are **N**eed) is a child at risk of having a developmental, behavioral, or emotional condition requiring health and related services of a type or amount beyond that generally required by children (see Box 15.1).

Epidemiology of CSHCN

Nationwide, about 1 in 7 children and youth meets criteria for a CSHCN, and more than 1 in every 5 households has at least 1 CSHCN.

Box 15.1 Causes of special health-care needs

Medical
- Prenatal and perinatal factors
  - Maternal illness or infection
  - Intrauterine exposure (e.g., toxin, drug, alcohol)
  - Prematurity complications (e.g., periventricular leukomalacia, intraventricular hemorrhage)
  - Hypoxic ischemic encephalopathy
- Postnatal
  - Kernicterus
  - Metabolic disorder
  - Seizure disorder
  - Meningitis
  - Other chronic illness

Genetic
- Chromosomal abnormality

Environmental
- Trauma (social, emotional, physical)
- Malnutrition
- Neglect or abuse
- Toxic exposure
- Effect of parental education

Idiopathic

Evaluation

Regular sequential stages in growth and skills acquisition follow remarkably predictable patterns and rates, although there is a wide normal range (see Table 15.1). Such milestones are grouped according to streams: cognitive, speech and language, motor, and social/emotional.

The Developmental Quotient (DQ) establishes the age-equivalent at which a child is functioning along individual developmental streams at the time of testing in children under 3 years of age. The DQ is not a valid measure of intelligence, and fails to consider psychosocial or environmental influences. A DQ can identify likely areas of functional involvement and help direct appropriate remedial and preventive interventions.

DQ = (Developmental Age [months]/
Chronological Age [months]) x 100

Note that a "corrected age" is often used during the first 2 years of life for children born prematurely.
- DQ interpretations:
  - 85 and above (normal)
  - 71–84 (mild to moderate delays)
  - 70 and below (severe delay)

Developmental patterns

- *Delay*: A significant lag in one or more developmental streams, but the order of milestone acquisition within each stream is typical
- *Dissociation*: A difference between the developmental rates of two streams of development, with one significantly more delayed
- *Deviancy*: The acquisition of milestones within a stream is out of sequence.

Key points

- Children present with a wide range in quality and severity of signs and symptoms in developmental and behavioral patterns.
- Difficulty in one stream of development can affect acquisition of milestones in other streams. A child with fine-motor skills difficulties may not be able to adequately explore objects in his or her surroundings, which then limits the ability to "test" textures, weights, and gravity and stimulate development of other cognitive skills.
- Development is an ongoing process. Routine clinical surveillance and periodic screening of milestones can help suggest patterns and rates in the direction of growth. Individual milestones do not predict a "developmental age."
- Acquisition of milestones in motor control proceeds in a head-to-toe direction and a midline-to-peripheral direction.
- Motor control progresses in a predictable sequence from primitive, mass-movement reflex patterns to voluntary controlled movement.

Typical development and behavior

The *medical home* is a model of delivering primary care, based on partnerships between the child and family and provider, so that care is accessible, continuous, comprehensive, family-centered, coordinated, compassionate, and culturally effective.

Health supervision

Surveillance and screening are fundamental in monitoring development and behavior.

Surveillance

This consists of skilled observations during child health care in consultation with families, specialists, and other providers. It includes determining parents' concerns, a relevant developmental history, and skillful observation of the child by means of standard instruments. When a concern is raised during surveillance, then screening or more specialized evaluation is indicated. A concerning surveillance outcome is not diagnostic.

Instruments

- Bright Futures (www.brightfutures.org)
- Child development charts (see Fig. 15.1 for the first 18 months, and Fig. 15.2 for a child's first 5 years)
- Visual–motor problem-solving developmental assessment instruments
  - Goodenough–Harris Draw-a-Person test assesses nonverbal cognition, organization of concepts, and reproduction of visual image via motor skills.
  - Gesell Figures are used to assess the ability to draw increasingly complex shapes and provide information on attention and temperament.
  - Block play assesses cognition, language, fine and gross motor skills

Screening

Screening of developmental and behavioral status periodically and whenever surveillance raises a concern enhances the surveillance process by using brief, objective validated instruments to identify children and youth at increased developmental and behavioral outcome risk. "Let's wait and see" is seldom the appropriate response to red flags discovered during surveillance or screening or to parental concerns about their child's development or behavior.

Instruments

- Capute Scales (CAT/CLAMS) (www.brookespublishing.com)
- Denver-II Developmental Screening Test (see Fig. 15.3)
- Ages & Stages Questionnaire (www.brookespublishing.com): Screens 4–60 months across all developmental streams
- Pediatric Symptom Checklist: Screens for psychosocial problems. Available in picture form (see Fig. 15.4)

Developmental and/or behavioral problems

Children and youth for whom screening reveals increased risk for delayed, atypical, or suboptimal developmental, behavioral, or social outcomes require further professional evaluation. Formal evaluations may take place in public school districts or academic medical centers, and/or with private providers and are individualized on the basis of identified risk factors.

Through the medical home, outcomes of such evaluations are incorporated to identify developmental and behavioral variations, problems, and disorders in the context of medical and psychosocial influences. Medical-home staff also coordinate ongoing appropriate services for prevention, accommodation, and remediation.

Evaluation

- History (see Developmental evaluation, Components of medical and social history, p. 23)
- Review of systems (see Developmental evaluation, Review of systems, p. 30)
- Examination (see Developmental evaluation, Examination, p. 632)

Key points

- Persistence of primitive reflexes and failure of emergence of postural reflexes suggest an upper motor neuron abnormality.
- The environment in which a child is examined (e.g., inpatient, clinic, school setting, accompanying family members or other caregivers) will influence behavioral and developmental manifestations.
- Hearing and vision impairments are often overlooked and can irreversibly impact all streams of development. Be sure appropriate screening is routinely performed.
- Visual language development (e.g., using spontaneous reciprocal eye gaze) is delayed in intellectual disability and in autism, and can help distinguish from other causes of language disorders.

Age	Language	Fine Motor	Gross Motor	Self-Help	Social
Birth	Cries. / Makes small throaty sounds.	Looks at objects or faces.	Wiggles and kicks. / Thrusts arms and legs in play.	Alert-interested in sights and sounds.	Quiets when fed and comforted. / Makes eye contact.
1 mo.	Cries in a special way when hungry.	Follows moving objects with eyes.	Lifts head and chest when lying on stomach.		Social smile.
2 mos.	Makes sounds—ah, eh, ugh.	Holds objects put in hand.	Holds head steady when held sitting.	Reacts to sight of bottle or breast.	Recognizes mother.
3 mos.	Laughs out loud.	Holds up hand and looks at it.	Makes crawling movements.	Increases activity when shown toy.	Recognizes other familiar adults.
4 mos.	Squeals.	Puts toys or other objects in mouth.	Pivots around when lying on stomach.	Reaches for objects.	Interested in his or her image in mirror; smiles, playful.
5 mos.	Makes sounds like "Ah-goo."	Picks up objects with one hand.	Rolls over from back to stomach.	Comforts self with thumb or pacifier.	Reacts differently to strangers.
6 mos.	Responds to voices; turns head toward a voice.	Transfers objects from one hand to the other.	Rolls over from back to stomach.	Looks for object after it disappears from sight—for example, looks for toy after it falls off tray.	Reaches for familiar persons.
7 mos.	Babbles. / Responds to his/her name; turns and looks.	Holds two objects, one in each hand, at the same time.	Sits alone, steady.	Feeds self cracker or cookie.	Gets upset and cries if left alone.
8 mos.	Makes sounds like da, ga, ka, ma. / Makes sounds like da-da, ma-ma, ba-ba.	Uses two hands to pick up large objects.	Moves forward somehow while on stomach.	Picks up small cup with two hands.	Plays "peek-a-boo."

Age	Social	Self-help	Gross motor	Fine motor	Language/Cognitive
9 mos.		Resists having a toy taken away.	Crawls on hands and knees. Pulls self to standing position.		
10 mos.	Plays "patty-cake."	Picks up spoon by handle.	Walks around playpen or furniture while holding on.		Imitates sounds that you make.
11 mos.	Waves "Bye-bye."		Stands alone briefly.	Picks up small objects using precise thumb and finger grasp.	Understands phrases like "No No" and "All gone."
12 mos.		Helps a little when being dressed.		Puts small objects in cup or other container.	Says "Mama" or "Dada" for parent. Hands you a toy when asked.
13 mos.	Plays with other children.	Lifts cup to mouth and drinks.	Stands alone, steady.	Turns pages of books a few at a time.	Points to things.
14 mos.	Gives kisses or hugs. Imitates simple acts such as hugging or loving a doll.	Insists on feeding self.	Walks without help.	Builds tower of 2 or more blocks.	
15 mos.	Greets people with "Hi" or similar.	Feeds self with a spoon.	Climbs up on chairs or other furniture.	Marks with crayon or pencil.	
18 mos.	Wants a doll, teddy bear or blanket in bed with him/her. Sometimes says "No" when interfered with.	Eats with a fork.	Runs.	Scribbles with crayon or pencil.	Says 2 or more words besides Mama or Dada.
21 mos.			Kicks a ball forward. Good balance and coordination.	Builds tower of 4 or more blocks.	Uses at least ten words. Asks for a drink or food, using words or sounds.

Figure 15.1 Infant development chart—first 18 months. Reproduced with permission. Material is copyrighted, and available in English and Spanish for purchase from ChildDevelopmentReview.com. Parent questionnaires are also available, and can be used with the chart.

Age	SOCIAL	SELF-HELP	GROSS MOTOR	FINE MOTOR	LANGUAGE
5-0 yrs.	Shows leadership among children.	Goes to the toilet without help.	Swings on swing, pumping by self.	Prints first name (fourletters).	When asked, for example, "What is an orange?" answers, "A fruit."
4-6	Follows simple rules in board or card games.	Usually looks both ways before crossing street.	Skips or makes running "broad jumps."	Draws a person that has at least three parts - head, eyes, nose, mouth, etc.	Reads a few letters (five+).
					Prints a few letters or numbers.
4-0 yrs.	Protective toward younger children.	Buttons one or more buttons.	Hops around on one foot, without support.	Draws recognizable pictures.	Counts ten or more objects.
		Dresses and undresses without help, except for tying shoelaces.			Follows a series of three simple instructions in order.
3-6	Plays cooperatively with minimum conflict and supervision.	Washes face without help.	Hops on one foot, without support.	Cuts across paper with small scissors.	Talks in long, complex sentences (10 or more words).
	Gives directions to other children.		Rides around on tricycle, using pedals.	Draws or copies a complete circle.	Answers questions like, "What do you do with your eyes? ears?"
					Identifies at least four colors by name correctly.
3-0 yrs.	Plays games like tag, hide and seek.	Toilet trained.	Walks up and down stairs - one foot per step.	Cuts with small scissors.	Asks questions beginning with "Why? When? How?"
		Dresses self with help.			Answers questions like, "What do you do with a cracker? a hat?"
2-6	Plays a role in "pretend" games like house or school - mom, dad, teacher.	Washes and dries hands.	Stands on one foot without support.	Draws or copies vertical (l) lines.	Speaks clearly - is understandable most of the time.
	Plays with other children - cars, dolls, building.		Climbs on play equipment - ladders, slides.		Talks in sentences at least four words long.
	"Helps" with simple household tasks.			Scribbles with circular motion.	Has a vocabulary of at least 20 words.
2-0 yrs.	Usually responds to correction - stops.	Opens door by turning knob.	Walks up and down stairs alone.	Turns pages of picture books, one at a time.	Follows two-part instructions.
		Takes off open coat or shirt without help.			

Social	Self-help	Gross motor	Fine motor	Language	Age
Shows sympathy to other children, tries to comfort them.	Eats with spoon, spilling little.	Runs well, seldom falls.	Builds towers of four or more blocks.	Names a few familiar objects in picture books.	18 mos.
Sometimes says "No" when interfered with.	Eats with fork.	Kicks a ball forward.	Scribbles with crayon.	Asks for a drink or food, using words or sounds.	
Greets people with "Hi" or similar.	Feeds self with spoon.	Runs.	Picks up two small toys in one hand.	Uses at least ten words.	
Gives kisses or hugs.	Insists on doing things by self such as feeding.	Walks without help.		Talks in single words.	12 mos.
	Lifts cup to mouth and drinks.	Stands without support.	Stacks two or more blocks.	Says "Mama" or "Dada" for parent, or similar.	
Waves "Bye-bye."	Picks up a spoon by the handle.	Walks around furniture or crib while holding on.	Picks up small objects - precise thumb and finger grasp.	Understands phrases like "No-no" and "All gone."	
Plays social games, "peek-a-boo," "patty-cake."		Crawls around on hands and knees.			9 mos.
Pushes things away he/she doesn't want.		Sits alone . . . steady, without support.	Uses two hands to pick up large objects.	Makes sounds like da-da, ma-ma, ba-ba.	
Reaches for familiar people.	Feeds self cracker.	Rolls over from back to stomach.	Transfers toy from one hand to the other.	Responds to name - turns and looks.	
				Babbles.	6 mos.
Distinguishes mother from others.	Comforts self with thumb or pacifier.	Turns around when lying on stomach.	Picks up toy with one hand.	Laughs out loud.	
Social smile.	Reacts to sight of bottle or breast.	Lifts head and chest when lying on stomach.	Looks at and reaches for faces and toys.	Makes sounds - ah, eh, ugh.	
				Cries in a special way when hungry.	
Birth					Birth

Figure 15.2 Child development chart—first 5 years. Reproduced with permission. Material is copyrighted, and available in English and Spanish for purchase from ChildDevelopmentReview.com. Parent questionnaires are also available, and can be used with the chart.

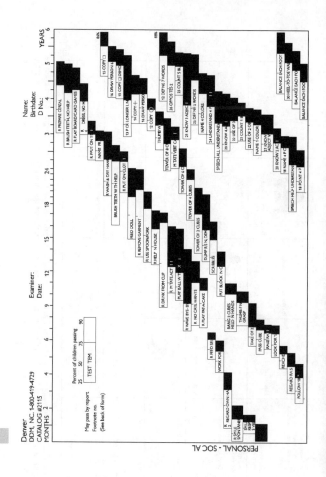

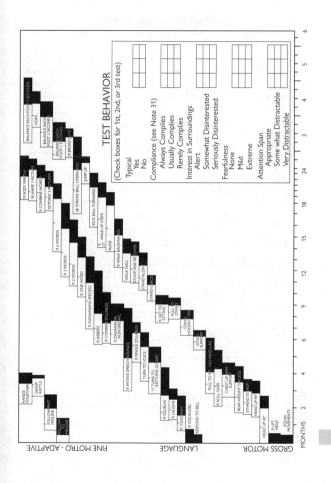

DIRECTIONS FOR ADMINISTRATION

1. Try to get child to smile by smiling, talking or waving. Do not touch him/her.
2. Child must stare at hand several seconds.
3. Parent may help guide toothbrush and put toothpaste on brush.
4. Child does not have to be able to tie shoes or button/zip in the back.
5. Move yarn slowly in an arc from one side to the other, about 8" above child's face.
6. Pass if child grasps rattle when it is touched to the backs or tips of fingers.
7. Pass if child tries to see where yarn went. Yarn should be dropped quickly from sight from tester's hand without arm movement.
8. Child must transfer cube from hand to hand without help of body, mouth, or table.
9. Pass if child picks up raisin with any part of thumb and finger.
10. Line can vary only 30 degrees or less from tester's line. |/
11. Make a fist with thumb pointing upward and wiggle only the thumb. Pass if child imitates and does not move any fingers other than the thumb.

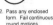

12. Pass any enclosed form. Fail continuous round motions.

13. Which line is longer? (Not bigger.) Turn paper upside down and repeat. (pass 3 of 3 or 5 of 6)

14. Pass any lines crossing near midpoint.

15. Have child copy first. If failed, demonstrate.

When giving items 12, 14, and 15, do not name the forms. Do not demonstrate 12 and 14.

16. When scoring, each pair (2 arms, 2 legs, etc.) counts as one part.
17. Place one cube in cup and shake gently near child's ear, but out of sight. Repeat for other ear.
18. Point to picture and have child name it. (No credit is given for sounds only.)
    If less than 4 pictures are named correctly, have child point to picture as each is named by tester.

19. Using doll, tell child: Show me the nose, eyes, ears, mouth, hands, feet, tummy, hair. Pass 6 of 8.
20. Using pictures, ask child: Which one flies?... says meow?... talks?... barks?... gallops? Pass 2 of 5, 4 of 5.
21. Ask child: What do you do when you are cold?... tired?... hungry? Pass 2 of 3, 3 of 3.
22. Ask child: What do you do with a cup? What is a chair used for? What is a pencil used for?
    Action words must be included in answers.
23. Pass if child correctly places and says how many blocks are on paper. (1, 5).
24. Tell child: Put block **on** table; **under** table; **in front of** me, **behind** me. Pass 4 of 4.
    (Do not help child by pointing, moving head or eyes.)
25. Ask child: What is a ball?... lake?... desk?... house?... banana?... curtain?... fence?... ceiling? Pass if defined in terms of use, shape, what it is made of, or general category (such as banana is fruit, not just yellow). Pass 5 of 8, 7 of 8.
26. Ask child: If a horse is big, a mouse is __? If fire is hot, ice is __? If the sun shines during the day, the moon shines during the __? Pass 2 of 3.
27. Child may use wall or rail only, not person. May not crawl.
28. Child must throw ball overhand 3 feet to within arm's reach of tester.
29. Child must perform standing broad jump over width of test sheet (8 1/2 inches).
30. Tell child to walk forward, heel within 1 inch of toe. Tester may demonstrate. Child must walk 4 consecutive steps.
31. In the second year, half of normal children are non-compliant.

OBSERVATIONS:

Figure 15.3 Denver-II Developmental Screening Test. For use of this form, see AR 600–75. © 1969, 1990 W.K. Frankenburg and J. B. Dodds © 1978 W.K. Frankenburg.

Child's Name _____   Record Number _____

Today's Date _____   Filled out by _____

Date of Birth _____

Pediatric Symptom Checklist

Please mark under the heading that best fits your child:

		Never	Sometimes	Often
1	Complains of aches/pains			
2	Spends more time alone			
3	Tires easily, little energy			
4	Fidgety, unable to sit still			
5	Has trouble with a teacher			
6	Less interested in school			
7	Acts as if driven by a motor			
8	Daydreams too much			
9	Distracted easily			
10	Is afraid of new situations			
11	Feels sad, unhappy			
12	Is irritable, angry			
13	Feels hopeless			
14	Has trouble concentrating			
15	Less interest in friends			
16	Fights with others			
17	Absent from school			
18	School grades dropping			
19	Is down on him or herself			
20	Visits doctor with doctor finding nothing wrong			
21	Has trouble sleeping			
22	Worries a lot			
23	Wants to be with you more than before			
24	Feels he or she is bad			
25	Takes unnecessary risks			
26	Gets hurt frequently			
27	Seems to be having less fun			
28	Acts younger than children his or her age			
29	Does not listen to rules			
30	Does not show feelings			
31	Does not understand other people's feelings			
32	Teases others			
33	Blames others for his or her troubles			
34	Takes things that do not belong to him or her			
35	Refuses to share			

Other comments

Figure 15.4 Pediatric symptom checklist. Scoring: 0 = not true; 1 = somewhat or sometimes true; 2 = very or often true. Minimum cutoff scores for positive indication of significant and psychosocial impairment:
—Children 6–16 years: 28 or above
—Children 2–5 years (the scores on items 6, 7, 14, and 15 are ignored; include only the remaining 31 items): 24 or above.
Reproduced with permission from JM Murphy and MS Jellinek.

Disability: definitions and specific problems and diagnoses

The World Health Organization (WHO) has developed the universal International Classification of Functioning, Disability and Health (ICF), a multipurpose tool that stresses health and functioning as a framework for disability. Disability with neurodevelopmental and behavioral problems may be expressed in cognitive, motor, communication, and/or social streams. Examples of problems in these streams and in associated academic and behavioral performances are presented below.

Cognitive

Intellectual disability is characterized by significant limitations in intellectual functioning and adaptive behavior.
• Streams most affected are all developmental domains.

Motor disability

This is a group of neurological conditions with atypical speed, quality, and/or ease of spontaneous movements and that do not result in weakness or paralysis. Broadly, these disorders are divided into excessive (hyperkinetic) and diminished (bradykinetic) movements.
• Streams most affected are gross and fine motor.

Cerebral palsy

CP is a nonprogressive disorder of movement and posture resulting from injury to the brain before, during, or shortly after birth. No cause is identified in about 1 in 4 cases, although prematurity is a known risk factor. The spectrum in presentation is wide, and often includes non-motor disability in any or all other streams of development.

Movement in CP is classified as
• *Spastic* (pyramidal, with increased muscular tone and a "clasp knife" resistance quality to passive movement)
• *Choreoathetoid* (extrapyramidal, with variable muscular tone, sudden involuntary movements, and a "lead-pipe," rigid resistance quality to passive movement)
• *Mixed* (both spastic and choreoathetoid qualities are present)

The Gross Motor Function Classification System (GMFCS) is a useful clinical instrument that categorizes individuals into one of five levels, based on functional abilities and limitations (www.canchild.ca/Portals/0/outcomes/pdf/GMFCS-ER.pdf).

Academic and behavioral problems

Inappropriate, delayed, or inefficient academic or social performance compared to that of typically developing peers is often associated with other primary and secondary problems in mood, anxiety, self-esteem, and behavior.

Attention deficit hyperactivity disorder (ADHD)

ADHD is a chronic condition apparent prior to 7 years of age, with problems in impulse control, attention, and hyperactivity observed in at least two environments (e.g., school and home). Other primary causes (e.g., learning disability, psychosocial, hearing loss) may also be present.

Standardized parent and teacher questionnaires that screen for ADHD and associated problems, such as the NICHQ Vanderbilt ADHD Diagnostic Rating Scales, should be completed as part of a thorough evaluation prior to making this diagnosis.

ADHD is classified according to three subtypes:

- Primarily inattentive
- Primarily hyperactive-impulsive
- Combined

Diagnostic criteria are available in the American Psychiatric Association's *Diagnostic and Statistical Manual of Mental Disorders, 4th edition, Text Revision (DSM-IV-TR)* (see Box 15.2).

Management must address educational accommodations, family-directed education and support, emphasis on strengths, and psychotropic medication use (typically a psychostimulant medication unless contraindicated or not tolerated after adequate trials). Community-based advocacy and education resources can be invaluable (see www.chadd.org).

Learning disabilities (LD)

These are disorders in one or more of the basic psychological processes involved in understanding or using language (spoken or written), resulting in an imperfect ability to listen, think, speak, read, write, spell, or do math calculations, *excluding* causes such as visual, hearing, or motor impairment, emotional disturbance, intellectual disability, cultural disadvantage, or some other primary cause.

School districts are no longer required to identify the presence of a statistically significant discrepancy between intellectual ability (based on IQ testing) and academic achievement (based on standardized academic testing) in one or more of seven specific areas (such as basic reading, oral expression, or math calculation) to qualify a child for special-education services.

Evaluations should include a variety of assessment tools, with input from parents as well as classroom observations.

Box 15.2 DSM-IV-TR criteria for ADHD

I. Either A or B:

A. Six or more of the following symptoms of inattention have been present for at least 6 months to a point that is disruptive and inappropriate for developmental level:

Inattention

1. Often does not give close attention to details or makes careless mistakes in schoolwork, work, or other activities
2. Often has trouble keeping attention on tasks or play activities.
3. Often does not seem to listen when spoken to directly
4. Often does not follow instructions and fails to finish schoolwork, chores, or duties in the workplace (not due to oppositional behavior or failure to understand instructions)
5. Often has trouble organizing activities
6. Often avoids, dislikes, or doesn't want to do things that take a lot of mental effort for a long period of time (such as schoolwork or homework)
7. Often loses things needed for tasks and activities (e.g., toys, school assignments, pencils, books, or tools)
8. Is often easily distracted
9. Is often forgetful in daily activities

B. Six or more of the following symptoms of hyperactivity-impulsivity have been present for at least 6 months to an extent that is disruptive and inappropriate for developmental level:

Hyperactivity

1. Often fidgets with hands or feet or squirms in seat
2. Often gets up from seat when remaining in seat is expected
3. Often runs about or climbs when and where it is not appropriate (adolescents or adults may feel very restless)
4. Often has trouble playing or enjoying leisure activities quietly
5. Is often "on the go" or often acts as if "driven by a motor"
6. Often talks excessively

Impulsivity

1. Often blurts out answers before questions have been finished
2. Often has trouble waiting one's turn
3. Often interrupts or intrudes on others (e.g., butts into conversations or games)
   i. Some symptoms that cause impairment were present before age 7 years.
   ii. Some impairment from the symptoms is present in two or more settings (e.g., at school/work and at home).
   iii. There must be clear evidence of significant impairment in social, school, or work functioning.
   iv. The symptoms do not happen only during the course of a pervasive developmental disorder, schizophrenia, or other psychotic disorder. The symptoms are not better accounted for

by another mental disorder (e.g., mood disorder, anxiety disorder, dissociative disorder, or a personality disorder).

Based on these criteria, three types of ADHD are identified:
1. ADHD, *combined type*: If both criteria 1A and 1B are met for the past 6 months
2. ADHD, *predominantly inattentive type*: If criterion 1A is met but criterion 1B is not met for the past 6 months
3. ADHD, *predominantly hyperactive-impulsive type*: If criterion 1B is met but criterion 1A is not met for the past 6 months.

Reprinted with permission from the *Diagnostic and Statistical Manual of Mental Disorders, 4th edition, Text Revision* (Copyright 2000). American Psychiatric Association.

Communication disorders

These disorders involve problems in speech and language. *Speech* refers to the mechanical aspects of sound production for communication, while *language* refers to the system of symbols (including speech) used to store and exchange information. Language is composed of visual or auditory *expressive* (output) and *receptive* (the decoding or interpretation of the output of others) components.

Communication disorders frequently present as delayed and atypical patterns in communication. Hearing should always be formally assessed. Speech and language screening instruments are useful.

Management focuses on decreasing child frustration through language enrichment exposure, patience, compensatory strategies in communication, and other means.

Speech disorders

These include any problem in speech production, such as dysarthria (poor speech articulation), that can be due to motor problems, anatomical malformations, or neurological impairment. The child may otherwise have normal language development.

Language disorders

Any primary problem in receptive or expressive communication constitutes a language disorder. While environmental influences can impact language development, these are seldom the root cause. Problems may result from primary (e.g., developmental language disorder) and/or secondary (e.g., hearing impairment, cognitive disability, autism) causes.

Atypical social perceptions (autism)

Pervasive developmental disorders (PDDs) include autistic disorder, Asperger syndrome, and, PDD–not otherwise specified, among others. Children with PDDs have problems in the quality of their reciprocal social interactions, expressed variably with stereotyped repetitive mannerisms, atypical communication skills, and impaired imaginative play.

About two-thirds of children with autism also have an intellectual disability. Intelligence and language are not delayed in Asperger syndrome but may be atypical in quality. A variety of genetic disorders are associated with autistic disorder.

Medical disorders and secondary complications are frequent (e.g., seizures, self-injurious behavior, gastrointestinal and sleep-related concerns). Increasing evidence suggests that early identification (see Fig. 15.5) and treatment with intensive behavioral interventions improve outcome.

Associated problems

Other developmental and behavioral problems may occur in isolation but are often primary or secondary problems in mood, anxiety, self-esteem, and nonspecific neurological maturation, such as tics, elimination disorders (encopresis and enuresis), and sleep disturbances. These problems must be equally considered, evaluated, and managed.

Sleep disturbances

Insufficient or disturbed sleep is negatively associated with multiple aspects of physical and mental health, especially in the control of behavior, attention, learning, and emotions, and is much more common among children with disabilities.

Cultural differences in child-rearing strongly influence sleep patterns and practices (e.g., co-sleeping, breast-feeding). Problems vary with age. The Child's Sleep Habits Questionnaire (www.kidzzzsleep.org/researchinstruments.htm) focuses on sleep disorders among children ages 4–12 years in three domains: *dyssomnias* (difficulty in falling or staying asleep); *parasomnias* (events occurring after falling asleep, such as sleepwalking, night terrors, or bedwetting); and *sleep-disordered breathing* (see Table 15.4: BEARS Sleep Screening Algorithm).

M-CHAT

Please fill out the following about how your child usually is. Please try to answer every question. If the behavior is rare (e.g., you've seen it once or twice), please answer as if the child does not do it.

1.	Does your child enjoy being swung, bounced on your knee, etc.?	Yes	No
2.	Does your child take an interest in other children?	Yes	No
3.	Does your child like climbing on things, such as up stairs?	Yes	No
4.	Does your child enjoy playing peek-a-boo/hide-and-seek?	Yes	No
5.	Does your child ever pretend, for example, to talk on the phone or take care of a doll or pretend other things?	Yes	No
6.	Does your child ever use his/her index finger to point, to ask for something?	Yes	No
7.	Does your child ever use his/her index finger to point, to indicate interest in something?	Yes	No
8.	Can your child play properly with small toys (e.g. cars or blocks) without just mouthing, fiddling, or dropping them?	Yes	No
9.	Does your child ever bring objects over to you (parent) to show you something?	Yes	No
10.	Does your child look you in the eye for more than a second or two?	Yes	No
11.	Does your child ever seem oversensitive to noise? (e.g., plugging ears)	Yes	No
12.	Does your child smile in response to your face or your smile?	Yes	No
13.	Does your child imitate you? (e.g., you make a face-will your child imitate it?)	Yes	No
14.	Does your child respond to his/her name when you call?	Yes	No
15.	If you point at a toy across the room, does your child look at it?	Yes	No
16.	Does your child walk?	Yes	No
17.	Does your child look at things you are looking at?	Yes	No
18.	Does your child make unusual finger movements near his/her face?	Yes	No
19.	Does your child try to attract your attention to his/her own activity?	Yes	No
20.	Have you ever wondered if your child is deaf?	Yes	No
21.	Does your child understand what people say?	Yes	No
22.	Does your child sometimes stare at nothing or wander with no purpose?	Yes	No
23.	Does your child look at your face to check your reaction when faced with something unfamiliar?	Yes	No

M-CHAT Scoring Instructions

A child fails the checklist when 2 or more critical items are failed OR when any three items are failed. Yes/no answers convert to pass/fail responses. Below are listed the failed responses for each item on the M-CHAT. Bold capitalized items are CRITICAL items.

Not all children who fail the checklist will meet criteria for a diagnosis on the autism spectrum. However, children who fail the checklist should be evaluated in more depth by the physician or referred for a developmental evaluation with a specialist.

1. No	6. No	11. Yes	16. No	21. No
2. **NO**	7. **NO**	12. No	17. No	22. Yes
3. No	8. No	13. **NO**	18. Yes	23. No
4. No	9. **NO**	14. **NO**	19. No	
5. No	10. No	15. **NO**	20. Yes	

Figure 15.5 Modified checklist for autism in toddlers (M-CHAT).
©1999 Robins, Fein, & Barton, reproduced with permission.

Developmental milestones

Table 15.1 Developmental milestones

Age	Cognitive/ Adaptive/Self-help	Speech & Language R = receptive E = expressive	Motor FM = fine motor GM = gross motor	Social/ Emotional	Red Flags
Birth	Fixates on face	R: "Prefers" human speech with high inflection; E: Body language showing positive and negative response	GM: Turns head while prone with nose touching surface of table; In ventral suspension, body is flexed around supporting hand; When supine, body generally flexed	Prefers facial conturs; Moves in cadence with sound	
1 mo	Follows face; Fixes on red ring	R: Alerts to sound; E: Cries; Throaty noises	FM: Hands tightly fisted; GM: Head up while prone; Turns head while prone with nose clearing the surface of table; In ventral suspension, lifts head to plane of body; When supine, head lags on pull to sitting	May smile	Speech/Language: Failure to alert to environmental stimuli may indicate sensory impairment
2 mo	Tracks horizontally past midline; Tracks vertically	R: Regards speaker; E: Attends to voice and coos; Vocalizes single vowel sounds	FM: Hands unfisted if placed in hand; Retains rattle if placed in hand; GM: Head and chest up while prone on table; Head bobs erect if held sitting; In ventral suspension, sustains head in plane of body	Smiles on social contact	Motor: Rolling prior to 3 months may indicate hypertonia

3 mo	Regards a 1-inch cube; Follows ring circularly; Visual threat	R: Listens to music E: Some vowel sounds: "aah, ngah"; Chuckles	FM: Hands unfisted most of the time; Bats at objects GM: Rests on forearms when prone on table; In ventral suspension, lifts head above plane of body with legs extended; When supine, partial head lag	Sustained social contact
4 mo	Reaches for and mouths objects; Shakes rattle; Regards objects while handling	R: Orients to voice E: "Ah-goo"; Silent and listens to speaker, then vocalizes when speaker stops	FM: Obtains rattle with open-hand reach; Reaches with open hand while supine GM: Head up to vertical axis and rests on hands while prone on table; When supine, hands come to midline and no head lag; Rolls front to back; Sits with truncal support	Laughs out loud; Active at sight of food; Displeasure if social contact broken
5 mo	Attains dangling ring; Regards pellet	E: Makes raspberries; Sing-song vocalizations that mimic speaker's voice	FM: Palmar grasp with thumb adducted; Transfers objects hand-mouth-hand GM: Rolls back to front; Lifts head when pulled to sit; Sits with pelvic support; Anterior protection	Smiles and vocalizes to mirror
			Motor: Poor head control General: Failure to reach for objects may indicate motor, visual and/or cognitive deficit	

Table 15.1 (Contd.)

Age	Cognitive/Adaptive/Self-help	Speech & Language R = receptive E = expressive	Motor FM = fine motor GM = gross motor	Social/Emotional	Red Flags
6 mo	Looks to floor when drops toy; Attains partially hidden object; Removes cloth covering face; Discriminates strangers	E: Repetitive vowel sounds; Babbles: "baba", "gagaga"; Consonant production without symbolic meaning or communicative intent	FM: Immature rake of pellet; Transfers objects hand-hand GM: Sits leaning forward on hands	Prefers parent; Responds to emotional content of interaction	Speech/Language: Absent babbling may indicate hearing deficit
7 mo	Bangs/shakes toys; Attends to grasp 2nd cube but drops first; Pats mirror image	E: Adult reinforcement begins to give meaning to random babbling	FM: Radial-palmar grasp of cube; Rakes object into palm GM: Sits without support; Commando crawls; Lateral protection		Motor: W-sitting may indicate adductor spasticity or hypotonia Social: Absent stranger anxiety may be due to multiple care providers (e.g., NICU)
8 mo	Pulls string to obtain ring; Inspects ring/bell; Seeks yarn ball after its silent fall/landing	R: Enjoys gesture games like peek-a-boo E: "Dada" inappropriately; Mimics sounds already in repertoire	FM: Scissors grasp of pellet-sized object between thumb and side of curled index finger. GM: Brings self into sitting position; Reaches with one hand while 4-point kneeling	Stranger anxiety	

9 mo	Rings bell; Bangs objects on table; Uncovers hidden object under cloth	R: Alerts to sound of own name; Associates words with meanings E: "Mama" inappropriately; Repetitive consonant sounds	FM: Radial-digital grasp of cube with thumb and fingertips GM: Pulls to stand. Creeps on hands and knees.	Plays peek-a-boo, pat-a-cake; Waves bye bye	Motor: Persistence of primitive reflexes may indicate neuromotor disorder.
10 mo	Bangs 2 cubes together; Isolates index finger and explores by poking; Looks at pictures in book	R: Comprehends "no" E: "Dada" and "Mama" appropriately	FM: Isolates index finger and pokes; Clumsy release of cube into box; Pincer grasp held between distal pads of thumb and index finger GM: Cruises around furniture; Walks with 2 hands held	Adjusts posture to dressing	
11 mo	Uncovers toy under cup	R: Looks for familiar family member when named E: First word; Imitates simple sounds	GM: Stands alone; Walks with 1 hand held		
12 mo	Looks selectively at round hold on form board; Removes lid to find toy	R: Follows command with gesture ("Give me.") E: One or more words with meaning besides mama/dada; Immature jargoning	FM: Fine pincer grasp of pellet between fingertips; Marks with crayon; Precise release of cube; Attempts tower of 2 cubes GM: Independent steps; Posterior protection	Indicates some wishes or interests with protoimperative pointing (single finger without verbal label)	Motor: Failure to develop protective reactions may indicate neuromotor disorder Cognition: Persistent mouthing may indicate lack of intellectual curiosity

Table 15.1 (Contd.)

Age	Cognitive/ Adaptive/Self-help	Speech & Language R = receptive E = expressive	Motor FM = fine motor GM = gross motor	Social/ Emotional	Red Flags
13 mo	Unwraps toy in cloth; Functional play	R: Looks appropriately when asked "'Where is (familiar object)?" E: Uses 2–3 words; "Oh-oh"			Speech/Language: Normal receptive language up to this point is not incompatible with hearing loss
14 mo	Combines 2 cubes into one hand to take 3rd; Dumps pellet after demonstration	R: Follows command without gesture E: Names one object; Says "no" meaningfully	FM: Tower of 2 cubes GM: Walks well independently	Indicates some wishes or interests with protodeclarative pointing (single finger with verbal label)	
15 mo	Places circle in form board; Symbolic play toward self	R: Points to a body part or favorite toy E: Uses 3–5 words; Mature jargoning		Hugs parent	Speech/Language: Lack of consonant production may indicate mild hearing loss
16 mo	Pellet in and out without demonstration; Finds toy hidden under layered covers	R: Points to 1 to 2 body parts; Fetches object from another room on request E: Uses 5–10 words	FM: Tower of 3 cubes; Imitates scribble GM: Creeps upstairs; Runs stiff-legged; Climbs on furniture; Walks backwards; Stoops and recovers		General: Lack of imitation may indicate deficits in hearing, cognition and/or socialization

18 mo	Round form in reversed board after searching; Matches pairs of objects; Feeds self	R: Points to 3 body parts; Points to self; Looks selectively at a book; Follows 2-directional commands E: Uses 10–20 words; Giant-words ("Thank you", "Stop it", "Let's go"); Names and points to one picture card; Names a test object (e.g., ball);	FM: Tower of 4 cubes; Scribbles spontaneously; Imitates single vertical stroke GM: Push/pulls large object; Throws ball while standing; Walks fast, seldom falling; Seats self in small chair	Symbolic play directed toward doll; Seeks help; Kisses parent with pucker	Motor: Hand dominance prior to 18 months may indicate contralateral weakness Social: Lack of protodeclarative pointing may indicate problem in social relatedness
20 mo	Places square in form board; Deduces location of hidden object (unwitnessed displacement)	R: Points to 6 body parts; Points to several clothing items on request; Selects 2 of 3 familiar objects; Knows 4-directional commands E: Uses two- to three-word sentences; Uses "I", "you", "me"; Names 3 picture cards; Names 2 test objects;	GM: Walks up stairs with hand held		
22 mo	Completes 3-piece form board	R: Points to 3 to 4 pictures E: Uses 25–50 words; Rapid vocabulary expansion;	FM: Tower of 6 cubes GM: Walks up stairs with rail marking time; Squats in play		Social: Advanced, noncommunicative speech (echolalia, rote phrases) may indicate autism

Table 15.1 (Contd.)

Age	Cognitive/ Adaptive/Self-help	Speech & Language R = receptive E = expressive	Motor FM = fine motor GM = gross motor	Social/ Emotional	Red Flags
24 mo	Adapts to form board reversal after 4 trials; Sorts objects; Matches objects to pictures; Solves problems by trial and error; Spills little with spoon; Attempts to fold paper; Uses utensils; Undresses; Pulls on simple garments; Refers to self by name	R: Points to 6 pictures; Understands "me"/"you"; Two-step commands ("Close the book and give the doll to Mommy"); E: Uses 50+ words; Uses 2- to 3-word sentences (noun-verb); Intelligibility = 50%+ to a stranger	FM: Train of 4 cubes without stack; Holds pencil with point down; Imitates single horizontal stroke; Turns pages one at a time GM: Jumps in place; Kicks ball; Walks down stairs with rail marking time; Runs well without falling; Throws overhand	Parallel play with peers; Offers toy; Symbolic doll or action figures; Mimics domestic activities; Listens to stories; Able to take turns some; Aggressive to get things	Motor: Inability to walk up and down stairs may be the result of lack of opportunity General: Absent symbolic play may indicate problems in cognitive and/or social development
30 mo	Knows name; Helps put things away		FM: Tower of 9 cubes; Adds chimney to train of cubes GM: Walks up stairs alternating feet; Stands on one foot momentarily;	Pretends in play	

3 yr	Identifies shapes; Pours some; Dresses with supervision; Unbuttons some; Asks "why" questions; Understands daily routines; Knows age and gender; Repeats 3 digits; Counts 3 objects correctly; Remembers and recites nursery rhymes	R: Understands 3-element commands E: Uses four- to five-word sentences; Tells stories; Uses plurals; Names most common objects; Intelligibility = 75%+ to a stranger	FM: Copies a circle; Holds pencil high and awkward; Tower of 9–10 cubes GM: Broad jumps 18 inches; Walks down stairs alternating feet without rail; Walks well on toes; Peddles tricycle	Takes on a role; Plays associatively with others; Simple fantasy play; Takes turns; Listens to stories; Shares some; Negotiates conflicts	Motor: inability to copy a circle.
4 yr	Identifies the longer line; Helps set table; Dresses all but tying; Counts 4 objects correctly; Goes to toilet alone	R: Understands 4-element commands E: Intelligibility = 100% to a stranger	FM: Copies a cross; Brushes own teeth; Dresses self including buttons; Tower of 8 cubes GM: jumps 32 inches with one foot leading; Hops on one foot; Balances on one foot for 5 seconds	Interactive games; Plays cooperatively with others; Elaborate fantasy play; Sings a song; Shares spontaneously; Follows rules in simple games; Wants to please friends	
5 yr	Prints letters; Counts 10 objects correctly; Repeats 10-syllable sentence; Asks [meanings of words	R: Understands 5-element commands; Can follow a story without pictures. E: Correct use of all parts of speech; Vocabulary of 5000 words; Corrects own errors in speech	FM: Copies a triangle; Ties a knot, Mature pencil grip; Tower of 10 cubes GM: Hops and skips; Balances on one foot for 10 seconds	Make-believe and dress up; Follows rules of the game.	

Reference sources:
American Academy of Pediatrics
Chapter published in Developmental-Behavioral Pediatrics, 3rd ed. Levine MD, Carey WB, Crocker AC, editors. The Preschool Years, pages 38-50, Copyright Elsevier, (1999).
Chapter published in Encounters with Children: Pediatric Behavior and Development, 4th ed. Dixon SD, Stein MT, editors. Two Years: Language Leaps, pages 382-409, Copyright Elsevier (2006).

Developmental evaluation

Components of medical and social history

History

Each component influences development and behavior
- Past medical history
  - Prenatal/pregnancy and delivery, including history of prematurity
  - Neonatal
  - Hearing assessment
  - Vision assessment
- Family history (including genetics; see Chapter 25)
- Nutrition, including iron deficiency
- Growth (review past charts)
- Education (past evaluations, individualized education program [IEP])
- Social
  - Parenting beliefs and approaches
  - Stressors (financial, parental, illness, other)
  - Environment (including drug abuse, toxins)
  - Integrative health care (values and adopted approaches)
  - Abuse or neglect (see Chapter 28)
  - Protective factors
- Neurodevelopmental (see Table 15.1)

Review of systems

- Careful neurological
  - Focal findings
  - Sleep
  - Seizures
  - Head injury
- Other organ systems
- Temperament
- Pain
- Elimination
- Sensory responses (see Chapter 24)
- Atypical developmental
  - Neurodevelopmental regression
  - Self-injuring behaviors
  - Tics
  - Stereotypies (e.g., hand-flapping)
  - Poor reciprocal eye contact
  - Pica

Examination

General observations

Observe attachments, caregiver–child interactions, self-regulation and activity, communication (speech and nonverbal, such as body posture, eye contact and facial expressions), and typicality.

Measurements

Measure length, height, weight, and OFC (ideally, include past measurements).

Physical examination

Conduct a complete examination, with attention to the following:
- Dysmorphology (deformations, major and minor malformations, disruptions)
- Skin (include Wood's lamp for neurocutaneous lesions)
- Neurological (see Chapter 14). Include assessment of
  - Primitive reflexes (automatic brain stem–controlled responses that are present at birth, but disappear and/or are suppressed sequentially during infancy by higher brain regions) (see Table 15.2)
  - Postural reflexes (higher brain-cortex automatic responses that emerge during infancy and control the position of the trunk and extremities) (see Table 15.3)
  - Tone, bulk, and strength

Surveillance and screening instruments

See Typical development and behavior (p. 632).

Table 15.2 Primitive reflexes

Reflex	Stimulus	Response	Age of Suppression	Clinical Significance
Moro	Sudden neck extension	Shoulder abduction, shoulder, elbow and finger extension followed by arm flexion abduction	4–6 months	Persists in CNS pathology, static encephalopathy
Startle	Sudden noise, clapping	Same as Moro reflex	4–6 months	Persists in CNS pathology, static encephalopathy
Rooting	Stroking lips or around mouth	Moving mouth, head toward stimulus in search of nipple	4 months	Diminished in CNS pathology, may persist
Positive support	Light pressure or weight bearing on plantar surface	Legs extend for partial support of body weight	3–5 months replaced by volitional weight bearing with support	Obligatory or hyperactive abnormal at any age, early sign of lower extremity spasticity, may be associated with scissoring
Asymmetric tonic neck reflex (fencer's posture)	Head turning to side. Neck flexion	Extremities extend on face side, flex on occiput side. Arms flex, legs extend	6–7 months	Obligatory response abnormal at any age, persists in static encephalopathy
Palmar grasp	Touch or pressure on palm or stretching finger flexors	Flexion of all fingers, hand fisting	5–6 months	Diminished in CNS suppression, absent in lower motor neuron paralysis; persists/hyperactive in spasticity

Plantar grasp	Pressure on sole distal to metatarsal heads	Flexion of all toes	12–14 months when walking is achieved	Diminished in CNS suppression, absent in lower motor neuron paralysis; persists/hyperactive in spasticity
Autonomic neonatal walking	On vertical support plantar contact and passive tilting of body forward side to side	Alternating automatic steps with support	3–4 months	Variable activity in normal infants, absent in lower motor neuron paralysis
Placement/Placing	Tactile contact on dorsum of foot or hand	Extremity flexion to place hand or foot over an obstacle	Before end of first year	Absent in lower motor neuron paralysis or with lower extremity spasticity
Neck righting or body derotational	Neck rotation in supine	Sequential body rotation from shoulder to pelvis toward direction of face	4 months replaced by volitional rolling	Non-sequential leg rolling suggests increased tone
Galant (trunk incurvation)	On prone suspension, stroke to paravertebral area from thoracic to sacral level	Trunk arches to side stroked	2–6 months	Absent in transverse spinal cord lesions

Reproduced with permission. Chapter published in Pediatric Rehabilitation 3rd ed. Molnar GE, Alexander MA. Growth and Development, pages 13–28, Copyright Elsevier (1999).

Table 15.3 Postural (support) reflexes

Reflex	Stimulus	Response	Age of Suppression	Clinical Significance
Positive support	In vertical upright suspension, feet touch table surface.	Leg extension, and: 3–4 months: attempts to support body weight 5–6 months: infant fully supports body weight 7 months: enjoys bouncing	3–4 mo	Allows correct posture for voluntary standing. Absence may suggest corticospinal disease
Landau	In horizontal prone suspension, head is gently pushed into flexion	Baseline, the infant's head extends above the plane of the trunk, and legs are extended, opposing gravity With head pushed into flexion, infant's legs drop into flexion With head flexion released, infant returns to baseline	4–5 mo	Allows independent sitting and walking
Derotational righting	Passive or active head turning	Body rotates in direction of head movement	4–5 mo	Allows independent rolling

| Propping; Anterior Lateral Posterior | In seated position, thorax is gently pushed Forward Laterally Backward | Arms extend in direction of being pushed to catch self. In lateral push, only the arm on the falling side extends | Anterior: 4–5 mo Lateral: 5–7 mo Posterior: 7–8 mo | Allows protective extension of arms for independent sitting |
| Parachute | Suspended at the waist in horizontal prone, upper body is suddenly tilted downward. | Arms extend forward and hands spread out to catch fall. | 8–9 mo | Allows protective extension of arms against falls |

Permission for adaptation granted from Paul D. Larsen, M.D., University of Nebraska School of Medicine. Source http://library.med.utah.edu/pedineurologicexam/html/home_exam.html

BEARS sleep screening algorithm

The "BEARS" instrument is divided into five major sleep domains, providing a comprehensive screen for the major sleep disorders affecting children in the 2- to 18-year-old range. Each sleep domain has a set of age-appropriate "trigger questions" for use in the clinical interview (see Table 15.4).

B = bedtime problems
E = excessive daytime sleepiness
A = awakenings during the night
R = regularity and duration of sleep
S = snoring

Table 15.4 BEARS sleep screening algorithm

	Toddler/preschool (2–5 years)	School-aged (6–12 years)	Adolescent (13–18 years)
1. **B**edtime problems	Does your child have any problems going to bed? Falling asleep?	Does your child have any problems at bedtime? (P) Do you have any problems going to bed? (C)	Do you have any problems falling asleep at bedtime? (C)
2. **E**xcessive daytime sleepiness	Does your child seem overtired or sleepy a lot during the day? Does he or she still take naps?	Does your child have difficulty waking in the morning, seem sleepy during the day, or take naps? (P) Do you feel tired a lot? (C)	Do you feel sleep a lot during the day? In school? While driving? (C)
3. **A**wakenings during the night	Does your child wake up a lot at night?	Does your child seem to wake up a lot at night? Any sleepwalking or nightmares? (P) Do you wake up a lot at night? Have trouble getting back to sleep? (C)	Do you wake up a lot at night? Have trouble getting back to sleep? (C)
4. **R**egularity and duration of sleep	Does your child have a regular bedtime and wake time? What are they?	What time does your child go to bed and get up on school days? Weekends? Do you think he or she is getting enough sleep? (P)	What time do you usually go to bed on school nights? Weekends? How much sleep do you usually get? (C)
5. **S**noring	Does your child snore a lot or have difficult breathing at night?	Does your child have loud or nightly snoring or any breathing difficulties at night? (P)	Does your teenager snore loudly or nightly? (P)

(P) Parent-directed question (C) Child-directed question. From Judith Owens, MD, MPH, with permission.

Management and prevention of behavioral and developmental problems

Management and prevention are highly individualized to the child's specific medical, psychological, social, educational, and other needs. Adherence to principles of medical-home health supervision is essential, and outcomes are optimized with efficient care coordination among all providers, resource services, and effective special education.

Special education

The Individuals with Disabilities Education Improvement Act (IDEA) is the federal law that secures special education services and ensures the rights of children and youth with disabilities from birth through high school and those of their parents. The overarching purpose is to protect equal access to education for all students.

Sources for advocacy and awareness in special education are invaluable, and available in all states through parent training and information projects, and community parent resource centers (www.taalliance.org).

Other resources

- Medical Home (www.medicalhomeinfo.org)
- Bright Futures (www.brightfutures.org)
- Developmental Behavioral Pediatrics online (www.dbpeds.org)
- Children and Adults with Attention Deficit/Hyperactivity Disorder (www.chadd.org)
- PACER Center (Parent Advocacy Coalition for Educational Rights) (www.pacer.org)
- National Dissemination Center for Children with Disabilities (www.nichcy.org)

Child, adolescent, and family psychiatry

Prevalence

The prevalence of child and adolescent mental health problems is similar across many Western countries (~14%–20%). Approximately 50% of patients also experience significant functional impairment, yet <20% children with mental health difficulty receive specialist care.

Applying the disability-adjusted life year (DALY) methodology, the burden of neuropsychiatric conditions affecting children is predicted to double by the year 2020.[1] In 2001, the U.S. Surgeon General David Satcher summarized, "the burden of suffering experienced by children with mental health needs and their families has created a health crisis in this country"[2]

Mental health problems are a potential affliction to all in society; however, adverse mental health is more commonly experienced by individuals from deprived or abusive backgrounds, from families that are financially or emotional troubled, and from single-parent families and members of ethnic minority groups. The latter may experience specific barriers to predominantly clinic- and hospital-based child mental-health care.

1. World Health Organization (1999). The World Health Report 1999: Making a Difference. Geneva: WHO.
2. U.S. Department of Health and Human Services (2001). Report of the U.S. Surgeon General's Conference on Children's Mental Health. A National Action Agenda. Washington, DC: USDHHS.

Classification, categories, and dimensions

The *Diagnostic and Statistical Manual of Mental Disorders* (DSM) classification system includes a section entitled "Disorders usually first diagnosed in infancy, childhood or adolescence." The system also allows children and adolescents to meet criteria for adult mental health disorders.

The DSM and International Classification of Diseases (ICD) are categorical nosological systems. The DSM system is the one most frequently used in the United States.

An alternate system suggests that child mental health presentations are on a continuum with developmentally normal youth. For instance, rather than diagnosing a child as having ADHD, the child may be considered to have more inattention and impulsivity relative to other children.

This dimensional view can be less stigmatizing for children, evoke a more holistic management strategy than a limited medical model, and for some presentations has more predictive validity than the categorical/diagnostic model. One frequently used dimensional system is the juxtaposition of externalizing problems (aggression and delinquency) versus internalizing (anxiety/depression) presentations.

Comorbidity and causation

The co-occurrence of conditions is common in child and adolescent mental health. Conditions A and B in examples 3 and 4 above are co-morbid. An example of 3 is sexual abuse as a nonspecific risk factor for later drug and alcohol use and deliberate self-harm. In example 4, the two conditions may co-occur but are etiologically unrelated. In 1, a condition may develop into another, e.g., the progression of oppositional defiant disorder to conduct disorder. Or in 2, the presenting condition, for instance, depression, may be secondary to earlier struggles with an eating disorder. Other potential relationships between A and B are possible.

1. Direct causation

2. Reverse causation

3. Shared causation

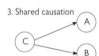

4. Co - occurrence but no causal relationship

Figure 16.1 Comorbidity and causation.

Developmental perspective

A cross-sectional understanding, a snapshot in time, rarely is informative about the child's pre-presentation strengths and vulnerabilities and has little predictive validity. In a developmental model, infant, child, and adolescent epochs are described, embedded within the emotional and material resources of the primary caregivers. These factors are in turn viewed within social and community resources and cultural factors such as a given group's typical way of expressing emotion, reaction to adversity, and morals about acceptable behavior.

Some factors such as a genetic vulnerability act across time. Family influences such as coercive parenting are also developmental continuities unless an active process of change is undertaken.

Children can be described as being on a normal or abnormal trajectory, globally or for a range of constructs such as regulation of mood, impulsivity, and emotional reciprocity. The usefulness of this perspective is that it provides an understanding of whether a recent presentation is a continuation of a long-standing behavioral or emotional state or a recent discontinuity from a normal trajectory. The former usually involves continuity of causative factors.

Such presentations require more complex interventions over longer periods and generally have a more guarded prognosis. The heuristic biopsychosocial formulation is another framework that helps the clinician avoid reductionistic and simple explanations for complex presentations.

Systemic thinking

No child is an island. No family should be one. Children and families present within the context of extended families and local and school communities, and are affected by regional and national phenomena such as employment, poverty gradients, and access to services.

Understanding the family system is essential—whether the parents work together or undermine the others' parenting; the function of sibling sub-systems; and whether there are typical alliances (i.e., father and son going to a baseball game) or "unholy" alliances (i.e., cross-generation grouping to remove someone from family activities).

- Has a child been elevated into a decision-making role?
- Has one parent been demoted?
- Is a child an "identified patient," for instance, presenting with withdrawn behavior when the real problem is an imminent parental separation?
- Have hospital staff been unwittingly triangulated by some family members to exclude others from caregiver roles?

Systemic thinking involves treating the child within the family and broader ecological system. Such understanding is especially important when treatment systems intersect around complex psychosocial presentations. The difficulties some physicians experience in caring for adolescents with anorexia nervosa is a good example. You must weigh the various inputs from mental health therapists, dieticians, schoolteachers and principals, the child, and the parents.

History taking

Why have multiple informants?

Children and adolescents may not see the whole picture. They may also withhold information from you. Which of us does not on occasion operate a need-to-know policy? As an example, the teenage girl with anorexia nervosa who wants to avoid admission may exaggerate the amount she is eating and minimize her level of exercise.

Parents may have a more objective report regarding the level of disruptive symptomatology, including aggression and property destruction. Children, however, are more likely to report anxiety and mood symptoms as well as suicidal ideation compared to the reports of their parents.

Who to get information from?

This is a balance between "the more sources the better" versus the demands of confidentiality and time.

- A good starting point is the referral details and information from the young person and members of the family.
- Information from the school should also be sought if possible, although this may not be practical in an emergency situation.
- Where relevant, others should be approached, e.g., social services, child and adolescent mental health services, or detention services.

An example is a child brought to the emergency room with an unexplained and suspicious injury. Collaboration with other agencies is essential if there are child protection concerns about child abuse. Local information-sharing protocols expedite this work (see p. 1142). Also, you may learn more information from one informant than from another.

Interviewing the family

To an extent, the family interview is an efficient way of hearing the views of the patient, siblings, and parents together. However, to see it this way only is missing the point; it is an opportunity to learn so much more.

- Are there obvious tensions or conflicts?
- Is tension between the parents diffused by the child's behavior?
- Are the children allowed appropriate autonomy, or do they rule the roost?
- Is one parent a "switchboard" through which all communication is routed?
- Are family members able to listen to each others' views?
- Is disagreement tolerated?
- Is there a family "story" that informs how they interact around the presenting problem? Examples include, "no one listens to us," "we have tried our best and can't do any more," "it is all this child's fault," and "our child cannot be helped, but at the same time someone has to do something about this child." This sort of mixed message around a scapegoated child can be very difficult to work with.

Family structures are variable. Often the interview is with one parent. Sometimes it can be illuminating if grandparents are also present. Are there coalitions across generations (e.g., grandparent and child) in effect combining forces to undermine one of the parents?

A further area to note is how the family responds to you. Are you treated as a threat, a messiah, a parent or grandparent, or just a doctor? Do you feel pulled to take sides in a dispute?

Communicating

See also p. 22.

Tips for communicating with children

- Young children's anxiety may be decreased if first interviewed with an adult they trust.
- Assume children do not fully understand why they are being seen.
- Often children assume they are "in trouble."
- Often children equate doctors with physical illness, or with painful procedures such as injections. Rarely have they met a "talking doctor."
- It can help to explain to a child your role as a doctor who talks to them about how they are feeling, acting, and thinking with the purpose to help them.
- Be prepared to see a child several times to gain trust and rapport.
- Learn and/or practice child-appropriate communication—i.e., drawing, storytelling, pretending, building and making things, exploring, appreciating tall tales, talking about current TV, technology, books. Do not take over play; follow the child's lead and behave like a sensible adult.
- Practice age-appropriate language.
- Do not undermine the parents' efforts by appearing too competent.

Tips for communicating with adolescents

- Don't assume they have chosen to be there.
- Understand that they may be ambivalent about recognizing they have a problem, dealing with or denying it, and seeing you as a source of help or as a threat.
- Discuss the context of your conversation—why are you meeting?
- As with children, adolescents may not understand the purpose of a psychiatric interview, and this may require a specific explanation.
- Discuss what you will do with what the adolescent tells you (confidentiality and its limits may be crucial).
- It may be helpful to ask about neutral areas first.
- Be prepared to ask closed questions, accepting a yes-or-no answer.
- Speak plainly. Avoid talking like an adult pretending to be a teenager.
- Convey your desire to understand by checking whether you are getting it right: "I am hearing that unless something changes pretty quick you are not going to be able to go to school any more. Have I got it right?"
- Ask the adolescent what she or he would like to happen but, as above, accept that they may have mixed feelings.
- Be patient. Unless it is an acute situation, consider continuing your assessment over more than one session.
- See the adolescent alone as well as with his or her parents.

Asking the difficult questions

About sexual abuse (see also p. 1136)

Sexual and other forms of abuse are common specific and nonspecific vulnerability factors for poor mental health and must be excluded as an etiological factor. The clinician's task is to find an approach to asking about abuse that they are comfortable with and that the child appears to be comfortable with. One approach is a hierarchical set of questions.

- Introductory comment: "I ask these questions to all children I see."
- Ask the child to respond to a broad, nonleading statement: "Some children tell me something has happened to them that they wish had never happened." The child's response may be verbal or nonverbal affirmation, denial, or looking perplexed; they may not understand the question at all.
- Ask more specific questions: "Some things are done by other people…" or "…. are touched in places where they wished they had not been touched."
- Ask very specific questions: "Some people are touched in places like their private parts, vagina, or penis (the language depends on age; you may also point or draw picture). Has this happened to you?"

Partial affirmation or nonverbal cues that are suggestive should be followed up during later appointments. One caveat is that there are differences between a purely forensic and a clinical interview. In both settings open, nonleading questions are preferable. Local protocols will also guide assessments.

About suicidal intent

Clinicians must ask about suicidal thinking, especially of adolescents with any depressive features. *Asking does not create or promote suicidal thinking.* Again, a hierarchical approach is used effectively by many clinicians.

- Introductory comment: "I ask these questions of everyone I see."
- Ask the adolescent to respond to a broad statement: "Some young people tell me that they feel life is not worth living anymore." Again, look for responses that may be verbal or nonverbal affirmation or denial.

Ask more specific questions:
- "Have you considered what it would be like to not be alive?" or "Some people think it would be better to be dead."

Ask very specifically to clarify risk and extent of planning:
- "Have you thought of killing yourself?" "Have you ever made a plan to kill yourself?" "Have you ever lost control and started your plan?"
- Are you thinking of killing yourself now?" "Do you have a plan to kill yourself now?"

As above, partial affirmation or nonverbal cues that are suggestive should be followed up during later appointments.

Treatment overview

As with all medical conditions, a decision needs to be made as to whether children and adolescents with psychiatric illnesses should be treated by primary-care providers or by specialists. Primary-care providers can be a significant component of a comprehensive care team. At a minimum, they must be able to recognize significant mental illness and make appropriate referrals.

Psychotherapy

Individual psychotherapy

All health professionals working with children talk to the children by themselves sometimes. All try to be helpful, and probably most are helpful at least some of the time. So in what way is psychotherapy different from an informal, helpful chat?

Perhaps the key element is that the treatment is delivered by a trained therapist who carries it out within a theoretical framework. A wide range of individual therapies exist, described below.

Behavioral therapy

This therapy is brief and is directed at encouraging desired behaviors and eliminating problem behaviors. Problems are dealt with in a behavioral framework rather than through focus on underlying thoughts, feelings, or past causes.

Cognitive-behavioral therapy (CBT)

CBT is like behavioral therapy but with a wider focus on thoughts and attribution of meaning, as well as behavior. This is one of the more well-researched therapies, although there remains a shortage of trained therapists. CBT involves the keeping of diaries and homework between sessions.

Psychodynamic psychotherapy

This longer-term treatment is directed at underlying problems and the presenting symptom. Central to treatment are theories of the unconscious mind. The patient uses the relationship with the therapist to play out dysfunctional patterns of behavior. The therapist is able to comment on these and help the patient to understand new ways of relating.

Therapy in the younger age-group may be based more on play materials such as animals, crayons, and paper. To complicate matters, there are also play therapists who are not necessarily psychodynamic in their orientation.

The inevitable question arises as to which therapy is better. This question is difficult to answer, as short therapies directed to diagnostic-related groups are easier to evaluate. There is a growing body of evidence in controlled trials to support the use of CBT in a range of conditions and less support for psychodynamic psychotherapy.

That being said, it is also probably true that well-motivated, intelligent, articulate patients without previous problems and from well-functioning families are likely to do better with any therapy modality. Nonspecific factors about therapists (e.g., empathy, good listening, and warmth) may be prerequisites to effective treatment, whatever the model.

Family therapy

This term covers a wide range of treatments with a similar diversity of theoretical underpinnings. They share the idea that problems are affected by the communication among family members and that such communication can serve to maintain or ameliorate difficulties.

One of the points of difference concerns understanding of the problem. Family therapy based on systems theory might identify recurring dysfunctional patterns of interaction and typically might hypothesize that the presenting problem in one family member is in fact a manifestation of these patterns. Such a view of pathology being located between rather than within people may be at odds with the Western focus on the individual.

An example of this approach is the school-refusing child who is being kept home to act as a buffer between parents who are in conflict. The child's presence may prevent dangerous escalation, but may also interfere with the parent's ability to resolve their differences. In this case, therapy might focus on helping the parents to address their difficulties without involvement of the child, and on helping the child to trust the parents to do this and get on with being a child, e.g., going to school.

An alternative is to help the family members reach an awareness that they are feeling overwhelmed by the problem, have lost confidence, and are not seeing that they have the resources to deal with it. They might, for instance, be helped to think of occasions when the parents managed their difficulties without the interference or help from their child. They may be helped to see how they do this and to do it more. The child may be helped to see that he or she at times overcomes fear and gets on with being a child, and can do this more often.

At the other end of the spectrum family therapy can be considered for multifactorial illnesses such as autism, which is not a product of any particular family pattern or dysfunction. The family can nonetheless be helped to manage this better. Such an approach is likely to focus on support, psychoeducation, and helping the family to address the developmental (independence) issues that any family will face but that are much more difficult when there is a child with chronic illness or disability.

Outcome

The heterogeneity of family therapy, the wide variety of problems it is used to address, and the sometimes overemphasis on complex theory, which can seem a long way from clinical practice, have contributed to a dearth of outcomes research. There is evidence, however, for effectiveness in treating a range of conditions, including anorexia nervosa, conduct disorder, and anxiety disorders.

Contraindications

Family therapy is not possible if the family cannot or will not attend. It is contraindicated in families where one member is being severely scapegoated. Unless there is reason to believe that such a family is open to the idea of doing things differently once this pattern is identified, family therapy should be discontinued.

Psychopharmacotherapy

Prescribing of psychotropics in children and adolescents should occur within the previously described theoretical framework. Also relevant are the following:

- Developmental factors, e.g., dosage by weight
- Systemic factors include the fact that any prescription is a complicated dynamic involving at least the child and their parents.
- Medication use in schools must also involve the teacher and school authorities.
- Mixed societal views exist about the use of medication for mental health in general and specifically for children.
- Not all mental health–allied professionals hold positive views that medication is effective; some nonprofessional groups are openly antagonistic.

Compliance can be a challenge. Current evidence-based medicine summaries do not comprise a comprehensive review of child and adolescent mental-health prescribing (see Cochrane Library). There are many listed protocols; over time it is hoped there will be more consistent coverage from completed reviews.

For specific prescribing information, indications, contraindications, precautions, side effects, and dosage regimens the reader should consult an up-to-date formulary. One reference text[1] offers the following useful headings in a section on general principles:

- First do no harm.
- Know the disorder and use drugs when indicated.
- Choose the best drug.
- Understand the drug and its properties.
- Minimize drug use and dosage.
- Keep things simple.
- Avoid polypharmacy.
- Don't be a fiddler or follow fads.
- Take particular care with children.
- Establish a therapeutic relationship.
- Compliance (adherence) with treatment

It should be noted that while some mental health presentations may respond to medication alone, for individuals with multiple comorbidities, impairment across domains, and distressed parents, medication is invariably adjunctive to or part of a comprehensive, overall management plan.[2]

---

1 Werry JS, Aman MC (1999). *Practitioners Guide to Psychoactive Drug for Children & Adolescents*, 2nd edition, New York & London: Plenum Medical Book Company.
2 Martin A, Scahill L, Charney D, Leckman J (eds.) (2003). *Pediatric Psychopharmacology: Principles and Practice*. New York: Oxford University Press.

Depression

Loose usage of the word *depression* causes much confusion. It can refer to a mood, which may be appropriate, to a symptom, or to a mental disorder.

Prevalence

Approximately 10% of 10-year-olds are reported by parents and teachers and 20% of 14-year-olds report themselves to be often sad and miserable. However, the rate of diagnosable depressive disorder in community samples of 11- to 16-year-olds is closer to 3%. The discrepancy is due to those who suffer low moods but do not meet diagnostic criteria. Depressive disorders, however, are much more common in children and adolescents who present to medical settings such as emergency rooms or pediatricians' offices.

Etiology

Genetic disposition, temperament, biological factors, and chronically poor life circumstances have all been implicated. Seligman's theory of learned helplessness is pertinent: Dogs given repeated electric shocks that they are unable to avoid eventually stop trying, even when escape is made possible. Some depressed children and adolescents seem to fit this pattern.

Clinical features

Diagnosis of depressive disorder requires that mood be persistently lowered and accompanied by a lack of pleasure. Among those referred to child psychiatric clinics comorbidity is common, e.g., conduct disorder, ADHD, and anxiety disorders. There also may be

• Weight change
• Sleep disturbance
• Agitation or psychomotor retardation
• Poor concentration
• Thoughts of death

Disorders may be divided into the following:
• *Major depressive episode*: With severe symptoms of at least 2 weeks duration (single episode, chronic, or recurrent)
• *Dysthymia*: Enduring depressed state of at least 1 year without the intensity of a major depressive episode)

Management

Medications

The most commonly used medications are the selective serotonin re-uptake inhibitor antidepressants (SSRIs). Recently there has been concern about side effects (including increased suicidal ideation and attempts) as well as efficacy. In the United States, fluoxetine is the only medication currently indicated for depression in children and adolescents, although there also have been positive trials with sertraline and citalopram. Tricyclics antidepressants appear to be ineffective.

Psychological therapies

Cognitive behavior therapy has the greatest evidence of efficacy. Most of the research has been done in adults. While children and adolescents do show short-term benefit, longer-term effects are still to be demonstrated. Intervention in the social context of the child or adolescent may also be indicated (e.g., family, parent mental health, school and friends).

Prognosis

While recovery from a depressive disorder is likely, this may take months or in some cases years. Prognosis is worsened by increasing severity of disorder and by the presence of comorbid oppositional defiant disorder. Even in those who have made a good recovery, recurrent depressive episodes are common (70% by 5 years). Prolonged follow up is, therefore, wise.

Suicide and nonfatal deliberate self-harm

Suicide is very rare in prepubertal children but rises in incidence through the teenage years; it is the third most common cause of death in the 15–19 year age group in the United States. Up to 20% of adolescents have suicidal ideation each year.

Nonfatal deliberate self-harm is common, affecting perhaps 500 per 100,000 15- to 19-year-olds per year. Some of those individuals who do kill themselves were ambivalent or did not intend to, and some of those who harm themselves without causing death did intend suicide.

Predisposing characteristics to completed suicide include the following:
- Psychiatric disorder (such as conduct disorder, depression, substance misuse, and psychosis)
- Social isolation
- Physical illness
- Low self-esteem

Relevant family factors include a family history of abuse and neglect or of psychiatric illness and suicide, and family dysfunction. The profile of those who nonfatally self-harm is in many respects similar. Notable differences include suicide being more common among males, and deliberate self-harm among females.

Methods of self-harm

Those who kill themselves use a range of methods, most commonly:
- Drug overdose
- Shooting
- Inhaling car exhaust fumes
- Hanging
- Suffocation

The vast majority of nonfatal deliberate self-harm is through overdosing, generally with analgesics or prescribed drugs such as antidepressants. Repeated scratching, picking at scabs, and burning are also common. Cutting is very common, particularly among adolescent girls.

Unless the cutting is particularly deep and over the site of major blood vessels, it should not be seen as necessarily linked to suicide or attempted suicide. Those who cut typically describe it as easing a buildup of bad feelings, resolving a state of emotional numbness, or sometimes as a form of self-punishment.

Management

The key to management is careful assessment. This should happen as soon as is feasible after the self-harm. Assessment should include the young person, the family, and, where relevant, information from other sources such as the family doctor or social services. Assessment should include the following:

• Details of the event (degree of isolation, potential lethality of the method, precautions to avoid detection, whether there was a suicide note)
• The presence of psychiatric disorder
• The degree of suicide intent
• The past history of self-harm

Focus management on alleviating the above factors. Psychiatric inpatient admission is occasionally required, although most of those who self-harm can be discharged home with outpatient treatment as appropriate.

Treatment interventions that have been tried include systems to make it easier for teenagers to access help rather than repeat their self-harm. Evaluation of these interventions has yielded encouraging but inconclusive results. Parental attitudes to behavior will also effect management and outcome.

Prognosis

Approximately 10% of those who self-harm will repeat the behavior within a year. A significant, though unknown, proportion will kill themselves within 5 years.

Bipolar disorder

Bipolar disorder in children and adolescents is a topic of considerable controversy in the United States. The traditional view in adults of onset in late adolescence to early adult life and of distinct periods of abnormal mood is not typically seen in children and adolescents with this diagnosis. Rather, they tend to have a more chronic state of irritability and don't have the cardinal symptoms of grandiosity or elated mood.

Epidemiology

There is a rising prevalence of this diagnosis being made. Whether there is an actual rise in prevalence or a change in diagnostic practice is currently a matter of intense debate.

Etiology

There is a strong underlying genetic vulnerability associate with bipolar disorder. Substance abuse may precipitate presentation, but it is not a primary etiologic factor.

Clinical features

The hallmark feature of bipolar disorder is a cyclical course. Frank mania is a distinct period of abnormally and persistently elevated mood, lasting at least 1 week or resulting in hospitalization.

Differential diagnosis

Distinction needs to be made from disruptive behavior disorders, including ADHD, and from other psychotic conditions, including schizophrenia.

Management

If bipolar disorder is truly present, the best treatment is a combination of supportive psychotherapeutic interventions including CBT, social-rhythms therapy, and psychoeducation in conjunction with mood-stabilizing medications.

Psychopharmacologic interventions include lithium, mood-stabilizing anticonvulsants, and atypical antipsychotics. There are prominent side effects with these medications, particularly weight gain. Their use should not be taken lightly. If substance abuse is present, it must be addressed as well.

Prognosis

There is some suggestion that bipolar disorder in adolescence is more serious than it is in adults.

Anxiety disorders

Diagnostic criteria

One anxiety disorder is uniquely described in children: separation anxiety disorder (SAD). Other diagnoses that may occur in children and adolescents are generalized specific anxiety disorder (GAD), panic disorder with and without specific agoraphobia, phobias, social phobias, obsessive-compulsive disorder (OCD), and post-traumatic stress disorder (PTSD). Specific physical and cognitive symptoms are described for each disorder. Developmental principles apply.

- Very young children experience "stranger danger" and later simple phobias and SAD with the beginning of the school years.
- Middle-childhood presentations include fears of animals, the dark, burglars, and anxiety-related abdominal pain.
- A recrudescence or first presentation of SAD may occur at the onset of secondary schooling.
- Adolescents may experience social phobia, OCD, and panic with or without agoraphobia.

Prevalence

Rates vary by disorder. SAD, GAD, and OCD are not uncommon presentations to tertiary clinics. Panic disorders are less common.

Differential diagnosis

Child abuse may present as an anxiety disorder. Anxiety and depression often co-occur. Truancy must be differentiated from separation anxiety. Acting-out behavior may be due to anxiety.

Prominent physical symptoms, especially without typical anxiety-related onset (e.g., Monday morning stomach pains) should be investigated. Occasionally, you must decide "who has the anxiety"—the child not wanting to go to school, the parent fearful for the child, or both.

Treatment

While anxiety disorders have specific treatments, general principles include the following:

- Clarity of diagnosis and psychoeducation of child and parents (over-investigation often causes more anxiety)
- Helping the child to face their fears, usually by hierarchical desensitization. Rapid-exposure techniques (flooding or implosion) are rarely used.
- Identification of unhelpful, distorted, or maintaining cognitions, challenging these cognitions, and practicing more functioning thinking
- Skills acquisition, e.g., progressive muscle relaxation, guided imagery
- Parents as motivators and behavioral coaches
- Early relapse identification

Medication

The best evidence for medical treatment of anxiety disorders is for OCD, for which three SSRIs have an FDA indication in the United States: sertraline, fluvoxamine, and fluoxetine. There also is an indication for the tricyclic antidepressant clomipramine. Comparatively less research has been done on medical treatment of other anxiety conditions, but there are some data on the benefit of treating SAD, GAD, and social phobia with SSRIs.

For children who are acutely anxious, it is appropriate to consider benzodiazepines, although the evidence for this is best for adults and not as substantial for children and adolescents. It is important to note in the treatment of anxiety conditions, particularly with the use of SSRIs or tricyclics, that initiation of pharmacologic treatment may be associated with increased anxiety. It is important to begin doses modestly and to advance dosage with careful attention to the development of side effects.

Special mention is necessary regarding clomipramine: it is a secondary medication for the treatment of OCD, as there are potential cardiovascular side effects that must be taken into consideration. Baseline electrocardiograms and vital signs are necessary, as is monitoring of blood levels to not exceed 400 ng/mL.

Prognosis

Anxiety disorders predict later internalizing conditions in girls and externalizing disorders in boys. Short-term outcome of treatment is positive, especially in conjunction with parental support.

Post-traumatic stress disorder (PTSD)

Prevalence

There is no unitary prevalence—all traumatic events vary in threat exposure, and individual responses vary by developmental stage, past experiences, and competencies. Prevalence varies, from 100% among children taken hostage, to 10% after natural disasters. Girls may report more PTSD symptoms.

Diagnostic criteria

A range of psychopathology may be experienced following an emotionally traumatic event, dependent on preexisting vulnerabilities, event exposure, and related loss and grief. PTSD has four symptom clusters:

A. Exposure to a traumatic event, threatened death, or serious injury and the response was horror, helplessness, or disorganized behavior
B. Re-experiencing phenomena, e.g., nightmares, flashbacks
C. Persistent avoidance, emotional numbing, and detachment
D. Persistent symptoms of increased arousal, e.g., hypervigilance

Age-specific symptoms

Younger children often present as regressing with altered sleep and feeding routines; exhibiting clingy, anxious, or aggressive behavior; or engaging in post-traumatic play. Young children may not be able to report emotional numbing or detachment; parents may report these symptoms as a "personality change."

Differential diagnosis

This consists of other anxiety disorders, including event-related phobias, GAD, OCD, or, if of lesser severity, an adjustment disorder. Comorbidity with depression is common. If trauma is repetitive, expect disruptive behaviors in boys and early evidence of personality dysfunction and interpersonal problems in teenagers.

Treatment

If the condition is severe, treatment can be complex and take time. Interventions include cognitive strategies such as identifying and modifying dysfunctional schema; behavioral strategies including prolonged re-exposure; skills acquisition such as relaxation techniques; and supportive therapy and family interventions to monitor for secondary impairment and altered family functioning.

The best evidence for psychotherapy is with trauma-focused cognitive–behavioral therapy. Eye movement desensitization and reprocessing (EMDR) may have a role.

Psychopharmacology may provide some symptomatic relief, typically with SSRIs. There have been no controlled trials, however, demonstrating benefit with medications for PTSD in youth, though benefit has been shown in adults.

Prognosis

Many children seem to be resilient to traumatic events, whereas others have long-term problems including symptom chronicity, generalization of fears, altered cognitive safety schema, and impairment in education and psychosocial domains, especially if parents have been unable to help the child manage their trauma. A history of chronic, repetitive trauma, such as sexual abuse, is overrepresented in other mental health presentations including drug and alcohol abuse, bulimia, and youth on borderline personality trajectories.

Attachment disorder

Developed by John Bowlby (1908–90), attachment theory describes attachment as a biological and adaptive two-way process. It provides an emotional connection, most obviously to members of the child's family, and serves the needs of the child for protection and nurture. Early attachment patterns can be categorized as follows:

- *Secure*: In the mother's presence the child feels safe enough to explore. On her return, the mother is able to comfort the child, who briefly seeks her reassurance before returning to play.
- *Anxious/resistant*: Initially the child does not feel safe enough to leave and explore. The mother's attempts to comfort may escalate the child's distress.
- *Anxious/avoidant*: The child explores easily and is quick to interact with a stranger with whom he or she is left. The mother's return evokes little interest in the child.
- *Disorganized/disoriented*: Return of the mother provokes confused and ambivalent feelings in the child who seems to want her, but is also angry or fearful.

A secure attachment is likely to result in the interaction of favorable infant characteristics (e.g., temperament) with favorable environmental conditions (e.g., well-functioning family). The children in the disorganized/ disoriented group are particularly at risk of unfavorable outcomes.

Disturbed attachment may be found among children with a range of diagnoses, e.g., conduct disorder, children with no disorder, or those identified as experiencing a primary attachment disorder. The criterion for a primary attachment disorder is that the child fails to make specific attachments to a small number of caregivers, despite having adequate intelligence.

The DSM classification system does not follow the dominant research paradigm (see above), but rather defines two phenotypes:

- *Inhibited type*: The child shows little or no interest in forming attachments. He or she is typically fearful, miserable looking, and may exhibit hyper-vigilance. Self-harm is common and there may be failure to thrive.
- *Disinhibited type*: The child is unduly friendly with strangers, does not seem to mind who looks after her or him, and forms superficial relationships easily. Such children may be overactive or aggressive, show emotional lability, or poorly tolerate frustration.

Attachment disorders of either type tend to be seen in children who have been severely neglected or raised in a series of institutions and foster homes.

Management

The principle of treatment is to support the child's caregivers (whoever they are) to
- Provide consistent warmth
- Set limits and improve communication and peer relationships

Removal of a child with an attachment disorder from an unsatisfactory home is not usually the end of the story. Further help is likely to be needed in the new environment. Working with a dyad (e.g., mother and child) is usually indicated.

Schizophrenia

Schizophrenia is characterized by disorders of thought, perception, mood, and sometimes posture. Peak onset is in young adult life. Prevalence in the mid-teens is ~0.25%, less in the prepubertal child, and higher among boys.

Etiology

There is a genetic contribution, with first-degree relatives of a patient with schizophrenia having a 12-fold increase in risk of developing the illness.

Clinical features

The features of schizophrenia are complex. Onset may be insidious or acute. Core features of schizophrenia include the following:

- *Thought disorder*: Thoughts are inserted or removed from one's head or broadcast to others.
- *Auditory or visual hallucinations*: External voices discuss the patient or comment on their behavior; the patient sees apparitions.
- *Delusions*: Fixed beliefs that are false, not open to reason, and not in keeping with the patient's cultural context
- *Disorders of posture*: Holding abnormal postures

Differential diagnosis

Important differential diagnoses include affective psychosis, drug-induced psychoses, and psychoses secondary to an organic state.

Assessment

Because a schizophrenia-type psychosis can be caused by organic conditions, it is essential that signs of these be sought. Include a full neurological examination and imaging, and check for thyroid, adrenal, or pituitary dysfunction and screen for drug abuse.

Management

Schizophrenia is often complex and difficult to treat. Psychiatric admission may be required to ensure the patient's safety. Antipsychotic medication, most commonly the newer atypical antipsychotics such as risperidone, olanzapine, quetiapine, ziprasidone, or aripiprazole, are agents of first choice with preferable side-effect profiles.

While the newer atypical antipsychotics are generally better tolerated, there are significant side effects, including weight gain, elevated prolactin levels, and possibly diabetes. Relapses are fewer when families are supportive but nonintrusive and not critical.

The acute phase can progress to a chronic state with poor motivation and inactivity. Clozapine (an atypical antipsychotic drug) may ameliorate this but can cause agranulocytosis and other serious side effects, so ongoing close monitoring is essential, including blood work.

Prognosis

Prognosis is relatively good for an acute episode in a previously well-functioning teenager. It is worse for insidiously developing illness, particularly in a child with preexisting developmental difficulties. The differentiation between schizophrenia and affective psychosis may be particularly difficult.

Somatoform disorders and typical consultation–liaison presentations

This is a broad area with a host of overlapping terms and confusion between description and implied etiology. Some of the terms are the following:

- *Psychosomatic*: A very general and rather unhelpful term that can include illnesses brought on by stress (e.g., tension headache). Physical symptoms due to psychiatric illness, e.g., hypothermia secondary to malnutrition in anorexia nervosa
- *Somatoform disorders*: Physical symptoms with no organic basis. These are subdivided into
  - Conversion disorders
  - Hypochondriasis
  - Pain disorders
  - Somatization disorder

While many of these terms are entrenched and thus unlikely to disappear, the concept of somatoform disorders has been much criticized on the grounds that

- It implies a cause that is not demonstrable and often intuitively does not appear to be correct.
- It is often unacceptable to patients and parents and is therefore an obstacle to forming a collaborative relationship.
- Its use may result in missing psychiatric or physical diagnoses.
- There seems little relationship between this term and other diagnoses commonly applied to the same patients in non-mental-health settings, e.g., irritable bowel syndrome, chronic fatigue.

Conversion disorder

This disorder is characterized by the presence of physical symptoms (e.g., paralysis, seizures, sensory deficits) or mental symptoms (e.g., amnesia) but without any evidence of physical cause. Previously it was called hysteria.

The proposed underlying mechanism is transformation of emotional conflict into mental or physical symptoms. The postulated splitting off of mental processes from each other is referred to as *dissociation*.

There may be secondary gain, e.g., when the child who is being bullied at school develops paralysis, which keeps him at home and thus not teased. Conversion disorders are rare in childhood, particularly before the age of 8 years.

Treatment

Principles of treatment include attempts to resolve any apparent emotional difficulties, avoidance of unnecessary physical investigation, removal of secondary gain, and help returning to normal life.

Prognosis

Prognosis is generally favorable.

Recurrent nonorganic abdominal pain

The child's complaints of recurrent abdominal pain are not found to have a physical basis (see also p. 364).

- Common, affecting ~10%–15% of children at some point, usually between ages 5 and 12 years (no gender or social-class bias)
- There may be associated symptoms of other pains, nausea, or even vomiting.
- Pains are usually episodic and relapsing, though they may be more persistent.
- An uncommon variant is the periodic syndrome, in which episodes of pain are associated with vomiting, headache, and low-grade pyrexia. This is thought by some to be a form of migraine.

Differentiation from organic pathology may be difficult. Features that may help include the diffuseness of the pain, the tendency not to be woken by it, pains elsewhere in the body, anxiety and depression in the child and parent, and the lack of positive findings on physical examination.

Treatment

Generally this consists of a combination of reassurance, education about the links between stress and the body, psychological treatment when appropriate, and avoidance of unnecessary physical investigation and treatment.

Prognosis

Short-term outcome is usually favorable, although it is not known whether this is due to treatment. In the longer term, further episodes of nonorganic pain are found in a large minority of cases.

Selective eating

This is a condition of younger children that in most, though not all, resolves in the teenage years. These children eat only a limited range of foods. In severe cases the restriction may be to only 3 or 4 foods. It is surprising that most children seem to ingest all the required nutrients in their very limited diet.

To treat this condition a mixture of reassurance and encouragement seems to be the best approach. More active intervention is indicated when the child is malnourished, and usually entails a gradual hierarchical desensitization program.

Anorexia nervosa

Epidemiology

Anorexia nervosa (AN) is a common chronic illness in teenage girls. Prevalence in the Western world is ~0.5%. While varying with age, a sex ratio of 9:1 girls/boys is fairly typical. Prepubertal cases are rare but do occur.

Etiology

This is often unclear in individual cases; however, genetic predisposition, a perfectionist personality, and low self-esteem seem to be implicated. Dissatisfaction with weight and shape is relatively common among girls as young as 8 years and is presumably a vulnerability factor.

The pathway to AN is through weight loss with a desire to lose weight. Onset may be associated with depression/anxiety, or viral illness.

Diagnostic features

- Dietary restriction (may be accompanied by vomiting, excessive exercise, laxative abuse, or other weight-control methods) leading to significant and unhealthy weight loss (e.g., to <85% of expected body weight for height or age) or to stunting of expected growth
- Intense fear of gaining weight even when severely underweight
- Disturbance of experience of weight and shape with feelings of being fat or bloated
- Amenorrhea (may be primary or secondary)

In younger teenagers, anorexic thoughts may often be either absent or hidden, e.g., the fear of becoming fat may be absent because they "know" they can control their weight. Individuals who exhibit significant weight-losing behaviors not explained by depression, a specific phobia, or physical illnesses may be referred to as having atypical eating disorders.

Treatment

The evidence base for treatment is small. Involvement of the family seems important. Correction of dangerous weight loss or complications such as hypokalemia, bradycardia, or cardiac failure may be urgent.

Treatment is likely to be lengthy and involve attention to anorexic behaviors, recognizing and not acting on anorexic thoughts and feelings, and returning to aspects of normal function such as school and home life. It is far preferable to work collaboratively with the young person. At times, compulsory treatment (requiring parental consent or involuntary mental-health treatment authorization) may be needed.

Patients who are unable or unwilling to manage adequate oral nutrition may need nasogastric feeding. In any rapid refeeding plan the risks of refeeding syndrome (p. 378) should be remembered. Medication (with SSRIs) may have a role if depression or OCD is present.

Prognosis

The prognosis for teenagers is variable, though generally better than for adults, with most patients making a full recovery. However, this can take years, and an interim step may be to learn how to live with the illness rather than be controlled by it.

Bulimia nervosa

- 2–3 times more common than AN in adolescents
- Affects girls predominantly
- Bulimic symptoms may occur as part of AN or during recovery
- Onset of bulimia nervosa is generally in adolescence.

Diagnostic criteria

- Recurrent episodes of binge eating
- During bingeing a lack of feeling of control
- Regular use of mechanisms to reduce weight gain from bingeing (e.g., vomit induction, laxatives, diuretics, appetite suppressants, excessive exercise)
- Persistent concern with fatness
- Body weight higher than that required for a diagnosis of anorexia

Repeated vomiting and/or laxative abuse may result in serious electrolyte disturbance, seizures, tetany, hematemesis, or stomach rupture.

Management

- Assess for a concurrent personality disorder.
- Cognitive–behavioral therapy including education on healthy eating, starvation, and bingeing
- Pharmacotherapy (e.g., SSRIs such as fluoxetine) may be helpful.

Oppositional defiant and conduct disorders

Oppositional defiant (ODD) and conduct disorder (CD) are related disruptive behavior disorders, typified by defiance, disobedience, and violation of social rules and the rights of others.

Epidemiology
- Both CD and ODD are overrepresented in males
- ODD is evident in younger children (under 10 years).
- CD prevalence increases with age: ~6% in children and 10% in adolescents.

Etiology
Longitudinal studies of delinquency suggest the cause is complex. Many individuals are likely to have an underlying genetic vulnerability and subsequent exposure to coercive parenting (intrusive parenting and subsequent reinforcement of child counterattack and parent withdrawal) early in life. Later involvement of these vulnerable individuals with a deviant peer group predicts a CD pathway.

Clinical features
The name ODD is highly descriptive—i.e., hostile, negativistic, and defiant, particularly to the parents. The defiant behavior pattern must last at least 6 months and cause impairment across a variety of domains. CD is usually obvious by early adolescence. Features are more serious aggressive behavior, rule violation, property damage, theft, arson, truancy, and running away.

Differential diagnosis
Comorbidity with other disruptive behavior disorders is common, e.g., ADHD (p. 700). Speech and language deficits may be comorbid or on a causal pathway: school failure, involvement with a less achieving and more deviant peer group, and modeling and reinforcement of delinquent behavior.

Management
Prevention is the best medicine. Early intervention with ODD in very young children, using universal parenting programs that target coercive parenting and parental abuse, is indicated.

If ODD and CD are established, programs that employ intensive interventions involving children, parents, and other participants in the child's social ecology have proved effective. Multisystemic therapy is an example of such an intervention.

Remedial education is likely to be needed and can also be helpful as self-esteem rises.

Psychopharmacology research on disruptive behavior disorders, other than ADHD, presently provides limited information.

- ADHD comorbidity should be treated.
- Planned, premeditated aggression is not an indication for drug therapy.
- Impulsive aggression or aggression in an individual with prominent affective symptoms may prove responsive to a novel antipsychotic such as risperidone or to mood-stabilizing anticonvulsants such as valproic acid. Further research is required.

Prognosis

Management of established disorders is difficult. Children often fail at school. Delinquent behavior, often displayed by individuals with conduct disorder, most commonly occurs in late adolescence and is surprisingly frequent; the cumulative conviction prevalence is 40% of all males by age 40 years.[1]

---

1 Farrington DP (1998). Predictors, causes and correlates of youth violence. In Tonry M, Moore MH (eds.). *Youth Violence*. Chicago: University of Chicago Press.

Attention deficit hyperactivity disorder (ADHD)

The conceptualization of ADHD has varied from 19th-century views of impulsive insanity and defective inhibition, to Still's description of hyperactive children, to biological formulations of brain damage and dysfunction, to the current operationalized criteria.

Recent advances in the genetic epidemiology of ADHD are counterpoised with ongoing controversy around diagnosis and treatment. Questions remain as to whether too many or too few children are being treated for ADHD; there are data to support either side of the argument.

Prevalence

Estimates of prevalence vary, but likely it is about 6%, being 2–3 times more common in boys, and decreases with increasing age.

Diagnostic criteria

Inattention

- Fails to attend to detail
- Difficulty sustaining attention
- Does not follow through
- Difficulty organizing tasks, easily distracted
- Reluctance at engaging if sustained mental effort is required

Hyperactivity

- Often fidgets
- Leaves seat in classroom
- Runs and climbs excessively
- Often on the go
- Acts driven

Impulsivity

- Often blurts out answer
- Difficulty waiting turn
- Interrupts

Symptoms must be present for at least 6 months, with onset before age 7 years plus evidence of impairment in two or more functional domains or settings. Inattentive, hyperactive-impulsive, and combined subtypes are described. It is essential to use appropriate developmental references in making the diagnosis.

Differential diagnosis

Difficulties occur in differentiating age-appropriate boisterousness and activity from ADHD. Inattention may be due to understimulation of children with above-average intelligence or seen in children in classroom settings too advanced for their mental age. ADHD symptoms are common in PTSD (p. 688) and PDDs (p. 702).

Common comorbidities
- Disruptive-behavior disorders
- Anxiety
- Depression
- Learning, speech, and language disorders are also overrepresented.

Treatment
Psychopharmacology
Psychostimulants (methylphenidate, dextroamphetamine, mixed salts of amphetamine, dexmethylphenicate) are the medications of first choice. Second-line medication includes atomoxetine and the α_2-agonists clonidine and guanfacine. Third-line medications include tricyclic antidepressants and modafinil.

Behavioral interventions
Integrated home and school behavior management, token economies, and parent effectiveness have shown some benefits in specific symptoms associated with ADHD, including social-skills relationships, social skills, and academic performance.

A multisite, randomized trial (NIMH-MTA) study of the combined subtype of ADHD found that over 14 months, expert management of medications was superior in treating core ADHD symptoms compared to treatment as usual in the community without benefit of additional sophisticated behavior treatment. However, other symptoms such as social skills, anxiety, and aggression were modulated by the addition of behavior management.

Prognosis
- 70%–80% continue to display symptoms as adolescents.
- 50%–65% display symptoms as adults.
- Only 10%–20% reach adulthood without any psychiatric diagnosis, functioning well and without symptoms of their disorder.

Pervasive developmental disorders (PDD)

Disorders in this cluster, also called *autistic spectrum disorders*, have common clinical features in the areas of communication, social relatedness, movement, and intrapersonal relations. Nosological issues include the diagnostic distinctiveness of syndromes and whether presentations can change over time.

The prevalence has reportedly increased over time. It is unclear whether this is a result of increased case finding or is an actual increase. PDDs include
- Autistic disorder
- Rett's syndrome
- Asperger's disorder

Etiology

It is likely that the PDDs are heterogeneous in etiology. Most believe there are underlying complex, genetic vulnerabilities with subsequent environmental influences and factors that trigger gene expression.

Recent functional neuroimaging studies have led to a wide variety of neurobiological hypotheses. It is likely that numerous neural systems are involved, with a focus on areas typically implicated in emotional regulation such as the limbic system.

Clinical features

- Usually identified in the preschool years but may be found later in individuals with above-average IQ.
- Problems with social interactions include appearing aloof, impaired nonverbal behaviors, difficulty establishing friendships, and poor or absent emotional reciprocity.
- Mental retardation, language delay, and medical complications such as epilepsy often coexist with a PDD diagnosis.
- Communication problems include marked delay of or lack of speech, inability to converse, and abnormal speech, including stereotypic speech.
- Behavior problems include preoccupied, stereotypic behaviors (e.g., hand flapping). In adolescence aggressiveness, mood variability, and sexually inappropriate behavior can be problematic.

Management

No single intervention appears superior. Psychosocial interventions, often with an emphasis on behavior management and parent involvement, can lead to increased child skills and have high parent satisfaction. However, such improvement does not usually lead to significant changes on standardized measures or improve the overall developmental trajectory.

Recent studies with atypical neuroleptics, particularly risperidone, hold much promise for improvement of global functioning. For an in-depth discussion of recent assessment, etiological, and treatment research see Volkmar FR, Lord C, Bailey A, Schultz RT, Klin A (2004). Autism and pervasive developmental disorders. *J Child Psychol Psychiatry* **45**(1):135–170.

Prognosis

Prognosis is quite variable, being better for Asperger's disorder than for autistic disorders, for which
- 70% remain severely handicapped,
- 50% develop useful speech, and
- 5% will lead independent adult lives.

Hematology

Peripheral blood smear

Table 17.1 Causes of complete blood count (CBC) blood smear abnormalities

Acanthocytes	Abetalipoproteinemia, protein kinase deficiency, chronic liver disease, hereditary acanthocytosis
Basophilia	Leukemia; inflammatory disorders, e.g., ulcerative colitis; drugs; infection
Burr cells	Renal failure
Elliptocytes	Hereditary elliptocytosis (p. 712)
Eosinophilia	Allergic syndromes, e.g., asthma; drugs; parasitic infection
Fragmented red blood cells (RBC)	Microangiopathic hemolytic anemia (p. 721), DIC (p. 731), HUS, renal failure
Heinz bodies (intracellular Hb precipitate)	G6PD deficiency (p. 713), hemoglobinopathies, post-splenectomy, hyposplenism
Howell–Jolly bodies (intracellular DNA fragments)	Hemoglobinopathies, post-splenectomy, leukemia, cytotoxic drugs, severe vitamin B_{12} or folate deficiency
Lymphocytopenia	Malignancy; infection, e.g., HIV; chemotherapy; liver or renal failure; aplastic anemia; congenital disorders, e.g., DiGeorge syndrome
Lymphocytosis	Leukemia (p. 754); lymphoma (p. 762); infection, e.g., EBV, CMV; trauma
Macrocytic RBC	Vitamin B_{12} or folate deficiency (p. 711), aplastic anemia (p. 722), normal neonatal blood picture (p. 194)
Microcytic RBC	Iron deficiency (p. 710), thalassemia (p. 718), anemia of chronic disease
Monocytopenia	Autoimmune disorders, e.g., SLE; drugs, e.g., corticoidsteroids; chemotherapy
Monocytosis	Malaria, typhoid, TB, infective endocarditis, post-chemotherapy, JMML
Neutropenia	See pp. 788
Neutrophilia	Infection, inflammation, chronic bleeding, post-splenectomy, drugs, e.g., corticosteroids
Polychromatic RBC	Recent blood loss, hemolysis, marrow infiltration
Reticulocytosis	Hemolysis, bleeding, response to iron, vitamin B_{12} or folate treatment, marrow infiltration

Table 17.1 (*Contd.*)

Sickle cells	Sickle cell anemia (p. 714)
Spherocytes	Hereditary spherocytosis (p. 712), isoimmune hemolytic disease, post-splenectomy
Target cells	Severe iron deficiency (p. 710), sickle cell disease, thalassemia, liver disease, post-splenectomy, asplenia syndrome
Thrombocytopenia	See p. 740
Thrombocytosis	See p. 739

Anemia

Red cell indices vary considerably with age. Hemoglobin (Hb) at birth may be as high as 20 g/dL but falls rapidly to about 10 g/dL by 2–3 months. A mild hypochromic, microcytic picture is common by age 3 years. Sex differences in red-cell indices do not appear until puberty.

Symptoms and signs of anemia
- Fatigue
- Dyspnea on exertion
- Poor growth
- Pallor
- Anorexia
- Rarely stomatitis or koilonychia

Diagnostic approach to anemia (see Table 17.2)

History
- Familial causes (sickle, thalassemia)
- Diet (cow's milk, vegan)
- Overt blood loss
- Duration of symptoms
- Drug history, e.g., NSAID

Examination
- Height and weight (failure to thrive [FTT], malabsorption)
- Jaundice (hemolysis)
- Adenopathy/organomegaly (underlying malignancy)

CBC and peripheral smear
- Mean cell volume (microcytic, macrocytic, normocytic)
- RBC (fragments, spherocytes)
- Other cytopenias

Table 17.2 Investigations for different types of anemia

Anemia type	Investigations
Microcytic anemia	Iron deficiency, thalassemias, anemia of chronic disease
Macrocytic anemia	Liver disease, B_{12}/folate deficiency, bone marrow failure syndromes (pure red-cell aplasia, aplastic anemia, Diamond–Blackfan anemia), myelodysplastic syndromes
Normocytic anemia	Combined iron and B_{12}/folate deficiency, anemia of chronic disease, recent bleeding
Hemolytic anemia	Suggested if there are RBC fragments or other morphologic abnormalities, with increased reticulocyte count Investigate as described on p. 709.

Hemolytic anemias

Hemolysis causes reduction in normal red blood cell (RBC) survival of 120 days. Causes can be intrinsic (RBC membrane defects, enzyme defects, or hemoglobinopathies) or extrinsic (immune or RBC fragmentation).

Diagnosis
History
- Symptoms (e.g., headache, dizziness, fever, chills, dark urine, back or abdominal pain)
- Possible precipitating factors (e.g., infection, medications, foods such as fava beans in G6PDdeficiency)
- Ancestry (e.g., African, Mediterranean, or Arabic ancestry is suggestive of G6PD deficiency in males)
- Family history (e.g., gallstones in spherocytosis)

Examination
- Temperature
- Splenomegaly
- Jaundice
- Gallstones
- Leg ulcers

Investigations
Specific tests include the following:
- *Increased RBC destruction* = Hb ↓, serum unconjugated bilirubin ↑, plasma haptoglobin ↓ (binds free Hb)
- *Increased RBC production* = reticulocytes↑, polychromasia, LDH↑
- *Abnormal blood smear*: Spherocytes or other RBC abnormalities, malaria parasites, features of RBC fragmentation (schistocytes, burr cells, or helmet cells)
- Thrombocytopenia and abnormal clotting suggest disseminated intravascular coagulation (DIC).
- Pancytopenia suggests hypersplenism.
- *Direct antiglobulin test* to establish if there is immune or nonimmune hemolysis. A positive direct antiglobulin test (DAT) = antibodies on RBC surface. A positive indirect test = antibodies in serum.
- *Hb electrophoresis*: Sickle cell anemia, thalassemias, unstable hemoglobins, e.g., Hb Koln
- *RBC enzyme assays*: RBC enzyme defects
- Intravascular hemolysis = free plasma Hb↑, hemoglobinuria, hemosiderin in urine
- *Red cell fragility test* for hereditary spherocytosis
- If DAT is positive, screen serum for red cell alloimmune antibodies, e.g., neonatal Rhesus or ABO hemolytic disease (see Chapter 6).
- If DAT is positive, IgG- and C_3-specific reagents suggest warm and cold antibody autoimmune hemolysis, respectively.
- *IgM* for mycoplasma; CMV, EBV, rubella for cold antibody autoimmune hemolysis
- *Immunophenotyping* (CD55 + CD59) for paroxysmal nocturnal hemoglobinuria

Deficiency anemias

Iron deficiency

This is the most common nutritional deficiency, occurring in 10%–30% of those at high risk:

- Preterm, low–birth weight infants; multiple births
- Exclusive breast-feeding >6 months, delayed introduction of iron-containing solids, excessive cow's milk (protein enteropathy)
- Adolescent females (growth spurt and menstruation)
- Low iron-containing diet due to poverty, fad diets, being strict vegans

Causes

- *Dietary*: This is the most common cause, e.g., exclusive breast-feeding >6 months, being strict vegans.
- *Infancy and early childhood*: Low levels of dietary iron (breast milk and cow's milk are low in iron), GI blood loss (cow's milk protein enteropathy)
- ↑ demand due to rapid growth, e.g., following prematurity or puberty
- *Malabsorption*, e.g., celiac disease, inflammatory bowel disease (IBD)
- *Blood loss*, e.g., Meckel diverticulum, angiodysplasia, esophagitis
- *Bleeding* (may be occult) secondary to drugs, e.g., NSAIDs, steroids
- Intestinal parasites

Presentation

- Most features are subclinical, as symptoms develop if iron deficiency is severe.
- Neurological effects of listlessness and irritability (infants), mood changes, and reduced cognitive and psychomotor performance can occur at levels at mild–moderate deficiency, i.e., before anemia develops.
- Insidious onset of symptoms of anemia
- Pica (eating unusual items, e.g., soil) occurs rarely.

Diagnosis

Iron deficiency anemia is a sign, not a diagnosis; always look for an underlying cause (usually GI or dietary).

- *CBC*: Hb ↓, mean cell volume (MCV) ↓ (<76 fL, depending on age), mean cell hemoglobin concentration (MCHC) ↓. Platelets are often increased.
- *Blood smear*: Microcytic, hypochromic anemia
- *Serum ferritin* ↓. It may be low before anemia; treatment helps with CNS effects. Check C-reactive protein (CRP), as ferritin may be falsely elevated due to acute-phase reaction (↓ serum iron and ↑ total iron binding capacity [TIBC] confirm iron deficiency).

Treatment

Give 3–6 mg/kg, depending on severity, elemental iron/day (as oral ferrous salt). Response in reticulocyte count is usually within 5–10 days. Continue for 3 months after Hb normalizes to replenish body stores. Prevention in high-risk groups:

- Iron supplementation in preterm infants and those solely breast-fed >6 months.

- Encourage an iron-containing diet, e.g., iron-fortified formulas and breakfast cereals, meat, green vegetables, beans, egg yolk, foods rich in vitamin C (↑ iron absorption).

Macrocytic anemia

B_{12} deficiency

Vitamin B_{12} (cobalamin) is usually sourced from animal products. Vegans or diets lacking meat are most at risk. Defective absorption is due to intrinsic factor deficiency (congenital-autosomal recessive or juvenile autoimmune pernicious anemia), defective B_{12} transport (transcobalamin II deficiency), intestinal disease causing malabsorption (e.g., ileal resection, IBD, celiac disease), and bacterial overgrowth in the small bowel.

Folate deficiency

This common nutritional deficiency occurs worldwide, brought on by the following factors:
- Malnutrition (marasmus, kwashiorkor), goat's milk feeding
- Malabsorption, e.g., celiac disease, IBD, other small intestinal disease
- Increased requirements, e.g., rapid growth, chronic hemolytic anemias, hypermetabolic states (infection, hyperthyroidism), severe skin disease
- Drugs, e.g., phenytoin, valproate, trimethoprim, nitrofurantoin
- Inborn errors of folate metabolism: Lesch–Nyan syndrome and orotic aciduria

Presentation

- Insidious onset, pallor, fatigue, anorexia, glossitis, developmental delay, hypotonia
- In severe cases, there is subacute combined degeneration of the spinal cord, with paresthesia of hands and feet, ataxic gait, and loss of vibration sense.

Diagnosis of macrocytic anemias

- Macrocytic anemia: Hb ↓, MCV ↑ (>110 fL, depending on age)
- WBC ↓, hypersegmented neutrophils, platelets ↓, ↑ bilirubin
- ↓ serum B_{12} or ↓ folate level (serum folate level reflects recent intake, red cell folate level is more reliable)
- Bone marrow shows megaloblastic appearance.
- Rarely, intrinsic factor autoantibodies or test of B_{12} absorption, e.g., Schilling test (no longer widely available)

Treatment

Improve diet or provide dietary supplements.
- B_{12} deficiency: IM cyanocobalamin usually produces response within 1 week. Watch K^+ level, as it may drop. Treat weekly until Hb is normal, then give 3-monthly if the underlying problem persists.
- Folate deficiency: Oral folic acid: response is prompt (within a few days) Again, look for underlying (usually GI) cause. Never treat with folic acid alone unless serum B_{12} level is known to be normal, as subacute combined degeneration of the spinal cord can be precipitated.

RBC membrane defect anemias

Hereditary spherocytosis (HS)

- Autosomal dominant (AD) in 75% of cases. Incidence is 1 in 5000 (Northern European).
- Various RBC membrane skeletal defects occur, the most common one involving ankyrin (~50%–60%).
- Mild to moderate anemia occurs in compensated cases, can be severe anemia with transfusion requirement.
- Splenomegaly is usually present.
- Infection accelerates hemolysis with jaundice.
- Aplastic crisis with erythema infectiosum (parvovirus B19 infection)
- Folate deficiency due to increased RBC turnover can occur; supplementation is needed for severe cases.
- Laboratory investigation includes ↑ RBC destruction, ↑ RBC production, ↑↑ spherocytes on blood smear, positive osmotic fragility test at or after 6 months of age (it may be false negative and show no spherocytes in the newborn), and negative direct Coombs test.
- Provide supportive treatment (e.g., folic acid supplementation, blood transfusion) if anemia is severe.
- Splenectomy is considered (after 5 years of age) for moderate to severe symptoms of anemia and persistent hyperbilirubinemia (leading to gallstones). This requires preoperative vaccination against *Haemophilus influenzae* type B (HiB), pneumococcus, and meningococcus, as well as postoperative 5-yearly boosters, annual influenza vaccination, and consideration of lifelong penicillin V prophylaxis.

Hereditary elliptocytosis (HE)

This is a heterogeneous group, with mainly AD inheritance. Incidence is 1:25,000.

- Varies from asymptomatic (majority of cases)
- Chronic compensated hemolysis to transfusion dependence
- Presentation and management are similar to that of HS.
- Blood smear shows elliptical RBC

Hereditary pyropoikilocytosis

- RBCs are extremely sensitive to raised temperature (they fragment after 10 minutes incubation at 45°C in vitro).
- Hb ~7–9 g/dL
- Jaundice and splenomegaly are present.
- Good response to splenectomy in those severely affected

Hereditary stomatocytosis

This condition has AD inheritance and is of variable severity.

RBC enzyme defect anemias

Glucose-6-phosphate-dehydrogenase (G6PD) deficiency

- Sex-linked recessive (disease in heterozygous males and homozygous females, variable expression in heterozygous females)
- Endemic in Southern Europe, South East Asia, West Africa, and the Middle East.
- There are over 400 enzyme variants—African (A-) (10%–60% enzyme activity) and Mediterranean (3% activity) are most clinically relevant.
- RBC G6PD levels fall rapidly as cells age, with impaired elimination of oxidants and reduced cell integrity.
- Intermittent acute hemolysis (spleen destroys less deformable RBC) is associated with oxidant drugs (antimalarials, sulfonamides, dapsone, aspirin, ciprofloxacin), foods (fava beans), chemicals (naphthalene—common in moth balls) or infections.
- May present as neonatal jaundice or chronic hemolytic anemia

Laboratory investigation

- Normal during nonhemolytic state.
- During hemolysis, findings of RBC destruction, increased RBC production, spherocytes, and Heinz bodies on blood smear, direct antiglobulin test (DAT) negative
- Definitive diagnosis is by measuring reduced G6PD enzyme activity (may be falsely normal during acute hemolysis; repeat 6 weeks later).

Management

Avoid oxidant drugs and foods, maintain good urine output with fluids, transfuse if required, give folate supplements in chronic hemolysis, treat hyperbilirubinemia in newborns.

Pyruvate kinase (PK) deficiency

- Chronic hemolytic anemia results from enzyme deficiency.
- Congenital autosomal recessive condition
- Enzyme deficiency leads to ↓ RBC ATP generation and ↑2,3-DPG (diphosphoglycerate) production (which shifts O_2 dissociation curve to the right).
- Variable severity
- May present in neonatal period or later
- Erythema infectiosum (e.g., parvovirus B19 infection) may cause an aplastic crisis.
- Laboratory findings are of ↑ RBC destruction and production, ↓PK enzyme level.

Management

- Oral folate supplements
- Blood transfusion if there is symptomatic anemia
- Support of aplastic crisis
- Splenectomy in severe cases

Sickle cell anemia

This type of anemia is a sickling disorder in homozygous sickle hemoglobin HbSS (most severe) or compound heterozygotes (HbSC, HbSD, HbSβ⁰, or HbSβ⁺ thalassemia). Single amino-acid substitution (valine for glutamine) occurs in the globin chain from mutation on chromosome 11 (autosomal recessive).

This condition is found throughout Africa, the Middle East, the Mediterranean region, and India. Incidence is highest in West Africa, at ~1:4; it is ~1:12 in the African-American population. Heterozygous carriers have ↑ resistance to malaria.

HbS is less soluble than HbA in deoxygenated state, forming rod-like crystals that cause permanent sickle-shaped red cells. Affected RBC ↑ blood viscosity and ↓ flow through small vessels, causing tissue infarction. Cells are also prematurely destroyed, resulting in a hemolytic anemia. The presence of HbF ↓ crystal formation reducing the severity.

Clinical features

There is a wide spectrum of disease, from asymptomatic to severe, with frequent crises and chronic multiorgan damage. It usually presents between ages 3 months and 6 years. Complications are age related:

- *Infancy*: High HbF is protective up to 6 months of age. The most common problems are dactylitis, infections, and splenic sequestration.
- *Young children*: Infection, vaso-occlusive crises in long bones, stroke, acute chest syndrome
- *Older children*: Vaso-occlusive crises, infections (pneumococcus, parvovirus).

Sickle crises and problems

- *Vaso-occlusive crises*: Excruciating pain in bones and joints, most commonly of hands and feet, becoming more central with increasing age. Dactylitis causing swollen, painful fingers and/or toes is a typical early manifestation of disease. It is precipitated by infections, cold conditions, and hypoxia.
- *Acute chest syndrome* mimics chest infection with shortness of breath, cough, yellow sputum, chest pain, and falling O_2 saturation. Chest X-ray changes may be late, and can progress within hours. This is a major cause of mortality, thus prompt treatment is essential.
- *Sequestration*: The organ acts as sponge with trapping of sickled blood. Splenic sequestration is more common in the first few years of life; later, liver and lung sequestration occurs. A rapid fall in Hb may be fatal. Recurrent episodes may warrant splenectomy.
- *Stroke*: Most common in 5- to 10-year-olds, this occurs in 7% of children. An additional 20% have asymptomatic infarcts. Untreated, mortality is 20%; recurrence rate is 70% within 3 years. Prompt treatment is with exchange transfusion to reduce HbS <20%. Prevent recurrence by serial transfusion to maintain low HbS rate.

- *Infections*: Patient is functionally hyposplenic by 1 year, resulting in a high risk of *Pneumococcus*, *Meningococcus* infections. Treat fever promptly.
- *Aplastic crises* typically occur after parvovirus infection. There is reticulocytopenia with a Hb drop. Spontaneous recovery usually occurs in 10 days. The patient may require transfusion.
- *Priapism*: ~50% affected. Acute fulminant (painful, lasting >6 hours) or "stuttering" priapism (shorter, self-limiting episodes) occurs. Untreated, this may lead to erectile dysfunction. Treat with IV hydration, analgesia, aspiration of blood from corpus cavernosa, and phenylephrine instillation. Exchange transfusion is not effective.
- *Avascular necrosis* most commonly affects the hip joint.
- *Renal impairment*: Hyposthenuria (urine concentration defect) results in high urine output and susceptibility to dehydration. Enuresis may occur. Papillary necrosis causes hematuria. Chronic renal failure.
- *Retinopathy*: Small-vessel occlusions are followed by neovascularization → vitreous hemorrhage → resorption, which results in fibrous strands → retinal detachment. Surveillance is needed (treat with photocoagulation).
- *ENT problems*: Adenotonsillar hypertrophy occurs in ~18%. This may lead to hypoxia at night, precipitating crises. Ask about snoring.
- *Leg ulcers* are uncommon in childhood.
- *Growth and developmental retardation* are uncommon; look for zinc deficiency.

Diagnosis

- *Clinical suspicion*: Pallor, hepatomegaly, splenomegaly, acute crises
- *Hematology*: Hb 5–9 g/dL, reticulocytes↑, sickled cells. Hemoglobin electrophoresis is the definitive test and distinguishes trait from disease.
- Routine screening of African-American children prior to anesthesia
- *Prenatal diagnosis*: Fetal red cells or amniotic (or trophoblastic) cells

Management of acute crises

- *Investigations*: Hb↓, reticulocytes↑, blood cultures, UA, creatinine, LFT, CRP (↑ with sickling/infection), O_2 monitoring, type and hold, chest X-ray if indicated
- *Hydration*: Aim for 100% normal maintenance (PO/IV) unless there are clinical reasons for increased fluid needs.
- *Analgesia*: Titrate to severity of pain. Initially, the patient is treated at home with simple analgesia (e.g., acetaminophen, NSAIDs), opiates if required.
- *Antibiotics*: Broad-spectrum cephalosporin, e.g., ceftriaxone, following blood cultures if fever >38°C. Add a macrolide, e.g., azithromycin, if there are signs of respiratory infection (to cover atypical pneumonias).
- *Oxygen* to maintain SaO_2> 95%. Keep warm.
- *Blood product support*: Simple transfusions for aplastic crisis, sequestration, or severe anemia; exchange transfusion for sequestration, acute chest syndrome, or stroke

Other treatments
- Avoid precipitating factors, e.g., hypoxia (air travel), cold, and dehydration.
- Vaccination (pneumococcal, hemophilus B, meningococcal) and oral penicillin V prophylaxis through age 5 against infection from hyposplenism
- Maintenance oral folate
- Hydroxyurea: ↑ HbF production and thereby ↓ sickling; lower WBC also likely contributes. Monitor CBC as drug is myelosuppressive. This reduces chest and vaso-occlusive crises.
- Hematopoietic stem cell transplantation may be curative.

Thalassemia

An inherited defect in synthesis of one or more globin chains (globin chain linked to heme group = hemoglobin) → imbalanced globin chain production → ineffective erythropoiesis → precipitated excess chains causing hemolysis → anemia of variable severity.

- Adult Hb is mainly HbA ($\alpha_2\beta_2$) with HbA$_2$ ($\alpha_2\delta_2$) comprising ~2.5% of the total.
- Two α globin chains are encoded on each chomosome 16 (i.e., each cell has four α globin genes), designated ($\alpha\alpha/\alpha\alpha$).
- There are only two β globin genes per cell, encoded on chromosome 11.

The severity of anemia and clinical picture is related to the number and nature of gene mutation and deletions and consequent imbalanced globin chain production. Thalassemia is common in malaria-affected regions of the world (the trait is probably protective), i.e., parts of Africa, the Mediterranean region, the Middle East, India, and Asia.

α-thalassemia

- Silent α-thalassemia ($\alpha\alpha/\alpha-$): One-gene deletion. Asymptomatic, may have hypochromic microcytic picture
- α-thalassemia trait ($\alpha\alpha/$——) or ($\alpha-/\alpha-$): Two-gene deletion. Asymptomatic. Hb may be ↓, MCV ↓, MCH ↓ (may mimic iron deficiency picture)
- Hemoglobin H disease ($\alpha-/$——): Three-gene deletion. Variable chronic anemia. Hepatosplenomegaly and jaundice. Hypochromic anemia with target cells and reticuloytes ↑. HbH inclusions (tetramers of β globin) are seen on special staining. Folic acid supplements are required, and occasionally transfusions. The patient may benefit from splenectomy.
- Hb Barts hydrops fetalis (——/——): Causes stillbirth or early neonatal death. Hb ~6.0 g/dL, nucleated RBCs, target cells, reticuloytes ↑, and polychromasia on smear. Hemoglobin analysis shows mainly Hb Barts ($\gamma4$). This is seen most often in South East Asia.

β-thalassemia

Loss of one β globin gene = thalassemia trait. Loss of both β globin chains = thalassemia major. The disorder is not obvious until γ chain production falls off around 6 months of age and HbF ($\alpha_2\gamma_2$) levels fall.

β-thalassemia trait

- Asymptomatic, mild Hb ↓, MCV ↓ and MCH ↓, RBC ↑ (a rough guide; if RBC >5.0 $\times$ 10^{12}/L with a normal red cell distribution width [RDW] and microcytic, hypochromic smear, then thalassemia trait is more likely than iron deficiency). Ferritin is normal.
- HbA$_2$ and or HbF characteristically ↑ on Hb electrophoresis.
- No treatment is required, but it is important to detect for genetic-counseling purposes, especially if the partner also has hemoglobinopathy.

β-*thalassemia major*

Presentation

- Presents in first year with anemia and recurrent infections.
- Growth and development failure
- Extramedullary hematopoiesis causes skeletal deformity (frontal bossing of skull, maxillary expansion) and hepatosplenomegaly.
- Severe anemia (3–9 g/dL), markedly ↓ MCV and MCH, ↑ reticulocytes, target cells and nucleated RBCs
- Mainly HbF present on Hb electrophoresis

Management

- Regular transfusions (every 3–4 weeks) to suppress extramedullary hematopoiesis and maintain Hb at a level to sustain growth and development
- Iron overload is major problem, with hemosiderosis affecting the heart, liver, and pancreas.
- Iron chelation when ferritin level >1000 µg/L (usually following 10–20 transfusions). Deferoxamine by subcutaneous infusion 5–7 nights per week. Side effects include cataracts, hearing loss, and *Yersinia* gut infections. Alternatively, give deferasirox (a new oral iron chelator) daily. Side effects include renal dysfunction, nausea, diarrhea, rashes, ocular and auditory abnormalities, and rare cytopenias.
- Splenectomy may help if there is massive splenomegaly or increased tranfusion requirements.
- Hematopoietic stem cell transplantation has been successful, but the procedure carries significant risks.

Thalassemia intermedia

This is less severe than thalassemia major in that patients do not require regular transfusions. There is variable severity of disease, from asymptomatic to moderately severe anemia with skeletal abnormalities similar to those seen in thalassemia major. This condition is usually due to co-inheritance of an ameliorating condition, e.g., ↑ HbF, α-thalassemia trait.

Immune hemolytic anemia

In this disorder, RBCs react with autoantibody ± complement, which leads to their destruction by the reticuloendothelial system. It can be divided into isoimmune and autoimmune forms

Isoimmune

Sensitization induces maternal antibodies that cross the placenta and affect fetal and neonatal red cells. Usually, direct Coombs test is positive.
- Rhesus hemolytic disease (p. 144)
- ABO incompatibility (p. 144)
- Other blood group incompatibilities, e.g., Kell, Duffy RBC antigens

Autoimmune

Warm antibody type—mostly IgG
- Rare
- Majority of cases are idiopathic
- Other causes: Drugs (e.g., penicillin), lymphoid malignancies, autoimmune diseases (e.g., SLE, IBD)
- Variable hemolytic anemia, mild jaundice, splenomegaly, DAT positive
- Warm autoantibodies—often nonspecific

Treatment
Give oral prednisone. If there is no response, consider intravenous immunoglobulin (IVIG) or other immunosuppressive agents (e.g., azathioprine). Perform splenectomy if condition is severe or poorly responsive to immunosuppression.

Cold antibody type—mostly IgM
- Common, but a very rare cause of hemolysis (mostly in the elderly)
- RBC antibody reacts most actively <32°C to cause intravascular RBC hemolysis.
- Idiopathic or secondary to EBV or *Mycoplasma* infection
- Acrocyanosis in cold, splenomegaly
- Chronic hemolytic anemia, DAT negative for Ig, positive for C3
- IgM autoantibodies react best at 4°C.

Treatment
Treatment is rarely needed in children. Warmth, immunosuppression, plasma exchange, and splenectomy may help. Usually the condition is self-limiting if there is an infectious cause.

Paroxysmal nocturnal hemoglobinuria
- Chronic intravascular hemolytic anemia, particularly at night. Acquired abnormality of RBC membrane results in complement-mediated lysis.
- High risk of venous thrombosis, e.g., sagittal sinus
- Immunophenotyping for low expression of CD55 and CD59 is diagnostic.

Treatment
- Immunosuppressives, e.g., steroids, hematopoietic stem cell transplantation (HSCT)

RBC fragmentation

Causes
- DIC
- Infection, e.g., malaria (black water fever), viral hemorrhagic fevers, *Clostridium perfringens*
- Burns
- Mechanical, e.g., prosthetic heart valves, March hemoglobinuria
- Microangiopathic hemolytic anemia (MAHA): Hemolytic uremic syndrome (HUS), thrombotic thrombocytopenic purpura, giant hemangioma, malignant hypertension
- Vasculitides, e.g., SLE, polyarteritis nodosa
- Hereditary acanthocytosis: Rare genetic condition of abetalipoproteinemia with mental retardation, ataxia, retinitis pigmentosa, and steatorrhea
- Envenomation from several of the world's venomous snakes, spiders

Clinical features
Features depend on the underlying cause and severity of anemia.

Laboratory investigations
- Hb ↓
- Blood smear: Reticuloytes ↑↑, RBC fragmentation, stomatocytes, spherocytes
- Possible ↓ platelets or clotting prolongation
- Malarial parasites on thick blood smear

Treatment
- Treat underlying disease.
- Correct hematological abnormalities, e.g., with blood or platelet transfusion, correct clotting abnormalities.
- Give oral iron or folate supplements if required.

Aplastic anemia

This is due to severe bone marrow suppression of RBC, WBC, and platelet precursors. Aplastic anemia is rare, and may be acquired or congenital.

Acquired aplastic anemia

Causes
- Idiopathic (most common)
- Radiotherapy, chemotherapy
- Idiosyncratic reaction to drugs or chemicals (chloramphenicol, carbamazepine, phenytoin, NSAIDs, mesalamine, several solvents)
- Viral (hepatitis A, B, and C; CMV; EBV; parvovirus)
- Bone marrow invasion (malignant cells, osteopetrosis)

Presentation
- Features of anemia are due to RBC ↓↓.
- Infection, particularly bacterial and fungal, due to WBC ↓↓, particularly if neutrophils <0.2 × 10^9/L.
- Mucosal bleeding, purpura, easy bruising are due to platelet count ↓↓.

Investigations
- CBC: Pancytopenia, reticulocytes ↓↓
- Bone marrow aspirate and biopsy: Severe reduction of all blood cell precursors, with (e.g., leukemia) or without cell infiltration
- CD55/CD59 immunophenotyping to exclude PNH (see below)
- Cytogenetics and chromosomal breakage studies to detect myelodysplastic syndrome (MDS) or Fanconi anemia

Treatment
- Remove or treat underlying cause, e.g., drug, malignancy.
- Depending on severity: RBC ± platelet transfusion, or antibiotics
- Stem cell transplant may be curative.
- Immunosuppression, e.g., anti-thymocyte globulin, cyclosporin ± filgrastim or treatment with androgens or danazol may be useful.

Prognosis
The prognosis depends on the underlying cause. Some patients will recover spontaneously. Otherwise, most will progress to more severe disease, PNH or acute leukemia. Long-term survival is unlikely in severe disease without successful hematopoietic stem cell transplant (HSCT).

Paroxysmal nocturnal hemoglobinuria (PNH)
- Rare, acquired RBC membrane defect resulting in complement-mediated lysis
- Low pH leads to hemolytic anemia, hemoglobinuria, nephropathy, anemia, and venous thrombosis.
- ↓ WBC and platelets
- CBC shows reticulocytosis.
- Bone marrow is hypoplastic with erthropoietic islands.
- Urine is positive for hemoglobin.
- Low CD55 and CD59 expression

Treatment

Iron replacement and immunosuppression (e.g., with steroids) may reduce severity. HSCT is curative. Otherwise, median survival is 8–10 years. Death is due to thrombosis or complications of pancytopenia.

Inherited aplastic anemia

Fanconi anemia

This rare, autosomal recessive condition leads to progressive bone marrow failure, affecting all three hemopoietic cell precursors. It is associated with chromosomal fragility and defective DNA repair.

Presentation

- May present at any age, including at birth, but typically at 4–10 years (boys earlier than girls)
- Usually presents with bruising and purpura or insidious-onset anemia
- *Associations*: Short stature (80%); skin hyperpigmentation (café-au-lait spots 75%); skeletal abnormalities, particularly upper limb and thumb (66%); renal malformations (30%); microcephaly (40%); cryptorchidism (20%); mental retardation (17%); deafness (7%), abnormal facies

Investigations

- CBC: Pancytopenia
- Bone marrow shows hypoplastic, dyserythropoietic or megaloblastic changes.
- Chemically induced lymphocyte chromosomal breakages
- Investigate to detect renal abnormalities or hearing loss.

Treatment

- Supportive, e.g., RBC transfusion, hearing aids, orthopedic
- Immunosuppression with corticosteroids and androgens (oxymetholone)
- Successful stem cell transplant is curative for hematological defects.

Prognosis

Most patients respond to steroids/androgens, but treatment is long term. Patients not responding to immunosuppression usually die within a few years due to complications of pancytopenia or acute leukemia.

Dyskeratosis congenita

This is a very rare condition with dystrophic nails, skin pigmentation, and mucous membrane leukoplakia. The bone marrow shows hypoplastic changes. Treatment is HSCT.

Shwachman–Diamond syndrome

Typically neutropenia occurs more than thrombocytopenia and anemia. Also, there is pancreatic enzyme insufficiency with diarrhea, FTT, and infection due to immunocompromise. Bone marrow examination is diagnostic ± pancreatic function testing. Consider SBDS genotyping.

Bloom syndrome

Phenotypically this syndrome appears like Fanconi anemia, but there is no aplastic anemia. Leukemia may develop, and lymphocyte chromosomal breakages are present.

Pure red-cell aplasia

Causes
- Transient erythroblastopenia of childhood
- Diamond–Blackfan syndrome
- Drugs
- Viral (e.g., parvovirus B19)
- Isoimmune hemolytic disease in newborn
- Severe infection or malnutrition
- Megaloblastic anemia (aplastic phase)

Diamond–Blackfan syndrome (congenital red cell aplasia)

This hereditary condition is of variable genetic inheritance. The defect is unknown; it leads to specific reduction in bone marrow RBC production.

Presentation
The syndrome presents in the first year of life (25% anemic at birth; 90% present in first year of life) with severe anemia. There is a positive family history in 10%–20% of cases. The syndrome is associated with the following features:
- Dysmorphic features
- Triphalangeal thumbs
- Turner syndrome–like phenotype
- Renal defects (>50%)
- Congenital heart disease
- Skeletal abnormalities

Investigations
CBC shows normochromic anemia with reticulocytes ↓ (<0.2%). WBC and platelet counts are usually normal. Bone marrow aspirate and biopsy show absent red cell precursors but are otherwise normal.

Treatment
Give oral prednisone 2 mg/kg/day; some recommend support with tranfusions until 10–12 months, then a steroid trial. Wean over several weeks. Some 70% of patients will respond, but most will continue to need a maintenance dose. Give serial RBC transfusion with iron chelation if unresponsive to steroids. HSCT can be curative.

Prognosis
Although 20% of patients with this syndrome spontaneously resolve, there is significant mortality and morbidity in the rest from steroid treatment and blood transfusion–related complications (e.g., iron overload).

Transient erythroblastopenia of childhood

This condition is idiopathic or secondary to bacterial or viral infection (e.g., parvovirus B19, EBV) drugs, malnutrition, or congenital hemolytic anemia (e.g., hereditary spherocytosis.) with equal incidence in both sexes.

It typically presents at <5 years age with insidious onset of anemic symptoms in the previously well child. Examination is usually normal except for signs of anemia. The patient may have preceding viral or bacterial infection. CBC shows normocytic, normochromic anemia, absent reticulocytes, and normal WBC and platelet count. Bone marrow is normal except for markedly reduced erythroid precursors.

Treatment
- Remove underlying cause (e.g., drugs)
- Blood transfusion if significantly symptomatic
- Spontaneously resolves, usually within weeks, but occasionally may take up to 6 months

Polycythemia

- Increase in total red blood cell mass (RCM) above age-defined normal
- Blood viscosity rises exponentially as the hematocrit (Hct) increases and risks pulmonary hypertension, congestive heart failure, thrombosis, and organ ischemia.
- Very rare in childhood
- Most common in the newborn: It exists when venous or arterial packed cell volume (Hct) >65%.

Box 17.1 Causes of polycythemia

Neonatal causes
- *Hypertransfusion*: Delayed cord clamping, twin-to-twin transfusion syndrome, maternal–fetal transfusion
- *Endocrine*: Infant of a diabetic mother, congenital adrenal hyperplasia, thyrotoxicosis
- *Chronic hypoxia*: Intrauterine growth retardation, placental insufficiency, high altitude
- *Maternal disease*: Pregnancy-induced hypertension, cyanotic heart disease
- *Syndromic*: Down syndrome, Beckwith–Wiedemann syndrome
- *Relative*: Reduced plasma volume due to dehydration, diuretic therapy

Causes in older children
- *Chronic hypoxia*: Cyanotic congenital heart disease, severe chronic respiratory disease, chronic obstructive sleep apnea, chronic alveolar hypoventilation, e.g., gross obesity, high altitude, abnormal Hb with high O_2 affinity
- ↑ erythropoietin production, e.g., pheochromocytoma, cerebellar hemangioblastoma, renal disease, renal dysplasia, postrenal transplant
- Relative: Dehydration or diuretic therapy

Presentation

- Asymptomatic plethora occurs in most patients, particularly newborns.
- Jaundice (newborn) is due to increased red cell turnover.
- Hypoglycemia (newborn) is due to increased red cell glucose consumption.
- *CNS*: Cerebral irritability, seizures, strokes, cerebral hemorrhage
- Respiratory distress, pulmonary hypertension, e.g., PPHN
- Congestive cardiac failure
- Necrotizing enterocolitis (NEC)
- Thrombosis, e.g., renal venous thrombosis
- *Miscellaneous*: Cyanosis (PaO_2 usually normal), hepatomegaly

Management

- Diagnosis is often obvious, e.g., cyanotic congenital heart disease
- *CBC*: ↑Hct, ↑RBC, blood smear
- Exclude ↓ serum glucose or calcium, or ↑ bilirubin (newborn)
- Investigate for cause if not obvious
- If symptomatic or Hct >70%, give partial (dilutional) exchange transfusion over 30 minutes with normal saline to reduce Hct <60%.

  Exchange volume (mL) = blood volume x (observed minus desired Hct)/observed Hct

Prognosis

Prognosis is generally good unless severe hypoglycemia or thrombotic complications occur.

Abnormal bleeding or bruising

Causes
- *Coagulation factor defects* are likely if there is frank excessive blood loss following surgery or dentistry, recurrent bruises >1 cm, muscle hematomas, or hemarthroses.
- *Platelet deficiency or dysfunction* presents as purpura or petechiae, mucosal bleeding (e.g., recurrent epistaxis), or GI or GU tract hemorrhage.
- *Microvascular abnormalities*: Palpable purpura suggestive of vasculitis

General approach
Detailed history
- Nature of bleeding
- History of recent trauma
- Concurrent disease
- Age, e.g., hemorrhagic disease of the newborn several days after birth
- Any maternal disease (if newborn), maternal idiopathic thrombocytopenic purpura (ITP)
- Diet
- Drug history
- Family history

Examination
- Is the child well or unwell?
- Hepatosplenomegaly, e.g., hemolysis, hypersplenism
- Dysmorphic signs, e.g., absent radius in thrombocytopenia–absent radius (TAR) syndrome
- Signs of anemia, e.g., leukemia
- Pattern of bleeding, e.g., extensor and lower limb pattern of HSP
- Associated features, e.g., arthritis (HSP), hemangioma (Kasabach–Merritt syndrome), eczema (Wiskott–Aldrich syndrome)
- Palpable purpura in vasculitis, e.g., HSP

Investigations
- Initially do coagulation screen (PT [INR], APTT, TT). CBC and smear, renal function, LFTs, CRP/ESR
- Depending on presentation also consider fibrinogen, FDPs (or D-dimers), bleeding time, platelet function studies, anti-platelet antibodies, autoantibody screen, specific coagulation factor activities, bone marrow aspirate and biopsy

Treatment
- Supportive, e.g., colloid/blood transfusion if patient is significantly hypovolemic or anemic
- Correct known coagulation or platelet abnormalities if required.

- If there is serious bleeding and an unknown bleeding disorder is likely, treat with fresh frozen plasma (FFP) (20 mL/kg) ± platelets (10–20 mL/kg) until the precise defect is known.
- Avoid IM injections, arterial puncture, NSAIDs.

The outcome depends on the cause, but generally, bleeding from whatever cause can be controlled by platelet or coagulation factor transfusion, resulting in a low risk of death or permanent morbidity.

Coagulation studies

- Activated partial thromboplastin time (APTT): Principally assesses intrinsic pathway of the coagulation cascade
- Prothrombin time (PT) or international normalized ratio (INR): Assesses extrinsic pathway
- Thrombin time (TT): Assesses final common pathway of coagulation cascade
- Plasma fibrinogen
- Bleeding time (rarely performed in children as cooperation is needed)
- Platelet function screen (PFA-100): In vitro test of platelet function
- Fibrinogen degradation products (FDPs)
- D-dimers: Similar to FDPs but more specific. However, raised levels may be found in healthy newborns.
- Specific tests, e.g., platelet autoantibodies, factor VIII activity

Table 17.3 Common causes of abnormal coagulation tests

PT ↑, APTT ↔	Deficiency of coagulation factor VII (liver disease, vitamin K deficiency, warfarin)
PT↔, APTT ↑	Deficiency of factors VIII, IX, XI, XII (hemophilia A or B, von Willebrand disease, heparin)
PT and APTT ↑	Deficiency of factors II, V, X, fibrinogen (DIC, liver disease, vitamin K deficiency, warfarin)
PT and APTT ↔	Normal child, platelet abnormality, vasculitis, e.g., HSP, LMW heparin
TT ↑	Fibrinogen defect, heparin, DIC
Fibrinogen ↓	DIC, severe liver disease, hypofibrinogenemia
FDPs or D-dimers ↑	DIC
Platelet function screen or bleeding time ↑	von Willebrand disease, platelet dysfunction

Note: Most clotting times are longer in healthy neonates, particularly in preterm infants.

Disseminated intravascular coagulation

Miscellaneous severe diseases cause inappropriate activation of coagulation pathways. All or some of the following may simultaneously occur:

- Activation of intravascular thrombosis with both macro- and microthrombi formation, leading to end-organ damage
- Consumption of platelets and clotting factors, → abnormal bleeding
- Widespread activation of fibrinolysis, leading to further bleeding
- Microangiopatic hemolytic anemia (RBC destroyed in fibrin mesh)

Causes in neonatal period

- *Common*: Severe asphyxia, sepsis
- *Less common*: Severe IUGR, respiratory distress syndrome (RDS), aspiration pneumonitis, NEC, rhesus isoimmunization, dead twin, severe hemorrhage, purpura fulminans profound hypothermia

Causes in older children

- *Common*: Septicemia (60%), severe trauma and burns
- *Less common*: Profound shock, hepatic failure, anaphylaxis, blood transfusion reactions, neoplasia (e.g., leukemia)

Presentation

- DIC may be acute (mostly hemorrhagic) or chronic (thrombosis predominates)
- Easy bruising
- Bleeding from venipuncture sites or wounds; GI, pulmonary, or GU hemorrhage
- Microthrombi causing renal impairment, cerebral dysfunction, localized skin necrosis
- Acute RDS (ARDS)
- Microangiopathic hemolytic anemia

Investigations

PT↑, APTT↑, TT↑, fibrinogen↓ (<100 mg/dL), FDP↑ or D-dimers (more specific than FDP but can be present in normal neonates), platelets↓.

Management

- Treat underlying cause.
- Supportive care: O_2, volume replacement for shock, blood transfusion
- Platelet transfusion to raise count >50 × 10^9/L
- Coagulation factor replacement, e.g., FFP, cryoprecipitate if fibrinogen <100 mg/dL
- ? Exchange transfusion may be beneficial, e.g., in sepsis, rhesus isoimmunization, or polycythemia (removes causative toxins or antibodies, replaces clotting factors).
- Consider heparin if there are large thrombi or significant organ damage from microthrombi predominates, e.g., chronic DIC.

Prognosis

There is high mortality with DIC, due to either underlying disease or DIC-related hemorrhage or thrombosis.

Hemophilia A

This is a congenital bleeding disorder due to the defective production of factor VIII, with sex-linked recessive inheritance. Incidence is 1:10,000–14,000 males. Carrier females are rarely symptomatic but may demonstrate a low factor VIII activity–von Willebrand antigen ratio. Genetic testing may be necessary to confirm carrier status. Severity depends on the degree of factor VIII deficiency:

- ≤1% activity = severe disease, with frequent serious bleeding and bruising.
- 1%–5% = moderate disease. Bleeding rarely occurs, but treat as severe disease when bleeding does occur.
- >5%–20% = mild disease. Rarely does the patient bleed spontaneously. This may present after surgery or trauma.

Presentation

- Rarely presents in the neonatal period; sometimes with circumcision
- Easy bruising
- Bleeding into joints. Knees > ankles > elbows > hips > wrists. There is a painful joint with localized tenderness, warmth, swelling, limitation of movement, erythema. Often bleeding takes days to weeks to resolve, leading to associated muscle wasting. Recurrent bleeding leads to degenerative joint disease.
- IM bleeds with pain and swelling. This may lead to compartment syndrome, nerve compression, or later ischemic contractures.
- Hematuria. Blood clots may cause ureteric colic.
- Intracranial bleeds. These usually follow minor head trauma. They may be extradural, subdural, or intracerebral (latter has poor prognosis).

Investigations

- INR ↔ APTT ↑, factor VIII ↓. von Willebrand factor and bleeding time are ↔.
- Perform cranial CT scan if there is any suspicion of intracranial bleed.
- Ultrasound scans are also useful for possible muscle hematomas, e.g., iliopsoas bleed leading to femoral nerve compression (groin pain, hip flexion, and femoral nerve distribution sensory loss).

Management

- *Major bleeds, major surgery, or severe disease*: Give factor VIII concentrate to raise plasma levels to 30%–100% normal, depending on the type or severity of bleed or procedure. Raise level to 100% with intracranial bleed. Generally 1 u/kg raises plasma level by 2%. Recombinant factor VIII is the preferred product. Normally, single doses are required only. $T_{1/2}$ = 8–12 hours.
- Give analgesia as appropriate. Generally, avoid NSAIDs (↓ platelet function) and avoid or minimize opiates as much as possible.
- *Minor bleeds*: Apply local pressure. Give a single dose of IV factor VIII if it persists.
- *Mouth bleeding*: Epsilon aminocaproic acid 50–100 mg/kg/dose every 6 hours until healed (max 3 g/dose)

- *Minor surgery or persistent bleeds*: IV, subcutaneous, or nasal DDAVP in mild hemophilia, if this has had demonstrated factor VIII response.
- Avoid IM injections, including vitamin K at birth, if disease is suspected.
- Rest, local ice packs, and limb splinting if there is joint or muscle bleeding
- Daily physiotherapy is important to avoid muscle weakness or contractures once joint bleeding has stopped.
- *Home treatment*: Families can be trained to give IV factor VIII concentrates, through either an indwelling central venous catheter or peripheral venipuncture, at home.
- *Prophylaxisis* is given in cases of severe disease, e.g., IV concentrate injections three times per week.

Complications
- Chronic arthropathy
- Transmission of hepatitis B, hepatitis C, and HIV. This was common in the 1980s but is now very rare in the pediatric population since virally inactivated plasma concentrates (since 1985) or recombinant factor VIII concentrate is now given.
- Factor VIII inhibitor development is suggested by bleeds not responding to treatment. Measure factor VIII inhibitor titer. This is difficult to treat; it may require increased factor VIII concentrate dosage or use of other products, e.g., FEIBA or recombinant activated VIIa.

Prognosis
Provided there is no viral infection or intracranial bleeding, the patient should have a normal life expectancy.

Hemophilia B

Previously known as Christmas disease, this is a sex-linked recessive disease caused by defective production of factor IX. It is clinically indistinguishable from hemophilia A and six times less common than hemophilia A.

Investigations are the same as for hemophilia A except that factor IX activity is deficient.

Management principles are same as for hemophilia A except that DDAVP is of no use. The cornerstone of treatment is recombinant factor IX concentrate IV (some patients use virally inactivated plasma-derived factor IX). Once-daily administration is sufficient, as the plasma half-life is longer. Generally 1 µ/kg raises the plasma level by 0.7%–1%, the lowest yields occurring in young patients receiving recombinant factor IX.

von Willebrand disease (vWD)

von Willebrand factor (vWF) functions as the carrier protein for factor VIIIC, protecting it from degradation, which facilitates platelet adhesion. Deficiency in vWF leads to impaired platelet function and reduced factor VIII activity.

- vWD is an inherited bleeding disorder due to deficiency of vWF.
- M = F
- Incidence ~1:5,000

There are many subtypes, but the disease is usually classified into three main types:

- *Type I*: Autosomal dominant. 70% of cases, mild–moderate severity
- *Type II*: Autosomal dominant/recessive. ~25% of cases, mild–moderate
- *Type III*: Autosomal recessive. Almost complete absence of vWF. <5% cases, severe.

Presentation

Presentation is very variable. Type III is clinically similar to hemophilia A. Other types may vary, from virtually asymptomatic to easy bruising with associated excessive bleeding from dental surgery, trauma, surgery, and menorrhagia.

Investigations

APTT is usually ↑ (if factor VIII activity is low), PT ↔, platelet count ↔, bleeding time and platelet function screen ↑, factor VIIIC ↓, vWF functions ↓.

Note: VWF is an acute-phase protein and may be normal immediately after birth and following trauma or illness.

Management

- Avoid NSAIDs.
- Minor bleeding may respond to local pressure or epsilon aminocaproic acid.
- More significant bleeds or minor surgery may respond to DDAVP (avoid if type IIB).
- Severe bleeding or severe disease requires factor VIII concentrate; mange as for severe hemophilia A.
- Consider oral contraceptives for chronic menorrhagia.

Complications

Complications are the same as those for hemophilia A. Acute joint involvement is rare, except in type III.

Prognosis

Patients with type I and II disease rarely have severe bleeds and generally have normal life expectancy and quality of life. Type III disease is similar to hemophilia A. Overall severity generally improves with age.

Other congenital coagulation factor deficiencies

- Deficiency of every coagulation factor exists, but individual incidence is very rare.
- All are of autosomally recessive inheritance.
- The most common defects are those of fibrinogen (e.g., dysfibrino-genemia or hypofibrinogenemia) and specific deficiency of factors VII, II prothrombin, V, XI, XIII, and X. Factor XII deficiency results in prolonged APTT but no bleeding tendency.

In general, the severity of bleeding tendency varies from that of mild hemophilia to a familial bruising tendency. Most cases present with bleeding after surgery, trauma, or dental extraction rather than with spontaneous bleeding or hemarthrosis. Cases rarely present as cord hemorrhage in the neonatal period. Congenital afibrinogenemia is clinically the most severe, and hemorrhagic manifestations usually appear within the first 2 years of life.

Depending on the specific deficient factor, PT and/or APTT will be increased (XIII deficiency excepted). The exact diagnosis depends on detecting low, specific factor activity. Treatment for an unknown coagulation defect is FFP.

Platelet function disorders

Congenital causes

All cases are rare and autosomal recessive. These disorders are due to

- Defective platelet membrane-specific glycoproteins, which cause defective adhesion to fibrinogen, e.g., Glanzmann disease (thrombasthenia), or to collagen, e.g., Bernard–Soulier syndrome (BSS)
- Defective or deficient platelet granules (normal release induces coagulation cascade, vasoconstriction, platelet aggregation), e.g., thrombocytopenia-absent radius (TAR) syndrome, Chediak–Higashi syndrome

Acquired causes

These cases may be secondary to renal disease, hepatic disease, or DIC or be drug-induced, e.g., NSAIDs, corticosteroids, penicillin, cephalosporins, β-blockers, antihistamines.

Presentation

- Easy bruising and purpura
- Mucocutaneous bleeding
- Menorrhagia
- Positive family history is common.

Investigations

- Normal platelet count (usually)
- ↑ platelet size, e.g., BSS
- Bleeding time >5 minutes; prolonged platelet function screen
- If congenital functional disorder is suspected, perform platelet function studies. These include platelet aggregation tests using agents such as ristocetin, collagen, adenosine 5-diphosphate (ADP), arachidonic acid, and adrenaline; platelet adhesion test to glass beads; and tests of platelet granule release. Interpretation is complex, so seek specialist opinion.

Treatment

- Control bleeding, e.g., apply pressure.
- Correct underlying abnormality or stop use of responsible drug.
- Epsilon aminocaproic acid for minor bleeding, especially oral
- Platelet transfusion if there is severe bleeding or to cover for surgery
- Avoid drugs that inhibit platelet function, e.g., NSAIDs.
- Many mild–moderate platelet function defects improve transiently with DDAVP.
- Consider oral contraceptives for menorrhagia.

Prognosis

Prognosis is generally good with normal life expectancy. Serious bleeding is rare.

Thrombocytosis

Normal platelet count is $<450 \times 10^9$/L; platelet counts $>1000 \times 10^9$/L may cause thrombosis or bleeding when platelets are dysfunctional.

Causes

Almost always, thrombocytosis is reactive.

Increased production—acute or chronic infection

- Acute or chronic hemorrhage
- Trauma or post-surgery
- Kawasaki disease
- Iron deficiency anemia
- Sepsis
- Malignancy, especially of bone marrow
- Any inflammatory disease, e.g., ulcerative colitis

Decreased destruction

- Post-splenectomy

On clinical examination, look for signs of iron-deficiency anemia, bruising or bleeding, splenomegaly, and general ill health.

Investigations

- CBC, e.g., WBC ↑ in infection or signs of iron deficiency anemia
- CRP/ESR: ↑ in inflammatory or malignant conditions
- Bone marrow aspirate if underlying cause is unclear

Treatment

- Treat underlying cause.
- Consider aspirin for Kawasaki disease (one of the few indications for aspirin in children).
- Most infection-associated thrombocytosis is benign and requires no treatment.

Prognosis

Generally, prognosis depends on the underlying cause unless significant thrombosis or hemorrhage occurs.

Thrombocytopenia

Thrombocytopenia is defined as a platelet count <150 × 10⁹/L: as platelet count decreases bleeding and bruising risk increase. Risk of bleeding is moderately high <20 × 10⁹/L, and likely if <10 × 10⁹/L.

Causes

Decreased bone marrow and platelet production

- *Marrow failure*: Aplastic anemia, severe IUGR, severe maternal preeclampsia
- *Marrow infiltration*: Leukemia, lymphoma, osteopetrosis
- *Marrow depression*: Radiotherapy, cytotoxic drugs, drug reaction
- *Hereditary thrombocytopenia*: Fanconi syndrome, absent radius (TAR) syndrome
- *Nutritional deficiency*: Vitamin B₁₂ or folate deficiency
- *Selective megakaryocyte depression*: Drugs, viral infection (HIV, parvovirus, Epstein–Barr virus), poisons

Increased destruction

- *Immune*: ITP (in child or maternal), neonatal alloimmune thrombocytopenia (NAIT), SLE, drug-induced (penicillin or heparin), infection (e.g., malaria or HIV), post-transfusion purpura
- *Non-immune*: DIC, giant hemangioma (Kasabach–Merritt syndrome), hemolytic uremic syndrome, TTP, cardiac disease (prosthetic valves or cardiopulmonary bypass)
- Hypersplenism (platelets consumed in enlarged spleen of any cause)
- *Hereditary*, e.g., Wiskott–Aldrich syndrome (X-linked recessive: boys present with early thrombocytopenia, eczema, immunocompromise due to immunoglobulin abnormalities), BSS

Investigations

- *History*: Drug history, family history, preceding viral illness
- *Examination*: Signs of bleeding, lymphadenopathy, hepatosplenomegaly, concurrent infection
- CBC and blood smear
- *Serology*: Anti-neutrophil antibody, DAT, monospot, anti-platelet antibodies (e.g., anti-HPA1 if NAIT is suspected), HIV, viral serology
- Renal function and LFTs
- Bone marrow aspirate and biopsy
- Cranial CT scan if any evidence of possible intracerebral hemorrhage

Treatment

- Treat underlying cause if possible.
- Platelet transfusion if very low platelet count or life-threatening or mucosal bleeding
- Immunosuppression, e.g., ITP, SLE
- Splenectomy, e.g., chronic ITP, hypersplenism
- Hematopoietic stem cell transplant may be helpful in some hereditary diseases, e.g., Wiskott–Aldrich syndrome.

Idiopathic thrombocytopenia (ITP)

ITP is caused by IgG autoantibody to platelet cell membrane antigens. It results in platelet destruction by the spleen and liver.

Presentation

- Preceding viral infection is common, particularly in younger children.
- Bruising and petechiae
- Mucosal bleeding, e.g., epistaxis, bleeding gums
- Menorrhagia
- Intracranial or intravisceral bleeds are very rare.
- Physical examination otherwise usually normal, e.g., no splenomegaly

Investigation

- CBC: Platelet count ↓↓, commonly platelet size ↑ due to compensatory megakaryocytosis. Otherwise, CBC is normal.
- Testing for platelet antibodies is not clinically useful.

Generally, bone marrow aspirate is not indicated if the child is otherwise well, unless there is concurrent pallor, hepatosplenomegaly, lymphade-nopathy, leucopenia, or ↑ blasts on CBC, as an alternative diagnosis is likely. Differential diagnosis includes acute leukemia, aplastic anemia, SLE (adolescent girls), hereditary thrombocytopenia. Bone marrow in ITP is normal marrow, usually with ↑ megakaryocytes.

Management

- Active treatment is only really required if the platelet count is <10 × 10⁹/L or there is mucosal bleeding or life-threatening bleeding. Some advocate no treatment unless there is "wet" bleeding.
- If there is severe, potentially life-threatening bleeding, give platelet transfusion urgently 10–15 mL/kg.
- ? If the platelet count is very low consider corticosteroids (↓ platelet antibodies and phagocytosis), e.g., prednisolone 4 mg/kg/day for 2 weeks, then wean dose over several weeks to months.
- ? If the platelet count is very low consider IV IgG (0.8 g/kg, usually for one dose). This acts as competitive inhibitor of anti-platelet IgG.
- ? If the platelet count is very low consider anti-D antibody (if patient Rh+) 50–75 µg/kg/dose; ensure adequate hydration, watch for excessive hemolysis.
- Splenectomy: If severe, chronic, and not responsive to steroids or IgG (primary site of platelet phagocytosis)
- Immunosuppression with cyclosporin, azathioprine, or other agents if there is no response to splenectomy (or if contraindicated). Cyclophosphamide/vincristine may be effective.
- Avoid contact sports or activities when the platelet count is low.

Use of corticosteroids, IgG, and anti-D is decreasing due to the unfavorable risk–benefit ratio and lack of evidence of clinically worthwhile effect.

Prognosis

Over 80% of cases spontaneously remit within 8 weeks. Presentation at >10 years of age or in girls increases the chance of chronic disease. However, >90% of patients recover.

Thrombophilia

These hemostatic disorders predispose to venous or arterial thrombosis.
- They may be inherited or acquired.
- Most inherited thrombophilias are asymptomatic or present in adult life. In children, most commonly present in the newborn period or following trauma or surgery.
- Inherited thrombophilia should be considered when there is an unexplained arterial or venous thrombosis, neonatal venous thrombosis, or positive family history.

Inherited causes

Activated protein C resistance

This is the most common inherited thrombophilia. Activated protein C (APC) limits hemostasis with cofactor protein S. More than 90% of APCR is due to factor V Leiden (FVL) deficiency (present in 3%–7% of population). Heterozygotes for FVL deficiency have a 5–10 times increased risk of thrombosis, homozygotes 30–80 times the risk. Because FVL defiency is so common, it is not rare for individuals to be also heterozygous for the prothrombin variant, protein C or S deficiency, leading to significant thrombophilia.

Prothrombin 20210 mutation

This is the second-most common inherited thrombophilia, present in 2%–3% of population. It results in a higher average prothrombin level. Heterozygotes have an ~3 times increased risk of thrombosis.

Protein C deficiency

Thromboembolism is rare in childhood but in homozygotes may cause life-threatening, massive thrombosis in the newborn, resulting in skin bruises that may become necrotic (purpura fulminans).

Protein S deficiency

This is clinically similar to protein C deficiency.

Antithrombin III deficiency

This deficiency is rare, but is associated with high thrombotic risk. It generally causes venous thrombosis.

Homocysteinemia

This may be secondary to a genetic defect or vitamin B_{12} or folate deficiency. Congenital homocysteinemia is associated with thromboembolism, e.g., stroke, mental retardation, and, in later life, arteriosclerosis.

Acquired causes

Acquired thrombophilia is most commonly associated with
- Polycythemia
- Septicemia
- Asphyxia
- Use of central lines
- Inflammation
- SLE, anti-phospholipid antibody

Newborns, especially if preterm, are most at risk. In the newborn, arterial or aortic thrombosis secondary to an umbilical arterial catheter (UAC) may lead to bowel infarction, NEC, buttock or leg infarction, or renal arterial thrombosis. The most common venous thrombosis involves the renal vein.

Investigation of thrombophilia

- CBC (polycythemia or infection)
- ESR/CRP (infection, inflammation)
- LFTs (proteins C, S, and prothrombin are vitamin K–dependent factors)
- Standard coagulation tests
- Thrombophilia "screen," including plasma levels of proteins C and S, antithrombin III, homocysteine, and factor V Leiden, prothrombin variant DNA testing, lupus anticoagulant screen, anti-phospholipid antibody panel, and factor VIII activity. Consider assay for APC resistance if other testing is negative.

Treatment

Acute thrombosis

Anticoagulate with heparin or low-molecular-weight (LMW) heparin and then warfarin. In emergency, e.g., neonatal purpura fulminans, treat with FFP at least every 12 hours.

Recurrent thrombosis

Treatment depends on the severity, presentation, coagulation defect, and risk factors. Long-term anticoagulation with warfarin may be appropriate (aim for INR of 2–3).

Major vessel or catheter related thrombosis

Consider treatment with fibrinolytic agents, e.g., TPA.

Prophylaxis

Give SC heparin during surgery or trauma. Alternatively, antithrombin III or protein C concentrate may be given if relevant.

Blood transfusion

Red blood cell transfusion

Generally, packed RBC are preferred (especially for cardiac, liver, or renal disease), except for special situations such as occasionally in the operating room, when whole blood may address both hypovolemia and reduced O_2 carrying capacity (e.g., acute blood loss). Small-volume QUAD packs or aliquots are preferred for newborns or infants to allow multiple transfusions from a single donor.

Formula for calculation of transfusion volume
- Packed cells (mL) = Desired rise in Hb (g/dL) × weight (kg) × 3 (this may overestimate actual rise in Hb achieved).

Platelet transfusion

This is indicated for prevention or reduction in bleeding due to significant thrombocytopenia (e.g., <10 × 10^9/L, or higher if patient is symptomatic or needs invasive procedure) or platelet function disorders. Platelet concentrate volume: Child weight <15 kg = 10–20 mL/kg; ≥15 kg = single apheresis unit/standard pool of 4 units.

Albumin

- 5% albumin traditionally is used as emergency treatment for shock, but use is decreasing, as 0.9% saline is preferred.
- 25% albumin is indicated to correct severe hypoproteinemia.

Fresh frozen plasma

Indications
- DIC
- Emergency therapy of nonspecific hemostatic failure
- Coagulation deficiencies for which no specific concentrate is available

  Volume = 10–20 mL/kg (guided by coagulation results)

Cryoprecipitate

This is rich in clotting factors VIII, XIII, fibrinogen, and vWF. The main indication is as support for clotting defects induced by massive transfusion or DIC, especially if fibrinogen <100 mg/dL: Volume = 5 mL/kg, or if child 15–30 kg = 5 units (1 unit = 1 bag), over 30 kg = 10 units.

Intravenous immunoglobulin

Normal immunoglobulin is predominantly IgG and is obtained from pooled plasma of >1000 blood donations. Indications include the following:
- Hypogammaglobulinemia, e.g., sex-linked hypogammaglobulinemia
- Prophylaxis following infection contact in immunocompromised patients, e.g., CMV, hepatitis A, measles
- Immunomodulation, e.g., ITP, neonatal alloimmune thrombocytopenia
- Prevention of potentially life-threatening chicken pox in previously noninfected immunocompromised patients

Special requirements

CMV-negative blood components

These are required in
- Intrauterine transfusion
- Neonates and infants up to 1 year
- CMV-seronegative recipients of allogenic HSCT (and potential recipients)
- Immunosuppressed patients, e.g., receiving chemotherapy

Irradiated blood products

These are required in
- Intrauterine and neonatal exchange transfusions
- Recipients of HSCT autografts (for at least 3 months) and allogenic HSCT (some say lifelong)
- HLA-matched platelets
- Directed donations from relatives
- Post-chemotherapy
- Hodgkin's lymphoma
- Congenital cellular immunodeficiencies
- Granulocyte transfusion

Leukodepleted blood components

These are required in
- Patients at high risk for alloimmunization, e.g., aplastic anemia, acute myeloid leukemia (AML)
- Patients with recurrent febrile transfusion reactions despite premedication with acetaminophen/diphenhydramine
- Patients requiring CMV-negative components when seronegative components are not available

Blood transfusion reactions

Incompatible blood

Signs or symptoms may appear after only 5–10 mL blood infused.

- Agitation, pain at venipuncture site, flushing, chest, abdominal, or flank pain
- Fever, hypotension, hemoglobinemia, hemoglobinuria, renal failure

Treatment

- Stop infusion.
- Keep line open with saline →.
- Monitor vital signs and urine output.
- Recheck patient and blood unit ID.
- Give supportive care (watch for hypotension, respiratory and renal failure).
- Inform blood bank.

Bacterial-infected blood

This is most like to occur with platelets. There is sudden hypotension, fever, rigors, hypotension, and DIC.

Treatment

Give IV broad-spectrum antibiotics and inotropic support.

Transfusion related acute lung injury (TRALI)

Rapid-onset cough and shortness of breath (may mimic fluid overload) occur. TRALI is caused by donor antibodies to recipient leukocytes. There is an ARDS-like picture, with bilateral infiltrates on chest X-ray. Respiratory support is required.

Febrile, nonhemolytic reactions

These are due to recipient anti-HLA or granulocyte antibodies, or cytokines in infused product. They occur less frequently with universal leukodepletion of products. Fever and rigors set in within few hours of starting or completing the transfusion. Slow the transfusion rate and give acetaminophen and antihistamines.

Circulatory overload

This is marked by pulmonary edema, dyspnea, headache, venous distension, and signs of cardiac failure. Slow the transfusion rate and give IV furosemide.

Transfusion-associated graft versus host disease (TaGVHD)

This occurs in patients with impaired cellular immunity. Lymphocytes in the donor unit "engraft," leading to rash, diarrhea, liver impairment, and bone marrow failure. There is no effective treatment. Mortality is ~90%.

Transfusion safety

The estimated U.S. rates of infection from blood products per transfused component are as follows (rates may change):

- Hepatitis B: 1 in 140,000
- Hepatitis C: 1 in 1 million
- HIV: 1 in 2.5 million
- Malaria: 0.5 in 1 million
- Bacterial infection: 2 in 1 million for RBC; higher (up to 1 in 2000) for platelet transfusion
- Variant Creutzfeld–Jakob disease (CJD): Unknown (2 cases reported in the U.K. up to 2005)

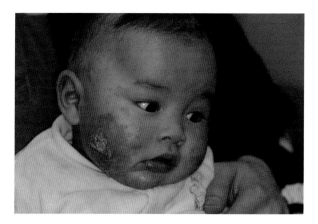

Plate 1 Atopic dermatitis.

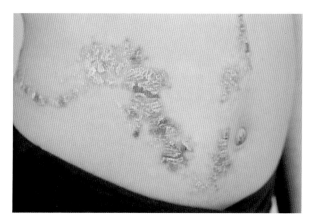

Plate 2 Psoriasis.

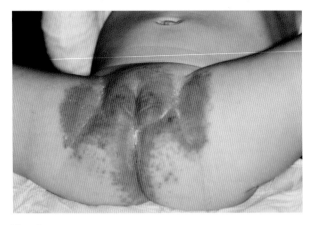

Plate 3 Irritated diaper rash with candidiasis.

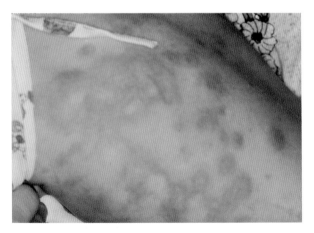

Plate 4 Urticaria.

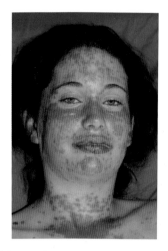

Plate 7 Stevens johnson syndrome.

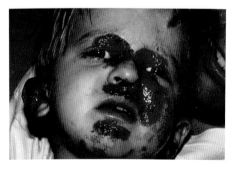

Plate 8 Epidermolysis bullosa.

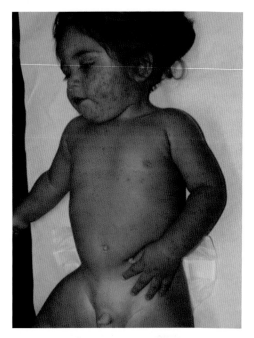

Plate 5 Viral rash—Gianotti Crosti syndrome.

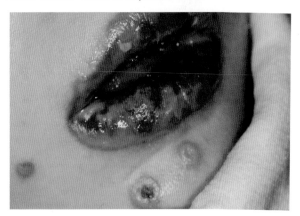

Plate 6 Erythema multiforme.

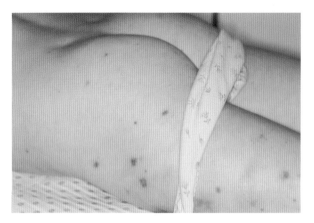

Plate 9 Henoch Schonlein purpura.

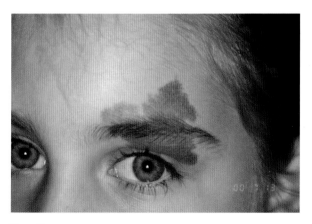

Plate 10 Capillary vascular malformation (port wine stain).

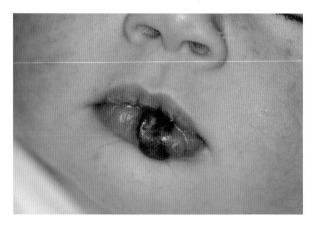

Plate 11 Superficial hemangioma.

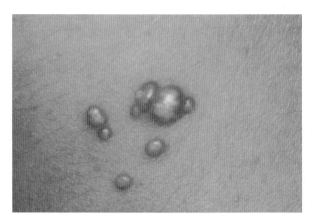

Plate 12 Molluscum contagiosum.

Oncology

Epidemiology of childhood cancer

- Childhood cancer (age <20 years old) accounts for 0.8% of all cancer.
- Approximately 12,400 new cases of childhood cancer occur in the United States every year.
- Childhood cancer is the most common cause of death in children aged 5–9 years and second to accidents in children aged 10–19 years.
- The annual incidence in children under 20 year of age is 1.5 in 10,000.
- One in 300 will have cancer before 20 years of age.

Causes of cancer in childhood

Environmental factors do not appear to be clearly linked with childhood cancer. An inherited predisposition applies to a minority of tumors.

The proportion of cases by diagnostic group (ages 0–14, Surveillance Epidemiology and End Results [SEER], 1992–2001):

- Acute leukemias   29%
- Lymphoma   10%
- CNS tumors   22%
- Neuroblastoma   8%
- Wilms tumor   6%
- Bone tumors   4%
- Soft tissue sarcoma   7%
- Germ cell tumors   3%
- Retinoblastoma   3%
- Liver tumors   1%
- Others   7%

Clinical assessment: history

Childhood

Include specific questions about the following:

- Fevers, night sweats, anorexia, weight loss, pallor, bruising and abnormal bleeding
- Family history, including malignancy and inherited conditions

Also be aware that childhood malignancy may present with a variety of clinical features and so special attention should be paid to symptoms described below.

Respiratory symptoms

New onset of wheeze (usually monophonic and fixed) may be caused by an intrathoracic mass. Treatment with oral steroids, based on a presumptive diagnosis of asthma, may lead to partial response in symptoms and therefore delay the diagnosis of leukemia or lymphoma involving mediastinal lymphadenopathy compressing the airways.

Bone and joint pain and swelling

Persistent back pain should not be dismissed as innocent in children. It may reflect bone pain of bone-marrow expansion (leukemia or bone marrow metastases), or a spinal tumor.

Abdominal mass

This may be

- Painless and isolated (e.g., Wilms tumor, ovarian teratoma)
- Associated with general malaise (e.g., B-cell lymphoma, neuroblastoma)
- Pelvic (rhabdomyosarcoma)

Raised intracranial pressure

The most common presenting features of brain tumors are the following:

- Headache (typically on waking)
- Vomiting
- Ataxia
- Papilledema
- Deteriorating conscious level

Growth and endocrine disturbances

Midline CNS tumors may result in disturbance in the hypothalamic–pituitary hormone axes and present with the following:

- Poor feeding or failure to thrive (diencephalic syndrome)
- Polyuria and polydipsia (diabetes insipidus)
- Poor growth and short stature (growth hormone deficiency)
- Hypoglycemia (ACTH deficiency)

Clinical examination

Conduct a thorough general examination including the following:

- *All lymph node sites*: Neck, axillae, inguinal regions
- *Skin*: Assess pallor, petechiae, bruising, mucosal bleeding, signs of infection.
- *Masses*: Measure dimensions of any mass and organomegaly.
- If leukemia or lymphoma is suspected, assess testes for swelling and optic fundi.

Specific diagnoses or concerns may be indicated by the findings discussed below.

Lymphadenopathy

Malignancy accounts for a small proportion of cases of persistent lymphadenopathy in children. Possible diagnoses include acute leukemia, non-Hodgkin's lymphoma, Hodgkin's disease, and metastases from neuroblastoma or sarcoma.

The following features of an enlarged lymph node should raise concern:
- Diameter >2 cm
- Persistent or progressive enlargement
- Non-tender, rubbery, hard, or fixed
- Supraclavicular location
- Associated with other systemic features, e.g., pallor, lethargy
- Hepatosplenomegaly

Unexplained mass on any site

The following features should raise suspicion of malignancy:
- Non-tender
- Progressive enlargement
- Diameter >2 cm
- Associated lymphadenopathy

Neurological signs

The following features should raise suspicion of a brain tumor:
- Cranial nerve deficits from direct tumor involvement
- False localizing signs—III and VI nerve palsies (mass effect from raised ICP)
- Cerebellar signs (e.g., ataxia)
- Visual disturbances or abnormal eye movements: Field and/or acuity defects (optic tract and suprasellar tumors); Parinaud's syndrome (paralysis of upward gaze) suggests pineal tumor
- Abnormalities of gait
- Motor or sensory signs
- Behavioral disturbances
- Deteriorating school performance or neurodevelopmental milestones
- Unexplained focal seizures
- Increasing head size (infants)

Key investigations

The most common reason for referral to specialist is the identification of an abnormality on blood film.

Pancytopenia

Not all cell lines are equally affected when the following problems occur, as leukemia or disseminated malignancy displaces

- Pallor, lethargy (low Hb)
- Bruising and/or petechiae (low platelets)
- *Unexplained fever*, recurrent or persistent infection (low WBC)

The following tests are used in diagnosis and assessment for prognosis, and as a baseline before starting treatment.

Laboratory tests

- Full blood count and differential
- Coagulation studies
- Type and cross-match blood
- Electrolytes, calcium, phosphorous, uric acid,
- Renal and liver profile, lactate dehydrogenase
- Blood cultures (if febrile)
- Urine catecholamines (neuroblastoma, pheochromocytoma)
- Lumbar puncture for cell count, cytology

Imaging

Sedation or general anesthetic may be needed in young children when performing these procedures. The choice of imaging depends on the likely diagnosis, and may include the following:

- Chest X-ray
- CT scan of chest and/or abdomen
- MRI scan (better than CT for soft-tissue swellings and brain)
- Bone marrow aspirate and/or biopsy
- Technetium (^{99}Tc) bone scan
- MIBG scan (neuroblastoma, pheochromocytoma)

Other investigations

These depend on the treatment being planned and may include

- EDTA glomerular filtration rate (nephrotoxic chemotherapy, nephrectomy)
- Audiology assessment (platinum chemotherapy, cranial radiotherapy)
- Echocardiogram (anthracycline, pulmonary radiotherapy)
- Lung function (bleomycin, pulmonary radiotherapy)
- Pituitary function (suprasellar tumors, CNS surgery or radiotherapy)

Acute lymphoblastic leukemia (ALL)

ALL is the most common malignancy in childhood. It arises from malignant proliferation of pre-B- (common ALL) or T-cell lymphoid precursors. The cause is unknown, but in a minority of patients it is associated with constitutional chromosomal aberrations.

Possible links to patterns of childhood infection acting as a trigger have been hypothesized.

- ALL accounts for 25% of all childhood malignancies.
- It commonly presents in young children aged 2–6 years.

Presentation

Typically patients present with a short history (days or weeks) and with symptoms and signs reflecting pancytopenia, bone marrow expansion, and lymphadenopathy. Symptoms include petechiae, bruising, pallor, fatigue, bone and joint pain and swelling, limp, lymphadenopathy, airway obstruction, and pleural effusion (see Box 18.1 for treatment).

Risk groups

- *Standard risk*: B-lineage, age 1–10 years, initial WBC <50,000
- *High risk*: B-lineage, age ≥10 years OR initial WBC ≥50,000
- *T-lineage*: Any age, any initial WBC
- *Infant*: age <1 year, any initial WBC

Specific diagnostic tests

- Bone marrow for morphology, immunophenotype, cytogenetics
- CSF for cytospin
- Clinical examination of testes in boys for inappropriate swelling
- Chest X-ray for mediastinal mass
- CT or MRI of head if there are CNS symptoms

Box 18.1 Outline of treatment of ALL

Induction (4 weeks)
- Steroids (dexamethasone or prednisone) throughout induction
- Weekly IV vincristine
- IM L-asparaginase (e.g., 9 doses in 3 weeks or 1 dose of pegaspar0067ase)
- IV daunorubicin (4 doses, in high-risk cases)
- Intrathecal (IT) cytarabine (day 1) and methotrexate (days 8 and 29, additional doses if there is CNS disease at diagnosis)

NOTE: Tumor lysis syndrome (p. 790) is a significant risk.

Consolidation or CNS-directed therapy (4–8 weeks)
- *Standard-risk cases*: 4 weekly doses of IT methotrexate and continuous oral mercaptopurine
- *High-risk cases*: IV cyclophosphamide, cytarabine, oral mercaptopurine
- CNS-directed radiotherapy for CNS-positive and selected high-risk cases

Interim maintenance (8 weeks)
- *Standard-risk cases*: Daily mercaptopurine, weekly oral methotrexate (doses titrated according to blood count); 4-weekly vincristine IV bolus and 5-day pulses of oral dexamethasone or prednisone
- *High-risk cases*: Every 10 days vincristine and methotrexate IV boluses, pegaspargase every 20 days
- IT methotrexate monthly

Delayed intensification (8 weeks)
Two blocks, prior to maintenance, with combinations of oral steroid, vincristine, doxorubicin, pegaspargase, cyclophosphamide, cytarabine, and thioguanine

Maintenance
Continuation treatment for a total duration of 2.2 years (3.2 years for boys)
- Daily 6-mercaptopurine (6-MP), weekly oral methotrexate; (doses titrated according to blood count)
- 4-weekly vincristine IV bolus and 5-day pulses of oral dexamethasone or prednisone
- 12-weekly IT methotrexate

Prognosis

Overall survival is approximately 80% with current treatment. Adverse prognostic factors include the following:
- Male gender
- Age <1 years or >10 years
- High white count at diagnosis
- Unfavorable cytogenetics: Philadelphia chromosome—t(9;22); MLL gene rearrangements (e.g., t(4;11) in infants)
- Slow early response to induction (assessed by bone marrow aspiration on days 8 and/or 15)
- Failure to achieve remission or high level of minimal residual disease (MRD) at 28 days of induction

Mature B-cell ALL (Burkitt type, L3 morphology)

Once considered a high-risk group, the outlook is similar to that for standard-risk ALL, now that patients are treated with intensive chemotherapy according to the strategy for B-cell non-Hodgkin's lymphoma (see p. 762).

Relapsed ALL

Extramedullary relapse (mainly CNS, testes) may present without bone marrow disease. Treatment is stratified according to risk factors:
- Time from first diagnosis (risk reduces with time)
- Extramedullary relapse (lower risk, particularly if isolated)
- MRD status after reinduction (negative status reduces risk)

Treatment
- Intensive reinduction and consolidation for all risk groups
- Low risk: 2 years of continuing conventional chemotherapy
- High risk: Allogeneic hematopoietic stem cell transplantation (HSCT)
- Intermediate risk: Offer HSCT, based on availability of a matched donor
- Radiotherapy for extramedullary disease is given as a boost for those receiving total body irradiation (TBI) for HSCT.

Prognosis
Long-term survival varies, at 30%–70% depending on risk (e.g., 70% is for those with isolated extramedullary relapse more than 2 years off treatment).

Acute myeloid leukemia (AML)

AML accounts for ~5% of all childhood malignancies and <20% of all acute leukemias. It is also known as acute nonlymphoblastic leukemia (ANLL), and AML results from malignant proliferation of myeloid cell precursors. AML can be subdivided into morphologically and cytogenetic abnormalities.

Acute myeloid leukemia with recurrent genetic abnormality

- Acute myeloid leukemia with t(8;21)(q22;q22), (*AML1/ETO*)
- Acute myeloid leukemia with abnormal bone marrow eosinophils and inv(16)(p13q22) or t(16;16)(p13;q22), (*CBF/MYH11*)
- Acute promyelocytic leukemia with t(15;17)(q22;q12), (*PML/RAR*)
- Acute myeloid leukemia with 11q23 (*MLL*) abnormalities

Acute myeloid leukemia with multilineage dysplasia

Acute myeloid leukemia and myelodysplastic syndromes, therapy related

- Alkylating agent/radiation–related type
- Topoisomerase II inhibitor–related type
- Others

Acute myeloid leukemia, not otherwise categorized

Classify as:
- Acute myeloid leukemia, minimally differentiated
- Acute myeloid leukemia without maturation
- Acute myeloid leukemia with maturation
- Acute myelomonocytic leukemia
- Acute monoblastic/acute monocytic leukemia
- Acute erythroid leukemia
- Acute megakaryoblastic leukemia
- Acute basophilic leukemia
- Acute panmyelosis with myelofibrosis
- Myeloid sarcoma

Presentation

- Symptoms and signs of bone marrow replacement
- Lymphadenopathy is less prominent than in ALL.
- Intrathoracic extramedullary disease is less common than in ALL.
- M3 may present with coagulopathy from proteolytic enzyme activity.
- Solid deposits (chloroma) are occasionally seen in M2, M4, or M5.

Cytogenetics

Cytogenetic analysis shows characteristic abnormalities:
- M1 and M2 AML: t(8;21) translocation is observed in 15% of all cases.
- M3 AML: t(15;17) translocation is observed in 100% of cases.
- M4Eo: inv(16) is frequently observed.

These translocations are regarded as good prognostic indicators. Monosomy 5, deletion 5q, and monsomy 7 are associated with poor risk.

Molecular alterations
Specific molecular abnormalities associated with AML
- *FLT3/ITD* observed in 15% of all cases
- *NPM* mutations observed in 10% of cases
- *CEBP* mutations observed in 5%
- These mutations are mainly observed in patients with normal karyotype. *FLT3/ITD* is a prognostic factor for poor outcome and *NPM* and *CEBP* are associated with improved outcome.

Treatment
In AML, prolonged continuation therapy is not used:
- 4 or 5 courses of intensive, nearly myeloablative chemotherapy
- Promyelocytic leukemia (PML): All-*trans*-retinoic acid and arsenic trioxide in addition to chemotherapy improve survival
- High-risk cases, i.e., failure to achieve complete remission after 2 courses, should have HSCT in the first remission.

Prognosis
Overall survival is 50%.

Relapsed AML
Most cases receive HSCT after intensive reinduction.

Leukemia and Down syndrome
The risk of developing acute leukemia is increased 20–30 times in children with Down syndrome. Most commonly this is either a pre-B (common) ALL or AML (especially M7).

Generally, response to chemotherapy is good and better relapse-free survival is found among those with AML. However, children with Down syndrome–associated leukemia experience more complications at treatment, particularly infection.

Other genetic conditions predisposing to AML
- Fanconi syndrome
- Bloom syndrome
- Ataxia–telangiectasia
- Kostmann syndrome (congenital severe neutropenia)
- Diamond–Blackfan anemia
- Klinefelter syndrome (47 XYY)
- Turner syndrome (45 XO)
- Neurofibromatosis
- Incontinentia pigmenti

Chronic myeloid leukemia (CML, adult type)

This is classically associated with Philadelphia chromosome–positive disease (t(9;22) translocation). It is rare in childhood.

The disease has a chronic phase with nonspecific symptoms (fever, night sweats, and hepatosplenomegaly). During this phase the only curative therapy is HSCT, although the advent of targeted therapy with imatinib (Gleevec) and other orally availably tyrosine kinase inhibitors may change the timing and necessity of HSCT. The chronic phase progresses to a blast phase that, typically, has a picture similar to acute leukemia (ALL or AML), and HSCT is required. Prognosis is worse if HSCT is delayed until blast crisis.

Juvenile myelomonocytic leukemia (JMML)

Classified with the myelodysplasias, JMML is also known as juvenile CML. It is rare (<1% childhood malignancy). Age of onset is mostly <2 years. It is associated with monosomy 7, NF1, and Noonan syndrome. The response to chemotherapy is poor and the disease is curable only with HSCT.

Lymphoma

There are two distinct disease entities that differ in natural history, presentation, and management. Both are more common in boys than in girls.

Non-Hodgkin's lymphoma (NHL)

The annual incidence of NHL is 10 per million. The majority of cases are high-grade tumors that are divided into categories, using histology, immunophenotype, and cytogenetics (see Box 18.2).

Box 18.2 Classification of NHL

- *Lymphoblastic* (90% T-cell, 10% pre-B-cell): 30% of all NHL. Most patients present with an anterior mediastinal mass. Disease may be present in bone, bone marrow, skin, CNS, liver, kidneys, and spleen. Cases with >25% blasts in bone marrow are conventionally regarded as leukemia (ALL). Terminal deoxynucleotidyl transferase (TdT) positivity is usually observed. Translocations t(1;14) or t(11;14) may be observed.
- *Mature B cell* (Burkitt or Burkitt-like): 30% childhood NHL. This type occurs in the abdomen, head and neck, bone marrow, and CNS. It may grow rapidly. Endemic or African Burkitt's is associated with early Epstein–Barr virus (EBV) infection and frequently affects the jaw. It expresses surface immunoglobulin and characteristic translocations t(8;14), t(8;22) or t(2;8).
- *Large cell lymphoma*: 15%–20% childhood NHL. Subtypes are diffuse large B-cell (BLCL), which presents like Burkitt, and anaplastic large cell lymphoma (ALCL), which involves extranodal sites (skin and bone). Lymphadenopathy is often peripheral and painful. CNS or bone marrow disease is rare. ALCL is characterized by CD30 expression and t(2;5).

NHL staging (St. Jude system)
- *Stage I*: Single site or nodal area (not abdomen or mediastinum)
- *Stage II*: Regional nodes, abdominal disease
- *Stage III*: Disease on both sides of the diaphragm
- *Stage IV*: Bone marrow or CNS disease

Investigations
- *Tissue*: Bone marrow aspirate; lumbar puncture; pleural and abdominal (peritoneal) fluid aspirate; excisional biopsy
- *Imaging*: CT and positron emission tomography (PET) scans

Treatment
Lymphoblastic (T-cell, pre-B-cell) lymphoma treatment is similar to that for ALL. Mature B-cell disease is treated with a short series of dose-intensive courses of chemotherapy. Risk of tumor lysis (p. 790) is high.

Prognosis
Survival is >70% (>90% in those with localized disease).

Hodgkin's lymphoma

The incidence of Hodgkin's lymphoma (HL) is very low before age 5 years and rises with age. It is more common in patients with previous EBV infection and ~25% of patients have EBV genome found within the tumor. The histology shows Reed–Sternberg cells surrounded by an inflammatory milieu within the affected lymph node infiltrate.

Presentation

There is painless lymph node enlargement, the most common sites being cervical (80%) and mediastinal (60%). Metastatic spread to extranodal sites is less common, and the most common sites of metastasis are lungs and bone marrow. Fever, night sweats, and weight loss (>10%) constitute "B" symptoms and are more common in advanced stages.

Subtypes

Hodgkin's lymphoma is divided into two subtypes, which are then further subdivided by histology. Classical HL includes nodular sclerosing (most common), mixed cellularity, and lymphocyte-depleted histology. Nodular lymphocyte–predominant HL is the other subtype, characterized by its histology.

Staging (Ann Arbor system)

- *Stage I:* Single site
- *Stage II:* More than one site but on one side of diaphragm
- *Stage III:* On both sides of the diaphragm
- *Stage IV:* Extranodal disease, such as lung or bone marrow

Investigations

- CT of neck, chest, abdomen, and pelvis
- FDG PET or gallium scan
- Bone marrow aspiration and biopsy
- Isotope bone scan (generally done with stage IV disease, evidence of bone pain, or stage II disease with B symptoms)

Treatment

Practices differ, but the balance between cure and adverse long-term effects should be considered.

While some patients, particularly those with stage I or II disease, may be cured by radiotherapy alone, studies have shown superiority to combined modality therapy with chemotherapy and radiotherapy. For all patients, chemotherapy generally includes alkylating agents, vinca alkaloids, and corticosteroids. Low-dose involved field radiotherapy is generally the standard of care. In the context of clinical trials, reduction or augmentation of these therapies is being explored to strike an appropriate balance between efficacy and toxicity.

Prognosis for initially treated patients

- 5-year overall survival is >90%, with event-free survival ranging from 80% to >90%.

Relapse

Cure is still possible with second-line therapy, including autologous HSCT.

CNS tumors (1)

Brain tumors are the most common solid tumors, accounting for 25% of all childhood malignancies.

> ## Box 18.3 Classification of CNS tumors
>
> - *Infratentorial tumors* (>50%) present with raised ICP, headaches and vomiting, and cerebellar ataxia.
> - *Supratentorial tumors* present with raised ICP, focal neurology, hypothalamic/pituitary dysfunction, and visual impairment.
> - *Primary spinal tumors* (rare): Differential diagnosis includes astrocytomas and ependymomas. They may present with cord compression
> - *CNS metastases* of extracranial tumors are rare.

- Involvement of a multidisciplinary team is central to management of CNS tumors.
- The presenting features vary and may delay the diagnosis. For every childhood brain tumor there are ~5000 children with migraine!

Initial management

Diagnostic imaging

- CT is quick and available. It provides essential information for emergency management of hydrocephalus.
- MRI gives better tumor definition. Combine it with spinal imaging for staging of disease.

Raised intracranial pressure

This requires prompt treatment:

- Referral and transfer to a pediatric neurosurgical unit
- Control tumor swelling with high-dose steroids (usually dexamethasone).
- CSF drainage: Initial surgery may involve CSF diversion only, biopsy, or complete resection, depending on location and the likely diagnosis.

Low-grade glioma (grade I, 45% CNS tumors)

Most of these are pilocytic astrocytoma in the cerebellum and optic pathway.

- Outcome depends on the site. Posterior fossa lesions can be cured with surgery alone, whereas optic-pathway tumors are relatively inaccessible and morbidity is high.
- Neurofibromatosis type 1 (NF1; see p. 1072)
- 50% of optic pathway low-grade gliomas
- Visual outcome is better.
- Radiotherapy is contraindicated because of risk of second tumors.

High-grade glioma (grade III / IV, 10% CNS tumors)
- Tumors are predominantly in older children and teenagers.
- Supratentorial sites predominate.
- These are difficult to manage since complete resection is difficult to achieve.

Brain-stem glioma
- Glioma is in the region of the pons, is usually high grade and inoperable.
- Radiotherapy is the primary treatment.
- Median survival is <1 year.

Primitive neuroectodermal tumors (PNETs, 25% CNS tumors)
- These are the most common malignant brain tumors of childhood.
- The majority occur in the cerebellum (medulloblastoma).
- Peak incidence is <5 years.
- Tumor metastases (mainly via the CSF) occur in 10%–15% of cases.
- 70% of localized cases can be cured, but expect significant long-term morbidity from radiotherapy.

Treatment
Treatment includes excision and craniospinal radiotherapy. Additional chemotherapy carries a survival advantage, allowing reduction in drug dose and/or field of radiotherapy, particularly in younger patients. Chemotherapy regimens include alkylating agents (e.g., CCNU, cyclophosphamide), platinum drugs (cisplatin, carboplatin), and vincristine. These are usually given after radiotherapy. High-dose chemotherapy may have a role in relapsed cases and in treating infants.

CNS tumors (2)

Ependymoma (10% of CNS tumors)
- Periventricular sites
- Usually present with obstructive hydrocephalus
- 10% metastasize to the spine
- Treated by surgical excision and involved field radiotherapy
- Chemotherapy treatment, depending age
- >70% survival if complete excision

CNS germ cell tumors (5% of CNS tumors)
- Rare and more commonly seen in teenage males
- Midline (suprasellar or pineal): 50% germinoma, 50% nongerminomatous secreting malignant germ cell tumors (e.g., embryonal carcinoma) or mature teratomas
- Secreting tumors are characterized by raised markers (AFP or HCG) in either serum or CSF (biopsy is marker in negative cases).
- Primary surgery for teratoma. Chemotherapy and radiotherapy for other tumor types
- Cure in 70% secreting tumors (>90% for germinoma/teratoma)

Craniopharyingioma (10% of CNS tumors)
- Slow-growing midline epithelial tumors in the suprasellar area from Rathke's pouch
- Treatment is complete resection in 80% of cases, partial resection with focal radiotherapy in the remainder. Complications include damage to the hypothalamic–pituitary structures, vision, and behavior.

Retinoblastoma (3% of all tumors)
- Sporadic or familial (40%) forms that are unilateral or bilateral (30%) on presentation
- *Peak incidence*: Unilateral disease is 2–3 years; bilateral disease is 0–12 months.
- *Presentation*: Absent or abnormal light reflex (leukocoria), squint, or visual deterioration
- *Treatment*: Surgery, chemotherapy, and focal therapy
- *90% 5-year survival*: The inherited form is at risk of second primary malignancy, with osteosarcoma being the most common.

Neuroblastoma

This is a malignant embryonal tumor derived from neural crest tissue with a wide spectrum of behavior. It represents 7% of all childhood malignancies. Median age of presentation is 2 years. Sites of involvement include the following:

- Adrenal glands (32%)
- Sympathetic chain (25%)
- Abdomen (28%)
- Thorax (15%)
- Pelvis (6%)
- Neck (2%)

The tumor may be locally invasive, surrounding rather than displacing vessels and other structures. Distant metastases to bone, bone marrow, liver, CNS, lungs, and skin (especially infants) occur.

Presentation

Presentation is nonspecific and variable. It depends on the site, spread, and metabolic effects:

- Palpable mass (may be painless)
- Compression of nerves (e.g., Horner's, spinal cord), airway, veins, bowel
- Bone pain and/or limp
- Lymphadenopathy and signs of pancytopenia
- Sweating, pallor, watery diarrhea, and hypertension

Specific diagnostic tests

- Urine catecholamine (VMA or HVA)-to-creatinine ratio is raised in >80% cases.
- ^{123}I-mIBG uptake scan is usually positive.

Treatment

- Biologic factors (such as *MYCN* amplification or tumor histology) and age strongly influence prognosis and treatment.
- Completely resected localized neuroblastoma with favorable biology may need no further treatment.
- Incompletely resected, stage III tumors require chemotherapy and possibly adjuvant radiotherapy.
- Stage 4 (disseminated) and *MYCN*-positive stage 3 tumors require induction chemotherapy, surgery, high-dose chemotherapy with autologous stem cell rescue, radiotherapy, and maintenance biotherapy with oral *cis*-retinoic acid.
- *Exception*: Young (<18 month old) stage 4 patients with favorable biologic features receive moderately intensive chemotherapy and surgery only.

Prognosis (see Box 18.4)

Disseminated neuroblastoma only is cured in 20%–30%, despite intensive treatment. Infants (<18 months old) are the exception, with >90% survival even with disseminated disease. Survival in low-risk cases (low stage, infants) is >90%.

> **Box 18.4 Poor prognostic factors in neuroblastoma**
>
> - Age >18 months
> - Stage 3 and 4 disease
> - Raised serum ferritin
> - Raised LDH
> - Raised neuron-specific enolase (NSE)
> - Unfavorable histology
> - *MYCN* oncogene amplification
> - 17q gain/1p loss

Relapse treatment

Options include further surgery, chemotherapy, and/or radiotherapy, depending on the primary treatment received. After previous high-dose chemotherapy and HSCT, cure is unrealistic and treatment is aimed at palliation.

Infant neuroblastoma (stage 4S)

Disseminated disease is restricted to the bone marrow, liver, and skin. Characteristically this usually resolves spontaneously. Chemotherapy is only for life-threatening symptoms. Resection (complete or partial) is usually sufficient for localized disease.

Wilms tumor (nephroblastoma)

This is an embryonal tumor of the kidney representing 6%–7% of all childhood malignancies. Up to 75% present at <4 years (90% <7 years). Most causes are sporadic, but 1% have an affected family member. Wilms tumor may be associated with the following conditions:

- Genitourinary abnormalities (e.g., horseshoe kidney, hypospadias)
- Hemihypertrophy syndrome
- Aniridia
- Beckwith–Wiedeman syndrome (BWS)
- WAGR complex (**W**ilms, **A**niridia, **G**onadal dysplasia, **R**etardation)
- Denys–Drash syndrome (nephropathy and genital abnormalities)
- Perlman syndrome

Mutations of the *WT1* tumor suppressor gene (located on chromosome 11p13) are detected in Wilms tumors, with only a minority of patients having germline mutations. Other genes involved in Wilms tumorigenesis include those found on chromosomes 1, 16, 17, and 11. Abnormalities of 11p15 are also implicated, associated with BWS.

Presentation

Mostly a visible or palpable abdominal mass is present, and it is usually painless. Hematuria and hypertension may also be seen.

Site

Bilateral cases are unusual and more often associated with genetic predisposition and younger age at presentation. Extrarenal Wilms tumors are very rare. Metastases occur in 10% of cases, most commonly to the lung.

Investigations

- Abdominal ultrasound
- CT scan of abdomen ("claw" sign in involved kidney)
- Chest X-ray or CT
- Urine catecholamines to exclude neuroblastoma
- Blood count and coagulation studies (a transient acquired von Willebrand–like syndrome is recognized and resolves with treatment)

Treatment

- Surgical excision is required.
- Chemotherapy is used for all tumors. Stage I or II disease (complete resection of tumor without or with breach of renal capsule) is curable with vincristine and dactinomycin. In higher-stage disease, doxorubicin is added. In bilateral (stage V) disease, the aim is to maximize the response to chemotherapy prior to performing bilateral nephron-sparing surgery.
- Local radiotherapy is required for incomplete-resection (stage III) disease or distant metastases (stage IV). Whole-lung radiotherapy is used for patients with pulmonary metastases. Carboplatin, cyclophosphamide, and etoposide are usually reserved for unresponsive or recurrent disease or with unfavorable histology.

- Most (90%) patients with Wilms tumor have favorable histology. Patients with unfavorable histology receive more intensive chemotherapy for all stages and radiotherapy even for stage I or II disease.

Prognosis

Overall survival ranges from ~70% for stage IV disease to >95% for stage I. Survival is worse for patients with unfavorable histology.

Relapse

- Follow-up should include a regular chest X-ray as well as abdominal ultrasound, as pulmonary relapse is twice as common as local recurrence.
- Surgery, second-line chemotherapy, and radiotherapy (if not previously received) may all be applied, depending on the stage. Cure is achievable following second remission.

Nephroblastomatosis

- Multiple foci of premalignant tissue, also known as nephrogenic rests, characterize this condition. They may be observed on renal ultrasound and CT scan.
- The condition is associated with Wilms tumor, but may exist without tumor formation (i.e., seen on 1% of routine postmortem examinations). Close monitoring is required due to risk of subsequent tumor formation.

Other renal tumors in childhood

Mesoblastic nephroma

This occurs in infants and is treated with surgery; chemotherapy is only indicated for incompletely excised cases.

Clear cell sarcoma

A bone-metastasizing renal tumor of childhood, it is more aggressive than Wilms tumor and accounts for about 6% cases.

Malignant rhabdoid tumor

This tumor is rare (<2% renal tumors) and occurs more commonly in infants. It can be associated with posterior fossa CNS tumors, and requires intensive multi-agent chemotherapy and radiotherapy.

Renal cell carcinoma

This tumor is rare (6% of childhood renal tumors). Treatment is almost exclusively surgical resection. Outcome is more favorable than that seen with adults, including patients with regional lymph node metastases.

Bone tumors

These tumors are rare in childhood (5% of all pediatric malignancies).

- Incidence peaks in the teenage years, when they are the fourth most common group of malignancies.
- Most cases are osteosarcoma (OS) or Ewing sarcoma (ES). They are histologically distinct, with different patterns of disease and response to treatment.
- Sarcomas are associated with Li–Fraumeni syndrome (familial mutation of *p53*), and patients cured of familial retinoblastoma are at high risk of osteosarcoma.

Osteosarcoma

Presentation

Localized pain and swelling occur, with pathological fracture and rarely erythema. Most cases affect the long bones around the knee (67%) and humerus. The metaphysis is a more common site than mid-shaft. Delay in diagnosis is common.

Metastases

- Seen at diagnosis in 15%–25% of patients
- Lungs are the most common site, followed by bones.

Diagnostic investigations

- Plain X-rays of bony lesion
- Biopsy (for definitive diagnosis)
- Lactate dehydrogenase and alkaline phosphatase
- MRI of primary site
- CT chest
- Isotope bone scan

Treatment

Chemotherapy is used, followed by surgery and then further chemotherapy. The aim is to perform limb-preserving surgery whenever possible.

Prognosis

Adverse outlook is associated with

- Inability to resect primary tumor site
- Poor response to induction chemotherapy
- Metastatic disease (especially extrapulmonary disease)

Relapsed osteosarcoma

Most recurrences are isolated pulmonary metastases. Surgical resection can result in long-term survival in 20%–30% of patients. The role of chemotherapy for recurrent osteosarcoma is uncertain.

Ewing sarcoma of bone and soft tissue

ES usually occurs in bone but may also occur in soft tissues. ES and peripheral PNETs share a common immunophenotype (CD99 or MIC2) and cytogenetic profile (t(11;22) in 85% and t(21;22) in 5%–10%). Both tumor categories belong to the Ewing family of tumors. (Peripheral PNET should not be confused with CNS PNET tumors.)

Presentation

Localized pain (often episodic) and swelling occur, with pathological fracture. The diaphysis is a more common site than ends of bones. Axial skeleton is involved in half of cases, with the pelvis being the most common single site.

Diagnostic investigations

- Plain X-rays of bony lesion
- Biopsy (for definitive diagnosis)
- Lactate dehydrogenase and alkaline phosphatase
- MRI of primary site
- CT chest
- Isotope bone scan
- Bone marrow aspirates and trephines (bilateral)

Treatment

Chemotherapy is used, followed by surgery and then further chemotherapy. For extremity sites, limb-preserving surgery is the goal when possible. Radiotherapy is an effective adjunct and an alternative to surgery, particularly in axial sites.

Prognosis

Adverse outlook is associated with

- Age >17 years
- Poor response to induction chemotherapy
- Metastatic disease

Bone and/or bone marrow metastases confer a particularly grave prognosis, with <20% long-term survivors.

Relapsed Ewing sarcoma

Salvage therapy is rarely successful and will depend on treatment previously received. Topotecan and cyclophosphamide may be used as second-line chemotherapy. Surgery and radiotherapy may have a role in treatment.

Rhabdomyosarcoma

Rhabdomyosarcoma (RMS) is the most common soft tissue sarcoma in childhood. It accounts for 6% of all childhood malignancies and is most commonly seen in children <10 years of age. Most cases are sporadic, and are either embryonal or alveolar (more aggressive) subtypes, with characteristic histological features and molecular pathology. Botryoid (good prognosis) and spindle-cell types are also recognized. A small numbers of cases are associated with Li–Fraumeni syndrome.

Presenting features

These are site dependent with palpable mass, local pain, and obstruction. The most common sites of involvement are the following:

- Bladder/prostate
- Parameningeal
- Orbit
- Pelvis
- Paratestis
- Extremity
- Intrathoracic

Regional lymph nodal involvement is common, with some primary sites (extremity) and alveolar histology. Distant metastases to lung, bone, and bone marrow are less common at diagnosis.

Diagnosis and staging

- Imaging of primary site: CT or MRI
- Biopsy for histological, molecular, and cytogenetic analysis. Alveolar RMS usually has t(2;13) or t(1;13).
- CT scan of chest
- Bone marrow aspirates and trephines
- Isotope bone scan
- Lumbar puncture (parameningeal primaries)

Treatment

- Chemotherapy for usually 24–28 weeks with cyclophosphamide, actinomycin, and vincristine
- Surgery is reserved for accessible sites (paratesticular, superficial head) at diagnosis or after 12 weeks of chemotherapy.
- Radiotherapy is used for almost all cases with residual tumor (microscopic or macroscopic) and for alveolar histology.

Prognosis

Prognosis ranges from <10% for bony metastatic disease to >90% for completely excised paratesticular tumors with embryonal histology. Favorable prognostic features include

- Age 1–10 years old at diagnosis
- Botryoid or embryonal histology
- Paratesticular, orbit, female GU, or superficial head and neck sites
- Absence of nodal involvement or distant metastases

Relapse
- Second-line chemotherapy
- Radiotherapy may be employed at sites not previously irradiated.

Outcome for metastatic relapse and local recurrence within a previous radiotherapy field is extremely poor.

Germ cell tumors (GCT)

GCTs comprise a heterogeneous group of neoplasms, often with mixed histology. They arise from primordial germ cells in gonads or, following aberrant germ cell migration, in midline extragonadal sites, including sacrococcygeal, mediastinal or CNS sites. GCTs are rare, occurring in 3–5 per million children under 15 years of age, with peak incidence seen in children <3 years. Ten percent of girls with ovarian GCTs are found to have an underlying intersex state.

The nomenclature of GCT is complicated.
- Mature teratoma is benign
- Immature teratoma may disseminate locally
- Malignant GCT
  - Germinoma (or seminoma, dysgerminoma, depending on site) is totipotent.
  - Teratoma, yolk sac tumor (YST), choriocarcinoma (CHC), and embryonal carcinoma (EC) represent more differentiated forms.
- Secreting tumors (YST, CHC, some immature teratomas, and mixed tumors) are characterized by secretion of AFP and/or HCG, which may be used for diagnosis, monitoring of treatment response, and detection of recurrence

Presenting symptoms

These are site dependent. Testicular masses are usually painless. Ovarian tumors present as either painful or painless abdominal mass. Metastases are rarely present at diagnosis (lungs are the most common site; bone and bone marrow).

Diagnosis and staging

- Measurement of AFP and β-HCG in serum (and CSF for CNS disease)
- Imaging of primary tumor: Ultrasound, CT, or MRI
- Biopsy of unresectable tumors, unless this is unsafe and/or imaging and markers are sufficient to make diagnosis
- CT scan of chest and abdomen
- Bone marrow and isotope bone scan to book for metastases

Treatment of extracranial tumors

- Surgery followed by observation for low-risk tumors (e.g., mature/immature teratoma and gonadal stage I)

Note: Testicular tumors should be removed via an inguinal approach. Sacrococcygeal teratomas should be removed together with the coccyx to reduce risk of malignant relapse. Chemotherapy is reserved for intermediate and high-risk disease.

Prognosis

Survival is >90% for malignant extracranial GCTs.

Primary liver tumors

- Hepatoblastoma (HBL) is the most common primary pediatric hepatic tumor (<1% all cancers), with two-thirds of cases occurring in the first year of life.
- Hepatocellular carcinoma (HCC) and embryonal (undifferentiated) sarcoma of the liver are rare in children.
- Serum AFP levels are raised in >80% of HBL.

Treatment

- Chemotherapy for HBL includes cisplatin, vincristine, and fluorouricil.
- HCC is less sensitive to chemotherapy than HBL.
- A good surgical result is critical for long-term survival. Liver transplantation is indicated if local resection is not possible.

Prognosis

- Long-term survival for HBL is >70%, even in the presence of lung metastases.
- Survival for HCC is significantly lower than that for HBL.

Other rare tumors

Up to 5% of malignancies in childhood are very rare and include
• Epithelial or adult-type tumors, (e.g., carcinomas and melanoma)
• Embryonal tumors (e.g., rhabdoid tumors)

Malignant melanoma

Risk factors include the following:
• Preexisting conditions
• Giant congenital nevi
• Dysplastic nevus syndrome
• Xeroderma pigmentosum
• Albinism
• Immunosuppressive diseases

Most cases arise on healthy skin and may be related to sun exposure. The overall incidence is increasing, but mortality is unchanged because thinner melanomas (with better prognosis) are being diagnosed early.

Surgery is the mainstay of treatment. Survival is ~90% for localized (most common) disease, 25% for metastatic disease.

Rhabdoid tumors

These are highly aggressive tumors that may arise in the kidneys or central nervous system and are known as atypical teratoid rhabdoid tumors.

In the CNS, they appear histologically similar to PNETs, but are sometimes associated with tumors outside the CNS.

Treatment may include surgery, chemotherapy, and radiotherapy. Long-term survival is rare.

Pheochromocytoma

These tumors arise in the adrenal medulla and sympathetic ganglia. They are usually sporadic but may be associated with von Hippel–Lindau disease and multiple endocrine neoplasia types 2a and 2b. They may present with endocrine manifestations (e.g., hypertension, excessive sweating) or a mass. Less than 10% of pheochromocytomas are malignant and they rarely metastasize.

Investigations
Plasma and urine catecholamine levels are usually raised

Treatment
Surgery is the definitive treatment after starting α-adrenergic antagonists to control endocrine (sympathetic) symptoms.

Nasopharyngeal carcinoma

This carcinoma accounts for up to one-third of pediatric nasopharyngeal tumors and is the most common epithelial cancer in children. It is mainly found in teenagers and is often associated with antibodies to EBV.
• Treatment involves a combination of cisplatin-containing chemotherapy and radiotherapy.
• Overall survival at 5 years ~70%.

Other carcinomas

These are rare:

- *Thyroid* (predominantly the papillary variant and occasionally associated with exposure to radiation). This type may present with asymmetrical nodular goiter (see p. 498).
- *Adrenal carcinoma* (seen in young adults with occasional occurrences in older children). It may present with precocious puberty, inappropriate virilization in females (see p. 518).

Langerhans cell histiocytosis (LCH)

LCH is a disorder of unknown cause with a wide range of presentations. Although not a malignant condition, it may behave like one in its severest forms and is therefore usually managed by pediatric oncologists.

Langerhans cells are normally found in skin, lymph nodes, and airways. LCH results from monoclonal proliferation and accumulation of histiocytes with the characteristics of Langerhans cells in skin, bone, pituitary, CNS, lungs, intestines, spleen, or bone marrow. It may manifest as single- or multisystem disease. Single-system disease is usually confined to bone, occasionally to skin, and seen more in older children. The natural history varies from spontaneous resolution to repeated recurrence or death.

Note: LCH was previously known as "histiocytosis X," which was subdivided into eosinophilic granuloma, Letterer–Siwe disease, and Hans–Schuller–Christian disease.

Approximately 1–2 per 1,000,000 children are affected each year.

Presentation
Presentation depends on the site of disease but may include
- Pain or lump associated with isolated bony disease (most common)
- Skin rash (widespread macular–papular or mimicking seborrhaic dermatitis of the scalp)
- Discharge from the ear
- Diabetes insipidus
- Systemic disturbance (fever, malaise, anorexia, and failure to thrive)

Diagnosis
Biopsy with confirmation of Birbeck granules (or positive CD1a or S100 immunohistochemistry) indicates LCH. Diagnosis can be made without biopsy based on characteristic pituitary, hypothalamic, or vertebral abnormality.

Further investigation
Suspected LCH should be fully staged to identify possible multisystem disease. Investigations should include skeletal survey, early-morning urine for osmolality, chest X-ray or chest CT if pulmonary symptoms are present, CT or MRI of pituitary, CBC (marrow aspirate if abnormal CBC), coagulation studies, and liver enzymes.

Treatment
- Single-system LCH, usually involving bone or skin, frequently resolves spontaneously or following biopsy or surgical curettage, but may require topical or intralesional steroids in persistent or recurrent cases.
- Multisystem LCH, seen mainly in young patients (under age 2), requires treatment with steroids and vinblastine.

Prognosis
More than 80% of patients survive long term without significant sequelae. Survivors of multisystem or CNS disease may have lasting disabilities.

Hemophagocytic lymphohistiocytosis

Hemophagocytic lymphohistiocytosis (HLH) is a rare condition that may be primary (familial hemophagocytic or erythrorphagocytic lymphohistiocytosis, FHL or FEL) or secondary to infection (sHLH). HLH is characterized by accumulation of phagocytic mononuclear cells rather than dendritic or antigen presenting cells, as seen in LCH.

- *Presenting features* include fever, splenomegaly, and cytopenia (two out of three cell lines: red cells, white cells, and platelets). Neurological symptoms relating to increased CSF monocytosis and protein are sometimes seen. There may also be lymphadenopathy, skin rash, jaundice and edema, and hepatic dysfunction.
- *Biochemistry* shows elevated triglycerides and low fibrinogen, sometimes elevated serum transaminases, LDH, and ferritin levels.
- Consider evaluation of natural killer (NK) function analysis (soluble IL-2 receptor, NK function analysis) and genetic studies (perforin, munc13-4, syntaxin-11) for primary HLH.
- Consider viral studies (EBV, CMV) for sHLH.

Treatment

Recovery may be spontaneous in sHLH with resolution of infection, but FHL is fatal without treatment. Steroids, etoposide, and intrathecal methotrexate may stabilize the disease. Allogeneic HSCT is required for cure. Overall survival is ~60%.

Chemotherapy

Chemotherapy may be given as adjuvant treatment (following surgery), or neoadjuvant treatment (before surgery). Combinations of drugs are used to increase efficacy, reduce development of resistance, and limit single-organ toxicity. Maximizing dose intensity (treatment frequency) increases efficacy.

- *Short-term side effects* include vomiting, myelosuppression, alopecia, and mucositis (inflammation of mucous membranes).
- *Long-term effects* on organ function (kidneys, gonads, hearing, heart) are variable, and in general less than effects of radiotherapy.

Antimetabolites

These are structural analogues of chemicals found in the intermediate steps in the synthesis of nucleic acids and proteins. They include

- 6-mercaptopurine (6-MP), 6-thioguanine (6-TG), cytarabine (ara-C), fludarabine (used in leukemia, NHL)
- Methotrexate (MTX) (used in leukemia, NHL, and osteosarcoma)

Side effects include renal toxicity (MTX), myelosuppression, hepatotoxicity, and mucositis.

Anti-tumor antibiotics

Originally isolated from bacteria and fungi, they have antibiotic and ant-tumor activity. They include the following:

- Anthracycline: Daunorubicin, doxorubicin, idarubicin, mitoxantrone (used in leukemia, NHL, Hodgkin's lymphoma, neuroblastoma, Wilms tumor, sarcoma). Side effects include myelotoxicity, alopecia, mucositis, and cardiotoxicity.
- Bleomycin (used in Hodgkin's lymphoma, germ cell tumors). Side effects include pulmonary toxicity.
- Actinomycin D (dactinomycin) (used in Wilms tumor and rhabdomyosarcoma). Side effects include myelotoxicity (mild) and hepatotoxicity.

Epipodophyllotoxins

These are semisynthetic analogues of podophyllotoxin. They stabilize normally transient DNA–protein complexes by inhibition of topoisomerase I or II.

- Etoposide (VP16), which inhibits topoisomerase II (used in leukemia, NHL, neuroblastoma, sarcoma, germ cell tumors, CNS tumors, palliative chemotherapy [low dose]). Side effects include hypotension, myelotoxicity, alopecia, hepatotoxicity, mucositis, secondary leukemia.
- Topotecan, irinotecan, new to pediatric practice, inhibits topoisomerase I (used in neuroblastoma, sarcoma, and CNS tumors)

Vinca alkaloids

These agents bind to tubulin, interfering with mitotic spindle.

- Vincristine (used in leukemias, NHL, Hodgkin's lymphoma, CNS tumors, Wilms tumor, sarcoma). Side effects include neurotoxicity.
- Vinblastine (used in Hodgkin's lymphoma, anaplastic large cell lymphoma). Side effects include myelotoxicity and mucositis.

Alkylating agents

Covalent binding to DNA prevents replication and transcription.
- Cyclophosphamide, ifosfamide (used for leukemia, lymphoma, sarcoma, neuroblastoma, high-risk Wilms tumor, CNS)
- Melphalan, busulphan (used for neuroblastoma, Ewing sarcoma)
- Lomustine (CCNU) (used for CNS tumors)

Side effects include myelosuppression, alopecia, mucositis, tubular nephropathy (ifosfamide), bladder toxicity (cyclophosphamide), encephalopathy (ifosfamide), late effects on fertility, secondary leukemia (CCNU).

Platinum compounds

These agents employ permanent cross-linking of DNA and inhibition of DNA synthesis.
- Cisplatin, carboplatin (osteosarcoma, neuroblastoma, CNS tumors)

Side effects include high emetogenicity, nephrotoxicity, ototoxicity, neurotoxicity (mainly cisplatin), and myelotoxicity (carboplatin).

Other agents

- Dacarbazine (DTIC) methylates nucleophilic sites (mucositis, myelotoxicity, hepatic dysfunction, local pain, flu like symptoms)
- Procarbazine was originally an MAOI but found to be anti-tumor; methylates once activated in vitro (myelotoxicity, reduced fertility)
- L-asparaginase, pegaspargase depletes the pool of asparagine, needed by some malignancies, e.g., ALL (hypersensitivity, coagulopathy, rarely pancreatitis)
- Hydroxyurea is an analogue of urea; it inhibits DNA synthesis.
- Steroids are used for symptom control, and direct anti-tumor effect in hematological malignancies.

Safe administration of chemotherapy

Chemotherapy should only be given by individuals fully trained in the avoidance and management of their complications, working in centers fully equipped and accredited to support chemotherapy.

Route

- *IV:* Central venous access preferred. Risk of extravasation from peripheral access is greatest with vinca alkaloids and anthracyclines.
- *Intrathecal:* Usually for treatment or prophylaxis of CNS disease in leukemia, NHL, and some CNS tumors. Safety arrangements for intrathecal treatment is paramount,

Dosage

This is usually calculated according to body surface area. Fluids are required with certain drugs (e.g., ifosfamide, cisplatin, methotrexate) to prevent nephrotoxicity or enhance renal excretion. Mesna is given with cyclophosphamide and ifosfamide to protect from bladder inflammation.

Monitoring

The type and level of monitoring depend on the agents used. This may include peripheral blood cell counts, GFR measurement, and echocardiogram before and between courses of chemotherapy.

Stem cell transplant

High-dose therapy

A conventional myeloablative transplant involves the delivery of high doses of chemotherapy and or radiotherapy, followed by rescue with hemopoietic stem cells. The latter may be autologous (from the patient) or allogeneic (from a sibling or unrelated donor, or haploidentical from a parent). Indications for use in treatment of childhood malignancy are selected high-risk leukemia and relapsed leukemia (from allogeneic donor) and high-risk solid tumors, including metastatic neuroblastoma. Nonmyeloablative transplants are being used for immunodeficiencies, aplastic anemia, inborn errors of metabolism, and some malignancies. These involve immunoablative doses of chemotherapy and radiation followed by infusion of stem cells.

Stem cells are harvested from bone marrow. They can also be collected from the peripheral blood (PBSC) by leukopheresis following "mobilization" with granulocyte colony stimulating factor (G-CSF). Stem cells can be collected from umbilical cords after delivery of the infant.

Marrow, cord, and PBSC are all used for allografts. PBSC are favored for autografts, offering advantages of less risk of tumor contamination, more rapid engraftment, less severe infections, and potential avoidance of anesthetic for marrow collection.

Outcome

Allografts carry a greater risk, with up to 10% procedure-related mortality. Morbidity and mortality from stem cell transplant are due to the following causes:
- Graft failure
- Infection secondary to profound immune suppression often required to suppress the graft-versus-donor disease
- Mucositis
- Veno-occlusive disease of the liver
- Multiorgan failure related to the conditioning regimen

Graft-versus-host disease (GVHD)

GVHD is a particular risk associated with allografts, in which immunocompetent donor cells mount an immune response against host organs, most commonly skin, liver, and the gastrointestinal system. Cyclosporin, methotrexate, or tacrolimus are given as prophylaxis. Steroids, monoclonal antibodies, and other immunosuppressants may also be employed in treatment.

Radiotherapy

In the use of ionizing radiation to kill cancer cells, dose and fractionation (number of treatments to deliver a total dose) vary according to the nature of the tumor and tolerance of the tissue.

Strategies to increase therapeutic success include the following:

- Conformal radiotherapy (matching beam to 3D shape of target) to spare surrounding tissue
- Targeted radiotherapy with specific isotopes (e.g., I^{131}mIBG for neuroblastoma)
- Radiosurgery (high-dose single fraction), brachytherapy (direct application of radionuclides to tumor). Proton beam radiotherapy (reduced dose to non-target tissues), currently limited availability in pediatrics

Indications

- Selected cases of Hodgkin's lymphoma, neuroblastoma, Wilms tumor, soft-tissue and Ewing sarcomas, most subgroups of CNS tumors
- Limited benefit in osteosarcoma, extracranial germ cell tumors, NHL
- In leukemia limited to treatment of CNS and testicular disease and to conditioning for HSCT
- Symptom control in palliative care (e.g., bony metastases, spinal cord compression)

Preparation for radiotherapy includes

- Planning, by combination of CT and MRI scanning
- Immobilization using masks/shells, tattoos as markers, sedation or general anesthesia for youngest children
- Protection of surrounding tissues (e.g., gonads, by means of lead shields)
- Play therapists have a central role in this process.

Side effects

- Acute effects include nausea and vomiting, cutaneous erythema and desquamation, diarrhea, myelosuppression, pneumonitis, and hepatitis. Toxicity is potentiated by dactinomycin or anthracyclines.
- Late effects on growth, CNS, heart, lungs, kidneys, liver (see p. 794)

Surgery

Surgical interventions for solid tumors include the following:

- *Biopsy only*: Chemotherapy and/or radiotherapy may be curative without further surgery (e.g., in Hodgkin's lymphoma, NHL, rhabdomyosarcoma, germ cell tumors).
- *Resection, primary, or following chemotherapy*: Completeness of excision influences subsequent adjunctive treatment (e.g., in bone tumors, Wilms tumor, rhabdomyosarcoma, hepatoblastoma and most CNS tumors).
- Management of the acute abdomen in neutropenic patients
- Raised intracranial pressure and spinal cord compression
- Central venous lines for chemotherapy

Acute care

All pediatric oncology treatment centers should have clear local guidelines for supportive management, which should be referred to for details. This section should not be regarded as a substitute for such guidelines.

Fever should be treated as an emergency. Immunocompromised children may succumb to overwhelming sepsis within hours. Greatest risk is associated with the nadir white cell count, typically at around 10 days after the beginning of a course of most cyclic chemotherapy regimens.

In the absence of neutropenia consider central venous line infection, particularly if symptoms (e.g., rigors) are associated with line flushing.

Febrile neutropenia

This constitutes fever (temperature >38°C) with a neutrophil count <1.0 x 10^9/L, leading to increased risk of bacterial infections. It complicates use of chemotherapy and spinal radiotherapy, bone marrow disease.

Causes
- Skin or GI bacterial flora
- Greatest risk from gram-negative organisms, including *Pseudomonas*
- Gram-positive organisms may be associated with central venous catheters.

Examination
Include inspection of the skin, mouth, intravenous line sites, surgical sites, and the perianal area.

Investigation
- CBC and differential count
- Culture of blood, urine, stool (if diarrhea), swabs of suspicious skin lesions or central line exit sites
- X-ray of chest or abdomen if indicated by symptoms or signs

Treatment
- *Broad-spectrum antibiotics* should be commenced <u>without delay</u> as infection with gram-negative bacilli may be <u>fatal within hours</u>.
- Antibiotic choice will vary by institution and local resistance patterns but must include adequate cover for *Pseudomonas* and gram-positive organisms. Include anaerobic cover in the presence of abdominal pain, diarrhea, or mucositis. Appropriate agents may include the following:
  - Ceftazidime, ciprofloxacin, meropenem, gentamicin, amikacin, piptazobactam (gram-negative coverage)
  - Vancomycin (gram-positive organisms, including coagulase-negative staphylococci)
  - Metronidazole, meropenem (anaerobic coverage)
- Antibiotic choice should be reviewed according to results of cultures.

Infection
Viral infections in immunocompromised patients
Varicella zoster virus (VZV)
- If patient is in contact with this and is nonimmune, give prophylactic acyclovir and/or immune globulin. Active chicken pox or shingles should be treated aggressively with intravenous acyclovir.

Herpes simplex virus (HSV)
- HSV may cause painful oral ulceration; treat early.

Other viruses
- Cytomegalovirus (CMV), adenovirus, respiratory syncytial virus (RSV), and adenovirus may all cause pneumonitis, associated with high morbidity and mortality, especially in HSCT patients.

Fungal infections
- Consider in prolonged febrile neutropenia and treat promptly. Mortality remains high, but is reduced with newer therapeutic agents.
- Clinical spectrum includes pulmonary aspergillosis, hepatic candidiasis, and abscess formation.
- Risk is highest during intensive chemotherapy, such as reinduction for relapsed leukemia and following bone marrow transplant.
- Treatment includes fluconazole (limited coverage), itraconazole, amphotericin B (liposomal formulation for reduced toxicity), voriconazole, and caspofungin. Prophylaxis is used in high-risk treatment regimens.

Pneumocystis carinii pneumonia (PCP)
- Interstitial pneumonitis associated with prolonged immunosuppression presents with tachypnea, dry cough, and low oxygen saturation readings.
- *Prophylaxis* (patients on chemotherapy causing lymphopenia): Co-trimoxazole, monthly pentamidine nebulizers or dapsone
- *Treatment*: High-dose trimethoprim/sulfamethoxazole, steroids in severe cases

Acute care: biochemistry

Tumor lysis syndrome

This syndrome involves lysis of malignant cells on starting chemotherapy, releasing intracellular contents and exceeding renal excretory capacity and physiological buffering mechanisms. Abnormalities include the following:

- Hyperuricemia
- Hyperkalemia
- Hyperphosphatemia and reciprocal hypocalcemia
- Dehydration
- Leads to risk of acute renal failure
- Mainly seen in ALL, NHL (especially lymphoblastic and Burkitt lymphoma), occasionally AML, rarely solid tumors (e.g., germ cell, neuroblastoma). The syndrome may occur spontaneously or be precipitated by a single dose of steroids.
- Risk is increased with a high white count, bulky disease, preexisting renal impairment, or infiltration.

Management

The key is prevention and monitoring.

- Hyperhydration (e.g., 5% dextrose in 0.45% saline at 3.0 L/m^2/day) 24 hours before starting treatment and continued for least 48 hours after treatment is started; *avoid added potassium*.
- Ensure good renal output, with diuretic (furosemide) if necessary.
- Allopurinol reduces urate production, urate oxidase in high-risk cases.
- Hyperkalemia may need treatment with Kayexalate, dextrose/insulin, or dialysis.
- Hyperphosphatemia/hypocalcemia: Increase fluids, use dialysis in extreme cases, avoid calcium unless symptomatic (tetany, seizures).

Other biochemical disturbances

Hypercalcemia

This rarely complicates disseminated malignancy (e.g., rhabdomyosarcoma). Manage it with hyperhydration (normal saline) and furosemide; biphosphonates are more effective than steroids or calcitonin.

Renal toxicity

This is due to use of chemotherapy or antibiotics:

- Cisplatin (glomerular function, Mg loss), ifosfamide (tubular losses of Mg, PO_4, bicarbonate), high-dose methotrexate
- Amphotericin B (glomerular toxicity and heavy potassium loss), aminoglycosides, vancomycin

Practice particular care when any of these drugs are used in combination.

The acute abdomen

Possible causes in the oncology patient include the following:

- *Gastric hemorrhage* secondary to gastritis or ulceration. Risk factors include high-dose steroids and raised intracranial pressure.
- *Pancreatitis* complicating treatment with steroids or L-asparaginase

- *Neutropenic enterocolitis or typhlitis* (Greek *typhlon* = caecum). Bacterial invasion (clostridium, pseudomonas) leads to inflammation, full-thickness infarction and perforation, sepsis, and bleeding. It is associated with leukemia. Symptoms of pain ± fever may be masked by concomitant steroids (e.g., in ALL induction). The key to management is early, appropriate antibiotic coverage on first suspicion and early involvement of surgeons.

Hematological support

Blood products may be leukodepleted to reduce allosensitization (which complicates future blood transfusions) and prevent transfusion reactions (treated with antihistamine and/or steroid premedication). Use irradiated products to prevent transfusion-associated GVHD (a rare but usually fatal complication secondary to immunocompromise in a transfusion recipient).

- *The threshold for blood transfusion* is usually a hemoglobin level of 7 g/dL, but teenagers are often symptomatic at higher levels. (Use caution if there is high-count leukemia, longstanding anemia, or heart failure).
- *Platelets* should be maintained above 10×10^9/L if the patient is well, 20×10^9/L for a minor procedure (e.g., LP), 30×10^9/L if there is a brain tumor, and 50×10^9/L after a significant bleed or for major surgery. These thresholds should be overridden where there is bleeding.

Nausea and vomiting

Chemotherapy varies in its emetogenicity: oral antimetabolites and vincristine require no prophylaxis; cisplatin and ifosfamide require multiple agents. Aim to prevent severe symptoms.

- *First line:* Ondansetron (5-HT antagonist)
- *Second line:* Metoclopramide
- Dexamethasone is a useful adjunct.
- In severe cases, lorazepam may be helpful, especially for anticipatory nausea.

Nutrition and mucositis

Good nutritional status is essential for recovery, but is compromised by the presence of malignancy, direct effects of treatment, and mucositis and infection.

A dietitian is central to successful nutrition. Support should include making appetizing meals available at all times, calorie supplementation, treatment of mucositis, and use of parenteral nutrition when an enteral route is inadequate

Chemotherapy-induced mucositis leads to oral ulceration, pain. and diarrhea. Good mouth care (involving basic oral hygiene and antiseptic mouthwash) helps prevent some infective complications. Prompt treatment with analgesia allows maintenance of oral intake for as long as possible.

Urgent care

Emergency treatment is needed for acute complication of tumors. For example:
- Leukemias with high peripheral white blood cell count, leading to hyperviscosity
- Superior vena cava (SVC) or airway obstruction caused by mediastinal masses
- Raised intracranial pressure
- Spinal cord compression

Hyperviscosity
- Risk of sludging of venous blood in cerebral vessels
- Associated with very high count ALL (WBC > 200 x 10^9/L)

Prevention
- Cautious transfusion,
- Prompt ALL treatment:
  - Hydration, allopurinol (urate oxidase for severe cases) due to risk of tumor lysis syndrome
  - Chemotherapy
- Leukopheresis may relieve symptoms

SVC and upper airway obstruction
- May present with dyspnea, chest discomfort, hoarseness, cough
- *Findings in SVC obstruction*: Plethora, facial swelling, engorgement of veins on upper chest wall, venous dilatation of optic fundi

Causes
SVC obstruction
- Upper mediastinal tumors (particularly T-cell NHL or ALL)
- Occasionally neuroblastoma

Airway compromise
- Thoracic Ewing sarcoma
- Lymphoma
- Rhabdomyosarcoma
- Malignant germ cell tumor

Management
- Sedation or anesthesia for diagnostic purposes is unsafe in SVC obstruction
- Empirical short-term steroid treatment based on imaging and non-invasive investigations may need to be used before biopsy confirmation of diagnosis.
- Presence of pleural effusion, common in T-cell NHL, exacerbates symptoms, but tap may relieve symptoms and provide diagnosis.

Spinal cord compression
- *Presentation*: Back pain; gait, sensory, bladder, and bowel disturbance
- *Causes*: Neuroblastoma, sarcoma, lymphoma, CNS tumors (also infection, osteomyelitis, abscess)
- *Multidisciplinary input is <u>vital</u>*: Urgent MRI and surgical biopsy and sometimes decompression. Perform other essential diagnostic procedures (e.g., LP, BM) under same anesthetic if possible.

Raised intracranial pressure (see p. 86)
This is a neurosurgical emergency. Give high-dose dexamethasone preoperatively.

Principles of follow-up

Follow-up after completion of treatment is focused on disease recurrence and long-term adverse effects of cancer and its treatment.

Monitoring for disease recurrence

This involves clinical review, combined with imaging or laboratory testing to pick up presymptomatic recurrence, which may be amenable to further attempts at curative treatment. For example:

- Chest X-rays: Hodgkin's lymphoma
- MRI scans: CNS tumors
- Urine VMA and HVA: Neuroblastoma
- Serum αFP and βHCG: Germ cell tumors
- CBC: Leukemia

Monitoring for long-term sequelae of treatment

With close to 80% of children cured from cancer, survivorship has developed into a discrete area of research and clinical care.

Long-term sequelae of radiotherapy

These may occur months or years after treatment has been completed. Sequelae will depend on sites, dose, mode of treatment, and age of patient at time of treatment. Organs in the field of radiotherapy are at risk of both abnormal function and subsequent malignancy. Common abnormalities include the following:

- CNS radiotherapy
  - Neuroendocrine complications (thyroid, hypothalamic, pituitary)
  - Neurocognitive complications
  - Visual or auditory loss (cataracts, retinal damage, hearing loss)
  - Neurological complications (cerebrovascular events, leukencephalopathy)
- Thoracic radiotherapy
  - Pulmonary fibrosis and diffusion abnormalities
  - Cardiomyopathy, coronary artery disease, cardiac valvular disease
- Abdominopelvic radiotherapy
  - Gonadal dysfunction or infertility
  - GI toxicity

Common second malignancies include solid tumors occurring in the field of radiotherapy, as well as non-melanoma skin cancers.

Late effects of chemotherapy

Sequelae depend on age at the time of exposure, drugs, and doses (see p. 782). Well-recognized long-term toxicities include

- Cardiotoxicity following anthracyclines
- Nephrotoxicity following platinum drugs
- Pulmonary fibrosis following bleomycin
- Impaired fertility following alkylating agents
- Ototoxicity following platinum agents

Second malignancies related to radiotherapy include secondary leukemia and myelodysplastic syndrome associated with topoisomerase II inhibitors and alkylating agents.

Psychosocial effects of cancer and its treatment

Cancer survivors and their family members are at increased risk for impaired psychosocial well-being. Risk is not clearly associated with a specific cancer type or treatment and likely is multifactorial in origin. This is an evolving area of clinical research.

Societal issues

Cancer survivors are also at increased risk for needing special education and, as they enter adulthood, unemployment and underemployment. These issues may be related to physical or psychosocial effects and may in turn lead to further physical or psychosocial dysfunction.

Palliative care

Approximately 30% of children with cancer will die, most of them from progressive disease. Death from complications of treatment is more likely to be swift, with limited opportunity for preparation. Palliative care is the active total care of patients whose disease is no longer curable. It needs to embrace physical, emotional, social, and spiritual needs of children and their families. Chemotherapy, radiotherapy, and surgery may still be used for palliation and control of symptoms.

Breaking bad news

It is extremely important to be honest, with an open approach, avoiding false hope. What to tell the child is always difficult, as many families tend to overprotect their child. Such overprotection risks loss of their child's trust when the truth can no longer be hidden.

Organization of care

There are few pediatricians specializing in palliative care.

Location

- Most children die at home, by family preference, but some prefer to be in the hospital's acute-care ward.
- A multidisciplinary approach is required and will vary according to needs.
- Bereavement support should be considered part of the role of the palliative care team and may be provided by various disciplines within the team, depending on local arrangements.

Symptom control

Anticipated symptoms will depend on the diagnosis. Symptom-control measures may be pharmacological or nonpharmacological. Aim to correct the underlying cause (e.g., constipation, infection). Good communication and consideration of psychosocial and spiritual factors will contribute to good symptom control.

Pain

- The oral route is effective for most children, until the terminal phase, when intravenous infusion, often in combination with antiemetics, sedatives, and anticonvulsants, may be preferred. The transdermal route is used for some agents.
- Different agents suit different types of pain—e.g., for inflammatory and neuropathic pain, muscle spasm, and raised intracranial pressure. Combining different agents is more effective than escalating the dose of one agent.
- World Health Organization (WHO) three-step analgesic ladder:
  - Step 1: Non-opioid ± adjuvants (e.g., paracetamol, NSAID)
  - Step 2: Weak opioid (e.g., codeine) + non-opioid ± adjuvants
  - Step 3: Strong opioid (e.g., morphine, fentanyl) + non-opioid ± adjuvants

- *Adjuvants* are additional drugs used in pain management:
  - Analgesics that relieve pain in specific circumstances, such as gabapentin for neuropathic pain, muscle relaxants (diazepam), corticosteroids, biphosphonates
  - Drugs to control adverse analgesic effects, e.g., laxatives, antiemetics

Other symptoms

- *Nausea, vomiting*: Ondansetron, metoclopramide
- *Convulsions, cerebral irritation*: Diazepam
- *Spinal cord compression*: Dexamethasone, radiotherapy, bladder and bowel management
- *Terminal restlessness*: Lorazapam
- *Dyspnea*: Nonpharmacological measures (position, play therapy, fan); opioids, benzodiazepines, oxygen, steroids
- *Excess secretions*: Scopolamine, glycopyrrolate
- *Anxiety, depression*: Diazepam, amitriptylline
- *Constipation*: Anticipate by prescribing laxatives when starting opioids, select the least constipating opioids (e.g., fentanyl); may need high enemas
- *Bowel obstruction*: Antispasmodics, stool softeners, rectal preparations to reduce impaction
- *Sweating* from advanced disease fever or drugs: Cimetidine, NSAIDs
- *Pruritus*: Cimetidine if due to disease, antihistamine if opiate induced
- *Hematological* (anemia, hemorrhage, bruising): Transfuse (blood ± platelets) only for symptomatic improvement and for quality of life; use topical tranexamic acid or adrenaline for troublesome mucosal bleeding

Infectious diseases

Introduction

Infection and infectious disease form a large part of clinical practice in pediatrics and child health. The list here shows the core areas that one should be familiar with:

- *The child with fever* (p. 801)
- *Common infections characterized by rash* (p. 816)
- *Bacteremia and shock*
  See also Emergency section (Chapter 5) for sepsis and shock (p. 82)
- *Mycobacterial infections*
  See also Respiratory section (Chapter 9) for pulmonary tuberculosis (p. 346)
- *Systemic infections*
  See also Renal section (Chapter 11) for post-streptococcal glomerulonephritis (p. 442)
- *Skin and soft tissues*
- *Nervous system infection* (p. 836)
- *Upper and lower respiratory tract infections*
  See also Respiratory section (Chapter 9) for the common cold, pharyngitis, bronchitis, bronchiolitis, pertussis, pneumonia, pleural effusion, and empyema (pp. 328)
- *Cardiovascular system*
  See also Cardiovascular section (Chapter 8) and Emergency section (Chapter 5) for endocarditis and myocarditis (pp. 286, 288)
- *Gastrointestinal system*
  See also Gastrointestinal section (Chapter 10) for gastroenteritis and viral hepatitis (p. 398)
- *Genitourinary system*
  See also Renal section (Chapter 11) for urinary tract infections (p. 412)
- *Musculoskeletal*
  See also Bone and Joints section (Chapter 20) for osteomyelitis and infective arthritis (p. 856)
- *The eye*
- *Special hosts*
  See also Neonatal section (Chapter 6) for infections in the fetus and newborn (p. 210); Oncology section (Chapter 18) for infections in children with malignancy and transplantation (p. 788)
- *Immunizations* (p. 846)
- *Tropical diseases* (p. 840)

The child with fever

In children aged 4 weeks to 5 years, body temperature should be measured using either a
- rectal thermometer,
- electronic thermometer in the axilla, or
- infrared tympanic thermometer (best over age 3 months).

Fever in infants ≤6 months is rare. Fever requiring further tests is classically defined as
- A temperature >38°C in infants ≤3 months
- A temperature ≥39°C in infants >3 months

Differential diagnosis

The majority of children with fever have a self-limiting viral infection that resolves without any problem. However, in the very young it is particularly important to consider the possibility of an underlying focus of infection. When there is no apparent cause of infection, the differential diagnosis of fever includes the following:
- Bacteremia (see p. 828)
- Urinary tract infection (see p. 412)
- Respiratory tract infection (see p. 328)
- Meningitis and encephalitis (see p. 836)
- Viral infection (see p. 812)
- Osteomyelitis (see p. 858)
- Bacterial gastroenteritis (see p. 394)
- Endocarditis (see p. 286)
- Rheumatic fever (see p. 284)
- Malaria (see p. 840)
- Tuberculosis (see p. 346)
- Post-vaccination fever

The signs and symptoms of diseases that require specific medical treatment are highlighted in Box 19.1.

Box 19.1 Features of illness needing specific treatment

Meningococcal disease (p. 836)
- Non-blanching rash
- Ill-looking child
- Purpuric lesions (>2 mm)
- Capillary refill time ≥3 seconds
- Neck stiffness

Meningitis (p. 836)
- Neck stiffness
- Bulging fontanelle
- Depressed level of consciousness
- Seizures

Herpes simplex encephalitis (p. 210)
- Focal neurological abnormalities
- Focal seizures
- Depressed level of consciousness

Pneumonia (p. 340)
- Tachypnea, nasal flaring, and chest recession
- Chest crackles on auscultation
- Pulse oximetery indicating oxygen desaturation

Urinary tract infection (p. 412)
- Vomiting, poor feeding, and abdominal pain or tenderness
- Lethargy or irritability
- Urinary frequency or dysuria
- Offensive urine or hematuria

Septic arthritis or osteomyelitis (p. 856)
- Swelling of limb of joint
- Not using an extremity, non-weight bearing

Kawasaki disease (p. 830)
Fever lasting longer than 5 days, and at least four of the following:
- Bilateral conjunctival injection
- Change in upper respiratory tract mucous membranes with injected pharynx, dry cracked lips, or strawberry tongue
- Extremity change, including swelling, erythema, or desquamation
- Polymorphous rash
- Cervical lymphadenopathy

Fever: examination and assessment

When assessing a child with a fever, a thorough history and examination is required. Key priorities include the following:

- *History*: Consider very seriously the parent's concerns and perception of a fever in their child. Check for ill contacts, immunization history.
- *Vital signs*: Make sure that temperature, heart rate, respiratory rate, blood pressure, and capillary refill time are measured, as this will determine the order of your priorities (see Chapter 5).
- *Signs and symptoms*: Assess the child for the presence or absence of symptoms and signs indicating serious illness.

Box 19.2, Box 19.3, and Box 19.4 summarize features of an illness that indicate low, medium, or high risk, respectively, of serious illness.

Box 19.2 Low risk of serious illness

Color
- Normal color of skin, lips, and tongue

Activity
- Responds normally to caretakers
- Is content and smiles
- Stays awake or awakens quickly if roused
- Strong, normal cry

Breathing
- Regular rate, unlabored

Hydration
- Normal

Other
- Well-appearing
- No fever at time of examination

Box 19.3 Intermediate risk of serious illness

Color
- Pallor reported by parent or caregiver

Activity
- Not responding normally and decreased activity
- Prolonged stimulation required to awaken child

Breathing
- Nasal flaring
- Tachypnea (respiratory rate >50/minute in 6- to 12-month old, >40 in >1 year old)
- Low oxygen saturation (≤95% in room air)
- Chest crackles

Hydration
- Dry mucous membranes
- Poor feeding
- Reduced urine output
- Capillary refill time >3 seconds

Other
- Fever ≥5 days
- Swelling of limb or joint
- Non-weight bearing or not using an extremity
- A new lump >2 cm

Box 19.4 High risk of serious illness

Color
- Pale, mottled, ashen, or blue

Activity
- Unresponsive, appears ill, and barely rousable
- Weak high-pitched or continuous cry

Breathing
- Grunting, severe distress

Hydration
- Reduced skin turgor

Other
- Non-blanching rash
- Fever at time of examination
- Bulging fontanelle
- Neck stiffness
- Seizures or focal neurological abnormality
- Bilious vomiting

Fever: management (low risk)

Children with features of low risk for serious infection generally do not need to be admitted to the hospital. However, other criteria for admission may include the following:

- Social and family circumstances
- Parental anxiety, instinct, or concerns
- Child's contact with serious illness
- Child's recent travel abroad to tropical or subtropical areas, or travel to any high-risk areas of endemic infectious disease

If a child is discharged home, the parents should be given clear instructions on what to look for and when to call for medical help (see Box 19.5).

Box 19.5 Advice to parents of a child with fever managed at home

Urgent problems

Check on your child, even during the night.

- Offer your child regular drinks; if breast-feeding, continue with breast feeds. *Seek medical advice if the child stops drinking.*
- Look for signs of dehydration—e.g., dry mouth, no tears, sunken fontanelle, decreased urine output. *Seek medical advice if these are present.*
- Look for a non-blanching rash: Use a glass tumbler and press it firmly against any rash. If the spots can be seen through the glass and they do not fade, this is a non-blanching rash. *Seek immediate medical advice if this is present.*
- Do not sponge your child with water.
- If your child has a convulsion *seek medical advice.*

Other advice

- Do not send your child to school or daycare if febrile.
- If the fever is present for more than 5 days, *seek medical advice.*
- If you are concerned about your child's health or if your child gets worse, *seek medical advice.*

Fever: management (moderate or high risk of serious illness)

Children with moderate or high risk of serious illness need hospital admission; those with high-risk features may have life-threatening illness and need *urgent* treatment (see Box 19.6).

In hypoxic children or those in shock, follow the emergency care outlined in Chapter 5.

If there is no apparent source of infection, despite fever, the investigations should include the following:

- *Blood*: Culture, complete blood count (CBC), C-reactive protein (CRP) or erythrocyte sedimentation rate (ESR), electrolytes
- *Urine*: Test for urinary tract infection
- *Lumbar puncture:* Consider if the clinical assessment dictates and there are no contraindications
- *Chest X-ray*: Consider if there are respiratory symptoms or a high white blood cell count

---

Box 19.6 Antibiotics for management of seriously ill children with fever of unknown origin

Immediate treatment

Third-generation cephalosporins (cefotaxime or ceftriaxone) should be given to children with fever AND

- Signs of shock or coma
- Meningococcal disease
- Age <1 month
- Age 1–3 months and unwell with WBC <5 or >15 x 10^9/L

Treatment for suspected bacterial infection

Give third-generation cephalosporin if any of the following are suspected:

- *Neisseria meningitidis*
- *Streptococcus pneumoniae*
- *Escherichia coli*
- *Staphylococcus aureus*
- *Haemophilus influenzae* type B

Special cases

Consider choice of antibiotics or route of administration carefully in the following instances:

- *Child <3 months*: Add antibiotic against *Listeria* (e.g., ampicillin)
- *Child with decreased level of consciousness*: Give parenteral antibiotics (also consider acyclovir for herpes simplex encephalitis)
- *Significant rates of antibiotic resistance*: Follow local guidelines

---

Antipyretics
Fever should be treated if the child is unwell with it.
- Do not use tepid sponging.
- Do not over- or underdress the child.
- Only use acetaminophen or ibuprofen if the child is distressed with fever.

Prolonged fever of unknown origin

Fever that has persisted for >21 days, without apparent cause, is a "prolonged fever of unknown origin." An explanation is found eventually in most cases—one-third of these will be infectious. The remaining cases are due to other causes:

- *Rheumatologic*: Juvenile rheumatoid arthritis, systemic lupus erythematosus (SLE), rheumatic fever, vasculitis (p. 912)
- Inflammatory bowel disease (IBD) (p. 388)
- Malignancy (p. 751)
- Drug fever
- Factitious illness (p. 1138)

Examination and assessment

A thorough history and physical examination is required. Consider other factors such as travel, geography, age, and significant exposures. Investigations include the following:

- *Blood*: CBC, CRP, ESR, liver and renal function tests, albumin
- *Serology*: Cytomegalovirus (CMV), Epstein-Barr virus (EBV), Brucella, and Q fever
- *Cultures*: At least three serial blood cultures, urine culture, stool culture, and maybe lumbar puncture and bone marrow culture
- *X-rays* of sinuses in the older child, and chest film
- *Bone scan* to exclude osteomyelitis
- *Echocardiography* to exclude endocarditis
- *Skin test* for tuberculosis and blood test for HIV after counseling

Treatment

Antibiotics

These are best avoided until a site of infection has been found. However, in many cases they will have been prescribed already. Remember that antibiotics may be the drug agent causing fever. If the child is critically ill, then empiric antibiotics are given.

Antipyretics

These are best avoided during the period of assessment of fever. Blood cultures should be taken when the patient is febrile. Determine whether there is a specific pattern to the fever.

Common respiratory tract infections

Fever in children is commonly caused by upper respiratory infections (URIs) including otitis media, sinusitis, and pharyngitis. Many of these are viral, and overuse of antibiotics with these infections may contribute to increasing antibiotic resistance.

Otitis media

Middle ear infection is a common disease of early childhood, with 90% of children having at least one episode by age 2 years. This diagnosis alone results in more than 20 million antibiotic prescriptions per year. Both viral and bacterial pathogens are common, so it is important to distinguish likely etiology and management based on signs and symptoms. When only nonspecific symptoms are used for diagnosis, only 50% of children may have positive bacterial cultures on tympanocentesis.

Specific signs and symptoms
- Middle ear effusion diagnosed by exam with tympanometry
- Earache, tugging at ear, bulging tympanic membrane

Nonspecific symptoms
- Fever
- Irritability

See Box 19.7 for a summary of the 2004 American Academy for Pediatrics (AAP) guidelines for the management of acute otitis media.

Sinusitis

It is estimated that up to 10% of URIs in children are complicated by acute sinusitis. Since children have frequent colds, sinusitis is commonly seen in pediatric practice.

Because both viral URIs and acute bacterial sinusitis may have nasal discharge and cough, it is important to distinguish between the two.

Distinguishing characteristics of acute sinusitis
- Persistent symptoms including nasal discharge and cough lasting more than 10 days and not improving
- Severe symptoms including high fever and purulent nasal discharge lasting more than 3 days
- Biphasic course with improvement followed by new or worsening symptoms after 1 week

Treatment
Give antibiotics directed against the most likely bacterial pathogens:
- *S. pneumoniae, H. influenzae, M. catarrhalis*

Surgical management is rarely required in acute sinusitis.

Box 19.7 Management of otitis media

Temperature >39 ℃ and/or severe otalgia

Day of diagnosis
- High-dose amoxicillin–clavulanate (90 mg/kg/day amoxicillin; 6.4 mg/kg/day clavulanate)

Clinical failure, day 3
- Ceftriaxone IM, 3 days

Temperature <39 ℃ without severe otalgia

Day of diagnosis
- Watchful waiting with analgesia OR treatment with high-dose amoxicillin (80–90 mg/kg/day)

Clinical failure, day 3
- If initial management was observation, give high-dose amoxicillin
- If initial management was antibiotics, give high-dose amoxicillin–clavulanate

This therapy is directed against the most likely pathogens:
- _Streptococcus pneumoniae_
- _Haemophilus influenzae_
- _Moraxella catarrhalis_
- Group A streptococcus

Penicillin-allergic patients should be managed with non-penicillin regimens.

Pharyngitis

Many bacteria and viruses can cause sore throat in children. There may be associated symptoms or isolated pharyngitis. The vast majority of cases in children are caused by viruses and are thus self-limited and benign, requiring only symptomatic treatment. However, group β-hemolytic streptococcus is an important bacterial cause that requires antibiotic treatment to shorten the course of symptoms and prevent the possible occurrence of rheumatic fever. In addition to common respiratory viruses, other potential viral causes of pharyngitis include EBV, Coxsackie virus, echovirus, and herpes simplex virus (HSV).

Diagnosis of group A streptococcal pharyngitis

The signs and symptoms of group A streptococcal pharyngitis (Box 19.8) overlap significantly with those of disease caused both by viruses and by other bacteria. Even the most experienced clinicians are not particularly accurate in making the diagnosis of group A streptococcus. Thus, diagnostic testing is indicated when group A streptococcus is considered. Rapid antigen tests are used frequently in the outpatient setting and are highly specific (95%) but not as sensitive as throat culture (70%–90%).

Treatment of group A streptococcal pharyngitis

Penicillin V is the drug of choice for treatment of group A streptococcal pharyngitis, unless the child is penicillin-allergic. Amoxicillin has no microbiological advantage, although it is often used because of ease of administration (single daily dose vs. three times daily dosing for penicillin V). Alternatives include

- Intramuscular benzathine penicillin G
- Oral macrolides (erythromycin, clarithromycin, azithromycin)
- Oral first-generation cephalosporin

The latter two are alternatives for penicillin-allergic patients.

Box 19.8 Features suggestive of group A streptococcal pharyngitis*

- Sudden onset
- Sore throat
- Fever
- Scarlet fever rash
- Headache
- Nausea, vomiting, and abdominal pain
- Exudative inflammation of the pharynx and tonsils
- Tender, enlarged cervical lymph nodes
- Patient 5–15 years of age
- History of exposure
- Lack of common URI symptoms (cough, coryza, conjunctivitis, hoarseness)

*It is important to note that even the most experienced clinicians find it difficult to clinically differentiate between bacterial and viral causes for pharyngitis, so these should not be considered diagnostic.

Common infections characterized by rash

Infections in childhood often have an associated rash (see Box 19.9). The skin lesion will give some clue to the potential cause (see p. 936 for definitions).

> ## Box 19.9 Types of childhood rash associated with infections
>
> *Macules and/or papules*
> - *Macules*: Red or pink discrete, flat areas that blanch on pressure
> - *Papules*: Small, raised lesions that blanch on pressure
> - **Infections**: Measles, rubella, roseola, and enterovirus
>
> *Purpura and/or petechiae*
> - Red or purple spots that do not blanch on pressure
> - **Infections**: Meningococcus, enterovirus, and *Haemophilus influenzae*
>
> *Vesicles*
> - Small, raised lesions that contain clear fluid
> - **Infections**: Chicken pox, shingles, herpes simplex virus, and hand, foot, and mouth disease
>
> *Bullae and pustules*
> - Large, raised lesions containing clear fluid or pus
> - **Infections**: Staphylococcal or streptococcal impetigo, and scalded skin
>
> *Desquamation*
> - Peeling skin, often of the hands and feet
> - **Infections**: Kawasaki's disease and subsequent to scarlet fever

An *exanthem* is a rash that "bursts forth or blooms" toward the end of incubating an infection. The six classic exanthems are characteristically
- Widespread, symmetrically distributed on the body
- Red, discrete or confluent macules or papules

Box 19.10 gives a summary of the exanthems. Look at the accompanying text that follows for more details.

Box 19.10 The six classsic exanthems

1st disease: measles
- Incubation: 8–12 days
- Duration: 6–8 days
- Infectivity: From 4 days before to 4 days after the rash appears
- Rash: Maculopapular rash starts on the face and spreads
- Features: Prodromal Koplik spots on the oral mucosa
- Treatment: Supportive

2nd disease: scarlet fever
- Incubation: 2–5 days
- Duration: 7 days
- Infectivity: Others can become colonized
- Rash: Fine, papular rash on flushed skin, sandpaper texture
- Features: Sore throat, strawberry tongue, rash, and lymphadenopathy
- Treatment: Penicillin V

3rd disease: rubella
- Incubation: 14–21 days
- Duration: 2–3 days
- Infectivity: From 7 days before to 7 days after the rash
- Rash: Maculopapular, rapidly spreads and fades
- Features: Enlarged lymph nodes at the back of the neck and ears
- Treatment: Supportive

4th disease: possibly Coxsackie virus
- No longer recognized as a disease entity

5th disease: parvovirus
- Incubation: 4–14 days
- Duration: 3–7 days prodrome then rash for 1–4 days; then evanescent rash over 1–3 weeks followed by arthropathy
- Infectivity: No isolation needed for children
- Rash: Slapped-cheek appearance, erythema infectiosum
- Treatment: Supportive

6th disease: roseola
- Incubation: 10 days
- Duration: 3–7 days
- Infectivity: Unclear
- Rash: Maculopapular
- Features: Temperature for 3 days, then as the rash appears, the temperature falls rapidly
- Treatment: Supportive

Exanthem: measles

Measles occurs typically in preschool-age and young children, with the peak incidence in late winter and spring.

Signs and symptoms

- *Prodrome*: Primary infection occurs in the respiratory epithelium of the nasopharynx and produces fever, coryza, cough, and non-purulent conjunctivitis. Koplik spots (which look like grains of sugar on the mucosa) are also a characteristic sign in the mouth, opposite the lower premolars. After 2–3 days there is viremia with infection of the reticuloendothelial system. During this phase patients are highly infectious.
- *Exanthematous phase*: A second viremia occurs 5–7 days after the initial infection with rash developing some 14 days after initial infection. The maculopapular rash starts on the face and lasts 6–8 days.
- *Other features*: Generalized lymphadenopathy, anorexia, diarrhea, and fever (may persist for 7–10 days).

Diagnosis

- *Clinical*: Koplik spots are pathognomonic.
- *CBC*: Leukopenia and lymphopenia
- *Liver function tests*: Elevated transaminases
- *Serology*: Measles IgM confirms the diagnosis and may be detected on the first day of the rash. There are false positive results.

Management

- *Acute treatment*: Generally supportive, but antibiotics are indicated for secondary bacterial infection (e.g., pneumonia, otitis media, tracheitis)
- *Prevention*: MMR (**M**easles, **M**umps, **R**ubella) vaccine at 12–18 months and a preschool booster to all children
- *Vitamin A*: In developing countries, vitamin A deficiency and malnutrition lead to a protracted course of illness with severe complications. The rash is dark red and is followed by desquamation and depigmentation. Consider supplements in children older than 6 months.

Complications

Complications commonly occur in young children, with almost 20% of cases having at least one additional problem. For example:
- Acute otitis media (10%)
- *Lower respiratory tract infection* (5%): Bacterial pneumonia, interstitial pneumonia, bronchiolitis, laryngotracheobronchitis
- *Encephalitis* (1 in 5000) occurs about 8 days after the onset of illness and starts with headache, lethargy, and irritability, followed by seizures and coma. Mortality is high and there are neurological sequelae in survivors.
- *Subacute sclerosing panencephalitis* (SSPE, 1 in 10,000): A rare and fatal neurological disease with progressive intellectual deterioration, ataxia, and seizures about 7 years after measles infection.

Scarlet fever

Scarlet fever is an erythematous rash that may occur with pharyngitis caused by group A streptococcus. Other patterns of infection caused by group A streptococcus include toxic shock syndrome and necrotizing fasciitis.

Signs and symptoms

- *Prodrome*: Infection is spread by respiratory secretions and droplets, or by self-infection from nasal carriage. During the incubation period (2–5 days) the child may have fever, vomiting, and abdominal pain.
- *Exanthematous phase*: Diffuse "sandpaper-like" rash in the neck and chest area (with perioral pallor), spreading to the flexor creases. The pharynx is erythematous and there may be exudative tonsillitis, palatal petechiae, uvular edema, and strawberry tongue.
- *Other features*: Tender anterior cervical lymphadenopathy.

Diagnosis

- *Clinical*: Group A streptococcus infection is unlikely if there is hoarseness, cough, conjunctivitis, diarrhea, or rhinorrhea.
- *Throat swab*: Culture and growth of the organism
- *Rapid tests*: Rapid antigen tests for group A streptococcus are an alternative to throat culture but have a lower sensitivity in pharyngitis. They are, however, highly specific.

Management

Antibiotics

Give penicillin V or amoxicillin for 10 days. Macrolides and oral first-generation cephalosporins are alternatives for penicillin-allergic patients. Appropriate antibiotic therapy will prevent development of rheumatic fever (but not glomerulonephritis) and may reduce the length of illness. Antibiotics should be started within 9 days of acute illness.

Isolation

Children should be isolated until 24 hours after the start of antibiotics.

Complications

These include peritonsillar abscess, retropharyngeal abscess, acute glomerulonephritis and rheumatic fever.

Rubella

Rubella is a mild disease in childhood, occurring in winter and spring.

Signs and symptoms
- *Prodrome*: The incubation period is 14–21 days, during which time the child may have a mild illness with low-grade fever.
- *Exanthematous phase*: Maculopapular rash starting on the face, then spreading to cover the whole body, and lasting up to 5 days
- *Other features*: Suboccipital and postauricular lymphadenopathy

Diagnosis
Serology
If there is a risk that a nonimmune pregnant woman might have been exposed to the child, the diagnosis should be confirmed by serology.

Management
- Supportive
- Prevention: Immunization with MMR (see Measles, Management, p. 846)

Complications
Very rarely, children may develop arthritis, myocarditis, encephalitis, or thrombocytopenia. (Remember fetal rubella syndrome if a nonimmune mother is infected early in pregnancy).

Enteroviruses

The majority of infections due to human enteroviruses (Coxsackie viruses, echoviruses, and polio viruses) produce nonspecific illness. They occur in the summer and autumn months, and occasionally there are characteristic features:

- *Meningoencephalitis*: Aseptic meningitis with an associated skin rash that can look like meningococcal septicemia (see p. 936)
- *Pleurodynia*: Febrile illness with pleuritic chest pain and tender thoracic muscles
- Myocarditis
- *Hand, foot and mouth disease*: Painful vesicles on the hands, feet, mouth, and tongue
- *Herpangina*: Vesicular and ulcerated lesions on the soft palate and uvula
- *Polio*: This condition should be eradicated with effective global immunization.

Parvovirus

Parvovirus B19 (fifth disease) induces immune-complex formation that deposit in joints and the skin, causing erythema infectiosum. It also infects the erythroblastoid precursors in the bone marrow. The infection occurs in all ages and is more common in the winter and spring.

Signs and symptoms
- *Prodrome*: Infection spread by respiratory secretions and droplets, then low-grade fever, headache, and coryza 7 days after exposure
- *Exanthematous phase*: A number of days long, bright red macules on the face with a "slapped-cheek" appearance (also, perioral pallor). The rash spreads to the limbs, sparing the palms and soles. It is more intense with exposure to sunlight, heat, exercise, and stress.
- *Other features*: Other patterns of illness include asymptomatic infection, aplastic crisis, and fetal hydrops (from maternal infection).

Diagnosis
- *Clinical*: Characteristic rash.
- *Serology*: If the diagnosis is in question, titers can be measured.

Management
Supportive treatment is with antipyretics for fever.

Roseola

Human herpes virus 6 (HHV-6) causes roseola, which is a benign, self-limiting exanthem commonly infecting children by the age of 2 years. It is also known as erythema subitum.

Signs and symptoms

- *Prodrome*: High-spiking fever up to 41°C lasting for up to 4 days. The fever typically stops once the rash appears.
- *Exanthematous phase*: The rose-colored maculopapular rash appears some days later, beginning on the trunk and spreading peripherally. It lasts for 2–5 days.
- *Other features*: Vomiting, diarrhea, pharyngeal injection without exudates, cervical lymphadenopathy, and febrile convulsions prior to rash (5%–10% of cases)

Diagnosis

- *Clinical*: Typical history and there may be associated neutropenia

Management

Supportive treatment is antipyretics for fever.

Complications

The most common complication is febrile convulsion, and HHV-6 probably accounts for a third of these cases in children under 1 year of age. Rarely, some children may develop aseptic meningitis, encephalitis, and hepatitis.

Rash: chickenpox and zoster

Varicella zoster virus (VZV) infection typically occurs between the ages of 1 and 6 years, with maximal transmission occurring during winter and spring.

Signs and symptoms

- *Prodrome*: VZV is spread by respiratory droplets or direct contact with lesions. The infectious period begins 2 days before vesicles appear and ends when the last vesicle crusts over (it is possible to retrieve virus from a crust).
- *Rash* usually starts on the head and trunk, then the rest of the body. Individual lesions start as red macules, then progress through stages (papule, vesicle, pustule, crusting). Different stages of the rash are seen at the same time and heal completely within 2 weeks.
- *Other features*: Headache, anorexia, signs of upper respiratory tract infection (i.e., sore throat, cough, coryza), fever, and itching

Diagnosis

- *Clinical*: Characteristic rash, its distribution and progression
- *Other*: Serology (VZV IgM), electron microscopy of vesicle fluid, Tzanck preparation or direct fluorescent antibody testing

Management

- *Symptoms*: Treatment of fever and itching
- *Antivirals*: Acyclovir is used in severe varicella, encephalitis, pneumonia, babies, and immunosuppressed patients (i.e., steroids, oncology, etc.). VZV immunoglobulin should also be considered.
- *Prevention*: Varicella vaccine at 12–18 months.

Complications

Secondary bacterial infection may occur with invasive group A streptococcus leading to necrotizing fasciitis or toxic shock syndrome. Other rare complications include purpura fulminant, cerebrovascular stroke, and encephalitis. Life-threatening pneumonitis may occur in the young infant and immunosuppressed child.

Herpes zoster (shingles)

A reactivation of latent infection may occur, leading to vesicular lesions in the distribution of a sensory nerve. Shingles is rare in childhood but occurs in the immunosuppressed, or in those who had primary infection in infancy.

Rash: infectious mononucleosis

Infectious mononucleosis is caused by Epstein–Barr virus (EBV) (90%) and cytomegalovirus (CMV). The source is oropharyngeal secretions. Virus infects B lymphocytes in pharyngeal lymphoid tissue and then spreads to the rest of the lymphoid system.

Signs and symptoms
- *Prodrome*: Flu-like illness (headache, low-grade fever and chills) for 3–5 days. The incubation period is 4–6 weeks.
- *Features*: Exudative pharyngitis; generalized, tender lymphadenopathy; hepatosplenomegaly; widespread erythematous macular rash, especially if treated with ampicillin; lethargy

Diagnosis
- *Classic triad*: Lymphocytosis (80%–90% of white blood cells); ≥10% atypical lymphocytes on peripheral blood film; positive serology for EBV
- *Monospot test*: A low-sensitivity test with false positives occurring in lymphoma and hepatitis
- *Serology*: IgM and IgG against viral capsid antigen (VCA) are elevated early in the disease; antibody against EBV nuclear antigen (EBNA) is not present until weeks to months after onset of infection.
- *Other*: Elevated liver function tests, mild thrombocytopenia

Management
- *Symptoms*: Supportive care.
- *Splenomegaly*: Patients with splenomegaly should avoid contact sports for 1 month.

Complications
- *Gastrointestinal and abdominal*: Hepatitis, splenomegaly, and splenic rupture
- *Central nervous system*: Aseptic meningitis, encephalitis, Guillain–Barre syndrome
- *Other*: Lymphoma, orchitis, myocarditis, pneumonia

Other infections: Lyme disease

Lyme disease is caused by the spirochete *Borrelia burgdorferi*. It is transmitted by the bite of the deer tick (*Ixodes scapularis* or *Ixodes pacificus*). Lyme disease occurs primarily in three distinct geographic areas of the United States (southern New England, eastern mid-Atlantic states, upper Midwest, and, less commonly, on the west coast).

- *Age group*: Any age
- *Incubation*: 4–20 days
- *Rash*: An erythematous macule at the site of the tick bite increases in size and forms a painless red lesion called erythema migrans.
- *Early time course* (weeks): The symptoms of fever, headache, myalgia, arthralgia, and lymphadenopathy fluctuate over several weeks.
- *Later time course* (months): Dissemination of infection leads to cranial nerve palsies, meningitis, arthritis, or myocarditis.
- *Diagnosis*: Clinical features and serology after 2–4 weeks
- *Treatment*: In the young child, amoxicillin or oral cefuroxime is used. In the child over 8 years use doxycycline. In those with persistent or recurrent arthritis and those with heart or central nervous system disease, use ceftriaxone.

Mumps

Mumps is a viral infection transmitted by respiratory droplets. The virus enters the parotid gland before systemic spread. The peak incidence is in children aged 5–9 years.

Signs and symptoms
- *Prodrome*: Myalgia, anorexia, headache, low-grade fever and chills. The incubation period is 14–21 days.
- *Features*: 20% of infections are asymptomatic. In 30%–40% of cases there is parotitis. In these patients there is often ear pain and tenderness over the gland.
- *Other features*: Headache, anorexia, signs of upper respiratory tract infection (i.e., sore throat, cough and coryza), and low-grade fever.

Diagnosis
- *Clinical*: Characteristic examination with glandular swelling
- *Other*: Serology (mumps IgM) in the first week of illness; viral culture of saliva or urine; blood shows lymphocytosis and increased amylase

Management
- *Symptoms*: Supportive care
- *Prevention*: MMR vaccine at 12–18 months and a preschool booster to all children

Complications
- Meningoencephalitis is the most common complication and it is usually asymptomatic.
- Orchitis results in testicular swelling, local pain, and later atrophy.
- *Other*: Oophoritis, pancreatitis, and myocarditis

Bacteremia and shock

Bacterial infection leading to "sepsis syndrome" and shock is discussed in the Emergency section (Chapter 5, p. 82). The most common cause of bacteremic shock is *Neisseria meningitidis*.

Meningococcal septicemia and shock

Meningococcal disease is rare, but it can be fatal in a previously well child. Unfortunately, at an early stage, the signs and symptoms are non-specific and the child may have features similar to a minor viral illness. In the acute presentation, it is important to identify a typical non-blanching purpuric or petechial rash.

Pathogenesis

In the United States, *Neisseria meningitidis* serogroups B, C, and Y each account for about 30% of reported cases. Asymptomatic colonization of the upper respiratory tract is not uncommon, but the trigger and mechanism of invasion is unknown. Once bacteremia occurs, bacterial autolysis leads to endotoxin release and systemic illness with disseminated intravascular coagulation, capillary leak, and distributive and cardiogenic shock.

Signs and symptoms

- *Nonspecific:* Fever, malaise, and thirst may be the first sign of shock, followed by poor urine output. Pain in proximal muscles, joints, and abdomen is very common.
- *Rash:* Initially maculopapular, then petechial, then purpuric
- *Central nervous system:* Meningitis or raised intracranial pressure (e.g., headache, neck pain or stiffness, irritability, and altered level of consciousness)
- *Respiratory:* Features of pneumonia or pulmonary edema

Diagnosis

Any febrile child who develops a purpuric rash should be considered to have meningococcal septicemia until proven otherwise.

Management

See Emergency section (Chapter 5, p. 82). Suspected cases should receive intravenous penicillin G at a dose of 250,000–300,000 U/kg/day, divided every 4 hours (maximum 12 million U/day). Cefotaxime, ceftriaxone, and ampicillin are acceptable alternatives. If there is a history of anaphylaxis to penicillin, use chloramphenicol.

Prevention is with tetravalent meningococcal conjugate vaccine at 11–12 years to all children.

Complications

Most survivors of meningococcal disease have few or no sequelae. However, there is significant mortality (2%–4%), and morbidity includes loss of digits and limbs due to peripheral vascular disease.

Kawasaki disease

Kawasaki disease is a systemic vasculitis that is important because approximately 20% of untreated children will develop coronary abnormalities, including aneurysms, thrombosis, myocardial infarction, and arrhythmias. Peak incidence in the United States is between 18 and 24 months, with 80% of children being less than 5 years of age.

Diagnostic criteria

The diagnosis can be made in children with fever (>38.5°C) present for at least 5 days, without other explanation, in the presence of four of the five following criteria:

- Bilateral nonpurulent conjunctivitis
- Erythematous mouth and pharynx, strawberry tongue and red, cracked lips
- Changes of the extremities with at least one of the following: induration and/or erythema of palms and soles; periungual desquamation of fingers and toes
- Polymorphous exanthem (92%): In young children, this may be most prominent in the diaper area.
- Acute nonsuppurative cervical lymphadenopathy >1.5 cm (42%)

Box 19.11 Differential diagnosis for Kawasaki disease

The differential diagnosis for Kawasaki disease includes

- Streptococcal and staphylococcal toxin-mediated diseases (including scarlet fever and toxic shock syndrome)
- Adenovirus and other viral infections (enterovirus, measles)
- Drug reactions or Stevens–Johnson syndrome
- Leptospirosis
- Rickettsial infection
- Juvenile rheumatoid arthritis

Associated features

In addition to the diagnostic criteria of Kawasaki disease, the other features of the condition include the following:

- *Renal*: Urethritis with sterile pyuria
- *Musculoskeletal*: Arthralgia and arthritis (35% of patients)
- *Central nervous system*: Aseptic meningitis, with mild CSF pleocytosis and normal CSF glucose and protein; sensorineural hearing loss—transient high-frequency loss or permanent loss.
- *Gastrointestinal*: Diarrhea and vomiting; hydrops of the gall bladder with or without obstructive jaundice
- *Cardiac*: Congestive heart failure, myocarditis, pericardial effusion, arrhythmias, mitral insufficiency, acute myocardial infarction within 1 year of disease
- *Coronary aneurysms*: Incidence of coronary artery aneurysms varies (15%–25% in untreated patients) and resolution varies with age at onset and size and shape of aneurysm.

Diagnostic testing

- *Hematology:* Leukocytosis with left shift common in acute phase; thrombocytosis peaks in the third to fourth week; normocytic, normochromic anemia present early and persists until inflammatory process begins to subside; reticulocyte count is low
- *Coagulation:* Increased coagulability, platelet turnover, and depleted fibrinolysis
- *Urine:* Mononuclear cells with cytoplasmic inclusions are abundant in the urine early in the disease; these cells are **not** detected by dipstick methods for white blood cells, which only detect polymorphonuclear leukocytes (PMNs).
- *Acute-phase reactants:* Elevated ESR persists beyond the acute febrile period and gradually returns to normal over 1–2 months. CRP may also be elevated.
- *Biochemistry:* Elevated liver transaminases; hypoalbuminemia
- *Immunology:* Marked activation of circulating monocyte/macrophages; B-cell activation elevated immunoglobulin production; T-cell lymphopenia
- *Cardiology:* ECG is usually normal, but strain, ischemia, and/or infarct can be present.
- *Echocardiography:* Aneurysms may first be seen from 7 to 21 days post-onset of fever.

Treatment

- *High-dose IV immunoglobulin* is the treatment of choice: 2 g/kg as a single infusion.
- *Aspirin* 80–100 mg/kg/day (divided q6h) reducing to 3–5 mg/kg as fever resolves
- The role of steroids is not clear.
- Follow-up is very important for cardiac monitoring.

Skin and soft-tissue diseases

Impetigo

- *Cause*: *Staphylococcus aureus* or group A streptococcus
- *Age group*: Infants and young children.
- *Features*: Erythematous macules (later vesicular/bullous) on the face, neck and hands—often associated with preexisting skin lesions such as eczema
- *Infectivity*: Nasal carriage is often the source of infection. Autoinoculation occurs and lesions are infectious until dry.
- *Antibiotics*: Topical for mild infection; systemic for severe infections

Boils (furuncles)

- *Cause*: *Staphylococcus aureus* (recent increase in methicillin-resistant *Staphylococcus aureus* [MRSA])
- *Age group*: Any age
- *Features*: Infection of hair follicles or sweat glands
- *Infectivity*: Nasal carriage is often the source of infection in recurrent boils.
- *Antibiotics*: Systemic

Periorbital cellulitis

- *Cause*: *Streptococcus pneumoniae* or *Haemophilus influenzae* type B (in unimmunized children); *Staphylococcus aureus* or group A streptococcus is more common when associated with trauma.
- *Age group*: Any age
- *Features*: Fever with unilateral erythema, tenderness, and edema of the eyelid, often following local trauma to the skin. It is important to rule out orbital cellulitis. Complications include local abscess, meningitis, and cavernous sinus thrombosis.
- *Diagnostic testing*: Cranial CT scan and lumbar puncture
- *Antibiotics*: Intravenous

Staphylococcal scalded-skin syndrome

- *Cause*: Exfoliative staphylococcal toxin
- *Age group*: Infants and young children
- *Features*: Fever and malaise with a purulent, crusting, localized infection around the eyes, nose, and mouth. Later, diffuse erythema and skin tenderness leading to separation of the epidermis through the granular cell layer. Nikolsky's sign is epidermal separation on light pressure with no subsequent scarring after healing.
- *Antibiotics*: Intravenous

Necrotizing fasciitis

- *Cause*: Staphylococcus aureus or group A streptococcus
- *Age group*: Any age
- *Features*: Subcutaneous infection involving tissue planes down to fascia and muscle. Accompanied by severe pain and systemic illness
- *Antibiotics*: Intravenous, and surgical debridement

Box 19.12 offers antibiotic choices for the management of MRSA skin and soft-tissue infections.

Box 19.12 Antibiotic treatment of MRSA soft-tissue infections

Topical agents
- Mupirocin

Oral agents
The choice of agents depends on susceptibility.
- Trimethoprim sulfamethoxazole
- Clindamycin
- Macrolide: azithromycin or clarithromycin
- Linezolid

Intravenous agents
- Vancomycin
- Linezolid
- Daptomycin
- Quinupristin–dalfopristin

Toxic shock syndrome

Toxic shock syndrome is a multisystem disease caused by toxin-producing *Staphylococcus aureus* or group A streptococcus.

Signs and symptoms
- Systemic illness with high fever
- *Gastrointestinal*: Vomiting, diarrhea
- Shock and hypotension
- *Neuromuscular:* Severe myalgia, altered consciousness
- *Skin rash:* Redness of mucous membranes and diffuse macular rash. Ten days after infection there is desquamation of the palms, soles, fingers, and toes.

Diagnostic testing
- *Hematology*: Thrombocytopenia, coagulopathy
- *Biochemistry*: Abnormal liver and kidney function tests

Treatment
- Intravenous fluids and resuscitation
- Antibiotics directed against staphylococci and streptococci, including a protein synthesis inhibitor, such as clindamycin or an aminoglycoside, to inhibit further toxin production
- Surgical debridement, as indicated

Box 19.13 lists the diagnostic criteria for staphylococcal and streptococcal toxic shock syndrome.

Box 19.13 Toxic shock syndrome (TSS)

Diagnostic criteria for staphylococcal TSS
- Temperature ≥39°C
- Systolic blood pressure <90 mmHg
- Rash with desquamation
- Involvement of three or more of the following systems: gastrointestinal, musculoskeletal, renal, hepatic, CNS, blood, and mucous membranes

Diagnostic criteria for streptococcal TSS
- Isolation of group A streptococcus
- Hypotension
- Involvement of two or more of the following: coagulopathy, adult respiratory distress syndrome, soft tissue necrosis, rash with desquamation, or renal or hepatic involvement (see above)

Meningitis

Three-quarters of cases of meningitis are believed to occur before 15 years of age. Three organisms (*Streptococcus pneumoniae, Neisseria meningitidis*, and *Haemophilus influenzae* type B) account for 80% of the cases. *H. influenzae* has declined very significantly following routine immunization in infancy.

There are two important practice points:

- Infants do not get symptoms of meningismus with meningitis. There should be an extremely low threshold for doing a lumbar puncture as part of the septic workup in infants with unexplained fever (see p. 142).
- Coexisting septicemia often causes the morbidity and mortality.

Pathogenesis

The sequence of pathology involves the following:

- Colonization and invasion of the nasopharyngeal epithelium
- Invasion of the blood stream
- Attachment to and invasion of the meninges
- Induction of inflammation with leak of proteins leading to cerebral edema
- Alteration in cerebral blood flow and metabolism
- Cerebral vasculitis

Symptoms and signs

In older children, headache followed by neck stiffness occurs 12–24 hours into the illness. Other features include the following:

- *General*: Fever, vomiting, and anorexia
- *Central*: Irritability, disorientation, altered mental status
- *Seizures* occur in 30%. Focal seizures suggest localized infarction or subdural collection.
- *Neck stiffness* is often present, but it may be absent in infants.
- *Neurology*: Focal cranial nerve signs are more common in children with tuberculous or cryptococcal meningitis.
- *Eyes*: Papilledema is a late sign and not a reliable indicator of raised intracranial pressure. Retinal hemorrhages (rarely present) may indicate sagittal venous thrombosis or coagulopathy.

Lumbar puncture

Lumbar puncture is needed to make the diagnosis of meningitis and identify the organism. It is generally safe. However, patients with bacterial meningitis may have raised intracranial pressure; thus, if there is clinical suspicion of this problem the procedure should be deferred. (The cellular and chemical changes of meningitis will remain in the CSF for several days). Contraindications to lumbar puncture include the following:

- Signs of raised intracranial pressure
- Infection of the skin at the lumbar puncture site
- Evidence of coagulopathy
- Cardiovascular instability
- Acute meningococcal disease before adequate stabilization

Treatment

The specific treatment of bacterial meningitis is dealt with in the Emergency section (see Chapter 5, p. 90).

Steroids

There is a clear benefit from the use of dexamethasone (but not methylprednisolone) in reducing the severity of neurological sequelae, particularly deafness, after bacterial meningitis. Most of the patients in these studies have had *H. influenzae* or *S. pneumoniae* meningitis. Patients with meningococcal meningitis have a similar pathophysiology and so steroids may also be beneficial in treating this infection. The benefit of dexamethasone is greatest if it is given early. Dexamethasone should be given in a dose of 0.15 mg/kg (6-hourly for 4 days) starting before, or simultaneously with, the first dose of antibiotics.

Mycobacteria

Pulmonary tuberculosis (see also p. 346)

Pulmonary tuberculosis due to *Mycobacterium tuberculosis* (an acid-fast bacillus) is discussed in the Respiratory section (see Chapter 9, p. 346).

Atypical mycobacterial infection could be the cause of the following:

- *Persistent lymphadenopathy*: This infection is diagnosed after histology of a surgically resected node.
- *Disseminated infection* in the immunocompromised patient. *Mycobacterium avium* intracellulare is an infection often seen in patients with advanced disease due to human immunodeficiency virus (HIV).

Tuberculous meningitis (TBM)

TBM is the most feared complication of *Mycobacterium tuberculosis* infection. It usually occurs within 12 months of the first infection. Most frequently TBM occurs in those under 5 years of age.

Pathology

The initial pathology is occult hematogenous dissemination to the cerebral cortex from a primary site (e.g., gut, lung). This increases in size until it reaches the meninges and subarachnoid space. A thick, gelatinous exudate is created especially around the brain stem so that cranial nerves III, IV, and VI are commonly compromised. Hydrocephalus is common.

Clinical course

The onset is insidious and is characterized by apathy or disinterest, then intermittent headaches and anorexia. Fever is almost always present. Vomiting occurs in 50% of cases. Focal neurological signs, seizures, or severely depressed conscious level may occur.

Diagnosis

Half of patients will grow mycobacteria from their CSF, and the Mantoux or PPD skin test is positive in 90% of cases. Some 40%–90% have chest X-ray changes of pulmonary disease. Typical CSF abnormalities (in HIV-negative patients) include elevated intracranial pressure, high protein, low glucose, and increased numbers of lymphocytes. MRI of the brain may reveal hydrocephalus, basilar meningeal thickening, infarcts, edema, or tuberculomas. PCR of the CSF is positive in 60%–70% of cases if performed by a qualified laboratory.

Prognosis

Most patients survive if treated in the early insidious stage. There is a very high complication rate, especially if the focal neurological signs are present at the start of therapy.

Treatment

Because of the importance of early intervention, treatment should be initiated when the clinical suspicion is high, since diagnostic tests have poor sensitivities and confirmatory cultures take weeks to be positive. Therapy is for at least 12 months and should be supervised by an infectious disease consultant. Corticosteroids are indicated with TBM because they decrease rates of mortality and long-term neurological impairment. They should only be given with concomitant anti-tuberculosis therapy.

Tropical infections

Tropical infections may be present in any child returning from the tropics (see p. 1168). A general evaluation in the febrile child should follow the process discussed in the section on Acute Fever (see p. 802).

Malaria

- *Agent*: *Plasmodium falciparum* (also *P. vivax*, *P. ovale*, and *P. malariae*)
- *Features*: Fever (may be cyclical), diarrhea, vomiting, flu-like symptoms, jaundice, anemia, and altered mental status (cerebral malaria)
- *Time course*: Onset is approximately 2 weeks after inoculation, but relapse is possible months to years after primary infection (*P. vivax* and *P. ovale*).
- *Diagnosis*: Thick and thin blood smears should be examined in all children with fever from an endemic area. Repeat daily for three samples if there is a high index of suspicion.
- *Treatment*: The choice of therapy is based on infecting species, possible drug resistance, and disease severity (see CDC Web site for current recommendations).

Typhoid

- *Agent*: *Salmonella typhi* or *S. paratyphi*
- *Features*: Initially fever, headache, nonproductive cough, abdominal pain, and myalgias. Later symptoms include diarrhea, splenomegaly, bradycardia, and classic rose-colored spots on the trunk. Complications include shock, gastrointestinal perforation, myocarditis, and hepatitis.
- *Time course*: Typical onset is between 1 and 3 weeks after exposure.
- *Diagnosis*: Blood and stool cultures
- *Treatment*: Third-generation cephalosporin or ciprofloxacin

Dengue fever

- *Agent*: Viral infection spread by mosquitoes
- *Features*: Primary infection produces high fevers, myalgias, arthralgias, and a fine erythematous rash (with secondary desquamation).
- *Shock*: Dengue shock syndrome occurs when a previously infected child has new infection with a second strain.

Viral hemorrhagic fevers

- *Agents*: Lassa, Marburg, Ebola, and other viruses
- *Features*: Fevers, coagulopathy, fulminant hepatic and renal failure, often lethal.
- *Management*: If suspected, strict isolation is required (there is a high risk of nosocomial spread) and infectious disease consultation is advised.

Immunodeficiency disorders

Immunodeficiency may be due to causes that are
- *Primary*: Intrinsic abnormalities (see Box 19.14)
- *Secondary*: Cancer, immunosuppressive agents, HIV infection, splenec-tomy, nephrotic syndrome, sickle cell disease, etc.

Box 19.14 Primary immunodeficiency

These conditions include defects in the following:

B lymphocytes and antibody production
- *X-linked agammaglobulinemia* presents in early childhood with severe bacterial infections primarily of the respiratory tract. B cells are low in number or absent.
- *Hyper-IgM syndrome* presents with bacterial infection and *Pneumocystis jiroveci* (*P. carinii*) pneumonia [PCP]). There is high IgM, low IgG.
- *IgG subclass deficiency* has a minor immunodeficiency that may cause recurrent respiratory infection.

Tests: Immunoglobulin levels, immunoglobulin responses, lymphocyte subsets and specific genetic testing.

T lymphocytes and cellular immunity
- *Severe combined immunodeficiency (SCID)* presents in the first few months with failure to thrive, PCP, and persistent infection due to viruses and fungi. T cells are low in number or absent. B cells and NK cells may or may not be present.

Tests: CBC with differential, immunoglobulin levels, and lymphocyte subsets and function

Neutrophil defects
- *Chronic granulomatous disease (CGD)* usually presents in childhood with recurrent bacterial and fungal infections including pneumonia, abscess formation, lymphadenitis, osteomyelitis, and skin infections. Catalase (+) organisms (*Staphylococcus aureus*, *Aspergillus* species, etc.) are the hallmark pathogens.
- *Leukocyte adhesion deficiency* presents in infancy with delayed separation of the umbilical cord and omphalitis, chronic skin ulcers, and bacterial and fungal infection involving lymph nodes, liver, and lung without pus formation.

Tests: CBC with differential, neutrophil oxidative burst (e.g., nitroblue tetrazolium test or dihydrorhodamine [DHR] assay for CGD), neutrophil surface adhesion molecules, and specific genetic testing

Opsonization deficiencies
- *Complement deficiency* presents with severe meningococcal disease.
- *Mannose binding lectin deficiency*: as above.

Tests: Total hemolytic complement testing: CH50 (tests classical pathway) and AH50 (tests alternative pathway)

Multisystem syndromes
- *Ataxia–telangiectasia (AT)*: Skin (telangiectasias), neurological (ataxia), and immune defects
- *Wiscott–Aldrich syndrome (WAS)*: eczema, thrombocytopenia with small platelet size, and immunodeficiency.
- *DiGeorge syndrome*: Hypocalcemia, branchial arch and heart defects, and immunodeficiency
- *X-linked lymphoproliferative disease (XLP; a.k.a. Duncan syndrome)*: Particular susceptibility to EBV infection causing fulminent mononucleosis and B-cell lymphoproliferative disease.

Tests: Chromosomal fragility and α-fetoprotein (AT), fluorescence in situ hybridization (FISH) test for deletion of 22q11 (DiGeorge syndrome), CBC and mean platelet volume (WAS), and specific genetic testing (WAS and XLP)

Investigation for these conditions in children with a history of recurrent or severe infection requires a set of tests that screen the four main compartments of the immune system: complement, phagocytic cells (neutrophils), B cells (including immunoglobulin production), and T cells. These tests should be directed by the type of infection that the patient is susceptible to (e.g., viral, bacterial, fungal).

Treatment

A variety of therapies are required for children with primary immunodeficiency, and they should be cared for in designated centers. Therapy includes the following:
- Supportive care and antibiotics, antifungals, or antivirals for acute infections
- Replacement immunoglobulins (IVIG) and immunization
- Prophylactic antibiotics or antifungals
- Bone marrow transplantation
- Gene therapy (in the future)

Acquired immunodeficiency syndrome (AIDS)

AIDS in children is a global issue. It is caused by the retrovirus HIV (human immunodeficiency virus) type1.

Vertical transmission of HIV (see p. 210)

The main group of children at risk of acquiring the virus is infants of HIV-positive mothers.

- Infants become infected in utero, peripartum, and through breast-feeding.
- The rate of vertical transmission is 15%–40% without antiviral management.
- Most of the sequelae of HIV infection can be explained in terms of loss of function of CD4 cells.

Prevention

Reduction of vertical transmission of HIV can be reduced to <1% by
- Use of antenatal, perinatal, and postnatal antiretroviral drugs
- Avoidance of labor and contact with the birth canal by elective caesarian section delivery
- Avoidance of breast-feeding
- Current guidelines for prevention of mother-to-child HIV transmission can be found at: http://aidsinfo.nih.gov/

Diagnosis

- *Infants and children <18 months of age*: Diagnosis should be based on specific viral assays (HIV DNA or RNA PCR), as maternal HIV antibodies may still be present.
- *Children >18 months of age*: HIV antibody tests (HIV enzyme immunoassay [EIA] with confirmatory Western blot).

Early signs of HIV disease in children:
- *Gastrointestinal*: Chronic diarrhea, failure to thrive
- *Central nervous system*: Delayed development
- Recurrent bacterial and viral infection
- Lymphadenopathy and hepatosplenomegaly
- *Dermatologic*: Oral thrush, atopic dermatitis
- *Pneumocystis jirovecii* pneumonia (PCP)

AIDS

Progression to AIDS occurs with continued CD4+ T-cell depletion. AIDS-defining conditions include the following:
- PCP
- Esophageal candidiasis
- *Mycobacterium avium* complex bacteremia
- HIV wasting
- HIV encephalopathy

Treatment
- Prophylaxis against PCP
- Avoidance of live vaccines, including oral polio vaccine and BCG
- Antiretroviral therapy to suppress viral replication
- Social, psychological, and family support
- Current guidelines for antiretroviral treatment can be found at:
  http://aidsinfo.nih.gov/

Immunizations

- Immunizations are an important part of child health in the community.
- An acute febrile illness is not a contraindication to immunization. However, immunizations should be delayed in a child who has a moderate to severe febrile illness at the time of scheduled immunization.
- In those for whom there is a family history of febrile convulsion, advice should be given about control of fever with antipyretics, and when to seek medical assistance.

Schedule

The recommended immunization schedule for children from the Advisory Committee on Immunization Practices, the American Academy of Pediatrics and the American Academy of Family Physicians, is as follows:

Hepatitis B (HepB)

- Birth, 1–2 month, 6 months in all infants

Diphtheria, tetanus, acellular pertussis (DTaP)

- 2, 4, and 6 months in all infants
- Booster at 15–18 months and 4–6 years
- Tdap booster at 11–12 years old (with catch-up in all adolescents who haven't had it)

Inactivated polio virus (IPV)

- 2, 4, and between 6 and 18 months in all infants
- Boosters at 4–6 years

Haemophilus influenzae type B (HiB)

- 2, 4 (6; variable depending on vaccine used), and 12–15 months in all infants

Pneumococcal conjugate vaccine (PCV)

- 2, 4, 6 and 12–15 months in all infants

Rotavirus live attenuated vaccine (Rota)

- 2, 4, 6 months (orally administered; first dose must be given between 6 and 12 weeks of age)

Influenza vaccine

- Live or inactivated vaccine annually for all children 6 months–18 years
- 2 doses first time for all children 6 m - 9 years of age
- Annual boosters in fall

Measles, mumps, rubella (MMR)

- 12–15 months in all infants
- Booster at 4–6 years

Hepatitis A (HepA)

- 1 year in all children
- Second dose at least 6 months later

Neisseria meningitidis (meningococcus) C (MCV)

- 11–12 years in all children

Human papilloma virus vaccine (HPV)

- 3 doses given at 0, 2, and 6 months beginning at 11 years, girls only

Live vaccines are contraindicated in children with immunodeficiency. Pertussis immunization is contraindicated in infants who have had a severe local or general reaction to a previous injection. MMR is contraindicated in children allergic to excipients such as gelatin and neomycin. Certain high-risk groups may be a priority for earlier immunization with the vaccines listed on the previous page or for administration of additional immunizations. As new vaccines or new data become available, these recommendations may change. Always consult the Advisory Committee on Immunization Practices Web site for the latest recommendations.

Web sites
- http://www.cdc.gov/vaccines/default.htm
- http://www.cdc.gov/vaccines/recs/acip/default.htm

Clinical assessment

History

This should focus on the following:

- Presenting complaint
  - *Pain*: Site, severity, onset, nature, duration and chronicity, exacerbating and relieving factors, rest pain, and radiation. Pain may not be the main complaint—children avoid doing things that hurt.
  - If the child presents with knee pain, *always ask about and examine the hips*. Pain is often referred one joint lower than its origin.
  - *Swelling*: Site, size, onset, duration, exacerbating and relieving factors
  - *Limp*: Refusing to weight bear and/or history of trauma or injury (painful or painless)
  - *Morning stiffness* that improves with heat or activity
  - *Deformity*: Static, worsening, or improving condition
- Associated systemic symptoms
  - Symptoms of systemic infection (fevers, rigors, night sweats, flu-like symptoms)
- Antenatal and birth history is important with congenital conditions.
- Neurodevelopmental milestones (see p. 630)
- *Past medical history*: Previous trauma, surgery
- Sports and activities
- *Drug history*: Response to nonsteroidal agents, glucocorticoid usage, previous antibiotics
- Preceding illnesses
- *Family history*: Hereditary conditions, including spondyloarthropathies and psoriasis
- Neurological screening is important in syndromic children.

Examination

Inspection

Observe the child walking and at play.

General

- Height, weight, proportion (long limbs, short trunk)
- Skin (scars, lesions, color, discharge), soft tissue (swelling, muscle wasting, contractures), skeletal (alignment, rotation, limb length)
- *Limb*: Amelia (absence), hemiamelia (absence of distal half), phocomelia (hand or foot attached directly to trunk), syndactyly (fused digits), polydactyly (many digits)
- *Gait*: Antalgic, Trendelenburg, high stepping, abnormalities of lower limb or spine

Skeletal alignment

- *Spine*: Normally there is a flexible kyphosis of the thoracic spine, and lordosis at the cervical and lumbar spine (not noticeable in neonates). Look also for plagiocephaly, torticollis, scoliosis, and asymmetry.
- *Lower limb*: Check rotational profile, symmetric range of movement, varus and valgus deformity. Always examine the hips.

- *Feet*: Babies have "flat" feet. The medial longitudinal arch develops during childhood. Look at foot shape and range of motion.
- *Elbows*: There is a mild valgus deformity when in extension, especially in females.

Mobility and gait

Toddlers have a wide-stepping, jerky gait. As the child matures (by age 7 years), the gait becomes more adult-like with the heel strike, stance phase (whole of foot to the ground), push-off phase, and arm swing.

- *Antalgic (painful) gait*: Short-stance phase (child does not want to put weight on affected limb), trunk shift over the sore limb
- *High-stepping gait* is usually due to foot drop (child lifts foot higher off the ground to avoid tripping over).
- *Trendelenburg gait*: Look at the pelvis—when weight is loaded on the ipsilateral side, the contralateral hemipelvis tilts downward (due to weak abductors or neurological, muscular, or hip joint disorder in the weight-bearing ipsilateral limb). The upper body is then used to counterbalance.
- *Toe walking*: Consider neurological causes (see p. 582).
- *Short leg gait* may mimic antalgic or Trendelenburg gait.

Trendelenburg test

Stand facing the child with your hands out, palms facing upward. Ask the child to rest their hands (palms down) on your hands. Then ask the child to lift one leg. Watch the pelvis tilt downward on the non-weight-bearing side (and feel the downward pressure on your hand of this side). Look for trunk shift over the standing leg.

Gower's sign

The child should be able to independently stand from a sitting position without using their upper limbs. With weak lower-limb muscles, the child may "crawl" their hands up the thighs in order to stand up, e.g., in muscular dystrophy.

Neurodevelopmental assessment (see p. 582)

- Can the child hop on either foot? (when age appropriate)
- Can the child climb onto the examination couch?

Feel

Feel for tenderness, warmth, swelling (firmness, fluctuant), pulses, leg-length discrepancy (true leg length: measure from the anterior superior iliac spine to the medial malleolus). Watch for joint irritability and guarding through range of movement.

Move

- *General*: Muscle tone, symmetric, full joint range of movement, hyperlaxity or stiffness, contractures (are they fixed or can they be overcome?)
- *Spine*: Fixed or correctable deformity?
- *Hip*: Ortolani and Barlow tests (newborn to 3 months)
- *Knee*: Patella instability; anterior drawer test (ACL integrity); patellar inhibition sign for chondromalacia

The limping child

Exclude trauma, infection, and malignancy before considering other disorders.

Examination

The lower limbs, back, and abdomen need to be examined. Observe
- Limb position of least pain (e.g., in hip septic arthritis, the hip is held in flexion, abduction, and external rotation)
- Gait

Movement and mobility
- Ability to weight bear passively and actively
- Ability to move the joints and limbs freely
- Palpate for tenderness, heat, and swelling around the joint, palpate the entire length of the extremity, the abdomen, and spine
- Leg length difference (ASIS to medial malleoli), femur and tibia (flex knees and hips and examine from the side)
- Range of movement (ROM) in individual joint and compare with other side
- Weakness getting up from the floor
- Neurological and vascular status. Abdominal examination

Beware of referred pain from the joint above or from the abdomen (consider appendicitis, inguinal hernia, UTI with hip pain). *Always* assess the joint above and below. Hip pathology may present as knee pain.

Investigations
- Temperature
- *Blood*: CBC, ESR (maybe normal), CRP, blood cultures, blood film, rheumatoid factor (RF) (only in children with multiple swollen joints), antinuclear antibody (ANA), anti-streptolysin (ASO) titer, Lyme titer, HLA- B27 if considering spondyloarthropathy. Check creatine phosphokinase (CPK) if patient is weak.
- *Urine*: Dipstick and/or midstream urine (MSU)
- *X-rays*: Anteroposterior (AP), lateral plain X-ray of entire bone involved, including joint above and below (e.g., if hip: AP pelvis and frog-leg lateral views)
- *Ultrasound* of muscle, bone, and joints (especially hip)
- *MRI* is very sensitive and specific; it is good for soft tissues and bone pathology.
- *Three-phase bone scan*: Use when pain is not easily located; this modality is sensitive but not specific.
- *CT scan* is the best imaging technique for bone shape, morphology, pathology, and joint anatomy.

The limping child: differential diagnosis

See Tables 20.1 and 20.2.

Table 20.1 Differential diagnosis according to area of lower limb

Age (years)	Back	Hip	Femur	Knee	Foot and ankle
0–5	Discitis	Developmental dysplasia of the hip Transient synovitis Septic arthritis	Toddler fracture	Septic arthritis	Idiopathic heel and contracture Arthritis
5–10	Tumors	Transient synovitis Perthes disease Septic arthritis	Osteoyelitis (consider with septic joint)	Juvenile arthritis (JIA) Discoid meniscus Septic arthritis	Kohler's disease Freiberg's disease Tarsal coalition Verruca
10–15	Vertebral osteomyelitis	Slipped upper femoral epiphysis Septic arthritis Spondyloarthroathies		Osgood–Schlatter disease Osteochondritis dessicans Patellofemoral pain syndrome Chondromalacia patella Spondyloarthropathies	Sever's disease Tarsal coalition Verruca Ingrowing toenails Plantar fasciitis Enthesitis

Table 20.2 Causes of limp

Age (years)	Tumor	Benign tumor	Hematology	Infection	Neurology	Rheumatology	Trauma	Congenital
0–5 5–10 10–15	Neuroblastoma Ewing sarcoma Osteosarcoma	Osteoid osteoma	Acute lymphocytic leukemia Lymphoma Sickle cell disease Thalassemia	TB Malaria Lyme disease Viral	Cerebral palsy Duchenne's muscular dystrophy Poliomyelitis Hereditary motor sensory neuropathy Spina bifida	Juvenile idiopathic arthritis Other inflammatory arthritides SLE Henoch–Schönlein purpura, vasculitis	Non-accidental Injury Trauma (open/closed fractures) Sprains/ contusions Ill-fitting shoes	Congenital deficiency Shorting/ deformity, Skeletal dysplasia

Infection: septic arthritis

This is infectious arthritis of a synovial joint. Frequency is highest in young children, with 50% of cases presenting in the first 2 years. It affects males more than females by a rate of 2:1.

Pathogenesis

Septic arthritis can develop from osteomyelitis, especially in neonates where infection spreads from the metaphysis via transepiphyseal vessels. It may also arise from hematogenous spread or by direct inoculation.

Etiology

- Age <12 months old: *Staphylococcus aureus*, group B streptococcus, gram-negative bacilli
- Age 1–5 years: *Staphylococcus aureus*, *Haemophilus influenzae* (even in immunized children), group A streptococcus, *Streptococcus pneumoniae*; *Kingella kingae*
- Age 5–12 years: *Staphylococcus aureus*, group A streptococcus
- Age 12–18 years: *Staphylococcus aureus*, *Neisseria gonorrhoeae*
- Host factors affect susceptibility, e.g., salmonella in sickle cell disease

Common joints affected

Most (75%) cases are in the lower limb: knee > hip > ankle. Other cases (25%) affect the upper limbs.

Differential diagnosis

This depends on age and the joint involved:
- *Hip*: Transient synovitis, Perthes disease, slipped capital femoral epiphysis, psoas abscess, proximal femoral or vertebral osteomyelitis, discitis
- *Knee*: Distal femoral or proximal tibial osteomyelitis. Pain is often referred from the hip.
- *General*: Cellulitis, pyomyositis, other infectious arthritis (viral, mycolasmal, mycobacterial, fungal, Lyme disease or *Borrelia burgdorferi* infection affecting large joints), sickle cell disease, hemophilia, trauma, collagen vascular disease, Henoch–Schönlein purpura, reactive arthritis from GI infections, streptococcal pharyngitis or viral hepatitis, salmonella
- *>1 joint involved*: Oligoarticular juvenile idiopathic arthritis, rheumatic fever, serum sickness, Henoch–Schönlein purpura, collagen vascular disease, sickle cell disease, Lyme arthritis
- *Hemophilia*: Increased risk of septic arthritis due to hemarthrosis (predisposes to infection with pneumococci)

Symptoms and signs

Infants often do not appear ill; 50% do not have fever. In the older child, onset is more acute, with fever; decreased range of movement with guarding; pain on passive motion; hot, warm, swollen joint; inability to weight bear; and systemic symptoms of infection. In <10% of cases more than one joint is affected (except gonococcal infections). The clinical picture may be less acute if the child has received antibiotics.

Investigations

These are often inconclusive in infants, but include the following:
- *Blood*: CBC, ESR, CRP, blood cultures; Lyme titers if exposure
- *X-ray of joint*: Usually normal early. Widened joint space, subluxation or dislocation is possible; erosive changes occur after 10–14 days.
- *Bone scan*: Hot spots
- MRI of joint if diagnosis is in doubt or there is osteomyelitis
- Ultrasound or fluoroscopic-guided joint aspirate
- Synovial fluid microscopy and culture (not always positive). PCR may be helpful. The hip should have open drainage to avoid avascular necrosis.
- Joint fluid analysis is most important and should not be delayed for imaging studies.
- Lumbar puncture if there is a septic joint with *Haemophilus influenzae* (increased incidence of meningitis)

Treatment

- *Medical*: Intravenous (IV) antibiotics AFTER aspirate is taken, for up to 3 weeks (until CRP normalizes); followed by oral antibiotics for a total of 4–6 weeks. Outcome of treatment is time dependent.
- *Surgical*: Early referral to orthopedic team, as there is a low threshold for irrigation and debridement of the affected joint (and drainage of any associated osteomyelitis), especially the hip
- *Physiotherapy* to avoid joint stiffness
- Immobilization is seldom needed and should be brief.

Prognosis

Prognosis is usually good unless the diagnosis is delayed. Recurrence of disease and development of chronic infection occur in <10% of cases. Long-term follow-up is needed, as growth-related sequelae may not become apparent for months or years. Hip joint infection has the worst prognosis for anatomical and functional impairment.

Complications

Chondrolysis, ongoing infection and bone destruction, joint incongruity and stiffness, and growth disturbance are some of the complications. Avascular necrosis of the hip can be encountered.

Infection: osteomyelitis

The frequency of osteomyelitis is greatest in infants, with 33% of all cases occurring in the first 2 years, and 50% occurring by 5 years. M/F = 2:1.

Pathogenesis

Infection is usually seen in the metaphyseal region of bones. Most infections spread via the hematogenous route from a primary site of entry (e.g., respiratory, gastrointestinal [GI], ENT, or skin sites). Infection may also occur by direct inoculation (open fractures, penetrating wounds) or local extension from adjacent sites.

In the infant, transphyseal vessels are patent; therefore, infection may spread to the adjacent joint, causing a septic arthritis.

In adolescents infection tends to spread through the medullary canal.

Types of osteomyelitis

- Acute
- Subacute (2–3 weeks duration)
- Chronic: may develop "equestrum" and "involucrum"
- Bone abscesses may become surrounded by thick, fibrous tissue and sclerotic bone (Brodie's abscess).

Etiology

The yield for bacterial growth from synovial fluid and bone aspirate is small, thus organisms are not always isolated. *Staphylococcus aureus* is most common in children in all age groups. Other organisms seen:

- Neonates: Group B streptococcus and gram-negative enteric bacilli
- <2 years: *Haemophilus influenzae* (rare)
- >2 years: Gram-positive cocci, *Pseudomonas aeruginosa*
- Adolescents: *Neisseria gonorrhoeae*

Consider salmonella in sickle cell disease. Tuberculosis is rare.

Symptoms and signs

Neonates characteristically do not appear ill and may not have fever.
Older children have pain, limping, refusal to walk or weight bear, fever, malaise, and flu-like symptoms.

Overlying bone may be tender (+ warm), with ± swelling. Long bones are principally affected: tibia > femur > humerus.

Differential diagnosis

This includes acute leukemia, neuroblastoma, and neoplasm (e.g., osteoid osteoma, osteosarcoma, Ewing sarcoma).

Investigations

- *Blood:* CBC, ESR, CRP, blood cultures (positive in 50%).
- *X-ray of bone:* Early stages may be normal, soft-tissue edema may be visible. Late stages reveal metaphyseal rarefaction or lytic lesions. Destructive changes in bone appear after 10 days.
- *Ultrasound* or fluoroscopic-guided aspiration for microscopy and culture
- *MRI:* Soft-tissue assessment: bone marrow involvement; abscess formation, joint effusion, subperiosteal extension
- *Bone scans* are good for acute osteomyelitis; they can identify up to 90% of joint involvement (seen as hot spots) and may differentiate joint from bone involvement. They are also good for assessing infections of the pelvis, proximal femur, and spine.
- Consider *immunologic evaluation* if atypical organism

Treatment

- *Medical:* IV antibiotics for a minimum of 2 weeks, followed by oral antibiotics for 4 weeks. Consultation with infectious disease specialist is recommended.
- *Surgical:* Drainage and debridement if there is frank pus on aspiration or a sequestered abscess or collection (not accessible to antibiotics)

Prognosis

Prognosis is usually excellent if treated early. Disease recurrence or progression to chronic infection occurs in <10% of cases.

Complications

- *Systemic:* May include septicemia
- *Local:* Pathological fracture, sequestration, growth disturbance

Spinal disorders

General management

- *History*: Pain, onset of deformity, family history, disability, other disorders

Examination

- *Inspection*: Asymmetry, scapular prominence, skin lesions (especially midline), café-au-lait spots (associated with neurofibromatosis), foot deformity, leg atrophy
- *Feel* for spinal tenderness.
- *Move*: Forward flexion, hamstring tightness
- *General*: Neurological examination
- *Investigations*: Radiographs, CT, MRI, bone scan

General spinal disorders

Back pain

Take it seriously! This is more likely to be caused by significant pathology than in an adult (e.g., osteoid osteoma, eosinophilic granuloma). Concerning findings, especially in young children, include several weeks of symptoms, night pain, increasing symptoms, neurological abnormality, and recent onset of scoliosis. Fevers and night sweats suggest underlying infection or malignancy. Pain may be referred to the spine from an intra-thoracic or intra-abdominal process. Investigate back pain thoroughly.

Discitis

This is inflammation (probably infection) of the disc space.

- *Age group*: Any age (infants and children rather than adolescents)
- *Symptoms*: Fever, irritability, unwilling to walk, back pain, symptoms may be vague or referred to hips or abdomen
- *Investigations*: Blood: ↑ CRP and ESR; MRI; bone scan
- *Treatment*: Antibiotics (based on local sensitivities), at least until inflammatory markers return to normal. An occasional brace or immobilization may also be needed.
- *Outcome*: These patients usually do well.

Congenital anomalies

Diastematomyelia: The spinal cord is split by a central cartilaginous or bony prominence.

- *Signs*: Other abnormalities are common (e.g., scoliosis, clubfoot, cavus foot); cutaneous lesions are seen in most children, positive neurology is seen in 50%.
- *Management*: Consider resection of the spur if neurology appears or is progressive.

Regional spinal disorders

Cervical spine
Torticollis (see p. 1019)

Thoracic spine
See Scheuermann's disease (p. 863)

Lumbar spine: spondylolysis and spondylolisthesis
These conditions constitute a defect of pars interarticularis (spondylolysis) resulting in anterior displacement of one vertebra upon another (spondylolisthesis). They are usually due a stress fracture through the congenitally dysplastic pars.
- *Incidence*: Uncommon, associated with spina bifida, metabolic disorder (e.g., osteopetrosis), connective-tissue disorder (e.g., Marfan syndrome), hyperextension sports (e.g., gymnastics)
- *Symptoms and signs*: Sudden and insidious onset of pain, tenderness, decreased forward flexion and straight-leg raise, pain on hyperextension.
- *Investigations*: X-rays with lateral and oblique spinal views: "Scotty dog" sign (see p. 883)—use oblique X-ray to delineate
- *Management*: Usually nonoperative. Rest and change of activities, consider short-term bracing, analgesia. Operative intervention is seldom required for stabilization.

Sacral spine: sacral agenesis
This is hypoplastic or absent sacrum, occurring most commonly in infants of diabetic mothers.
- *Signs*: Abnormal pelvic ring affecting lower limbs with associated neurology
- *Management*: Tailor according to severity of agenesis and neurology

Spine: kyphosis

Kyphosis is increased curvature of the spine in the sagittal plane, visible from the side. Normally there is a 20°–40° curvature of the thoracic spine.

- *History*: Site, age of onset, rate of progression, associated scoliosis, pain, neurological symptoms; family history

Examination

Assess
- *Flexibility*: Have patient stand, bend forward, and bend backward (hyperextension).
- Ability to lie flat is associated with lumbar lordosis (more prominent with greater severity of kyphosis).
- Hips for tight hamstrings: Limited straight-leg raising
- Full respiratory (pulmonary function) and neurological examination

Investigation
- PA and lateral standing X-rays of entire spine

Diagnosis

Three major causes are identified by answers to the following questions:
- Is it flexible?
- Is it painful?
- When did it start?

Postural kyphosis

This is the most common form, being usually painless in a patient with flexibility. Onset is at <10 years of age.
- *Other findings*: Affects tall girls more than boys; poor physical development
- *Investigations*: Supine hyperextension lateral radiograph confirms complete correction.
- *Treatment*: Physiotherapy to improve posture and provide exercises for dorsal spine
- *Outcome*: Corrects spontaneously by end of adolescence

Congenital kyphosis

This is a rigid form with occasional pain. Onset is at <10 years of age.
- *Other findings*: Severe deformities are recognized at birth, associated with congenital spinal abnormality, e.g., spina bifida, tethered cord.
- *Cause*: May be secondary to failure of vertebral formation and/or segmentation during the first trimester
- *Treatment*: Brace or fusion to prevent paraplegia
- *Outcome*: Can progress rapidly and lead to paraplegia

Adolescent or Scheuermann's disease

This disorder consists rigid kyphosis with aching pain. Onset is at age 12–15 years (previously normal spine). Incidence is unknown; it occurs in up to 7%–8% of the population in cadavaric studies.

Other findings

Type 1

Type affects boys more than girls. Initially patients have a painless rounded back; later they have aching pain around the apex (usually eighth thoracic vertebra) with corresponding "flattening" of the chest and compensatory lumbar lordosis, ± scoliosis. There is normal neurology.

Type 2

Type 2 is less common, affecting boys closer to maturity; 25% of cases have associated family history. Pain is often associated with strenuous activity, standing (may initially be alleviated by lying down), and progressively more rigid thoracolumbar or lumbar kyphosis. Percussion over interspinous ligaments and spinous processes produces pain. Hamstrings are tight. Rarely, neurological signs secondary to disc herniation or extradural spinal cysts may develop.

Investigations

These include AP and lateral spine X-rays: >45° kyphosis with >5° anterior wedging at three sequential vertebrae = radiographic definition of Scheuermann's disease. The patient may have vertebral body end-plate changes (Schmorl's nodes: vertical herniations of the intervertebral discs into the vertebral end plate), spondylolysis (30%–50%), or scoliosis (33%).

Treatment

- *Physiotherapy* (hyperextension program): Bracing may be considered.
- *Medical:* NSAIDs
- *Surgical* correction if there is severe kyphosis (>70°), the patient is skeletally mature, or the condition is painful.

Outcome

There is little evidence that patients with kyphosis <70° experience late progression, disabling pain, or neurological compromise.

Spine: scoliosis

Idiopathic scoliosis

Lateral curvature (usually >10°) and/or rotation deformity of the spine occur without an identifiable cause. Description of the curvature is based on direction of apical convexity. There are three types, based on age.

Infantile

Patients are under 3 years old, with more males than females affected. The left side is affected more than the right. Associated plagiocephaly (skull flattening), hip dysplasia and other congenital defects are seen. The condition may be secondary to underlying spinal abnormality.

Juvenile

The scoliosis affects 3- to 10-year-olds and may be secondary to underlying spinal abnormality. There is a high risk of curve progression (70% of patients require treatment, with 50% needing a brace and 50%, surgery).

Adolescent

The adolescent form is most common in 11- to 16-year-olds and affects more females than males.

Incidence

- Curves >10°: 2% incidence.
- Curves >30°: 0.2% incidence
- Right thoracic curves > double major (right thoracic and left lumbar) > left lumbar > right lumbar

Risk factors

A positive family history is associated; daughters of affected mothers are more likely to be affected.

Disease progression

Three-quarters of children with curves of 20°–30° will progress at least 5°. Risk factors for curve progression are age <12 years, skeletal immaturity, females > males, and curve magnitude >20°. The spine is at greatest risk of curve progression during puberty. Severe curves (Cobb angle >100°) are associated with pulmonary dysfunction, early mortality, pain, and poor self-image

Symptoms

The scoliosis is recognized with onset of symptoms and rate of progression. The main question to ask is: IS IT PAINFUL? Ask about respiratory and neurological symptoms.

Signs

- Inspect child standing.
- Describe scoliosis as the side to which the spine is convex (shoulder on the convex side is elevated).
- Inspect pelvic height for limb length difference; waistline asymmetry, trunk shift, spinal deformity, rib rotational deformity (rib hump).
- Have the patient bend to touch their toes: IS IT FIXED?

- *Adam's forward test* for assessing asymmetry of the posterior chest wall on forward bending. If scoliosis disappears it is postural (80% of scoliosis).
- Full neurological examination to exclude spinal cord disorder
- Look for presacral dimple, hair patch, and pigmentation.
- Lower limb examination (other causes of postural scoliosis: unilateral muscle spasm, unequal leg length)

True idiopathic scoliosis

This form is painless, convex to the right in the thoracic spine, and not associated with any neurological changes.

Investigations
- Standing PA and lateral X-rays of full spine
- MRI if there is pain, neurological changes, rapidly progressive curve, excessive kyphosis, or left thoracic/thoracolumbar curves, or if considering surgery

Treatment
Treatment is based on maturity of patient, magnitude of deformity, and curve progression. The aim is to prevent further progression.

Nonoperative
- Close observation (6-monthly X-rays for curves <25°)
- Bracing is controversial, although it may slow or halt curve progression. The more the brace is worn, the more effective it is; consider for children with curves <40°.

Operative
- AP spinal fusion with instrumentation for severe deformities (>45°)

Congenital scoliosis

This is the most common congenital spinal disorder.

Etiology
There is abnormal vertebral development in the first trimester.

Associations
The scoliosis is an Isolated deformity or is associated with other congenital abnormalities: spinal (40%) > genitourinary (20%) > heart disease (10%–15%), and intraspinal pathology. It is also associated with syndromes e.g., VACTERL syndrome (p. 984).

Disease progression
Risk of progression depends on morphology and growth potential of the vertebrae. The greatest risk is during periods of rapid growth (<2 years and >10 years old).

Treatment
Early diagnosis is important, with patients often needing surgery.

Secondary to neuromuscular disorders

Symptoms and signs

These progress more rapidly and may continue after maturity. There are longer curves involving more vertebrae, with compensatory curves less likely to occur.

Associations

- *Skeletal*: Pelvic obliquity, bony deformities, cervical involvement
- *Pulmonary*: More frequent, ↓ lung function, pneumonia
- *Neurological*: Brain stem, proprioception, Klippel–Feil syndrome
- *Upper motor neuron disease*: Spinocerebellar degeneration, syringomyelia, spinal cord tumor or trauma, tethered cord, diastematomyelia
- *Lower motor neuron*: Poliomyelitis, spinal muscular atrophy, (myopathic: Duchenne muscular dystrophy)
- *Syndromes*: Neurofibromatosis, Marfan syndrome

Hip disorders: developmental dysplasia of the hip (DDH)

DDH was previously known as congenital dislocation of the hip. A disorder of hip joint development results in hip instability, subluxation, or dislocation ± acetabular dysplasia.

- *Incidence:* 2:1000 (but up to 20:1000 newborn hips are unstable; 90% of cases stabilize by 6 weeks)
- *Risk factors:* Family history (1:5), F>M (5:1), L>R (1.5:1), racial predilection
- *Etiology:* Capsular laxity (increased type III collagen, maternal estrogens), decreased intrauterine volume (breech position, first born, oligohydramnios)
- *Associations* include other "packaging" disorders: Torticollis (20%), metatarsus adductus (10%), talipes calcaneovalgus, teratologic dislocation
- *Teratologic dislocation:* A distinct form of hip dislocation associated with neuromuscular syndromes (e.g., myelodysplasia, arthrogryposis, chromosomal abnormalities, myelomeningocele, lumbosacral agenesis, diastrophic dwarfism). The hip is dislocated before birth and is more difficult to treat.

Disease progression

Capsular laxity + shallow acetabulum → instability, subluxation, or dislocation → muscle contracture → progressive acetabular dysplasia with fibrofatty filling (pulvinar); the femoral head becomes hypoplastic.

History

Usually there is an uneventful pregnancy. Parents may notice limited abduction, delayed walking, or a painless limp in the child, who is prone to falls. DDH may be an incidental finding.

Examination

All newborn infants should be screened for DDH by physical examination before discharge and then at well-baby visits. Ultrasound screening for high-risk infants should be done.

Neonate

1. Is the hip dislocated (i.e., <u>out</u>)? If so, is it reducible?
Ortolani's test: Gently elevate (anteriorly) and abduct the dislocated hip to reduce it (you'll discern a subtle, palpable clunk)
2. If the hip is not dislocated, can I dislocate it (i.e., is it dislocatable)?
Barlow's test: Gently adduct and depress (posteriorly) the femur; a vulnerable hip dislocates.

These two provocation maneuvers become unreliable after 6–8 weeks.

Infant

An infant will have asymmetric gluteal folds, limited abduction, and leg length discrepancy.

- *Galeazzi sign*: Flex knees with feet together. A positive sign = affected femur appears short due to a dislocated hip joint (*Note*: it is also positive if the femur is congenitally short, and negative with bilateral DDH).

Older child

On walking you may see a limp and positive Trendelenburg test. With bilateral dislocations, the only signs may be an exaggerated lumbar lordosis and limited hip abduction.

Investigations

- *Age <6 months*: Hip ultrasound (before ossification, operator dependent)
- *Age >6 months*: AP pelvis radiograph. A shallow acetabulum with increased acetabular index, and a hypoplastic femoral head in super-olateral position are demonstrated.

Treatment

This depends on the age of the child (see Table 20.3). An urgent referral to a pediatric orthopedic surgeon is needed to start treatment as soon as possible. The aim is to achieve and maintain concentric hip reduction to encourage early acetabular development, thus reducing the risk of future degenerative joint disease.

Table 20.3 Treatment of DDH at different ages

Age of child	Treatment
<6 months	Pavlik harness (maintain hip in flexed position with some hip abduction)
6–18 months	Manipulation and closed reduction (+/ adductor tenotomy) + hip spica plaster cast
	Open reduction (medial approach if <12 months old, anter-olateral approach if >12 months old) + hip spica
18–24 months	Trial of closed reduction
	Open reduction (anterolateral approach) +/ pelvic osteotomy + hip spica plaster cast
2–6 years	Open reduction (anterolateral approach) +/ femoral shortening +/ pelvic osteotomy + hip spica plaster cast

Complications

- *Early*: Inadequate reduction and redislocation
- *Intermediate*: Residual acetabular dysplasia, avascular necrosis
- *Late*: Early osteoarthritic changes

Prognosis

Any residual acetabular dysplasia is more likely to lead to early degenerative changes in the hip.

Perthes disease

Perthes disease is also known as Legg–Calve–Perthes disease. It is due to an idiopathic osteonecrosis (avascular necrosis) of the femoral head of unknown etiology. Incidence is 1:10,000.

Risk factors

Boys are affected more than girls (4:1), at age 4–10 years. Less than 20% of cases are bilateral (usually staged + asymmetric), and 10% have a family history. Low birth weight is a factor, as is delayed skeletal maturity; 4% of children with transient synovitis are at risk.

Etiology

The etiology is unknown, although several risk factors lead to avascular necrosis: trauma, endocrine (e.g., hypothyroidism, renal disease, steroids) and metabolic factors, and hypercoagulability (blood dyscrasia, protein C or S deficiency, thrombophilia).

Differential diagnosis
- Multiple epiphyseal dysplasia
- Spondyloepiphyseal dysplasia
- Hypofibrinolysis
- Septic arthritis
- TB of the hip
- Trauma
- Sickle cell disease
- Hypothryoidism

Pathological stages
Ischemia and necrosis stage
Cessation of epiphyseal growth occurs over the first 6–12 months. X-ray findings include smaller femoral head with medial joint space widening (presence of effusion). Fragmentation with resorption results in the femoral head appearing partly cystic and partly sclerotic.

Re-ossification stage
This occurs 12–18 months after clinical onset.

Healed or residual stage
This is usually within 24 months of onset, and results in residual deformity or healed bone with remodeling.

Symptoms
Symptoms are mild to intermittent anterior thigh, groin, or referred knee pain with limp; there is also a classical "painless limp". With knee pain, watch for hip pathology.

Special signs

- *Look*: Proximal thigh atrophy, mild short stature, limp or Trendelenburg or antalgic gait is common
- *Feel*: Effusion (from synovitis), groin or thigh tenderness
- *Move*: Decreased hip range of movement (especially abduction and internal rotation) with muscle spasm
- Radiology
- Catterall's "head at risk" sign and Herring's lateral pillar classification, Gage's sign, lateral subluxation of femoral head with lateral calcification, whole head involvement, metaphyseal cysts

Investigations

- AP and lateral pelvic X-rays. There are several different classification systems based on the amount of femoral head involved (Catterall and Herring).
- MRI may help diagnosis, especially in the early stages.
- Technetium 99 bone scan: Decreased uptake in femoral epiphysis due to poor vascular supply
- Dynamic arthrography to delineate hip joint and plan surgery

Prognosis

This is a local self-healing disorder. Prognosis depends on bone age and X-ray appearance during the initial phase. A poor prognosis is associated with bone age >6 years old and with female gender.

Treatment is controversial

The aims are to relieve symptoms and signs by eliminating hip irritability and maintaining hip range of movements. These iare achieved by

- *Maintaining* sphericity of femoral head
- *Containing* femoral head in acetabtulum while remodeling occurs
- *Preventing* epiphyseal collapse and secondary osteoarthritis

Nonoperative treatment

This includes observation and activity modification, as well as NSAIDs and physiotherapy. Bracing is controversial.

Operative treatment

Femoral or pelvic osteotomy can be performed to contain the femoral head in acetabulum.

Slipped femoral capital epiphysis

SFCE is displacement of the upper femoral epiphysis on the metaphysis through the hypertrophic zone of the growth plate. The femoral neck displaces anteriorly and the head remains in the acetabulum. This is the most common adolescent hip disorder (3:100,000); 25%–60% of cases are bilateral.

Risk factors include African-American descent, >50% obese (weight >95th percentile), positive family history, and puberty. Boys (12–16 years) are affected more than girls (10–14 years).

Etiology is unknown, but SFCE is associated with the following factors:

- *Endocrine*: Hypothyroidism, hypogonadism, renal osteodystrophy
- *Mechanical*: Retroversion of femoral neck or vertical growth plate
- *Other*: Down syndrome, radiotherapy and chemotherapy

Symptoms and signs

There is groin, thigh, or knee pain, as well as antalgic gait, limited hip flexion and abduction, flexion into external rotation, and thigh atrophy. Passive hip flexion causes obligatory external rotation.

Always consider hip pathology in a child presenting with knee pain.

Presentation

SFCE is characterized by occurrence in two broad types of children:

- *Obese hypogonadal* (low circulating sex hormones): Delayed skeletal maturation
- Tall, thin children, often boys, after the growth spurt (younger age in girls). There is an overabundance of growth hormones.

Diagnostic classification

This is based on the duration of symptoms:

- *Preslip*: Wide epiphysis; mild discomfort but normal examination; often seen on contralateral hip
- *Acute slip*: Mild symptoms <3 weeks, then sudden slippage, usually without trauma. The pain is so severe that the child is unable to weight bear and is usually unstable.
- *Acute on chronic*: Acute slip on preexisting chronic slip. Usually children have previous symptoms (pain, limp, out toe gait) for several months, and are unable to weight bear and are usually unstable.
- *Chronic*: Most common type, with history for several months. Symptoms worsen as slip progresses (usually there are not severe symptoms because of continuity between femoral neck and epiphysis). The child is able to walk with mildly antalgic, externally rotated gait, and is usually stable.
- *"Unstable slip" (Loder)*: The child is unable to weight bear and cannot straight-leg raise actively.

Investigations

These include X-rays; MRI may detect early slip and avascular necrosis. X-rays of the hips are in AP pelvis and frog lateral positions. Perform endocrine tests if appropriate.

Treatment

The aim is to prevent further slippage and to minimize complications.

Operative

Usually a pin in situ (to encourage the proximal femoral physis to close, hence preventing further slippage) is placed; usually reduction is not used, as manipulation may increase the incidence of avascular necrosis. Prophylactic pinning of the opposite hip is controversial. It is recommended in younger children and those with endocrinopathy.

Complications

- *Chondrolysis* (degeneration of the articular cartilage of the hip with narrowed joint space, pain, and decreased motion) is associated with more severe slips, occurs more frequently among African-American children and females, and is associated with pins protruding out of the femoral head.
- *Osteonecrosis/avascular necrosis* (higher incidence in unstable hips) is due to injury to retinacular vessels (at the time of slip or manipulation) or compression from intracapsular hematoma. Commonly this leads to degenerative joint disease. Avascular necrosis is uncommon in stable disease.

Knee disorders

Anterior knee pain

This type of pain is common in the growing child and is usually due to overuse. Pain is worse with load-bearing, going downstairs, and prolonged sitting with the knee flexed.

Common causes are detailed below.

Osteochondroses: Osgood–Schlatter disease

See p. 881.

Sinding–Larsen–Johannnsson disease

See p. 881.

Patella maltracking

Several causes include dysplasia of the femoral condyles, malalignment of the quadriceps mechanism with relatively weak vastus medialis, genu valgum, tibial torsion, and increased laxity. The disorder presents with vague anterior knee pain, instability, and/or episodes of patella dislocation. Treatment is physiotherapy, but some patients may need surgery.

Chondromalacia patellae

This is a pathological defect of the articular cartilage, which may progress to osteoarthritis (X-rays may be normal).

Bipartite patellae

This disorder is usually bilateral and a normal variant of ossification. There is a risk of developing an avulsion fracture, thus the child should rest, and stop sports, and the knee should be splinted. NSAIDs may help. Once resolved, a gradual return to activities is possible.

Genu recurvatum

Congenital hyperextension

This disorder is most common in breech presentations. It is associated with arthrogryposis, spina bifida, DDH, and talipes equinovarus. Severity varies from mild hyperextension to dislocation.

For management look for other abnormalities. Treatment involves gentle stretching, serial casting, and quadriceps lengthening at 1–3 months if necessary.

Acquired recurvatum

This is physiological "curved" knee occurring in girls, due to joint laxity. The condition may be familial and predispose to sprains or patella instability. Consider neurological causes if it is not bilateral. Clinical features include a hyperextended knee and generalized lax joints. It may be caused by trauma to the proximal anterior tibial physis, bringing about a progressive deformity with growth.

Genu valgum (knock knees)

Genu valgum is defined by position of knees such that when standing with knees together the medial malleoli are not touching (thus it is a frontal-plane deformity). It is commonly observed between ages 2 and 7 years.

Causes

Bilateral

- A physiological cause is most common.
- Metabolic: Renal osteodystrophy, rickets, hypophosphatemia
- Skeletal dysplasia: Kniest's syndrome, congenital dislocation of patella, mucopolysaccharidoses (MPS)
- Neuromuscular: Cerebral palsy
- Hematological: Myelodysplasia

Unilateral

Asymmetric growth is from trauma to, infection of, or tumor in, the tibia.

Presentation

The child walks knock-kneed. Establish rate of progression, diet, and family history.

Examination

General

Measure height and body proportions. The child may be overweight or have dysmorphic features. Conduct a full lower-limb examination (standing and lying), look for flat feet (pes planus), and measure knee angle and intermalleolar distance.

Specific signs

Assess the tibiofemoral angle. The angle at which the long axis of tibia bisects the long axis of femur can be measured clinically and radiologically. A widened intermalleolar distance (distance between medial malleoli of ankles) will be found.

Investigations

No X-rays are required until >18 months age, then AP and lateral, standing full-leg length views should be obtained.

Treatment

- *Nonoperative* treatment is the mainstay for physiological genu valgum.
- *Operative*: Epiphysiodesis (physeal stapling) of the medial side or corrective osteotomy in children >10 years old with an intermalleolar distance >10 cm or >15°–20° valgus

Prognosis

In children, 95% of physiological valgus resolves with growth; normal adult alignment is achieved by age 7–8 years.

Genu varum (bowed knees)

Genu varum is bowing of the knees if the patient stands with ankles together. Normally, genu varum (15°) at birth progresses to physiological genu valgum by 4–5 years. Genu varum is common in children <3 years of age (especially obese children who start walking at <1 years old).

Causes

- *Physiological*: In utero (curled up) fetal position results in a bowed appearance due to
  - A tight posterior hip capsule, which causes external rotation of the hips
  - Internal tibial torsion
- *Structural*: Osteogenesis imperfecta
- *Metabolic*: Vitamin D deficiency (nutritional rickets) or resistant rickets, hypophosphatemia
- *Skeletal dysplasia*: Metaphyseal dysplasia, achondroplasia, enchondromatosis
- *Local asymmetric growth*: Blount's disease (abnormal growth of medial aspect of proximal tibial epiphysis), osteochondromas, physeal injury (e.g., trauma, infection), dysplasia

History

Parents will notice that the child is walking bowlegged or with in-toeing of the feet. Establish developmental milestones and rate of progression, family history, diet, social history, etc.

Examination

General examination consists of height and weight, and full lower-limb examination including rotational profile and widened intercondylar distance (distance between medial femoral condyles).

Investigations

On weight-bearing AP and lateral lower-leg views look for symmetrical physiological bowing, and flaring of the tibia and femur. You can also measure the tibiofemoral angle and metaphyseal–diaphyseal angles.

Treatment

No treatment is required if the cause is physiological. Braces and splints are ineffective. Refer patient to an orthopedic pediatric surgeon.

Prognosis

95% of physiological varus cases resolve with age.

Osteochondritis dissecans of the knee

This disorder occurs when an area of subchondral bone becomes avascular, fragmenting and separating from the underlying bone. This may involve the overlying cartilage, leading to mechanical problems (e.g., loose bodies) and joint incongruity. Most commonly it involves the lateral aspect of the medial femoral condyle. It may progress to early degenerative osteoarthritis.

Risk factors

Adolescents (10–15 years) and boys more than girls are affected. This disorder is often secondary to trauma, ischemia, and abnormal epiphyseal ossification.

Clinical features

Features include nonspecific knee pain, and/or locking an/or stiffness. There is knee swelling after activities but no history of acute trauma or injury. You may be able to palpate the affected articular cartilage of medial femoral condyle if the knee is fully flexed.

Disease progression

The overlying articular cartilage is usually intact in younger children and the bone heals as revascularization occurs. The risk of articular fracture with separation and loose body formation increases with increasing age (closed physes), larger lesions, and a weight-bearing location.

Investigations

Obtain X-rays of the knee in AP, lateral, and notch views to assess femoral condyles. MRI may be useful for determining the integrity of articular cartilage and defining whether synovial fluid is behind the lesion.

Treatment

Treatment depends on the patient's age, and size and stability of the fragment. Usually a short treatment with rest, anti-inflammatory drugs, and splinting will suffice; however, some patients may require surgery.

- *Nonoperative* treatment is as above, along with observation with periodic X-rays and MRIs to assess the degree of healing. Bracing and restriction of weight-bearing and activities are controversial.
- *Operative* treatment is indicated in an adolescent with minimal growth left or when there is a loose lesion: (arthroscopic) drilling with multiple holes to promote revascularization and healing. Fixation of large fragments and microfracture can also be done.

Prognosis

There is worse outcome with large lesions in lateral femoral condyle in older children.

Note: Osteochondritis dessicans may occur in other major joints, including the elbow (capitellum) and, less often, the lateral condyle of the patella.

Orthopedic trauma

Trauma is the most common cause of childhood deaths. While most fractures occur in the home environment (others: sports > school), these are usually single-bone injuries. Motor vehicle accidents (MVA) (car > bike > pedestrian) are the leading cause of death. Nonaccidental trauma (NAT) should be considered (see p. 1134).

Fractures

Generally, boys suffer more fractures than girls, with a peak incidence at 12 years of age (although specific injuries peak at different ages—e.g., NAT = 1 year, femoral fractures = 3 years, pedestrian versus car = 6 years, lateral condyle and supracondylar fractures = 7 years, physeal injury = 11–12 years). 4% of fractures are multiple fractures. Children's fractures usually occur in summer more than winter.

Principles of management
- Stabilize according to resuscitation principles (see p. 54).
- Full history (including nature of injury, left- or right-handedness) and examination.
- Is the fracture open or closed?
- Is the limb neurovascularly intact? Is there a compartment syndrome?
- Is the associated joint dislocated?
- Splint limb for comfort, give analgesia, and elevate limb.
- X-ray the affected bone ± the joint above and below.
- Liaise with the orthopedic team.

Complications
Early
- *Neurovascular problems*: E.g., median nerve paraesthesia with distal radius fractures, median/ulnar nerve paraesthesia with supracondylar fractures, radial nerve in humeral shaft fractures, common peroneal nerve with proximal fibula fractures
- *Compartment syndrome* is especially associated with closed, low-energy mid-shaft tibia fractures.

Intermediate
- *Joint stiffness* occurs especially with fractures around the elbow.
- *Malunion* is usually well tolerated if it is within the plane of motion; it may be compensated in younger children with remodeling.

Late
- *Overgrowth*: Overcompensation of growth in long bones is due to physeal stimulation (from hyperemia). Femoral fractures in children may overgrow by 1–3 cm.
- *Deformity*: If the epiphysis is damaged, the child may develop progressive deformity several months later.
- *Nonunion* occurs rarely, in the shaft of the tibia or ulna.

Common fracture patterns

The most common fracture pattern is a complete fracture of both cortices (e.g., spiral, transverse, oblique, multi-fragmentary). However, the following fractures are specific to children.

Buckle or Torus fractures

These occur in children <10 years of age and are usually caused by a fall on an outstretched hand (causing compression of one cortex, resulting in "buckle" on the X-ray). This results in a metaphyseal distal radius fracture. It is inherently stable.

- *Treatment*: Immobilize limp in a splint, plaster of Paris, or backslab.
  Fracture clinic follow-up should occur within 2–3 days. Remove plaster in 3–4 weeks and mobilize.

Plastic deformation or bend fractures

These result from traumatic bending or bowing of bone, but with insufficient energy to produce a fracture. No fracture is seen on X-ray (the limb may appear "bent"). Commonly the ulna is involved (watch for radial head dislocation), occasionally the fibula. Treat as for torus fracture.

Greenstick fractures

Like bending a young twig, the cortex will break on the tension side and bend on the compression side. The energy is insufficient to result in a complete bicortical fracture. It may require manipulation under anaesthesia.

Salter–Harris fractures (physeal injuries)

Some 20% of all children's fractures involve the physis (most commonly, the distal radius). It is usually extra-articular, but fractures in the proximal femur or humerus, radial neck, and distal fibula may be intra-articular.

Some fractures may indicate nonaccidental pathology (e.g., spinal, scapular, or rib fractures or femoral shaft fracture in the nonambulant child). These children should be referred for full investigation.

Osteochondroses

These make up a spectrum of conditions that affect primarily the epiphyses but may also involve cartilage and bone. Despite the term *osteochondritis*, the condition is not always due to inflammation and may be due to trauma, overuse, or vascular irregularities or may be a normal variation. The affected devascularized bony region undergoes spontaneous healing with revascularization, resorption, and reossification. Symptoms are worse with activity and relieved with rest. It is usually a self-limiting condition, with clinical outcomes ranging from normal to serious disability. Investigations include radiographs of the affected region, which may demonstrate fragmentation or collapsed sclerotic bone. An MRI scan will confirm the diagnosis. The conditions can be classified anatomically.

Physeal (growth plate) osteochondroses

These disorders often require treatment.

Madelung deformity

The defect occurs in the volar and ulna side of the distal radial physis, resulting in a shortened tilted distal radius and a prominent ulna. It occurs in teenage girls. Features include pain, decreased range of movement, and abnormal wrist joint. It is treated with analgesia and surgery. Consider dyschondrosteosis (autosomal dominant, bilateral).

Scheuermann disease

This disorder affects the vertebra; see Spine: kyphosis (p. 863).

Blount disease

This disorder affects the tibial physis. There is progressive bowleg, unilaterally or bilaterally. Obesity and African-American descent are risk factors, and there are juvenile and adolescent forms. Bracing in early childhood may be effective. Surgery is usually required.

Articular osteochondroses

These disorders have a great potential for disability.

Freiberg disease

This disorder consists of infarction of the second metatarsal head or epiphysis in teenagers (females > males), presenting with pain on running and dancing. There is joint tenderness with decreased range of movement, and pain on tiptoe standing. The disease is managed with change of activities, analgesia, intra-articular corticosteroids, and/or surgery.

Perthes disease

See p. 870.

Panner's disease

Osteonecrosis of the capitellum may be due to overloading of the elbow (e.g., overhand throwing, batting by children 10 years of age) with accentuation of any valgus deformity. Clinical findings include mechanical block ± flexion contracture, and general lateral elbow pain and swelling. An AP X-ray with the elbow flexed 45° may demonstrate irregular joint surface.

Treatment includes rest with avoidance of exacerbating factors, anti-inflammatory agents, and arthroscopic removal of loose bodies.

Radial head

This disorder is similar to Panner's except the radial head is affected. The child is prone to developing overgrowth and joint incongruity.

Nonarticular osteochondroses

At tendon attachments

Osgood–Schlatter disease

Failure of the tibia tubercle apophysis is due to repetitive traction stress from the extensor mechanism in boys (aged 12–14 years), more than in girls (aged 10–12 years). This is usually a self-limiting condition with complete resolution through physiologic healing (physeal closure) of tibia tubercle within 12–24 months. It presents with painful swelling over a prominent tibial tubercle (usually unilateral), associated with running and jumping. An irregular fragmented tibial tubercle may be seen on X-ray.

Treatment includes nonoperative (activity modification, rest ± ice ± knee brace), physiotherapy (isometric hamstring and quadriceps exercises), medication (NSAIDs), and operative (occasionally, excision of separate ossicles may improve symptoms after skeletal maturity).

Sinding–Larsen–Johansson syndrome

This is a related condition arising at the distal end of the patella.

At ligament attachments

Adam's disease (medial epicondyle)

This is a repetitive injury to the elbow following throwing or serving in sports (e.g., racquet sports). It results in medial epicondylar fragmentation or avulsion and delayed closure of the growth plate. It may have ulnar nerve involvement and point tenderness over the medial epicondyle. It is treated with rest and change of activities, splinting, analgesia (NSAIDs), and gradual return to activities once the symptoms have settled. Some patients may need surgery to excise loose bodies.

At impact sites

Kohler's disease

Infarction of the navicular bone presents as medial mid-foot pain and a limp in young children (males > females), especially with load-bearing sports. It is treated with rest from load-bearing sports, in soles or casts. If symptoms are severe, the child may need to be non-weight bearing, with gradual return to activities depending on the symptoms.

Sever's disease

This involves microfracture (with subsequent inflammation and healing) of the fibrocartilaginous insertion of the tendo-achilles to the calcaneum during the pubertal growth spurt. Symptoms vary according to the level of activity and improve with skeletal maturation. There may be a bony prominence at the tendon insertion due to overgrowth during the healing response. Treatment is with symptomatic NSAIDs, and heel cord stretching.

Osteogenesis imperfecta

This is an inherited condition affecting collagen maturation and organization (see also p. 883). Incidence is ~1 in 20,000. Osteogenesis imperfecta (OI) is due to mutation in type I collagen gene that predisposes to fracture formation. Following a fracture, initial bone healing is normal, but there is no subsequent remodeling and the bone heals with deformity.

Clinical features

There are seven clinical subtypes; 10% are clinically asymptomatic. Signs are common in all subtypes:

- Bones
  - Low birth weight and short length for gestational age
  - Short stature
  - 50% scoliosis
- Joints have ligamentous laxity, resulting in hyperextensible joints
- Specific signs and X-ray features (see Table 20.4)

Investigations and diagnosis

- Prenatal ultrasound scan may detect severe forms in fetus
- Molecular genetic testing (pre- or postnatal)
- Biochemistry is normal or shows increased   alkaline phosphatase (ALP)
- Skin biopsy to assess collagen in cultured fibroblasts
- Bone biopsy histology shows increased Haversian canal + osteocyte lacunae diameters, increased cell numbers
- DEXA scan: Low bone mineral density Z scores

Treatment

There is no curative treatment. Aim to prevent and manage fractures with long-term rehabilitation.

Prevention strategies to decrease fracture frequency include

- Oral calcium supplements
- Bisphosphonates
- Synthetic calcitonin

Surgical interventions

Intramedullary rods (fixed length, telescoping) are used to prevent bowing of long bones, especially for fractures in children >2 years old. Corrective surgery is needed for scoliosis deformities 50°.

Prognosis

In severe OI, a good predictor of future walking is being able to sit by age 10 months. The patient may develop cardiopulmonary or neurological complications. Usually they develop progressive shortening and deformity caused by multiple fractures, e.g., "sabre" tibia, "accordion" femora.

Table 20.4 Osteogenesis imperfecta: subtype classification

Type	Intrauterine fractures	Eyes (sclera)	Bones	X-ray features: thin cortice, osteopenia
Type I[a] Mild; AD; 60%–80%; presenile hearing loss in 30%–60%, often with aortic valve regurgitation		Blue	Frequency of Z recurrent fractures ↓ after puberty; diaphyseal > metaphyseal fractures, usually ambulatory	Wormian bones on scull X-ray (occipital)
Type II Perinatal lethal (stillborn or death within first year); AD	√	Blue	Relative macrocephaly, large fontanelles, micromelia, triangular facies with beaked nose, bowed limbs, legs abducted 90°	"Beaded" ribs – respiratory insufficiency
Type III Progressive and deforming (most severe non-lethal type); AD germ-line mutation	√	White	Pectal deformity, triangular facies, relative macrocephaly, abnormal teeth, easy bruising, severe osteoporosis (fractures), progressive shortening deformity	"Popcorn" metaphyses, flared lower ribs, vertebral compression
Type IV[a] Moderately severe; AD; usually able to attain community ambulation skills	√	White	Bowed long bones, relatively infrequent fractures (frequency ↓ after puberty) Moderately short stature	Osteoporotic, metaphyseal flaring, vertebral compression
Type V Moderately deforming; AD		White	Mild/moderate short stature	Interosseous calcification Hyperplastic calus
Type VI Moderately to severely deforming		White	Short stature, scoliosis	"Fish scale" bone lamellation
Type VII Moderately deforming; AR		White	Short stature Short proximal limbs	

[a] Type A: no teeth involvement; type B: dentinogenesis imperfecta present; AD, autosomal dominant; AR, autosomal recessive.

Osteopetrosis

Also known as marble bone disease or Albers–Schönberg disease, this is a rare chromosomal condition defined by failure of osteoclastic bone resorption and, hence, failure of remodeling.

Classification
- *Malignant/infantile type*: Autosomal recessive. Severe skeletal deformity presents at birth or shortly thereafter. Poor prognosis. Bone marrow transplantation may help in some cases.
- *Benign type*: Autosomal dominant. Later childhood or adulthood benign presentation. Patient is prone to frequent fractures.

Clinical features
- *Face*: Macrocephaly, hydrocephalus, "abnormal eyes" (optic atrophy, partial oculomotor nerve paralysis), compression of other cranial nerves resulting in deafness, facial nerve palsy. Teeth have late eruption and early caries. Osteomyelitis leads to necrosis of the mandible.
- *Limbs*: Generalized osteosclerosis, fragile bones (due to failure to form lamellated bone in stress areas) with fractures that are difficult to fix and prone to delayed union, dwarfism.
- *Hematological*: Encroached marrow cavities leading to anemia, pancytopenia, spontaneous bleeding and bruises. Extramedullary hemopoesis leads to hepatosplenomegaly.
- *Kidneys*: Distal renal tubular acidosis (type 1 RTA)

Investigations
- *Blood*: Pancytopenia and leukoerythroblastic picture (increased primitive cells on blood film). Perform dry bone-marrow tap.
- *X-rays* show dense, "marble" bone (generalized increased density with loss of normal trabecular pattern). The skull has underdeveloped mastoid air cells and paranasal sinuses.
- *Long bones*: Widened ends ("Erlenmeyer flask" proximal humerus/distal femur)
- *Phalanges*: Dense transverse band in metaphysis close to the epiphyseal line, condensed bone proximal and distal to ends of phalanges
- *Metacarpals* have a bone-within-a-bone appearance—sclerotic cortex is separated from the central part of the bone by an area of more normal calcification.
- *Vertebral bones* have a "sandwich" or "rugby jersey" appearance, with relative sclerotic upper and lower plates.
- *Bone scan* shows increased uptake in epiphyseal ends of long bones, normal elsewhere.

Treatment
Treatment depends on the severity of disease and is mainly supportive. Medical therapy includes glucocorticoids. Bone marrow transplant may help. Treatment of fractures is difficult due to dense bone quality.

Prognosis
The malignant type is usually terminal within the first 10 years of life. In the benign form lifespan is unaffected.

Cleidocranial dysplasia

Also known as cleidocranial dysostosis, this disorder is characterized by deficient ossification of the clavicle (cleido) and bone of skull (cranial). It is a rare congenital, autosomal dominant condition.

Clinical features

- *General*: Proportionate mild short stature. No mental retardation
- *Cranium*: Large skull, frontal and parietal bossing, delayed imperfect ossification of sutures and fontanelles. Premature closing of the coronal suture
- *Face*: Underdeveloped or deficient facial bones, resulting in prominent forehead, pseudoexothalmos, and hypertelorism (due to small, wide nasal bridge and widely spaced shallow orbits), protruding mandible
- *Dental*: High arched/cleft palate, late loss of deciduous teeth with slow, disordered eruption of secondary teeth (leading to extra or absent teeth)
- *Ears*: Hearing loss and/or frequent ear infections
- *Upper limb*: Mobile drooping shoulders, completely or partially absent clavicle (especially lateral part, usually unilateral), occasional recurrent dislocation of the shoulder or elbow, short middle and distal phalanges, long second metacarpal
- *Torso*: Narrow thorax and pelvis
- *Spine*: Delayed vertebral ossification, scoliosis or lordosis, kyphosis, prominent cervical transverse processes
- *Lower limbs*: Tubular phalanges of feet

Investigations

X-ray is the primary investigation.

- *Skull*: Multiple imperfect ossification centers (wormian bones); large, open anterior fontanelle; absent or delayed development of sinuses; hypoplastic maxilla
- *Clavicle*: Total or partial absence of lateral-aspect clavicle (most common) or bipartite clavicle
- *Shoulder*: Subluxation of humeral heads
- *Pelvis*: Delayed ossification of pelvic bones with widened symphysis pubis, coax vara of hips
- *Spine*: Failure of union of neural arches

Treatment

Usually abnormalities cause little functional disability. The lateral part of the clavicle may cause brachial plexus problems (if so, for excision). Recurrent dislocations of the shoulder may require stabilization. Dental anomalies should be treated by a maxillofacial surgeon.

Prognosis

Patients have a normal lifespan.

Skeletal dysplasias

This is a heterogeneous group of conditions characterized by abnormal growth of bones. They can be classified according to the region of bone involved or by their genotype (see Table 20.5). Skeletal dysplasias fall into two broad clinical types: short-limb dwarfism and short-trunk dwarfism. Disproportionate short stature is the hallmark. Angular deformity of the limbs and spinal curvature require orthopedic management; the associated abnormalities (deafness, myopia, cervical–cranial stenosis, sleep apnea) and issues with social integration require the most care. The most common skeletal dysplasia, achondroplasia, has an incidence of 1:20,000 live births. Prenatal diagnosis of all dysplasia necessitates careful genetic testing.

Radial dysplasia

An absent or hypoplastic radius causes abnormal radial deviation of the hand. This is the most common form of longitudinal upper-limb deficiency and is often accompanied by a congenitally absent thumb. Anomalies of other systems may also be associated:

• TAR (thrombocytopenia absent radius syndrome)
• Fanconi anemia
• Holt–Oram syndrome: Autosomal dominant, with cardiac anomalies and radial dysplasia
• VACTERL syndrome (**V**ertebral anomalies, **A**nal atresia, **C**ardiac malformations, **T**racheo**E**sophageal fistula, **R**enal and **L**imb anomalies)

Management
• Serial castings or splinting

Surgery is usually required to place the hand in position to maximize function. If a thumb is absent, pollicization (plastic surgery) of the index finger could improve function. The index finger is reconstructed and radially positioned to form a functional "thumb."

Table 20.5 Classification of skeletal dysplasia

Region		Example of hypoplasia ("failure of")	Example of hyperplasia ("excess of")
Epiphysis	Articular cartilage	Spondyloepiphyseal dysplasia	Dysplasia epiphysealis hemimelica (Trevor's)
	Ossification center	Multiple epiphyseal dysplasia	
Physis	Proliferating cartilage	Achondroplasia	Marfan syndrome
	Hypertrophic cartilage	Metaphyseal chondrodysplasia (Schmid, McKusick, Jansen)	Enchondromatosis
	Type 2 collagen	Spondyloepiphyseal dysplasia	
	Proteoglycan metabolism	Kneist syndrome	
Metaphysis	Intramembrous bones	Cleidocranial dysostosis	
	Formation of primary spongiosa	Hypophosphatasia	
	Absorption of primary spongiosa	Osteopetrosis (functionally deficient osteoclasts)	
Diaphysis	Diaphyseal aclasia		Multiple exostoses fracture
	Periosteal bone formation		Engelmann disease
	Endosteal bone formation		Hyperphosphatemia (vitamin D–resistant rickets)

Juvenile idiopathic arthritis (JIA)

JIA is a common chronic childhood disorder (prevalence 1 per 1000; incidence: 1 per 10,000). It is a diagnosis of exclusion in children <16 years old with a history of at least 6 weeks of persistent arthritis. JIA is divided into seven subsets for research purposes (see Table 20.6 and Table 20.7). These are not diagnostic categories but are useful clinical groups. As a child's symptoms evolve with time (e.g., the appearance of a psoriatic rash), they may change subtype.

Table 20.6 International League of Association of Rheumatology (ILAR) classification of juvenile idiopathic arthritis (JIA) with relative frequency

Systemic arthritis	(10%–13%)	p. 894
Oligoarthritis (persistent or extended)	(40%)	p. 896
Polyarthritis (rheumatoid factor positive)	(3%)	p. 898
Polyarthritis (rheumatoid factor negative)	(27%)	p. 900
Psoriatic arthritis	(2%–15%)	p. 901
Enthesitis-related arthritis	(1%–7%)	p. 902
Undifferentiated arthritis	(2%–15%)	

Table 20.7 Differential diagnoses of childhood arthritis

Infection	*Bacterial:* Septic arthritis, osteomyelitis (staphylococcal, pnemococcal, *Hemophilus*, *Kingella*, other)
	Viral: Rubella, parvovirus B19, Cocksackie, infectious mononucleosis
	Lyme, Brucella, tuberculosis, gonorrhea, mixed organisms from penetrating injury
Post-infection	Reactive arthritis (especially after gastrointestinal or viral infections)
	Post-streptococcal reactive arthritis
	Rheumatic fever
Malignancy	Leukemia or lymphoma
	Neuroblastoma
	Primary bone tumors—benign or malignant
	Metastatic disease

Orthopedic	Perthe's disease and other osteochondritides
	Slipped capital femoral epiphysis
	Hip dysplasia
	Chondromalacia patellae
Systemic inflammatory diseases	Crohn's disease,
	Ulcerative colitis
	Celiac disease
Hypermobility	Benign hypermobility—local or generalized
	Marfan, Ehlers–Danlos syndromes
Metabolic disorders	Gout (inborn errors, polycythemia, renal disease)
	Mucopolysaccharidoses
Immunodeficiency syndromes	Most immunodeficiency syndromes cause arthritis
	IgA deficiency
	IgG deficiency
	Common variable immunodeficiency
	DiGeorge syndrome
Hematological	Sickle cell disease
	Other hemoglobinopathies
	Hemophilia
Rheumatic diseases	Systemic lupus erythematosus (SLE)
	Juvenile dermatomyositis
	Systemic sclerosis—localized or systemic
	Vasculitis:
	Henoch–Schönlein purpura
	Polyarteritis/microscopic polyangiitis
	Kawasaki disease
	Takayasu arteritis
Other inflammatory disorders	Sarcoid
	Chronic recurrent multifocal osteomyelitis
	SAPHO (**S**ynovitis, **A**cne, **P**ustulosis, **H**yperostosis and **O**steitis)
Idiopathic pain syndromes	Reflex sympathetic dystrophy
	Fibromyalgia
	Widespread regional-pain syndromes
	"Nonorganic pain"—a cry for help

General clinical principles for JIA

Before labeling a child with diagnosis of JIA, it is imperative to exclude the differential diagnoses, the most important of which are sepsis, malignancy, and trauma (see p. 751). Persistent objective signs of joint inflammation must be present for at least 6 weeks.

History from caretaker and child

- Limp, stiffness and loss of function, pain or malaise
- Onset is usually gradual. Beware of misleading history of trauma, as young children frequently fall without significant injury.
- History of non-use, or change in use
- Child may not complain of pain. Infant may be "irritable"
- Inflammatory symptoms being worse after rest or inactivity
- Stiffness is rarely volunteered. Parents sometimes describe the child as "like a little old person in the mornings." Toddlers' behavior may be perceived as being difficult and uncooperative (e.g., refusing to move in the morning, then running in the afternoon).
- History of associated rash, fever, and weight loss
- History of sore throat, URI, antecedent infections, and travel
- Family history of arthritis, psoriasis, inflammatory bowel disease, rheumatic fever, or acute iritis

Examination

- Observe the child before they become self-conscious.
- Watch them playing and walking.
- Examine all the joints and spine for swelling, warmth, and pain on movement or limited range of movement.
- Measure for leg length inequality and pelvic tilt.
- Examine muscle bulk around the affected joints.
- Assess general muscle strength.
- Examine the skin, hair, and nails for rashes and psoriasis.
- General examination: Vital signs, height, weight, and blood pressure
- Examine the mouth and palate for ulcers, dentition, and asymptomatic tonsillitis, and the heart for murmurs and bruits. Examine for hepatosplenomegaly and adenopathy.

Investigations

- CBC may show mild anemia and thrombocytosis.
- Neutrophilia suggests sepsis or systemic JIA.
- Severe anemia, leukopenia, or thrombocytopenia can indicate leukemia.
- ESR/CRP may be normal or mildly elevated; they are markedly elevated in systemic-onset disease. Very high levels suggest infection or malignancy.
- High ESR plus thrombocytopenia; elevated LDH suggests leukemia.
- Infection screen: Throat culture, urinalysis, blood for ASO, viral serology (CMV, EBV, parvovirus B19, hepatitis if indicated), culture if febrile
- Rheumatoid factor (RF): Nonspecific test but significant in polyarthritis (>5) joints. RF is the exclusion criterion for oligoarticular JIA.

- Anti nuclear antibody (ANA): Nonspecific (5% of normal children are ANA positive). In oligoarticular JIA, ANA is a limited prognostic determinant for iritis.
- Muscle enzymes (CK, LDH, aldolase) are raised in dermatomyositis but can be normal. High LDH or uric acid suggests malignancy.
- Imaging: *Radiographs* exclude fracture or tumor. In early JIA, films may be normal or show soft-tissue swelling and juxtaarticular osteopenia. Later, joint-space narrowing and erosions are evident.
    - *Ultrasound* is helpful for confirming synovitis and joint effusion.
    - *MRI* is useful for detecting atypical monoarthritis. Gadolinium-enhanced MRI is best for diagnosis of synovitis but does not differentiate from infection.
- Synovial fluid aspirate: Culture for sepsis; white cell counts are usually lower in inflammation than in infection.

Management
General
- Establish diagnosis and counsel child and parents.
- Start treatment as soon as possible.
- Most children will need regular examination to look for presence or reappearance of thickened synovium or effusions.
- Exercise: Regular, daily aerobic and range of motion (ROM) exercises
- Psychological support for children and caretakers: Education and support groups (e.g., Arthritis Foundation)
- Ask about school performance and support at school.
- Adolescents need counseling about contraception and alcohol if taking methotrexate (MTX) or leflunomide (see p. 920).
- Amyloidosis is a rare complication of severe, prolonged disease.

Joints
- Minimize pain and stiffness with NSAIDs: all should be given with food.
    - Ibuprofen (40–50 mg/kg/day, divided into 3 doses)
    - Diclofenac (2–3 mg/kg/day, divided into bid doses)
    - Naproxen (15–20 mg/kg/day, divided into bid doses)
    - Piroxicam (0.4 mg/kg/day once a day)
- Prevent deformity with regular daily exercises and night splints.
- Control inflammation with intra-articular steroid injections (triamcinolone), which may control inflammation for months.
- Systemic medications: Methotrexate (MTX) 0.5–1 mg/kg (max 25 mg) oral or subcutaneously weekly; give with daily folic acid
- Anti-tumor necrosis factor (TNF) agents (etanercept, infliximab, or adalimimab) if unresponsive to NSAIDs and subcutaneous MTX

Eyes
- Screen for uveitis. The patient must undergo regular screening by an experienced ophthalmologist (see Table 20.8). Treat with topical steroids and midriatics and, sometimes, systemic anti-inflammatory medications such as steroids, MTX, and TNF blockers. The course is independent of joint disease severity. The disorder is potentially blinding.

Table 20.8 Frequency of ophthalmologic examination in patients with juvenile idiopathic arthritis (JIA)

Type	ANA	Age at onset (years))	Duration of disease (years)	Risk category	Eye exam frequency (months)
Oligoarthritis or polyarthritis	+	≤6	≤4	High	3
	+	≤6	>4	Moderate	6
	+	≤6	>7	Low	12
	+	>6	≤4	Moderate	6
	+	>6	>4	Low	12
	−	≤6	≤4	Moderate	6
	−	≤6	>4	Low	12
	−	>6	NA	Low	12
Systemic disease (fever, rash)	NA	NA	NA	Low	12

ANA, antinuclear antibodies; NA, not applicable. Recommendations for follow-up continue through childhood and adolescence. Reproduced with permission from Cassidy J, Kivlin J, Lindsley C, Nocton J, the section on Rheumatology and the section on Ophthalmology, "Ophthalmologic examinations in children with juvenile rheumatoid arthritis," Pediatrics May 2006;**117**:1843–1845, copyright 2006 by the AAP.

Growth and nutrition
- Measure growth velocity; check nutritional status; muscular atrophy
- Most children are low in vitamin D and calcium.

Dental
- Dentition: Watch for caries

Once the diagnosis is established, the child should be looked after by a pediatric rheumatologist for specialist drugs and multidisciplinary support.

Systemic-onset arthritis

Systemic-onset arthritis makes up 10%–20% of JIA cases and affects males and females in equal numbers.

Clinical features

- Fever is essential, is typically quotidian fever (up to 39°C), and must return to normal or lower between daily attacks.
- Rash (present in 80%) is salmon pink, macular or urticarial on chest, trunk, and intertriginous regions. It is present during fever or when the patient is warm (e.g., during bath) and disappears within minutes (evanescent). May exhibit the Koebner phenomenon
- Myalgia, arthralgia, and arthritis. Arthritis can be oligo- or polyarthritis.
- Generalized lymphadenopathy and hepatosplenomegaly
- Polyserositis with pericarditis, pleuritis, and sterile peritonitis in about half of patients. Silent pericardial effusions. Myocarditis + tachycardia, cardiomegaly, and congestive cardiac failure is rare.
- Growth retardation is secondary to disease, steroids, or joint damage.
- Late complications include amyloidosis, which is difficult to treat.
- Macrophage activation syndrome (MAS) is rare but life threatening; it is sometimes precipitated by intercurrent infection or a change in drugs. Hemaphagocytic bone marrow with falling WBC, platelets, ESR, and fibrinogen, and elevated d-dimers and very high ferritin indicate MAS.

Investigations

- CBC (normocytic/hypochromic anemia; leukocytosis; thrombocytosis)
- ESR/CRP can be very high; use levels to monitor disease course during treatment.
- Hypoalbinemia is multifactorial, with poor diet, general ill health with catabolism, rarely, proteinuria is secondary to renal amyloid.
- ANA and RF are usually negative.
- Viral titers and blood cultures
- Malignancy screen: LDH, uric acid, chest X-ray, ultrasound of abdomen; consider bone marrow
- ECG and echocardiogram

Management

- NSAIDs for initial management of pain, fever, and serositis. Indomethacin 2–3 mg/kg/day is often used for pericarditis.
- Pulsed IV corticosteroids (20–30 mg/kg/day max 1 g) are needed for serious systemic disease (after infections and malignancy are excluded).
- Oral steroids (consider if no dramatic improvement after 1 week of NSAIDs), initially at a dose of 1 mg/kg in divided doses until fever settles and inflammatory markers are normal. Taper dose to minimize side effects, particularly growth retardation. Use alternate-day doses and add steroid-sparing agent.
- Methotrexate is used, but is not as effective as in other JIA subsets.
- Intra-articular corticosteroid for flares of single joints
- Biologic therapy: Anti-TNF and anti-IL-1 in resistant cases; new drugs such as anti-IL-6 are being investigated.

Prognosis

There are three groups: monocyclic (11%), recurrent or polycyclic (34%), and persistent (55%). Those with monocyclic disease do well with no significant disability. Historically, more than a third of patients have permanent disability with active disease into adult life. Death can occur from infection, MAS, or amyloidosis.

Oligoarticular JIA (previously pauciarticular JRA)

- Absence of systemic findings and fewer than five joints affected
- Duration at least 6 weeks
- Girls > boys 6:1
- Most common subtype occurring in 40% of patients with JIA
- Two subsets are recognized: persistent and extended. If the number of joints increases to more than 4 after the first 6 months of illness, it is termed extended oligoarticular.
- Children may develop silent, blinding iritis (anterior uveitis). ANA is positive in 40%–75% of cases. (ANA-positive patients are more likely to develop chronic iritis.)

Clinical features

- Diagnosis of exclusion: rule out infection.
- Milder symptoms than reactive arthritis; no constitutional symptoms
- Often present with joint swelling or limping rather than pain
- Two-thirds of cases have a single joint affected; in one-third only two joints are affected. Disease occurrence is often asymmetrical; knees, ankles, elbows, and wrists are common—any joint is possible.
- Careful examination may reveal more extensive disease, as the child may be too young to express pain.
- Elbows and knees may lack full extension but are not painful.
- The affected leg may overgrow; measure leg lengths and check that pelvis is level.

Investigations

- CBC: CRP (often normal); ANA (prognostic value for uveitis)
- X-ray: Exclude fracture and tumor; look for overgrowth and damage.

Management

- Regular review to assess joints, eyes, and general growth
- NSAIDs for pain and stiffness: full dose for 8 weeks (ibuprofen, diclofenac, naproxen, or piroxicam)
- Intra-articular steroid injections may settle inflammation for months to years
- If pain is not controlled with oral NSAIDs and intra-articular steroids, then MTX oral or subcutaneously is used in resistant cases.
- Rarely is anti-TNF therapy needed.
- Screen for uveitis, initially 3-monthly, by an ophthalmologist.

Disease course and prognosis

- 60% of patients are normal at 15 years, but disease may flare up at any time. An extended subset has a worse prognosis.
- Uveitis is the most important extra-articular complication.

Rheumatoid factor (RF)–positive polyarthritis

This is adult-type rheumatoid disease beginning in childhood. It accounts for~10% of juvenile idiopathic arthritis. Presentation is a chronic symmetrical inflammatory polyarthritis (at least 5 joints, often 20+) with positive RF on two occasions at least 3 months apart (see Box 20.1). Typically the disease affects teenage girls, although any age is possible. This is generally a very aggressive disease.

> **Box 20.1 American Rheumatism Association (ARA) criteria for diagnosis of rheumatoid arthritis (1987)**
>
> 1. Morning stiffness >1 hour at peak illness
> 2. Arthritis in at least 3 joints, witnessed by a physician
> 3. Hand arthritis—wrists, MCPs, or PIPs
> 4. Symmetrical arthritis
> 5. Rheumatoid nodules
> 6. Rheumatoid factor positive
> 7. Erosions on X-ray

All symptoms need to be present for at least 6 weeks. Four or more criteria need to be fulfilled for diagnosis of rheumatoid arthritis (RA). These are primarily classification criteria (90% sensitivity and specificity).

Clinical features
- History of early-morning and immobility stiffness
- Symmetrical arthritis affecting large and small joints associated with rheumatoid nodules. Wrists and finger joints are affected early.
- Tenosynovitis is common around the fingers and ankles.
- Systemic features include low-grade fever (differential diagnosis for systemic JIA), hepatosplenomegaly, lymphadenopathy, serositis (pericarditis and pleurisy)
- Eyes: Uveitis is rare, dry eyes are relatively common (10%–35%); other eye complications are possible.
- Rarely, other extra-articular features, such as lung disease, vasculitis

Investigations
- CBC; CRP; LFTs; RF, CCP (may be more specific than RF); ANA
- Renal function and urinalysis
- X-rays of affected joints and chest X-ray

Management

- Monitor disease activity and aim for good control of arthritis.
- Conduct regular, meticulous assessment for tender and swollen joints, muscle wasting, joint damage, and loss of joint function.
- Monitor growth development and nutritional status. Exercise should include range of motion and aerobic.
- Psychosocial development can be severely affected and needs addressing.

Treatment

- Start early aggressive treatment to prevent joint damage.
- NSAIDs provide relief from pain, stiffness, and swelling.
- All children will need disease-modifying antirheumatic drug (DMARD) therapy.
- MTX is the least toxic and most well established medication, orally or subcutaneously. Other medications, such as sulfasalazine and hydroxychloroquine, have been used in combination with MTX or alone.
- *Steroids:* Intra-articular steroids are used to settle synovitis in individual joints; give oral steroids as an adjunct to DMARDs; pulsed intravenous steroids for flare of disease. Aim to minimize total steroid load.
- *Biologic agents:* Anti-TNF agents (etenercept, infliximab, adalimimab) have been shown to reduce joint erosions and prevent progression of disease.

Prognosis

Historically, most children survived into adulthood, though with poor functional outcome because of aggressive, unremitting disease, early erosions, and a high incidence of joint replacement. The use of aggressive, early systemic MTX and biologic therapies has greatly improved this outcome.

RF-negative polyarthritis

This type of arthritis comprises 30% of JIA cases. Previously it was known as polyarticular-onset JRA. It is characterized by five or more affected joints within the first 6 months. Girls are affected 4 times more than boys.

Clinical features

- Diagnosis of exclusion: IgM RF should be negative 3 months apart
- Systemic features: Low-grade fever and transient rashes are possible but mild.
- Any joint can be affected, including the jaw, cervical spine, wrists and fingers, and subtalar joints.
- Joint swelling leads to flexion contractures, limited mobility. and muscle wasting.
- Chronic hyperemia leads to accelerated bone growth and premature epiphyseal fusion. Common sites are carpus, subtalar, jaw (micrognathia, dental malocclusion), and cervical spine (apophyseal joint fusion or instability).
- Tenosynovitis and bursitis develop around the fingers and feet.

Investigations

- *Blood*: CBC, CRP, ANA
- X-Ray or MRI of affected joints

Treatments

- Start treatment as soon as possible.
- NSAIDs for 4–6 weeks in adequate dose, plus intra-articular steroids to target joints
- Start DMARDs early to try and induce remission with MTX.
- Remission: Continue NSAID for 6 months and DMARD for 1 year.
- Persistent arthritis: Intraarticular steroids into target joints + combination DMARDs
- Anti-TNF therapy if patient is intolerant of or unresponsive to MTX

Prognosis

This heterogeneous group of conditions has variable prognosis. Prognosis has dramatically improved in recent years with the aggressive use of MTX and anti-TNF therapy. However, up to a third of patients suffer persistent deformity and disability. Many have continuing disease activity into adult life.

Psoriatic arthritis

This is a recently recognized, underdiagnosed subset of JIA. It affects 2%–15% of children with JIA. Although the etiology is unknown, there is a background of strong genetic predisposition (up to 50% of cases).

International League of Associations for Rheumatology (ILAR) criteria for diagnosis of psoriatic arthritis

Diagnostic criteria are inflammatory arthritis occurring in the presence of psoriasis, or inflammatory arthritis occurring with dactylitis or psoriatic nail changes, plus a first-degree relative with psoriasis.

- *Exclusions*: RF positive; HLA B27 in males >6 years; any enthesitis-related arthritis or uveitis in a first-degree relative; systemic arthritis

Clinical features

- Arthritis and rash rarely present simultaneously. Rash often precedes arthritis.
- *Arthritis*: The most common form is asymmetrical large joint (knees or ankles). Small-joint polyarthritis of fingers and toes (metacarpal phalangeal [MCP], proximal interphalangeal [PIP], and distal interphalangeal [DIP] joints) and dactylitis are also common. Some children have tendonitis or tenosynovitis, especially around the ankles.
- *Skin*: Predominantly plaque psoriasis (examine extensor surfaces of elbows and knees, hairline, behind the ears, umbilicus, groin, and natal cleft)
- *Nails*: Pitting, ridging, onycholysis, subungual hyperkeratosis
- *Uveitis* needs regular screening like JIA.

Investigations

- No specific tests; need exclusion bloods (see p. 940).
- Often there is evidence of chronic inflammation: Raised CRP, ESR, thrombocytosis, and low-grade normocytic anemia. The ANA may be positive.

Radiographs

- Periarticular osteopenia and soft-tissue swelling
- Periosteal new-bone formation, particularly in dactylitis

Treatment

It is important to diagnosis dactylitis. NSAIDs are the initial treatment. Intra-articular steroid injections often help settle inflammation. Methorexate and anti-TNF agents are effective for persistent disease.

Prognosis

Arthritis can be episodic and continue into adult life. A few patients have a very destructive course, with arthritis mutilans.

Enthesitis-related arthritis

This recently introduced ILAR terminology and category was previously known as juvenile ankylosing spondylitis or seronegative spondyarthropathy. This form is characterized by arthritis with enthesitis (inflammation in any tendinous, ligamentous, or muscular insertion onto bone) or arthritis alone or enthesitis alone with two of the following features:
- Sacroiliac joint tenderness (usually seen in older patients)
- Inflammatory spinal pain
- HLA B27 positive
- First-degree relative with a family history of acute uveitis
- Age of onset 6 >years
- *Exclude*: RF positive; systemic arthritis; psoriasis in the patient or first-degree relative

Clinical features
- Commonly, occurs in adolescent or preadolescent boys (M:F: 10:1)
- Oligo- or polyarthritis predominantly in lower limbs
- Enthesitis, especially around the foot (heel pain, plantar fasciitis), sometimes for many years before spinal symptoms develop
- May progress to sacroiliac joint tenderness, inflammatory spinal pain, or buttock pain (worse at night plus early-morning stiffness)
- Systemic features: Low-grade fever, weight loss, and fatigue
- Acute anterior uveitis (10%–15%): Acutely painful red, photophobic eye—this is different from the uveitis seen with other JIA
- Associated inflammatory bowel disease or celiac disease (monitor growth, abdominal symptoms)
- Reactive arthritis

Examination
- *Examine affected joints* for synovitis, effusions, associated muscle wasting, and range of movement.
- *Spine examination is essential*. Test for cervical rotation, thoracic rotation, and lateral flexion and document the Schober test (mark 10 cm above and 5 cm below the dimples of Venus and note the increase gained by forward flexion). Normal is at least 21 cm—this varies little with age and gender. Look for loss of normal lumbar lordosis. There tends to be ascending disease.
- Chest expansion may be limited with reduced lung volumes in advanced disease.
- Examine commonly affected enthesis sites around the heel—Achilles insertion and calcaneous.
- Can mimic Osgood–Schlatter disease at patellar tendon insertion

Investigations
- CBC (normochromic anemia, mild leukocytosis, and thrombocytosis)
- If there is microcytic anemia, low albumin, think of occult inflammatory bowel disease.
- CRP may be raised.
- RF and ANA negative
- HLA B27 positive in 90%, but also positive in 8%–10% of normal population

Radiology
- X-ray changes lag behind clinical symptoms by up to 10 years. Interpretation is difficult in children. MRI may show changes earlier.

X-rays
- Affected joints: Soft-tissue swelling, periarticular osteopenia, erosions, joint-space narrowing, bony ankylosis (late)
- The heel may show calcaneal spur or fluffy exostoses on Achilles.
- Sacroiliac joints may show erosions, sclerosis, and fusion (late).
- The thoracolumbar junction may show syndesmophytes (late).

Treatment
- Start early, aggressive treatment to prevent bone and joint damage.
- NSAIDs provide relief from pain and stiffness.
- MTX is effective for some patients. Other medications such as sulfasalazine have been used alone or in combination with MTX.
- *Steroids*: Intra-articular steroids reduce synovitis in individual joints; give a brief course of oral steroids as adjunct to DMARDs.
- *Biologic agents*: Anti-TNF agents (etenercept, infliximab, adalimimab) have been shown to be very effective.
- Physical therapy to maintain spine, joint, and chest mobility

Prognosis
Some children will have progressive disease into adulthood. Aggressive treatment, especially with TNF blockers, has improved outcome.

Systemic lupus erythematosus (SLE)

SLE is a complex, multisystem autoimmune disorder affecting adolescents (it is rare in younger children; the female-to-male ratio is 8:1). It is more common and more severe in African-American, Hispanic, and Asian girls.

The ARC criteria (Box 20.2) are helpful (90% sensitivity, 97% specificity), but are less reliable in detecting early disease. SLE is one of the great mimics of other conditions.

Box 20.2 Revised ACR criteria for classification of SLE

SLE is diagnosed if 4 out of 11 features are present simultaneously or serially:

1. Malar rash
2. Discoid rash
3. Photosensitivity
4. Mucus membrane ulcers (hard palate, nasal septum)
5. Arthritis (non-erosive)
6. Serositis: Pleuritis or pericarditis
7. Renal disease: Persistent proteinuria >0.5g/24 hours or cellular casts
8. Neurological disorder: Psychosis or seizures in absence of known precipitants
9. Hematological abnormality: Hemolytic anemia or leukopenia <4.0 × 10^9/L × 2 or thrombocytopenia <100 × 10^9/L
10. Immunological: Raised anti-DNA-binding antibody, anti-Sm antibody; positive antiphospholipid antibodies
11. Antinuclear antibody

Clinical features

The presenting complaint may affect any organ system.

- *Nonspecific constitutional symptoms* include common low-grade fever, weight loss, fatigue, anorexia, and lymphadenopathy.
- *Mucocutaneous problems* include malar "butterfly" rash over the bridge of the nose and sparing the nasolabial folds; discoid lesions; hair thinning or loss (scarring and nonscarring alopecia); mouth and nasal ulcers; photosensitivity (50%); livido reticularis; urticarial rashes; purpuric rashes; and digital vasculitis.
- *Musculoskeletal* (90%): Polyarthritis resembling rheumatoid arthritis (non-erosive); tendonitis; arthralgia; myalgia; myositis (5%), aseptic necrosis
- *Cardiovascular*: Raynaud's phenomenon (white, blue, red sequence); pericarditis (silent or rapidly constrictive); myocarditis, valvulitis with endocarditis (Libman–Sachs)
- *Pulmonary*: Pleurisy, pleural effusions, hemoptysis from pulmonary vasculitis, interstitial fibrosis, pneumonitis
- *Renal*: Hypertension, proteinuria; nephritis; nephrotic syndrome, renal failure

- *Hematological*: Anemia (normochromic normocytic, Coombs-positive hemolytic, renal failure, drug-related); leukopenia and lymphopenia are common (80%); thrombocytopenia (20%); thrombotic episodes from antiphospholipid antibodies
- *Neurological*: Migraine (40%), mood disorders (anxiety, depression, emotional lability [70%]); psychoses (rare); seizures (rare); transverse myelitis peripheral neuropathies (10%)
- Take a careful drug history, especially for tetracyclines for acne (positive antihistone antibodies).

Investigations
- BP measurement
- Urinalysis
- CBC; LFTs; renal function; ANA (98%). Remember that not every positive ANA means lupus.
- dsDNA and Smith (RNP) antibodies (40% but specific for SLE); RF
- Coagulation screen
- Anticardiolipin and antiphospholipid antibodies
- ESR is often raised; CRP is low unless there is serositis or infection.
- Check CH50 to look for complement deficiencies in children.
- C3 and C4 are low in active disease and useful for monitoring.

Screen major organ systems, e.g., thyroid, heart, lungs, kidney regularly. Perform a kidney biopsy to determine the type and severity of renal lesion if indicated.

Management in a specialist clinic
- *General*: Patient should avoid sun exposure and use sunscreen. Treat hypertension and minimize long-term cardiovascular risks. Give ACE inhibitors for nephroprotection for proteinuria.
- Treat targeted organ systems aggressively.
- Give NSAIDs for musculoskeletal symptoms (note increased risk of renal and CNS complications).
- Hydroxychloroquine for fatigue, rashes, arthritis, and hyperlipidemia
- Prednisone and steroid-sparing drugs (azathioprine [AZA], MTX, mycophenylate mofetil [MMF]) for other severe manifestations
- Methylprednisolone pulses and cyclophosphamide for active, diffuse proliferative nephritis, then MMF or azathiaprine. For milder disease you may start MMF.
- Experimental treatments for refractory cases: Rituximab; autologous stem cell replacement
- Give calcium and vitamin D routinely, as well as nutrition consultation.
- Counseling regarding contraception, pregnancy, and childbirth risks

Prognosis
- Very variable between ethnic groups. Overall 5-year survival is 90%, with death resulting from unremitting active disease or complications of immunosuppression (infections).
- Prognosis is worse for those with nephritis (60% after 15 years).
- There is a bimodal survival curve with markedly increased long-term risk of premature cardiovascular disease.

Juvenile dermatomyositis (JDM)

JDM is an inflammatory disease of skin and muscles. The causes are unknown, although host predisposition with infectious and environmental triggers is likely. The diagnostic criteria are presented in Box 20.3.

Box 20.3 Diagnostic criteria for JDM

1. Symmetrical weakness of proximal muscles
2. Periorbital edema with heliotrope discoloration; scaly rash over MCPs, PIPs (Grottron's papules); knees, elbows, and malleoli
3. Elevation of one or more muscles enzymes: Creatine kinase, AST, LDH, aldolase
4. EMG changes of myopathy and denervation
5. Muscle biopsy evidence of necrosis and inflammation
6. MRI (MRI has largely superceded EMG)

Modified from Bohan A, Peters JB (1975). Polymyositis and dermatomyositis (part 2). *N Engl J Med* **292**(8):403–407.

Clinical features

- Onset varies from insidious to very acute, rash may precede muscle weakness.
- Rash: Periorbital edema with heliotrope discoloration of upper lids; facial rash may include nasolabial folds (unlike SLE); erythematous maculopapular rash over extensor surfaces nail fold vasculitis. Often it is photosensitive.
- Muscles: Typically symmetrical proximal muscle weakness with fatigability of arms and legs; truncal weakness (unable to sit from lying); Gower's sign (p. 612). Palatal and respiratory muscles are affected in severe cases with nasal speech, poor swallowing, and decreased lung volume.
- Arthritis (60%): 2/3 oligoarthritis, 1/3 polyarthritis
- Lung disease (uncommon): Interstitial fibrosis; pulmonary vasculitis
- Vasculitis, especially gastrointestinal involvement (pain, bleeding, perforation), correlates with nail fold capillary changes.

Diagnosis

Diagnosis is usually made by typical rash, proximal muscle weakness, raised muscle enzymes, and typical MRI changes.

Differential diagnosis

Infectious myositis (usually viral) overlaps with autoimmune disorder (SLE and mixed connective tissue disease).

Late complications

Calcinosis

This is linked with active and prolonged myositis; it occurs in skin, fascia, subcutaneous fat, and muscle. Superficial lesions may erupt and discharge. Sheets of calcification may prevent movement but may resolve with time (no specific treatment). Tumoral deposits can be surgically removed.

Lipodystrophy

This is generalized or partial, and painless. The generalized form is associated with insulin resistance, diabetes, liver disease, and short stature.

Investigations

- *Muscle enzymes:* CK; LDH, aldolase; AST; ALT
- *ANA* (6%–60%) may be raised. Myositis-specific antibodies rarely present in children.
- *ESR and CRP* are variable. Check CBC for anemia, as there is concern about GI blood loss.
- *Swallowing study* to look for pharyngeal and upper esophageal dysfunction
- *Chest X-ray and pulmonary function tests (PFTs):* Look for aspiration, adequate ventilation, and hemorrhage.
- *MRI* (STIR or T2 fat suppressed) shows a diffuse white signal throughout affected muscles.
- *EMG* (seldom needed): Low-amplitude, short-duration polyphasic potentials with early recruitment, fibrillations, and repetitive discharges
- *Muscle biopsy* can show histological evidence of necrosis and inflammation.

Monitoring

Regular examination includes muscle strength testing and muscle enzymes. Aim to maintain function, rapidly normalize muscle enzymes, and limit steroid effects on growth.

Course and treatment

The condition may be uniphasic, polyphasic, or chronic. The goal is to control inflammation quickly to prevent permanent muscle loss and other complications.

Corticosteroids are the mainstay of treatment, with pulses if there is moderate to severe disease (GI absorption is not reliable), otherwise orally. Methotrexate is effective and frequently used as a steroid-sparing drug.

Hydroxychloroquine is helpful for skin and vasculitic disease; MMF and cyclosporine may have a role. Cyclophosphamide is used in some centers for vasculitis.

Rituximab and TNF blockers may be helpful in treating resistant disease.

Sunscreen and vitamin D and calcium supplementation should be routine.

Treat for 18 months after remission is induced. There is evidence that aggressive treatment minimizes calcinosis.

Mixed connective tissue disease–overlap syndromes

These syndromes show combined features of SLE, progressive systemic sclerosis, and/or dermatomyositis with positive RNP antibody.

Prognosis and management are determined according to the major disease features. These disorders usually require steroids and steroid-sparing agents.

Clinical features

- Raynaud's phenomenon (common)
- Swollen hands and fingers (common)
- Polyarthritis—symmetrical peripheral joint disease, nodules
- Rashes are similar to SLE or JDM rash; tight, non-elastic skin of hands
- Muscle weakness and myositis
- Restrictive lung disease and pulmonary hypertension
- Renal disease is less common.

Differential diagnosis

- RF polyarticular JIA
- SLE
- JDMS

Investigations

- Characteristic anti-RNP (ribonucleoprotein) antibody
- Other autoantibodies: ANA positive (90%); RF positive (often)
- CBC: Leukopenia; thrombocytopenia
- Chest X-ray and PFTs; possibly CT of lungs
- Renal function
- Echocardiogram: Screen for right ventricular hypertrophy secondary to pulmonary hypertension in established disease.

Scleroderma

Scleroderma causes hard, tight, inelastic skin and subcutaneous tissue. It occurs twice as often in females than in males, as two distinct syndromes, localized and systemic.

Localized scleroderma (morphea, linear scleroderma)

- Lesions confined to the skin are termed *morphea*.
- Lesions that involve the underlying tissues, sometimes down to bone, are termed *linear scleroderma* (LS).
- In both types there is an initial inflammatory phase with single or multiple flesh-colored or erythematous plaques. These evolve into firm, waxy, yellow–white shiny lesions sometimes with a violaceous border.
- Growth of the region under LS is affected and can result in flexion contractures, localized growth abnormalities, and cosmetic deformities.
- Linear lesions across the forehead to the nose are termed *en coup de sabre*. These lesions may extend down to the brain and be associated with seizures and iritis.
- Oligoarthritis (10%) can precede skin changes.
- Esophageal involvement is not infrequent but there are rarely other systemic changes.
- May need biopsy or MR confirmation of extent of lesion

Treatment and management
- Trials of UVA1, methotrexate steroids, and topical agents have all been tried with variable success.
- Physical therapy to conserve range of movement, help with skin flexibility
- Occasional surgical correction of contractures and deformities is required.

Systemic sclerosis (SSc) or progressive systemic sclerosis (PSS)

- Raynaud's phenomenon is often the presenting symptom; severe attacks can result in digital ischemia, ulceration, and bony resorption.
- Skin changes follow with edema and inflammation. There is symmetrical involvement with loss of range of the MCP and PIP joints.
- Finger edema lasts for several weeks and is replaced by taut, waxy, shiny, thickened skin, which eventually becomes atrophic. Fingertip skin may crack ("mechanics' hands").
- Facial involvement: Initial loss of nasolabial folds and small mouth. Late findings include pinched nose and tight, expressionless face.
- Nail folds are ragged with telangectasia.
- Joints are stiff from overlying scleroderma. There is occasional oligoarthritis.
- Dysmotility and bowel wall thickening can occur throughout the bowel, leading to malabsorption, wasting, bloating, abdominal cramps, diarrhea, or severe constipation.
- Pulmonary fibrosis and pulmonary hypertension are initially asymptomatic. When more severe they lead to dyspnea, syncope, and death.
- Myocarditis, pericarditis, and arrthymias are reported.

- Renal disease with crisis used to be the most common cause of death.
- Sjogren's syndrome is often associated (dry eyes, dry mouth).

Investigations

- CBC, ESR; LFTs, renal function including BP; ANA, anti-centromere and anti-topoisomerase antibodies (Scl-70)
- Chest X-ray; ECG; echocardiogram to screen for pulmonary hypertension
- Lung function tests and high-resolution computerized tomography (HRCT) if there is fibrosis or pulmonary hypertension
- Barium swallow to look for lower esophageal involvement and reflux

Treatment and management

No treatment is consistently effective in slowing or preventing fibrosis and sclerosis in severe, progressive cases. MTX, mycophenolate, cyclosporin, and low-dose steroids have been used in the inflammatory phase. (Steroids and cyclosporine may precipitate scleroderma renal crisis; check for hypertension and treat with ACE inhibitors).

Symptomatic treatment depends on organ involvement:

- *Raynaud's disease*: Hand warmers, double gloves, biofeedback training; oral or topical vasodilators, prostacyclin for severe attacks and digital gangrene
- *GI tract*: Avoid NSAIDs. Metoclopramide aids gut motility; proton pump inhibitors reduce gastritis and complications of reflux.
- *Lung disease*: Cyclophosphamide may delay the progression of pulmonary fibrosis.

Prognosis

Localized scleroderma

This form generally has a good prognosis. Cosmetic and functional deformities may occur if there is bone involvement with linear scleroderma.

SSc/PSS

This syndrome has poor prognosis, with 5-year survival of 34%–73%. Death results from pulmonary hypertension or fibrosis and renal crisis.

Vasculitis

This group of conditions is characterized by inflammation of blood vessels and may be primary, or secondary to underlying diseases (e.g., SLE, dermatomyositis). Some cases appear to be precipitated by infections, e.g., streptococcus.

Classification is defined by the size of affected vessels:

- *Small-vessel vasculitis*: Henoch–Schönlein purpura (HSP), microscopic polyangiitis (MPA), Wegener's granulomatosus (WG)
- *Medium-sized vessel vasculitis*: Polyarteritis nodosa (PAN)
- *Large-vessel vasculitis*: Takayasu arteritis (TA)

Henoch–Schönlein purpura

HSP is small-vessel vasculitis associated with IgA immune complexes. Symptoms include palpable papular, purpuric rash, arthritis, colicky abdominal pain, and nephritis. HSP affects prepubertal boys more than girls.

Clinical features

- *Skin rash*: Palpable purpura over buttocks and lower legs; edema over dorsum of hands and feet, scrotum, and periorbital region
- *Arthritis*: Typically short-lived, affecting large joints (knees, ankles. or elbows)
- *Gastrointestinal*: Colicky abdominal pain (most common), melena, hematemesis, intussusception, perforation
- *Renal*: Dipstick hematuria and proteinuria are present (50%). Severe glomerulonephritis and nephrotic syndrome are rare.

Investigations

- CBC, and coagulation studies, renal function, dipstick urinalysis, and full renal investigation with biopsy if there is evidence of renal involvement (crescentic IgA glomerulonephritis)
- Skin biopsy is rarely necessary. IgA-mediated leukocytoclastic vasculitis
- Abdominal investigations as per symptoms (p. 364)
- In older patients or severe disease, consider MPA and WG mimicking HSP.

Treatment and prognosis

Most cases have a benign course with complete resolution of symptoms within 6 weeks. NSAIDs help lessen arthritis symptoms. Use of corticosteroids for abdominal pain and arthritis may speed symptom resolution and prevent renal disease. Test for hematuria because nephritis carries a worse prognosis for long-term hypertension and decreased renal function.

Wegener's granulomatosis (WG)

WG is a triad of antineutrophil cytoplasmic antibodies (c-ANCA, PR3 antibody) positive for small-vessel vasculitis, respiratory tract granulomata, and renal disease. WG is a rare disorder that is usually diagnosed in adolescents.

Clinical features

- Subacute disease can be present for years, but may become acute. Transformation into systemic disease (malaise, fever, weight loss, vasculitis) occurs.
- *ENT* (90%): Nasal crusting, obstruction and ulceration; nosebleeds; serous otitis media, and sinusitis. Nasal septum and sinus wall destruction (saddle nose deformity late)
- *Pulmonary* (80%): Subglottic stenosis (stridor); hemoptysis (25%); lower bronchial obstruction with atelectasis and pneumonia; pulmonary hemorrhage; asymptomatic nodules
- *Renal* (90%): Features range from mild, asymptomatic (more common, microscopic hematuria; mild renal impairment) to fulminant diffuse, pauci-immune, necrotizing crescentic glomerulonephritis and renal failure.
- *Arthritis* (50%): Non-erosive polyarthritis; muscle and joint pains are common (60%).
- *Skin* (40%): Palpable purpura of leukocytoclastic vasculitis; livido reticularis, pyoderma gangrenosum
- *CNS* (30%): Mononeuritis multiplex and sensorimotor peripheral neuropathy
- *Eye lesions*: Episcleritis; uveitis; orbital pseudotumor

Investigations

Blood

- CBC (normocytic, normochromic anemia, leukocytosis, thrombocytosis). ESR and CRP are raised (differential diagnosis is infection)
- Antiphospholipid antibodies in about half of cases (with risk of thrombotic events)
- Renal screen with blood pressure measurement and urinalysis at each visit. Perform renal biopsy if there is active sediment and declining renal function.
- cANCA (proteinase 3) positive in 90% of patients with generalized WG (high specificity)

Lungs

- Chest X-ray, sputum culture and cytology; CT of lungs; PFTs (increased DLCO suggests hemorrhage), bronchoscopy
- CT sinuses ± nasendoscopy and biopsy

Histology

- Necrotizing, giant cell, granulomatous, medium-vessel vasculitis in respiratory tract

Course and treatment

Systemic disease

This is treated with oral or pulsed intravenous cyclophosphamide and steroids to induce remission. Remission is maintained with MMF, MTX or AZA. Rituximab is helpful in treatment failures. Aim to minimize total steroid load. Give vitamin D and calcium supplementation. Stop only after patient is at least 12 months disease free.

- The patient may need intubation and high PEEP for pulmonary hemorrhage; provide renal support including dialysis for severe disease.

Subacute and limited disease

These forms have a variable (milder) course, and may respond to MTX alone or with low-dose steroids. Long-term cotrimoxazole in remission reduces pulmonary infection and relapse rates. With 10-year survival is 75% and morbidity is considerable.

Microscopic polyangiitis (MPA)

This small-vessel necrotizing vasculitis targets skin, the brain, and kidneys. It affects males twice as frequently as females.

Clinical features
- Antecedent systemic illness with unexplained fevers, abdominal pains, and arthralgia of up to 1 year
- Vasculitic or purpuric skin rash
- Arthritis (30%) in large joints
- Renal: Hypertension; hematuria, proteinuria; renal failure
- GI involvement
- CNS: seizures and strokes, mononeuritis multiplex; peripheral neuropathy
- Pulmonary hemorrhage

Investigations
- CBC; LFTs may be elevated
- Check renal function; urinalysis for active sediment
- p-ANCA positive (MPO) is not specific; this is also seen in IBD, autoimmune hepatitis, and other autoimmune diseases.
- Vascular imaging is not helpful, as resolution is inadequate.
- *Histology*: Inflammatory changes are evident in pre- and post-capillary vessels; pauci-immune features are seen in the skin, kidneys, and lungs.

Course and treatment
If treated promptly, with pulsed cyclophosphamide and high-dose steroids, prognosis is good.

Polyarteritis nodosa (PAN)

PAN is a rare medium-vessel necrotizing vasculitis with aneurysm formation. It occurs twice as often in males than in females.

Clinical
- Antecedent systemic illness with unexplained fevers, abdominal pain, and arthralgia of up to 1 year
- Testicular pain in males (often mistaken for torsion)
- Vasculitis or purpuric skin rash
- Arthritis (30%) in large joints: Exquisite bony tenderness from peripheral vasculitis and periosteal new bone formation
- Renal: Hypertension; hematuria, proteinuria; renal failure; intrarenal aneurysms
- GI involvement (50%): Abdominal pain; pancreatitis; bowel infarction
- CNS: Mononeuritis multiplex; peripheral neuropathy; seizures, strokes

Investigations
- CBC; LFTs may be elevated
- Check renal function; urinalysis for active sediment
- MRI; MR angiography (MRA) or angiography to reveal multiple aneurysms
- *Histology*: Panarteritis with fibrinoid necrosis, thrombosis, infraction, weakening of artery walls, and aneurysms. Segmental lesions are evident at bifurcations of small- and medium-vessel walls.

Course and treatment
Without treatment this condition may be fatal. It is often underrecognized and undertreated in children. If treated promptly with pulsed cyclophosphamide and high-dose steroids prognosis is improved.

Takayasu's arteritis (pulseless disease)

This is a rare, chronic granulomatous panarteritis affecting the aorta and large arteries. Adolescent Asian (Japanese) girls and young women are most susceptible.

Clinical features

- *Subclinical prepulseless phase* may last years: Anorexia, fatigue, poor growth, unexplained fevers, and episodic arthritis (50%)
- *Pulseless phase*: Diagnoses are often made incidentally:
  - Diminished peripheral pulses and aortic dilatation on chest X-ray or hypertension and renal artery stenosis
  - Dramatic presentation with severe hypertensive encephalopathy and seizures; congestive cardiac failure; aortic valvulitis and aortic regurgitation; pulmonary stenosis
  - Syncope secondary to paroxysmal hypertension or paroxysmal tachycardia with facial-flushing headaches, chest pain, dyspnea, and palpitations
  - Ischemia, e.g., in extremities, intestines

Investigations

- *CBC* (normochromic normocytic anemia, thrombocytosis); ESR and γ-globulins are very elevated even in the prepulseless phase.
- *Imaging*: High-resolution carotid ultrasound, angiography, or MRA show characteristic arterial dilatation, post-stenotic dilatation, aneurysm, thrombosis, and occlusion of the proximal branches of the aorta.

Treatment

- Manage hypertension with β-blocker and ACE inhibitors. Avoid vasodilators.
- Treat vasculitis initially with high-dose steroids (1 mg/kg/day), with MTX or AZA as steroid-sparing drugs. Use cyclophosphamide or anti-TNF agents in resistant cases.
- Surgery ranges from angioplasty to bypass grafting.

Prognosis

The 10-year survival rate is 90%, although most patients (75%) have some impairment of daily living, and 50% are disabled. Prognosis depends on hypertension and aortic incompetence.

Adolescent health

Communication

One of the primary goals of providing care to the adolescent, regardless of the presenting complaint, is to establish a relationship of trust. Achieving effective and efficient communication with the adolescent may be very difficult and challenging.

When adolescents are undergoing rapid psychological and social change they may not have the adult perspective of health issues and society. Adolescents should be seen with and without the parent or caregiver. Parents should not be excluded, but it is important to emphasize that the adolescent is the priority of the visit.

Communication of information should be in a manner appropriate for developmental stage of the adolescent (see also p. 22).

Have a style of communication that is

- Open
- Sensitive
- Empathic
- Nonjudgmental

A sensitive and positive respect for any differing values and practices should be openly promoted. There must be repeated reassurances about confidentiality.

- Use an open-ended questioning style.
- Avoid medical jargon and inappropriate reassurance of normality.
- Alleviate fears and anxieties.
- Abstract concepts should be avoided.

The HEADS (expanded to HEAADSSS) protocol (Box 21.1) is a psychosocial history toolkit specifically designed for adolescent health-related consultations.

Box 21.1 HEAADSSS protocol

H   Home life including relationship with parents
E   Education or employment, including financial issues
A   Activities including sports (also note friendships and social relationships, especially close friendships)
A   Affect (mood, particularly whether mood is responsive to situations)
D   Drug use, including illegal substances, cigarettes and alcohol
S   Sex (information on intimate relationships and sexual risk behaviors may be important in both acute and chronic illnesses in adolescents)
S   Suicide, depression, and self harm
S   Sleep

Adapted from Goldenring JM, Cohen E (1988). Getting into adolescent heads. *Contemp Pediatr* **5**:75–80.

Adolescence: overview

Adolescence is the transition period between childhood and adulthood. A wide array of physical and psychological developmental tasks is achieved.

Physical and psychological objectives of adolescence
- Achievement of physical maturation
- Achievement of sexual maturation
- Attainment of personal identity
- Establishment of independence
- Establishment of autonomy
- Development of sexuality and sexual relationships

Adolescence is therefore filled with major changes that need to be taken into account when caring for adolescents with health-related problems.

Management of adolescents: keys areas for consideration
Communication issues
- Decision-making ability on and appreciation of adolescent-relevant issues
- Sexuality, substance use and abuse, tobacco use
- Mental health concerns

Physical examination
- Privacy and respect
- Personal integrity
- Pubertal assessment

Psychosocial issues
- Personal identity
- Adherence
- School achievement

Ethical and legal issues
- Consent
- Competence
- Confidentiality

All individuals working with adolescents need to acquire the appropriate skills to manage and communicate effectively with young people.

Psychological development
Adolescence marks the beginning of the development of more complex thinking processes:
- The ability for abstract thinking (thinking about possibilities)
- The ability to reason from known principles (form own new ideas or questions)
- The ability to consider many points of view according to different criteria (i.e., compare or debate ideas or opinions)
- The ability to think about the process of thinking.

During adolescence, young people acquire the ability to think systematically about logical relationships within a problem. Adolescents progress at varying rates in developing their ability to think in more complex ways. Some adolescents may be able to apply logical operations to schoolwork long before they are able to apply them to personal dilemmas and visa versa.

Emotional, family, or health issues often interfere with an adolescent's ability to think in more complex ways. The ability to consider possibilities, as well as facts, may influence decision making. Interactions between puberty and psychological development are important in the context of developing a sense of self, body image, and sexuality, as well as aspirations.

Social development

A gradual shift in the balance between dependence on others to a position of independence occurs during adolescence. This process is variable and will depend on the social and cultural context and environment.

There may be an early onset of adult behaviors as well as other behaviors that threaten the continued development of an adolescent into a healthy adult. Adolescents can display resilience to threats moderated with strong protective factors in self, family, or environment as they move toward independence.

Physical development

Psychological and social changes occur against a background of physical changes of puberty.

Adolescent health concerns

Adolescence is the period between 10 and 24 years of age. In the United States this accounts for 30% of the population.

Adolescent health status has not enjoyed the same progress as other age groups, reflecting fragmented health-care delivery to young people and lack of a systematic, evidence-based approach to adolescent health care. Access to best health-care practices for a culturally diverse adolescent population must also be addressed.

Adolescent mortality

Mortality rates in adolescents have not improved in recent years. The top three causes of death in this age group are accidents, homicide, and suicide.

Adolescent health problems

The pattern of adolescent illness is distinct. Common concerns of adolescents are summarized in Box 21.2.

Adolescent health problems that are largely preventable and/or treatable are often the result of early acquisition of adult behaviors:
• Substance misuse
• Sexual health problems
• Mental health problems (see Chapter 16)
• Obesity (see Chapter 12)

Box 21.2 Common adolescent-related health concerns

- Acne
- Chronic fatigue

Chronic illness
- Diabetes mellitus
- Asthma
- Cystic fibrosis
- Cancer
- Rheumatologic disorders

Somatic symptom disorders
- Chronic pain
- Headache
- Recurrent abdominal pain

Constitutional delay in growth and puberty
Substance abuse
- Alcohol
- Tobacco
- Illicit drugs
- Cannabis
- Prescription drug abuse
- Over-the-counter drug abuse

Psychological problems
- Attention-deficit hyperactivity disorder
- Anxiety disorders
- Conduct and behavior disorders
- Depression
- Eating disorders
  - Anorexia nervosa
  - Bulimia nervosa
- School phobia
- Stress-related symptoms

Gynecological disorders
- Oligomenorrhea, dysmenorrhea
- Menometrorrhagia
- Polycystic ovarian syndrome
- Structural abnormalities

Sexual health
Contraception
- Teenage pregnancy
- Sexually transmitted infections

Obesity
Sports-related injuries
- Overuse sports injuries
- Female athletic triad

Substance misuse

Substance abuse and/or misuse begin for most individuals during adolescence and is the cause of significant health and social problems. It can lead to years of loss of productivity that extend into adulthood.

Alcohol and tobacco are by far the most commonly used substances by adolescents and are thought to account for 95% of the morbidity and mortality in this age range. Most adolescents who use alcohol or tobacco regularly do not progress to using illegal or illicit substances. Most users of illicit drugs will have used alcohol and tobacco.

Only 20%–25% of the 1.4 million adolescents in the United States who are estimated to need substance abuse or dependence treatment actually receive any treatment.

- *Alcohol*: By the 12th grade of high school, 75% of adolescents will have had alcohol. Binge drinking is an increasing problem, with at least 25% of adolescents admitting to at least 5 drinks in a row over the last 30 days.
- *Tobacco*: 54% of adolescents state that they have tried cigarettes; 13% have used cigarettes daily and 16% began to use cigarettes before age 13.
- *Illicit drugs*: Cannabis is the most commonly used illicit substance worldwide. 31% of high school adolescents report using cannabis in the last year.

Prescription drug use for nonprescription purposes

Over the last decade there has been a steady increase in use of prescription drugs for nonmedical purposes. Currently, OxyContin, Vicodin, amphetamines, and dextromethorphan are some of the most commonly abused substances.

As many as 30% of adolescents have reported use one or more of these substances.

Management of suspected substance abuse and dependence

Risk factors for substance misuse
Psychosocial and behavioral disorders
- Behavioral problems
  - Conduct disorder
  - Depression
  - Post-traumatic stress
  - Eating disorders
- Familial factors
  - Favorable attitudes to substance use
  - Poor or inconsistent parenting practices
- Early-age experience of substance misuse
- Peer group pressure
- Poor social environment and relationships
  - Chronic illness

Signs of substance misuse

Nonspecific
- Emotional changes
- Personality changes
- Depression
- Mood swings
- Social difficulties
- Decline in school attendance and performance
- Behavior changes
- Physical changes, e.g., increased fatigue
- Parental anxiety

Specific
- Signs of drug usage
  - Pupil constriction
  - Skin changes: venipuncture marks, skin abscess
  - Blood pressure changes
  - Weight loss
- Withdrawal effects
  - Fatigue
  - Agitation, irritability
  - Tremor
  - Dilated pupils

Assessment of signs of substance dependence
- Difficulty controlling, ceasing, or limiting substance use in the face of unwanted consequences
- Tolerance—the need for greater amounts to achieve the same effect
- Signs and symptoms of withdrawal when substance is unavailable
- Treatment goal
- Attempt to decrease ambivalence around ceasing substance use and move adolescent through stages of change toward abstinence. Ultimately, a return to full function and continued development into a mature productive adult
- Sexual health (see also p. 928)

Further resources
- University of Michigan (2006). Monitoring the Future Study. Ann Arbor: University of Michigan,
- Substance Abuse and Mental Health Services Administration (2004). The National Household Survey on Drug Abuse (NHSDA) Report 2003–2004. Washington, DC: U.S. Department of Health and Human Services.

Sexual health

Promotion of good sexual health is a priority for adolescent care. Adolescents must have access to confidential health care for sexually related concerns.

The mean age of first sexual intercourse in the United States is estimated to be around 16.5 years of age. Among minority youth, this mean age is younger.

While the rate of vaginal intercourse among high school youth is declining, other sexual behaviors that increase risk for sexually transmitted infections (STIs) may be rising, such as oral and anal sexual behaviors. It is important to ask about these behaviors in history taking. Substance misuse may cause an adolescent to engage in high-risk sexual behaviors.

It is important to counsel young people regarding the risks of unprotected sexual contact and about the use of condoms and "safer" sexual practices.

Pap smear screening

Annual pap screening for young women should begin 3 years after becoming sexually active or by the age of 21. See the American Society for Colposcopy and Cervical Pathology 2007 guidelines for management of abnormal screening tests.

HPV vaccine

The human papillomavirus (HPV) vaccine is recommended for young women ages 9–26 years in a three-shot series at 0, 2, and 6 months. It is preferable that the vaccine be given prior to initiation of sexual activity or contact with the wart virus.

It is also recommended in women who may have been exposed to one or more genital wart types, as these women will still be protected against the other vaccine subtypes. The vaccine prevents vaccine type–related genital warts and cervical changes that can lead to cervical cancer.

Adolescent pregnancy

The United States still leads the fully industrialized world in teen pregnancy. The vast majority of teenage mothers never finish high school. Risk factors associated with teen pregnancy include the following:
- Poverty
- Low parental monitoring
- Having a sibling who is a teen parent
- Family history of teen parenting
- History of sexual abuse
- Low cognitive ability and low educational achievement
- Younger onset of sexual activity
- Older male partners
- Frequent office visits for pregnancy tests that are negative

Discussion of ambivalence about the desire for pregnancy may help teens make conscious decisions regarding contraception.

After a pregnancy is diagnosed, the teen should receive options counseling and an appropriate referral for continuation of care. Pregnant teens should be cautioned about avoiding tobacco, drug, and alcohol use, should be cautioned about avoiding tobacco, drug, and alcohol use, as well as about use of over-the-counter medications.

Sexual transmitted infections (STIs)

Sexually active women under 20 years of age have two to three times the chlamydial infection rate of adult women and should be screened annually. Teenage girls infected with *Chlamydia trachomatis* or *Neisseria gonorrhoeae* are at risk for developing upper reproductive tract infection or pelvic inflammatory disease, with subsequent complications of infertility, chronic pelvic pain, and ectopic pregnancy. When an STI is found, the provider should look for other infections, including syphilis and HIV.

Adolescents: risk factors for sexually transmitted infections
- Avoidance of barrier contraception methods
- Multiple, sequential, or concurrent partners
- Mental illness
- Substance misuse
- History of sexual abuse

The clinical symptoms and signs of STIs are similar to those experienced by adults, although in young teenage girls *Chlamydia* infection may present with vaginal discharge.
- Males
  - Asymptomatic—50%
  - Urethritis, dysuria, or discharge
- Females
  - Asymptomatic—70%
  - Vaginal discharge (especially early adolescence), dysuria
  - Pelvic inflammatory disease

For further information on the evaluation and up-to-date treatment of STIs, see the Web site of the Centers for Disease Control and Prevention (CDC) and the following sources:
- http://www.cdc.gov/STD/stats05/chlamydia.htm
- http://www.cdc.gov/STD/treatment/default.htm
- Centers for Disease Control and Prevention (CDC) (2005). National Youth Risk Behavior Survey. Atlanta: CDC,

Adolescence and chronic illness

A chronic illness is defined as a condition lasting 6 months. The number of young children surviving into young adulthood with a congenital or chronic health problem is increasing. The prevalence of certain chronic, lifelong conditions (e.g., type 2 diabetes) is increasing. It is estimated that 20%–30% of young people may have a chronic illness.

Impact on the adolescent

Compared to peers, teenagers with a chronic illness are disadvantaged in terms of their physical, psychological, emotional, and social development and well-being.

Consequences of chronic illness on adolescent development
Physical
• Constitutional delay in growth and pubertal development

Psychological
• Poor self-esteem
• Negative body self-image
• Sense of alienation
• Depression
• Anxiety, including concerns about sexual function and sexual relations
• Behavioral problems

Social and educational
• Poor school performance
• Social isolation and integration

Impact on the family

Parents must allow additional time for care and support of the teenager with a chronic illness, often suffering financial consequences. Parents may experience guilt, frustration, and anxiety. In this context, the frequency of parental mental health problems may be increased. Siblings are also disadvantaged, often missing out on parental time and attention.

Specific support agencies and child and adolescent psychology services are often required and may be helpful.

Impact on health professional relationships

Young people are usually more concerned about short-term issues and are less interested in the long-term consequences of their treatment. This often results in a conflict of priorities between health professionals (and parents) and the adolescent, and may lead to problems with treatment adherence. The following strategies may help with adherence.

Treatment discussions
• Make sure language is developmentally and cognitively appropriate
• Conduct discussions alone and in confidence
• Use a nonjudgmental approach
• Explore understanding of illness and treatment; correct misunderstanding and educate

- Identify potential barriers to adherence
- Use shared decision-making model
- Look for opportunities for agreed-upon small changes
- Avoid medical jargon
- Encourage treatment routine

Treatment goals

- Relevant to (current) adolescent issues—e.g., to appearance; socializing; recreational opportunities
- Include adolescent in negotiations
- Short-term (weeks–months)
- Use the simplest regimen possible
- Tailor to daily routine

Treatment application

- Provide written instructions
- Suggest simple reminder strategies, e.g., sticky notes, calendar
- Enlist support and help from parents, family, and peers
- Discussions of limit setting may be necessary, with recommended limits changing over time in response to both patient adherence and the stage of adolescent development.

Transition to adult health services

Adolescents requiring ongoing specialist hospital care will eventually need transfer to adult health-care services. This transition requires more than a simple transfer of medical records from one service to another. There are many different models of transition of care (e.g., direct pediatric to adult service or indirect via an intermediary adolescent or young-adult service).

A discussion of the eventual need for transition should start early (perhaps as soon as 14 years of age) and be planned so the adolescent patient and the family have time to consider it and prepare for it. The transition should take place when the adolescent is ready and has the necessary coping skills to deal with the adult clinic, rather than at a specific age.

Personalized transition plans are needed for each patient and careful communication, coordination, and organization are required between the pediatric and adult teams. Ensure that the reproductive health needs of these adolescents are addressed prior to or as part of this transition, including fertility and genetic counseling.

Adolescent health care: consent and confidentiality

In many ways, adolescents represent a unique population within pediatrics, particularly in terms of legal issues surrounding consent and confidentiality. The Society for Adolescent Medicine suggests that "Adolescents should be able to receive confidential services based on their own consent whenever limitations on confidentiality would serve as an obstacle impeding their access to care."[1]

Though adolescents under age 18 are still legally minors, there are situations in which teens can provide consent or are able to procure confidential care. An understanding of these situations is essential for any provider caring for adolescents (see also Chapter 31).

Consent

Issues of consent typically involve determining who is authorized and/or required to give consent for care.[2] The law generally requires parental or guardian consent before medical care can be provided to minors.

The HIPAA Privacy Rule is an example of a federal law that governs issues of consent of minors for health care. Under this rule, minors are considered "individuals" and allowed to exercise rights for themselves in three different situations.[3,4]

The first is when the minor has the right to consent and has consented. Examples of this include: emancipated minors, married minors and minors who are serving in the military.

There also are specific services that adolescents can often receive legally without parent or guardian consent. These services may include contraception, prenatal care, abortions, treatment for sexually transmitted infections, treatment for substance abuse and/or mental health services.

Laws governing the right of a minor to consent to these services vary from state to state. All practitioners working with adolescents should familiarize themselves with the relevant state and local laws and statutes regarding which services are available to adolescents without parent/guardian consent. One resource to identify state-specific policies regarding the above services is the Guttmacher Institute Web site (www.guttmacher.org).[5]

The second situation is when the minor may legally receive care without the consent of the parent, and the minor or another individual or a court has consented to the care. An example is when a court has allowed an adolescent to have an abortion without parental consent.

The third situation is when a parent has assented to an agreement of confidentiality between the health care provider and the minor. In the absence of a specific statute or law allowing a minor to consent for care, "mature minors" may also have the legal capacity to give consent for their own care. Practitioners should become familiar with the interpretation of the mature minor doctrine in their area.[2]

Confidentiality

Issues of confidentiality typically involve determining who has the right to control the release of confidential information about the care and who has the right to view this information.[2] Protecting adolescents' confidentiality encourages adolescents to seek necessary care and provide complete health information.

The HIPAA privacy rule states that an adolescent's adult guardian may access medical information about health services when the minor has not given consent or there is no agreement of confidentiality.[6] It is generally thought that when a minor can consent for care, the information regarding this care is to be kept confidential.

Under the HIPAA Privacy Rule, an adolescent minor would be able to access records for that care. The Health Insurance Portability and Accountability Act (HIPAA) Privacy Rule defers to state or other applicable law on the question of whether a parent can access records when a minor under the age of 18 has consented to care, or if there is an agreement of confidentiality.

Other laws may forbid access, require access, or allow providers discretion in the matter. Some states have adopted health privacy laws that explicitly specify when minors have authority over their own information and records, both confidential and nonconfidential.[3]

It is important to note that even when a minor is able to provide consent for confidential health care under the HIPAA privacy rule, certain legal and ethical limits apply. These limits are generally thought to include when an adolescent expresses intent to hurt themselves or others, or if child abuse has occurred.[2]

Practical issues and recommendations

- Practitioners should be aware of the laws and statutes governing minor consent and confidentiality in their area.
- When possible, practitioners should meet with adolescents alone for part of the visit and should make certain that the adolescents are aware of their rights with respect to confidentiality and consent.
- Although access to confidential health care is essential for appropriate health care of adolescent patients, this does not mean that parents should always be excluded. It is frequently beneficial to teens to work with them on including their parents when dealing with difficult issues, even if the law does not require it.

1 Society for Adolescent Medicine (2004). Access to Health Care for Adolescents and Young Adults: Position Paper for the Society for Adolescent Medicine. *J Adolesc Health* **35**(4):342–344.
2 English A (2002). Understanding legal aspects of care. In Neinstein LS (ed.), *Adolescent Health Care*. Philadelphia: Lippincott Williams and Wilkins, pp. 186–196.
3 English A, Kenney KE (2003). *State Minor Consent Laws: A Summary*. Chapel Hill, NC: Center for Adolescent Health and the Law.
4 Wibbelsman CJ (1997). Confidentiality in an age of managed care: Can it exist? *J Adolesc Health* **8**(3):427–432.
5 Boonstra H, Nash E (2000). *Minors and the Right to Consent to Health Care*, The Guttmacher Report on Public Policy. New York: The Guttmacher Institute.
6 Health Insurance Portability and Accountability Act of 1996 (HIPAA).

Dermatology

Assessment of a rash

History
- When did the rash start?
- Any exacerbating and relieving factors?
- Any contacts with the same rash?
- Recent medications or skin treatments?
- Family history?
- Where did the rash start?
- Is it itchy?
- General drug history?
- Past medical history?
- Any recent foreign travel?

Examination
Have the child undress, and inspect all the skin.
- Describe primary lesion morphology:
    - *Macule*: Flat, circumscribed lesion <1 cm diameter
    - *Papule*: Raised, palpable, circumscribed lesion <1 cm diameter
    - *Nodule*: Palpable mass >1 cm diameter
    - *Plaque*: Large, raised, disc-shaped lesion >1 cm diameter
    - *Patch*: Flat, circumscribed lesion >1 cm diameter
    - *Vesicle*: Blister containing clear fluid <0.5 cm diameter
    - *Bulla*: Blister containing clear fluid >0.5 cm diameter
    - *Pustule*: Visible blister containing pus
    - *Erythematous*: Blanching and red
    - *Purpura*: Red–purple nonblanching discoloration of the skin (due to extravasation of red cells)
    - *Petechiae*: Purpuric lesions <2 mm diameter
    - *Telangiectasia*: Permanently dilated visible, small blood vessels that blanch on pressure
    - *Wheal*: Raised, itchy, white papule surrounded by red flare
    - *Scaly*: Dry, flaking skin

Describe distribution of primary lesion, e.g., diffusely scattered, linear.
- Look for and describe the following:
    - Secondary changes, e.g., excoriation (scratch marks)
    - Pigmentation
    - Scarring
    - Atrophy (thinning of the skin)
    - Lichenification (skin thickening)
    - Sclerosis (induration of skin, often due to increased collagen production)
    - Erosion (partial-thickness loss of epidermis)
    - Ulceration (full-thickness loss of epidermis and possibly dermis)
    - Crusting (due to dried exudates)
- Palpate. The lesion may be impalpable, hard, firm, soft, tender, or hot. If the lesion is red, test whether it blanches on pressure.
- Conduct general examination, taking care to examine the nails, scalp, and mouth.

Atopic dermatitis (eczema)

The terms *atopic dermatitis* and *eczema* are interchangeable.
- 15%–20% incidence during childhood in developed countries
- M=F occurrence
- 60% of cases present during infancy (85% before age 5 years)

The cause is multifactorial and includes the following factors:
- *Genetic*: 70% have a positive family history of atopy.
- *Immune*: Hyperresponsive epidermal Langerhans cells, T-cell activation
- *Allergic*: Raised serum IgE level is present in ~80% of cases and various allergens such as animals or foods may exacerbate eczema.
- *Infection*: Endotoxins from *Staph. aureus* skin colonization.

Presentation (see Plate 1)
Early
- Erythema
- Scaling
- Itching
- Excoriation
- Weeping
- Rarely vesicles
- Sleep disturbance
- Secondary infection

Late
- Skin lichenification; pigmentation changes
- Distribution of typical skin involvement is age-dependent.
    - *Infancy*: Face, trunk, perineum, and limb extensor surfaces
    - *Childhood*: Antecubital fossa, knee flexures, and neck
    - *Adolescence*: Hands, feet, and limb flexural surfaces

Treatment
- *Avoid irritants*: Avoid soap, bubble baths, shampoo, overheating, itchy clothing (recommend cotton).
- *Allergens*: Avoid allergens, e.g., pets, foods.
- *Topical emollients*: Apply at least 4 times daily, e.g., aqueous cream. Consider emulsifying ointment soap-substitute ± bath oil.
- *Topical steroids*: Intermittent use (hydrocortisone 1% initially, increase potency as required) for acute exacerbations. Steroid ointments are preferred over creams. Occlusive steroid dressings may be required if rash is severe.
- *Topical steroid-sparing agents*: Treatments such as topical tacrolimus should be considered as a second-line therapy in children requiring frequent topical steroid use (in children >2 years).
- *Sedatives*: Oral antihistamines ± cotton mittens to ease nighttime itching and allow sleep
- *Oral antibiotics*: Antistaphylococcal/antistreptococcal agent for secondary infection. Antiseptic washes may prevent recurrent infection.
- *Hospitalization* for severe cases needing IV antibiotics for diffuse secondary infection and aggressive skin therapy

Complications
- Sleep disturbance
- Emotional upset
- Secondary infection, e.g., staphylococcal (may lead to scalded skin syndrome)
- Eczema herpeticum

Prognosis
Over 60% of cases resolve by age 13 years. The remaining patients may develop chronic relapsing adult disease.

Prevention
In those with a strong family history, incidence may be reduced by
- Breast-feeding
- Use of hypoallergenic milks if formula is required, e.g., Nutramigen
- Delayed introduction of common food allergens in infancy, e.g., cow's milk protein

Eczema herpeticum
This type of eczema results from herpes simplex virus (HSV) type I infection in a child with active atopic dermatitis. HSV can be detected in vesicular fluid by viral culture or immunofluorescence.

The initial widespread vesicular rash becomes pustular and crusts over. The patient may develop
- Fever
- Severe systemic illness
- Lymphadenopathy.
- HSV keratitis

Treatment
Treatment is unnecessary if the eczema is localized and the child is well. Give IV aciclovir if it is widespread or unwell or involving the eyes. Generally resolves within 4 weeks. This condition is rarely fatal.

Red scaly rashes

Atopic dermatitis (see p. 938)

Psoriasis

Psoriasis is a common, chronic, relapsing and remitting disease. it may affect any age but usually >5 years. It is characterized by epidermal proliferation, hyperkeratosis, and T-cell-driven inflammatory infiltration of the epidermis and dermis. Although its cause is unknown there is an important genetic component (30% of patients have a parent affected). Infections (guttate psoriasis secondary to streptococcal infection) or drugs (β-blockers, antimalarials) can trigger disease. It is associated with IBD.

Presentation (see Plate 2)
- Multiple, discrete, large, red patches and plaques with overlying thick silvery scales
- Particularly affects extensor limb surfaces, scalp, and anogenital area
- Mild pruritus is common.
- Nails are often involved with pitting, distal nail separation from the nail bed (onycholysis), and thickening, ridges.
- Psoriatic arthropathy may develop (p. 901).
- Variants include
  - Generalized guttate (small) psoriasis of the trunk (lasts 3–4 months)
  - Pustular psoriasis (microabscesses and scaling of palms or soles)
  - Koebner phenomenon (psoriasis along site of skin trauma)

Treatment
In stepwise manner:
- Remove any precipitating triggers.
- Apply simple emollients 3–4 times daily.
- Use topical steroids.
- Use tar-based/salicylic acid creams and shampoos for the scalp.
- In older children only, apply topical calcipotriol (vitamin D derivative).
- Severe cases may require tar baths; ultraviolet radiation ± oral psoralen (PUVA); topical dithranol pastes (side effects include burning, skin staining); oral etretinate; oral cytotoxics, e.g., methotrexate, cyclosporine; or newer biologics, e.g., etanercept.

Prognosis
Prognosis may be life-long or spontaneously remit.

Contact dermatitis

This skin disorder may be irritant or allergic (delayed hypersensitivity type IV reaction). Diaper dermatitis is caused by the caustic effect of irritant ammonia released from urine and feces by bacteria, as well as increased wetness and skin pH, and frictional damage.

Common causes of allergic contact dermatitis include the following:
- Plants (e.g., poison ivy)
- Nickel
- Chromium
- Rubber
- Colophony (e.g., in sticking bandages, glues)
- Drugs (e.g., topical antibiotics)

Presentation (see Plate 3)
- Itchy eczematous rash, usually localized. Skin patch testing can be used to identify the offending allergen(s).

Treatment
- Irritant and allergen avoidance
- Emollients
- Topical steroids (severe)

Prognosis
Recovery occurs once the offending agent is removed.

Seborrheic dermatitis (see p. 12)

Pityriasis rosea

This is a self-limiting condition that is common between ages 1 and 6 years.

Cause
It is probably a secondary reaction to viral infections (possibly human herpes viruses 6 or 7).

Presentation
- Distinctive initial truncal (usually) oval, red, scaly "herald patch" (2–5 cm diameter)
- Several days later, generalized smaller, scaly, yellowish-pink patches develop over the trunk and proximal limbs.
- Characteristic "Christmas tree" distribution is common: the patches follow lines parallel to the ribs.
- Pruritus, malaise, and lymphadenopathy may occur.

Treatment
Treatment is offering reassurance. Antipruritics may be required.

Prognosis
The condition resolves after 4–6 weeks.

Tinea infections (see p. 962)

Papular rashes (1)

Urticaria (hives)

Acute urticaria affects 10% of the population at some time.

Pathophysiology

Adverse stimulus → mast cell degranulation → histamine release → localized vasodilatation and capillary permeability.

Causes

These rashes are usually idiopathic or triggered by viral infection. Other causes include the following:

- Allergens (e.g., drugs, foods, inhalants, insect bites)
- Trauma (physical urticarias), e.g., dermographism due to light skin trauma (most common), pressure, cold, heat, and sunlight

Chronic urticaria (acute urticaria not resolving after 2 months) is idiopathic in >90% of cases but may be caused by

- Chronic bacterial, fungal (e.g., oral candida), or parasitic infection
- Ingested food dyes (rare)

Presentation (see Plate 4)

- Rapidly developing erythematous eruption with raised, central white wheals and occasionally local purpura
- Any part of body can be affected and is often itchy.
- Lesions last 4–24 hours.
- The patient may have associated fever and arthralgia (serum sickness).

Investigation

Apart from a good history investigation, other tests are usually not necessary. Skin prick testing is rarely helpful. If the condition is chronic, consider the following:

- CBC
- Throat swab (streptococcus)
- Urine culture
- Exclude pinworms
- Food and symptom diary

Treatment

- Oral antihistamines, e.g., chlorpheniramine
- Oral prednisolone, give short course if condition is severe
- Avoid triggering factors, e.g., ingested food dyes and drugs.

Angioedema

Angioedema is a variant of urticaria with significant swelling of subcutaneous tissues, often involving the lips, eyelids, genitalia, tongue, or larynx. If severe, it may cause acute upper or lower respiratory tract obstruction and may be life threatening.

Causes

Causes are the same as those for urticarial. Hereditary angioedema is a rare autosomal dominant condition caused by C_1-esterase inhibitor deficiency or dysfunction.

Investigations and management

These are the same as those for urticaria. If hereditary angioedema is suspected, measure serum C4 complement level initially.

Treatment

For severe angioedema:

- Give oxygen by mask
- IM 0.01 mg/kg epinephrine 1:1000
- IM/IV hydrocortisone 12 hourly
- Nebulized albuterol

For prophylaxis in severe and recurring cases of hereditary angioedema, use tranexamic acid (not currently available in the U.S.) or anabolic steroids (e.g., danazol boosts liver production of C1-esterase inhibitor). The latter is rarely used in childhood because of its androgenic effects.

Molluscum contagiosum

This is a common pox virus infection that affects infants and young children.

Presentation

Multiple discrete pearly-pink papules with central depression affect mostly the trunk, face, and anogenital areas. It is exacerbated by active eczema or topical steroids.

Treatment

There is none if the condition is uncomplicated, as it usually resolves spontaneously within a year.

If symptoms are problematic:

- Treat any associated eczema.
- Topical cantharidin, washed off in 2–6 hours
- Topical tretinoin cream (good for facial lesions)
- Topical salicylic acid
- Topical 5% potassium hydroxide
- Liquid nitrogen cryotherapy
- Lesion curettage if the child is able to tolerate this

Scabies (see p. 964)

Viral warts (see p. 960)

Papular rashes (2)

Papular urticaria

Hypersensitivity reaction to insect bites results in itchy small, red papules or vesicles evolve into 1- to 5-mm papules ± surrounding urticaria or surface crusting, usually on the limbs and buttocks. They may last for weeks and be exacerbated by new bites elsewhere. Secondary infection is common.

Treatment
• Prevent new bites
• Antipruritics (e.g., oral antihistamines, topical steroids)
• Antibiotics for any secondary infection.

Keratosis pilaris

This is very common and occurs at any age. Horny plugging of follicles causes asymptomatic, rough papular rash ± erythema. It affects the upper outer arms, thighs, and cheeks.

Treatment
Treatment consists of reassurance, as well as emollients, especially urea-based creams.

Papular acrodermatitis (Gianotti–Crosti syndrome) (see Plate 5)

Acute, non-itchy, red papules appear over the face, limbs, and buttocks, sparing the trunk. The condition can be asymptomatic or accompanied by malaise, hepatomegaly, or lymphadenopathy.

Causes
• Enteroviruses
• Epstein–Barr virus
• Adenovirus
• Mycoplasma

Treatment
• Reassurance

The rash spontaneously resolves after a few weeks.

Vesiculobullous rashes

Erythema multiforme

Cause

This is an immunologically mediated syndrome. It may be idiopathic but is usually precipitated by infection (e.g., mycoplasma, herpes simplex, or other viruses) or drugs (e.g., sulfonamides, penicillin).

Presentation (see Plate 6)

- Crops of characteristic symmetric "target" lesions develop with a pallid or purple center surrounded by an erythematous ring.
- There may also be hemorrhagic, red macules, or large bullae.
- Lesions last 2–3 weeks and affect the hands, feet, elbows, and knees.
- Typically, mucous membrane ulcers occur (oral, eye, genitalia).

Treatment

If precipitating infection recurs, treat it early, as it tends to cause rash again, e.g., with topical or oral acyclovir for recurrent HSV.

- Fluid maintenance
- Analgesic mouthwashes
- Lip emollient ointment
- Oral antihistamines.

Prognosis

There is complete recovery, but the condition may recur.

Stevens–Johnson syndrome/toxic epidermal necrolysis

This syndrome consists of severe and overlapping conditions.

Presentation (see Plate 7)

- Widespread blisters/bullae over erythematous, purple macular, or hemorrhagic skin
- Mucous membranes are often affected with hemorrhagic crusting.
- Rubbing may cause skin separation at the dermoepidermal junction (positive Nikolsky sign).
- Also possible are fever, arthralgia, myalgia, prostration, renal failure, pneumonitis, conjunctivitis, corneal ulceration, and blindness.

Treatment

- Supportive, as for severe burns (e.g., hydration, airway protection)
- Identify causative antigen and remove it or treat it.
- Frequent emollient ointment
- Specialist eye care
- ? Systemic corticosteroids or immunoglobulin used in the first 2–3 days may be helpful if the condition is life threatening.

Prognosis

This disorder can be life threatening. Recovery usually occurs in 3–4 weeks.

Staphylococcal scalded-skin syndrome

This syndrome consists of exotoxin-mediated epidermolysis from *Staphylococcus aureus* infection (which may be trivial). It occurs in children <5 years.

Presentation
- Extensive tender erythema with flaccid blisters or bullae ("scalded appearance")
- Erosions and positive Nikolsky sign
- Crusting around the eyes and mouth, fever

Treatment
- Supportive treatment and analgesia
- IV antistaphylococcal antibiotics
- Gentle skin care, emollient ointments

Prognosis
- Rapid recovery without scarring

Impetigo

Impetigo is a highly contagious *Staphylococcus aureus* or β-hemolytic streptococcal superficial skin infection. It may be primary or complicate other skin disease (e.g., HSV infection, eczema, scabies). Risk factors include overcrowding and poor hygiene.

Presentation
- Superficial, rapidly spreading, initially clear blisters or erythematous oozing areas that rapidly develop into straw-colored "dirty"-looking lesions with yellow crusting
- It often starts around the nose and face; neonates may develop bullous impetigo.
- Risk of staphylococcal scalded-skin syndrome (*Staphylococcus*) or acute glomerulonephritis (*Streptococcus*)

Investigation
- Skin swabs for bacterial culture and sensitivity

Treatment
Impetigo rapidly resolves with the following:
- Bathe crusts off, using antiseptic (they contain infectious bacteria).
- Give antibiotics (e.g., topical mupirocin 2% ointment or oral cephalexin).
- Treat any predisposing condition.

Eczema herpeticum (see p. 939)

Traumatic blisters

These are caused by friction, burns, or insect bites. Sterile aspiration of the blister within 12 hours after appearance and pressure dressing may be curative.

Epidermolysis bullosa (see p. 974 and Plate 8)

Red blanching (erythematous) rashes

The causes for these rashes vary with age. Viral causes are most common in younger children. In older children, eczema, psoriasis, and drug reactions (e.g., reaction to ampicillin in mononucleosis) predominate.

Viruses (exanthem) (see p. 816)

Culprits include the following:
- Adenovirus
- Coxsackie
- Echovirus
- Epstein–Barr virus
- Influenza
- Parainfluenza
- Human herpes virus 6 (roseola infantum)
- Parvovirus B19 (erythema infectiosum)
- Rubella
- Measles

These rashes are usually associated with fever and a widespread non-specific erythematous rash that may be macular or macular–papular. If the child is significantly unwell or lethargic or peripheral perfusion is reduced, admit the child and investigate their condition (may be bacterial sepsis). Otherwise, provide reassurance and advise symptomatic treatment.

Drug eruptions

Erythematous macular–papular rash is most common (e.g., to penicillins, cephalosporins, anticonvulsants). Drugs may also cause the following:
- Urticaria (e.g., opiates, ACE inhibitors, penicillins, cephalosporins, NSAIDs)
- Exfoliative dermatitis (e.g., sulfonamides, allopurinol, carbamazepine, gold)
- Erythema multiforme or Stevens–Johnson syndrome/toxic epidermal necrolysis (e.g., anticonvulsants)

Treatment
- Discontinue offending drug (prick or patch testing may be required to identify it).
- Symptomatic treatment (e.g., antihistamines and/or emollients for pruritus)

Erysipelas and cellulitis

These conditions overlap. Erysipelas is a superficial skin infection whereas cellulitis involves deeper subcutaneous tissues. They are usually due to *Strep pyogenes* or *Staph. aureus*; occasionally *H. influenzae* type B is the cause in young children.

Presentation
- Tender, spreading, sharply marginated erythema with edema
- May also have ascending red streaks of lymphangitis
- Regional lymphadenopathy, fever, malaise
- Deeper infection may coexist, e.g., osteomyelitis.

Management
- Blood culture
- If erysipelas occurs alone, give IV penicillin (erythromycin if patient is penicillin-allergic).
- *Cellulitis*: Raise the affected part (e.g., limb); consider IV penicillin or nafcillin depending on the suspected organism. If MRSA is suspected, you may need to start with IV vancomycin. Consider cefotaxime instead of penicillin if the child is <5 years of age and not immunized against *Haemophilus*.

Erythema marginatum

Crops of prominent, evanescent, pink truncal rings (lesions fading within hours, only to recur) are caused by rheumatic fever. Lesions are seen more easily in the afternoon. No treatment is required.

Erythema nodosum

This typically affects older children. It is caused by an immunological reaction to the following:
- Tuberculosis
- Streptococcal infection
- Mycoplasma infection
- IBD
- Sulfonamides, oral contraceptive pills, penicillins
- Viruses
- Pregnancy
- Idiopathic (30%)

Presentation
Multiple discrete, large, red, hot, tender nodules appear on the shins, occasionally the thighs and forearms. They appear over 10 days before resolving over 3–6 weeks, with color changes similar to fading bruises. Fever, malaise, and arthralgia, particularly of the knees, may also occur.

Treatment
Treat the underlying disease; use analgesics.

Sunburn

Sunburn is caused by excessive UV light exposure. Midday sun avoidance, skin covering, hats, and water-resistant high-factor sunscreens are preventative! Fair-skinned individuals, infants, and those with preexisting hypopigmented disorders are at particular risk.

Presentation
- Painful, tender erythema ± blistering over exposed area. Resolves with skin peeling

Treatment
- Cool compresses or cool tub baths
- Antipyretics
- Analgesics
- Topical calamine lotion
- Topical corticosteroids if severe

Intertrigo

Cause
- Excessive friction between skin surfaces
- Obesity is a predisposing factor.

Presentation
- Moist, erythematous eruption typically affects the groin, axillae, neck, and submammary areas.
- Secondary *Candida* infection is common.

Treatment
- Treat associated infection, e.g., with topical antibiotic.
- Improve general hygiene.
- Expose affected area to air.
- Talc application or topical steroid may be helpful.

Kawasaki disease (see p. 830)

Septicemia

Meningococcal disease, as well as other bacterial pathogens, can present with an erythematous rash (see p. 836).

Pruritus

Pruritis is the sensation provoking a desire to scratch. If severe it leads to excoriation, papules or nodules (localized skin thickening), and lichenification.

Generalized pruritus

Causes

- Skin diseases (see below)
- Hepatic disease (bile salts)
- Food or drug reaction or allergy (e.g., penicillin)
- Underlying malignancy, particularly lymphoma
- Chronic renal failure
- Hypo- or hyperthyroidism
- Parasites (e.g., scabies)
- Iron deficiency anemia

Investigation

In the absence of obvious underlying skin disease:

- CBC
- Blood smear
- CRP/ESR
- Ferritin
- LFTs
- BUN
- Creatinine
- Urinalysis
- Glucose
- TFT

Treatment

- Treat causative disease.
- Bland topical emollients
- Emollient bath oils
- Nighttime sedative, e.g., antihistamines

Localized pruritus

Causes

- Atopic dermatitis (cheeks, hands, and limb flexures)
- Contact dermatitis
- Urticaria
- Insect bites
- Fungal infection (e.g., tinea capitis)
- Head lice (pediculosis capitis)
- Scabies (finger webs, wrists, groin, buttocks)
- Psoriasis
- Dermatitis herpetiformis (elbows, shoulders, genitalia, perineum, buttocks)
- Pityriasis rosea
- Chicken pox
- Dermatitis artefacta (!)

Investigation

In the absence of obvious underlying skin disease, investigate as for generalized pruritus.

Treatment

- As for generalized pruritis

Pruritus ani

- Localized perianal itching

Causes

- Pinworms
- Anal disease (e.g., anal fissure, hemorrhoids, Crohn's disease)
- Poor hygiene
- Chronic fecal soiling
- Chronic diarrhea
- Localized skin disease (e.g., candidiasis, psoriasis)
- Contact dermatitis (e.g., to toilet paper)
- Idiopathic

Investigation

Pinworms may be seen during anal inspection or their eggs seen on microscopy of cellophane tape applied to the anus; get skin swab culture.

Treatment

- Treat underlying disease.
- Improve perianal hygiene.
- A mild topical steroid may relieve symptoms once the infective cause is excluded.

Pruritus vulvae

This involves localized perivulval itching.

Causes

- Idiopathic
- Poor hygiene
- Infection (e.g., candidiasis, trichomoniasis)
- Diabetes mellitus
- Pinworms
- Contact dermatitis
- Localized skin disease (see pruritus ani), e.g., lichen sclerosus et atrophicus

Treatment

- As for pruritus ani

Pustular rashes

Generalized pustulosis is unusual. When the child is <2 years old, immunodeficiency, particularly phagocyte dysfunction, should be excluded. Local causes in older children include the following:

- Acne vulgaris
- Folliculitis
- Impetigo (p. 832)
- Scabies (p. 964)
- Perioral dermatitis
- Pustular psoriasis (p. 940)

Acne vulgaris

This is an inflammatory disorder that affects teenagers and is characterized by pilosebaceous follicles of the face, neck, upper chest, and back.

Cause

The cause of acne is a combination of sebum production resulting from a pubertal androgen surge, abnormal keratinization and desquamation causing follicle blockage (comedones—"blackheads" or "whiteheads"), anaerobic *Propionibacterium* acne proliferation within the follicle, and a subsequent localized inflammatory response. Maternal androgens (neonatal acne) or corticosteroids (medication or excess endogenous production) can also induce acne (investigate if acne develops before puberty).

Presentation

"Blackheads," "whiteheads," papules, pustules, nodules, cysts, and scarring can occur.

Treatment

Treat in stepwise fashion:

- Topical keratolytic, e.g., benzoyl peroxide 2.5%–10%, salicylic acid, azelaic acid
- Topical antibiotic, e.g., clindamycin, erythromycin, sulfacetamide
- Topical retinoid, e.g., tretinoin, adapalene, tazarotene
- 6 months oral antibiotic, e.g., tetracycline, doxycycline, minocycline, erythromycin (moderate severity only)
- Hormonal therapy, e.g., oral contraceptive pill, spironolactone
- 4–6 months oral isotretinoin if case is severe or unresponsive to above treatment (side effects are teratogenic, headaches, myalgia, dry skin or mucous membranes, sun photosensitivity, possible depression)
- Avoid teen pregnancy. Regulated through national "iPLEDGE" program

Prognosis

Acne resolves but may persist for years. Include psychological support.

Purpuric rashes

Causes
- Viral infections, most commonly enteroviral
- Septicemia, most commonly meningococcal (p. 82)
- Thrombocytopenia, platelet or clotting disorders (p. 740)
- Vasculitis, e.g., Henoch–Schönlein purpura (HSP) (p. 913 and Plate 9). Lesions are painful.
- Trauma, including nonaccidental injury
- Drug reactions
- Vasomotor straining, e.g., strenuous coughing or isometric exercise

Management
If the patient is well and there is an obvious benign cause, reassure the patient that this will resolve spontaneously. If the cause is unclear, initial investigations should include the following:
- CBC
- Blood smear
- Clotting studies
- Blood cultures
- Check blood pressure, urinalysis, blood electrolytes, BUN and creatinine, and ASO titer (if HSP is likely).
- Consider a skin biopsy if the diagnosis is unclear.

If sepsis is suspected, admit the patient and start IV antibiotics. Stop any drug likely to be causative.

Lymphedema

Diffuse soft-tissue edema is caused by inadequate lymphatic drainage, which in turn may be due to a developmental defect, e.g., congenital lymphedema (isolated or part of Turner's syndrome) or cystic hygroma (which also commonly has a vascular component). Secondary causes include surgical lymphatic destruction, malignant infiltration, irradiation, recurrent lymphangitis, and parasitic infestation (in the tropics, filariasis or elephantiasis).

Presentation

- Pitting, firm swelling
- ± Hypertrophy of affected limb
- Lymphangiography may be helpful to identify the area of obstruction.

Treatment

Treatment is often difficult. Limb elevation, massage, pressure garments, or diuretics may be helpful. Give oral penicillin prophylaxis against increased risk of erysipelas.

Blood vessel disorders

Telangiectasia

Telangiectasias are permanently dilated small vessels, the most common ones being spider angiomas (e.g., dilated capillaries radiating from the central arteriole). Less than 5 is considered normal. Laser or cautery of the central vessel is sometimes required. Five or more telangiectasias may be part of

- Hereditary hemorrhagic telangiectasia (autosomal dominant genetic disorder with telangiectasia on lip, tongue, and nasal epithelium, risking recurrent epistaxis ± GI hemorrhage)
- Ataxia telangiectasia (p. 622)
- Hereditary benign telangiectasia

Vascular malformations

Superficial capillary nevi

These are characterized by salmon patches and stork bites (see p. 122).

Port wine stain (nevus flammeus) (see Plate 10)

Developmental capillary malformation is evident at birth, with a vivid red or purple patch. It may affect any site, but the face and neck are the most common sites. Involvement of the eye is associated with glaucoma, ophthalmic division of trigeminal nerve with Sturge–Weber syndrome (seizures, hemiplegia, and mental retardation).

Klippel–Trenaunay syndrome

This syndrome comprises a triad of vascular malformations, venous varicosities, and hyperplasia of soft tissue ± bone. The lower limb is the most common location.

Treatment

Treatment is with repeated laser therapy, cosmetics, and surgery. Lesions may become darker and hypertrophic with age.

Infantile hemangiomas

These may be superficial (e.g., "strawberry" hemangioma), deep, or mixed (e.g., combined superficial and deep). Most present after birth anywhere on the body, and are more common in females and ex-preterm infants (see Plate 11). Superficial hemangiomas start as erythematous macules that rapidly grow into bright red papules. Deeper lesions appear as bluish subcutaneous lesions with an indistinct border. Superficial and deeper hemangiomas grow for ~9 months before resolving over several years.

Treatment

Provide reassurance. Laser treatment, intralesional or systemic corticosteroids, interferon therapy, embolization, and surgery are restricted to lesions that cause ulceration, deformity, or interference (e.g., airway or nasal hemangiomas).

Perniosis (chilblains)

This is an abnormal reaction to cold with local, inflammatory, red–blue lesions on the extremities (e.g., digits, ears). On rewarming, pain or itching occurs. Lesions may ulcerate. They resolve spontaneously. This reaction is prevented by warm clothing and housing!

Raynaud's syndrome

Episodic artery spasm causes digital ischemia. The syndrome is precipitated by cold, finger constriction (shopping bags), or emotion. Most cases improve with age. The syndrome may be idiopathic (Raynaud's disease) or secondary (Raynaud's phenomenon) to

- Systemic sclerosis
- Arterial occlusion (e.g., cervical rib)
- Occlusive arterial disease

Presentation

Fingers ache, burn, or tingle with color changes of pallor (ischemia)—blue (cyanosis) and red (reactive hyperemia).

Treatment

- Treat underlying disease.
- Local warmth
- Nifedipine; sympathectomy (if severe and recurrent)

Skin infection: viral and bacterial

Viral

Warts

Warts are very common. They usually resolve spontaneously within 3 years. They are caused by infection with papilloma virus. Warts may affect individuals of any age, but mainly school-aged children. They are painless, firm papules with a rough, hyperkeratotic surface. Capillary ends can usually be seen superficially. Typically they affect the hands, knees, face, and feet.

- Plantar warts (verrucae) may be painful due to pressure-induced ingrowing.
- Genital or perianal warts (condyloma acuminata) may occur and, although sexual abuse should be considered, causation is commonly innocent.

Treatment

Treatment is not usually needed. If they are painful or embarrassing:

- Keratolytic agent (e.g., salicylic acid)
- Liquid nitrogen cryotherapy
- Immunotherapy
- Surgical removal or laser therapy (rarely used in children)

Molluscum contagiosum (see p. 816 and Plate 12)

Herpes simplex (HSV)

Most cases are due to type I HSV. Type II HSV typically causes genital herpes. Coinfection with active atopic dermatitis causes eczema herpeticum (p. 939).

Primary infection

Typically this occurs in preschool children, with sore throat, stomatitis, vesicles or ulceration involving the mouth, lip, and face, and fever. It resolves within 2 weeks.

- Secondary bacterial infection frequently occurs.
- Treat with antipyretics, analgesic mouthwashes or throat lozenges, and topical acyclovir cream. Consider intravenous fluids if the child becomes dehydrated due to reluctance to swallow. Treat bacterial secondary infection.

Secondary reactivation

This manifests initially as an itch or tingling, followed by localized vesicles, which then break down. Typically they are perioral (cold sores). The reactivation may be idiopathic but can be precipitated by illness, immunosuppression, or menstruation. Early topical acyclovir cream aborts the episode or reduces its severity.

Chicken pox (varicella) (see p. 824)

This is a very contagious infection due to varicella zoster virus. Chicken pox starts with fever, followed by pruritic vesicular eruption over the trunk spreading to the face, mouth, and limbs. Lesions evolve at different rates so that macules, papules, vesicles, and pustules will all be present at once. Secondary bacterial skin infection may occur. Illness may cause life-threatening pneumonitis in congenital infection, older teenagers, or immunosuppressed patients. Infectivity lasts until the FINAL vesicle crusts over.

Treatment
- Antipyretics
- Oral antihistamines
- Cooling baths
- Topical calamine lotion.
- IM human-specific varicella zoster immunoglobulin (VZIG) should be given early if there is a risk of severe illness (IV acyclovir in severe illness).

Reactivation (shingles)
Shingles can occur in childhood, particularly when varicella occurs at <1 year old. It may be severe in immunosuppressed individuals. It presents with localized unilateral pain, itching, or hyperesthesia, followed by vesicular eruption in the distribution of the affected dorsal root ganglia. Treat with oral acyclovir if disease is severe and with topical antibiotics if there is secondary bacterial infection.

Hand, foot, and mouth disease
Infection is with Coxsackie or enterovirus 71, usually in preschool children. Painful, small vesicles (may be linear or oval) affect the mouth (stomatitis), palms, and soles and occasionally the diaper area. Lesions spontaneously resolve within 10 days. Treatment is symptomatic.

Bacterial
Impetigo (see p. 832)
Erysipelas/cellulitis (see p. 832)
Furuncle (boil)
A confluence of furuncles = a carbuncle. Hair-follicular abscess is usually due to *Staphylococcus aureus* infection. Boils are common in postpubertal males. A tender superficial, red papule develops into a large, painful, inflamed pustule that ultimately discharges superficially. They affect mainly hairy areas such as the back, axilla, and buttocks. They can be associated with diabetes mellitus, obesity, and poor hygiene. Chronic carriers of *Staph. aureus* are particularly predisposed. Treatment is with warm, moist compresses several times a day. Recurrent or severe furuncles require surgical drainage, oral cephalexin or flucloxicillin, and daily chlorhexidine baths to decrease *Staph. aureus* skin colonization.

Fungal and other agents

Dermatophyte infection

Tinea corporis (ringworm)

Ringworm produces a circular scaly lesion with sharp edge on the trunk, face or limbs. It slowly grows outward with central clearing. Investigation includes skin scrapings for microscopy and culture.

Treatment
- Topical antifungals, e.g., an imidazole cream, terbinafine cream

Tinea capitus (scalp ringworm)

Red, scaling scalp lesions are associated with localized hair loss with short hair stumps. They may present as a tender erythematous inflammatory patch covered with pustules (kerion). This infection is human or animal acquired. Investigation is as for *Tinea corporis*. Skin lesions will sometimes appear as fluorescent green under Wood's light.

Treatment
- Topical antifungal and 6–8 weeks oral griseofulvin 20 mg/kg/day (plus oral steroids if kerion exists)

Tinea pedis (athlete's foot)

This consists of itchy, irritable skin between the toes ± sole of foot. It mainly affects adolescents, and is uncommon in young children.

Treatment
- Topical antifungal

Tinea unguium (onychomycosis)

Nail infection causes discolored, friable, and deformed nails. Diagnosis is by microscopy and culture of nail clippings.

Treatment
- If mild, debridement and antifungal lacquer applied to the nail. If extensive, use an oral antifungal for 3 months (e.g., terbinafine).

Candida albicans infection

Predisposing factors

Moist body folds, treatment with broad-spectrum antibiotics, immunosuppression, and diabetes mellitus are predisposing factors. Variants include the following:
- Cutaneous candidiasis (e.g., diaper rash; see Plate 3): Well-demarcated macular erythema, slight scaling and small outlying "satellite" lesions, worse in body folds
- Chronic paronychia
- Chronic mucocutaneous granulomatous candidiasis (secondary to congenital immunodeficiency disorder)

Investigations

- Skin scrapings for microscopy and culture

Treatment

- Oral or topical anticandidal drugs, e.g., nystatin, fluconazole as appropriate

Tinea versicolor (pityriasis versicolor)

Malassezia yeast infection occurs in postpubertal children, producing hypo- or hyperpigmented small macules with fine scaling on the trunk or upper limbs. The condition may be asymptomatic or may mildly itch. Recurrences are common.

Treatment

- Topical selenium sulfide 2.5% shampoo for 10 minutes prior to rinsing for 1–2 weeks; ketoconazole 2% shampoo daily for 3 days; oral therapy if severe

Parasitic skin infections

Scabies

Scabies is caused by infestation with the *Sarcoptes scabiei* mite. It is common in all ages. It produces an itchy papular rash with visible burrows affecting the finger and toe webs, palms, soles, wrists, groin, axillary folds, and buttocks (truncal in infants). Excoriation, eczematization, urticari, or impetigo may develop. Diagnosis is confirmed by microscopy of the mite removed from the burrow.

Treatment

- Treat the whole household and close contacts simultaneously with 12 hours topical application below the head (in children <2 years old the entire body except the face) with permethrin cream (5%); repeat in 1 week if necessary.
- Simultaneously, launder bed linen and underwear.
- Antihistamines or calamine lotion is useful for itching, which may last for 10 days after treatment.
- Apply topical corticosteroids if scabies nodules are present.

Lice

Infestation with *Pediculus capitus* (scalp "nits"), *Pedicularis corporis* (body), or *Phthirus pubis* (pubic area "crabs") is very common in children of all ages, particularly young children. It presents with localized pruritis, occasionally secondary impetigo or regional lymphadenopathy. Although lice are difficult to see, small white eggs (nits) are easily seen attached to hair shafts.

Treatment

Treatment consists of daily thorough combing with a fine-toothed comb, combined with permethrin 1% cream rinse; apply 10 minutes before rinsing. Consider a second application 1 week later. Other treatments include pyrethrin and piperonyl butoxide for a 10-minute application; malathiom 0.5% lotion for ~12 hours is approved for children ≥6 years.

Other insects

Many insects (e.g., fleas, bedbugs, gnats, midges, mosquitoes) can cause erythematous macular lesions with central punctum or papular urticaria.

Treatment

- Avoid bites, e.g., treat infested pets.
- Antihistamines
- Topical steroids
- Antibiotics if there is secondary bacterial infection

Protozoal skin infections

Cutaneous leishmaniasis

Infection with flagellate protozoa of the *Leishmania* species is endemic in hot climates (e.g., Mediterranean, South America). It is spread by sand-flies. A large reddish-brown papule, nodule, ulcer, or granuloma develops on exposed skin after several months' incubation. This usually resolves within 1 year but often leaves a scar.

Treatment

• Intralesional or IV antimony compound if severe

Hair disorders

Hair absence or loss

Alopecia areata

- This is the most common cause of hair loss.
- This is an autoimmune disease.
- Hairless, smooth areas are most often on the scalp. At the margin short remnants of broken hairs are visible ("exclamation marks").
- All of the scalp (alopecia totalis) or the whole body (alopecia universalis) may be involved.
- Hair typically regrows after 6–12 months but may be recurrent.
- The larger the area of hair loss, the poorer the prognosis.

Traumatic hair loss

Hair loss may be unintentional (e.g., chronic hair twisting due to ponytail or rubbing of occiput in babies) or intentional (trichotillomania) due to hair pulling, twisting or cutting as part of habit or secondary to anxiety, chronic social deprivation, or a psychological disorder. Characteristically there is an irregular margin, along with bizarre patterns without complete hair loss and broken hairs of different length. Hair regrows once the behavior is modified.

Scalp infection

This involves tinea capitis, ringworm (see p. 962).

Scarring alopecia

The most common cause is aplasia cutis: Circumscribed areas of the skin are absent, usually on the scalp, which presents at birth with a raw, red ulcer that heals with scarring and later has no hair growth. There is a significant incidence of other abnormalities (e.g., trisomys). Irreversible absent, localized hair growth will also follow other causes of trauma (e.g., burns, skin disease, trauma).

Congenital diffuse alopecia

This is a rare autosomal recessive condition. Hair is present in the newborn period but total hair loss occurs over the next few months and does not regrow. It may be associated with other anomalies.

Systemic disease

Hair loss can be secondary to hypothyroidism, diabetes mellitus, severe systemic disease, iron or zinc deficiency, and chemotherapy.

Management of hair absence or loss

- History: Include general health, recent illnesses, drug history, family history of alopecia, and age of onset.
- Examination: Pattern of hair loss; scalp and general examination
- Investigations: Hair M,C&S; Wood's light (tinea capitis); scalp biopsy
- Treat any underlying condition.
- Wigs may be helpful.
- Topical or intralesional steroids may be helpful for alopecia areata.

Excessive hair

Hypertrichosis

Hair growth is in areas not normally hairy in either sex. Causes:

- Racial
- Familial
- Certain rare syndromes (e.g., Cornelia De Lange syndrome, mucopoly-saccharidosis)
- Drugs (e.g., diazoxide, cyclosporine, minoxidil)
- Anorexia nervosa
- Protein-energy malnutrition
- Persistence of fetal lanugo hair at birth

Localized hypertrichosis may be associated with pigmented nevi, spina bifida occulta, inflammatory skin diseases, or topical steroids.

Treatment

Provide treatment if required. Remove or treat underlying cause if possible; use depilatory creams or waxing for hair removal.

Hirsutism

This is a male pattern of hair growth in females. Causes:

- Racial
- Familial
- Androgen excess (adrenal hypoplasia or tumor, Cushing's disease, polycystic ovary syndrome)
- Turner's syndrome
- Drugs (e.g., anticonvulsants, progesterones, anabolic steroids)

Investigate if there is any suggestion that this is not racial or familial (e.g., virilization evident)

- CBC
- Plasma free testosterone
- Plasma dehydroepiandrosterone sulfate
- Plasma 17-OH progesterone
- Serum cortisol
- Urine steroid profile
- Skull X-ray (pituitary tumor?)

Treatment

Treat any underlying disease; reassure patient if the cause is racial or familial. Remove hair using depilatory creams or waxing.

Hair diseases

All diseases are rare and include the following:

- Menke's kinky hair disease: Wiry, woolly hair (p. 1112).
- Monilethrix is a rare autosomal dominant condition that causes brittle hair that fails to grow and breaks at 1–2 cm.
- Pili torti: Hair repeatedly twists over 180°, leading to brittle hair that "flickers" under direct light.
- Woolly hair syndrome: Wiry, woolly African American–like hair in Caucasians

Nail disorders

Paronychia

Acute paronychia is common, particularly in newborns. It presents as acute inflammation and tenderness of nail folds and surrounding skin.

Treatment
• Topical antiseptics, and, if severe, oral antibiotic, e.g., cephalexin

Chronic paronychia is associated with nail dystrophy. It is usually caused by chronic wetness (e.g., thumb sucking, resulting in infection with mixed bacteria and *Candida*).

Treatment
• Keep nail dry; apply topical nystatin and antiseptics.

Tinea unguium (onychomycosis)

See p. 962.

Nail biting

This is a common habit. Permanent nail damage may occur if the nail matrix is damaged.

Treatment

Gentle dissuasion is best. Proprietary topical nail solutions that impart a very unpleasant taste may be effective.

Ingrowing toenail

This most commonly involves the hallux. The spicule of the nail grows into the lateral nail fold, resulting in pain, bacterial paronychia, and granulation tissue.

Treatment
• Local antiseptic
• Careful trimming of nail spicule
• Education on correct toenail cutting
• Silver nitrate cauterization of granulation tissue or radical surgery is required when severe

Subungual hemorrhage

This is caused by trauma leading to hemorrhage under the nail. Perforation of the nail with a hot needle is curative and relieves pain immediately.

Nail abnormalities secondary to generalized disease

• *Congenitally abnormal nails* (usually atrophic) may be due to rare inherited conditions, e.g., ectodermal dysplasia.
• *Clubbing*: Chronic pulmonary suppuration, e.g., cystic fibrosis; fibrosing alveolitis; bacterial endocarditis; cyanotic congenital heart disease; malabsorptive states; IBD; hepatic cirrhosis
• *Onycholysis*: Premature separation of the nail from the nail bed due to psoriasis, trauma, eczema

- *Koilonychia*: Spoon-shaped nails due to chronic iron deficiency anemia (Koilonychia is normal in the first few months of life.)
- *Nail pitting*: Psoriasis, eczema, alopecia areata
- *Beau's line*: Transverse groove in the nail caused by severe systemic illness
- *Splinter hemorrhages*: Bacterial endocarditis, trauma
- *Yellow nail syndrome*: Defective lymphatic drainage (also affects the lungs)
- *Nail-patella syndrome*: Rare autosomal dominant condition with small rudimentary patella, elbow deformities, and reduced or longitudinally split nail formation. Rarely, chronic glomerulopathy develops.

Pigmentation disorders

Hyperpigmented lesions

Generalized hyperpigmentation (hypermelanosis)

Causes
- Racial
- Sun
- ACTH (e.g., hypoadrenalism)
- Chronic renal failure (MSH)
- Malabsorption
- Drug reaction

Localized hyperpigmentation (hypermelanosis)

Causes
- Pigmented nevi (see below)
- Freckles
- Lentigines
- Café-au-lait macules
- Neurofibromatosis (before puberty ≥6 café-au-lait macules >0.5 cm diameter, axillary freckles)
- Viral warts
- Polyostotic fibrous dysplasia (McCune–Albright syndrome)
- Peutz–Jegher syndrome (perioral brown macules)
- Post-inflammatory skin disease or trauma

Pigmented nevi

Melanocytic nevus (mole)

This is a developmental anomaly of melanocyte migration. It may be brown, black or pink, macular, papular, hyperkeratotic or smooth, hairy or hairless. Moles are almost universal, appearing commonly on the face, neck, or back. They occur after birth throughout childhood, particularly at puberty.
- *Treatment*: Surgical removal for cosmetic reasons, recurrent trauma, e.g., from bra straps, or malignant change (rare in childhood). If congenital, moles can be extensive; refer patient to a dermatologist or plastic surgeon for treatment and follow-up.

Halo nevus

This is the area of depigmentation around a mole due to production of autoimmune antibodies to melanocytes.
- *Treatment*: Reassurance alone

Mongolian blue spot

This macular blue–black lesion is present at birth, and is common in dark-skinned races, particularly over the sacrum, buttocks, back, and shoulders. Most spots fade spontaneously by age 10 years.

Spitz nevus (spindle-cell nevus)

This benign melanocyte tumor has a red–brown dome-shaped nodule.
- *Treatment*: Simple excision and histology (spindle cells evident)

Malignant melanoma

This condition is rare in childhood. The risk increases with increased sun exposure. It occurs in older children, those with giant congenital pigmented nevi, immunosuppressed individuals, those who have undergone previous chemotherapy, and those with albinism or xeroderma pigmentosum. Change in mole color, shape, or size (unless in proportion to child's growth), ulceration, itch, or hemorrhage requires urgent specialist excision biopsy and histology.

Hypopigmented lesions

Generalized hypomelanosis

Causes

- Hypopituitarism (ACTH and MSH)
- Oculocutaneous albinism (see below)
- Protein-energy malnutrition
- Poorly controlled phenylketonuria (phenylalanine acts as a competitive inhibitor of tyrosinases)

Oculocutaneous albinism is an autosomal recessive disorder of melanin synthesis. It presents with hypopigmented skin, blonde hair, pink irises, photophobia, reduced visual acuity, and nystagmus.

Treatment

Restrict sunlight exposure, e.g., use protective high-level sunscreen; provide ophthalmology referral.

Localized hypomelanosis

Vitiligo

This is a common autoimmune disease (anti-melanocyte antibodies present) resulting in sharply demarcated, often symmetrical white patches.

- *Treatment*: Reassurance; topical steroids; cosmetics; sun protection; phototherapy if severe. Lesions usually persist.

Tinea versicolor (Pityriasis versicolor)

See page 962.

Pityriasis alba

This is common in prepubertal children. It represents low-grade eczema with post-inflammatory hypopigmentation. Hypopigmented 1- to 2-cm patches ± fine scale appear on the face or upper body.

- *Treatment*: Topical hydrocortisone 1%, frequent moisturizing. The condition resolves in 2–3 weeks.

Post-inflammatory hypopigmentation

Tuberous sclerosis "ash leaf" macules

These are small, oval, hypopigmented macules that are more easily seen under Wood's light examination.

Photosensitivity and light eruptions

Photosensitivity
Reactions to sunlight can be precipitated by drugs, e.g., thiazide diuretics, nalidixic acid; soaps; perfumes; plant pollens; and plant contact, e.g., giant hogweed plant. Most common is a dermatitis-like reaction, but it may also be erythematous or blistering.

Porphyria
Some forms are photosensitive, e.g., erythropoietic protoporphyria (skin burning, redness, swelling, serous crusting ± subsequent scarring). Treatment is that of the underlying porphyria together with sun protection (see also p. 1110)

Juvenile spring eruption
Red papules and herpetiform vesicles or blisters develop, usually in the spring, over light-exposed skin, particularly ear helices. They occur more often in boys than in girls. They heal without scarring. Topical steroids hasten healing.

Polymorphous light eruption
Itchy, erythematous, papular rash occurs in sun-exposed areas 6–48 hours after exposure, most commonly among adolescent girls. Treatment is with high-factor sunscreen.

Actinic prurigo
This uncommon condition is precipitated by sunlight. Irritant papules, exudation, and excoriation develop on both exposed and unexposed skin areas. Treatment is with sun protection. The condition generally resolves after several years.

Xeroderma pigmentosum
This is a rare autosomal recessive disease in which hypersensitivity to sunlight causes marked erythema followed by dry skin, freckles, hyperpigmentation, atrophy, and scarring. Solar keratoses and skin cancers eventually develop due to the decreased ability to repair DNA damaged by UV radiation.

Collagen and elastin disorders

Collagen disorders

Ehlers–Danlos syndrome (EDS)

EDS comprises a group of several rare genetic (mostly autosomal dominant) disorders of collagen (see p. 973). In classical EDS the skin is soft, hyperextensible, and easily bruised and heals poorly with thin, atrophic, "cigarette paper" scars. Hypermobile EDS is characterized by soft skin with hypermobility of large and small joints. There is no specific treatment.

Striae (stretch marks)

Striae are due to linear growth exceeding the capacity of new collagen production (e.g., during pubertal growth spurt, with glucocorticoids). Linear reddish-purple marks develop. They are common on the lower back and outer thighs. There is no treatment. Marks slowly fade.

Keloid

This is an excessive fibrous-tissue response to skin trauma. Its cause is unknown but it is often familial and is more common in African-American children. Skin trauma results in a well-demarcated raised, smooth, scar that extends beyond the original injury.

Treatment

Repeated intralesional triamcinolone injections are helpful if given early in keloid development. Radiotherapy may also be helpful if given early or before surgery.

Osteogenesis imperfecta

This is a group of several rare genetic diseases, mostly autosomal recessive, in which there is inadequate or defective collagen production (see p. 882).

Presentation

There are frequent skeletal fractures and multiple deformities; thin skin; defective teeth; hypermobile joints; and blue sclera.

Treatment

There is no specific treatment. Supportive therapy, including use of wheelchairs, orthotics, etc. may be required, and analgesics for fractures. Severe forms are lethal in infancy. Less severe forms lead to short stature, multiple or recurrent fractures, and deformities.

Elastin disorders

Cutis laxa

This rare congenital disorder of defective elastin presents with loose skin folds and easily stretched skin that only slowly returns to its original position. It is associated with later hernia, large vessel rupture, and emphysema.

Miscellaneous skin conditions

Ichthyoses
This is an inherited group of disorders with underlying abnormal keratinization. Variants include the following:
• Ichthyosis vulgaris
• X-linked ichthyosis
• Lamellar ichthyosis
• Non-bullous congenital ichthyosiform erythroderma (NBCIE)
• Epidermolytic hyperkeratosis

Some types (e.g., lamellar ichthyosis, NBCIE) present as "collodion" baby, due to lamellar desquamation associated with eye ectropion and lip eclabium, respiratory distress, and inability to suck normally. Otherwise, the disorder presents in the first few months of life with dry, scaly skin ± erythema.

Investigation
Obtain skin biopsy and histology.

Treatment
Avoid soap and detergents; use bath oils; apply regular urea-containing emollients or mild keratolytics (e.g., 1% salicylic acid in aqueous cream). If severe, oral retinoids are justified.

Prognosis
Most forms improve with age, (except X-linked ichthyosis).

Dermatitis herpetiformis
This rare, chronic, autoimmune disease is secondary to IgA antibody directed against dermoepidermal junctional antigen. It occurs in celiac disease and affects ages 6–12 years. The initial itchy rash of knees, elbows, buttocks, and perineum evolves into vesicles or blisters.

Treatment
Treat with a gluten-free diet; oral dapsone. Prognosis is good.

Epidermolysis bullosa
In this group of genetically distinct disorders the epidermis separates from the dermis. It often presents at birth with sloughing of skin (± mucous membranes) following minor skin trauma; blister or bulla formation; and positive Nikolsky sign. The level of epidermal /dermal cleavage differs between disorders, with the more severe form resulting in scarring, finger pseudosyndactyly ("mitten deformities"), esophageal strictures, and limb contractions. Nails, hair, and teeth may be affected. Biopsy for immunofluorescent mapping determines the precise diagnosis.

Treatment
Treatment is supportive (e.g., minimal handling, skilled nursing on silk sheets, foam padding, IV fluid with protein or electrolyte replacement as needed, antibiotics for superficial infection, nutritional support, topical protective petrolatum and nonadherent dressings of blistering areas). Referral to a specialized unit is recommended.

Prognosis

Prognosis is variable and depends on the exact disorder. Generally, auto-recessive forms are more severe, result in scarring, and present at birth. Severe forms are frequently lethal in the newborn period. Prognosis improves with skilled input.

"Adult" seborrheic dermatitis

This condition affects the postpubertal child.

- *Cause*: Yeast overgrowth, e.g., *Malassezia ovalis*
- *Presentation*: Erythema with overlying scaling affecting scalp (dandruff), eyebrows, nasolabial folds, cheeks, and joint flexures
- *Treatment*: Mild topical steroid or antifungal, antiseborrheic shampoos

Zinc deficiency

Causes

These include dietary deficiency, e.g., breast-fed very preterm infants, and acrodermatitis enteropathica (rare autosomal recessive defect in zinc absorption).

Presentation

Infants develop demarcated areas of erythema, scaling, and pustules around the mouth, ears, fingers and toes, and anogenital regions; diarrhea; and FTT. Investigation is of low plasma zinc levels.

Treatment

Oral zinc supplements restore health.

Ectodermal dysplasia

There are many forms, the most common one being hypohidrotic ectodermal dysplasia (X-linked recessive).

Presentation

Sparse sweat glands, dry skin, sparse hair, thin eyebrows, characteristic facies (prominent frontal ridges in the chin, saddle nose, sunken cheeks, thick lips, large ears), and defective peg-shaped teeth are characteristic features. The patient is prone to hyperthermia and heat stroke due to reduced or absent sweating.

Treatment

Treatment is supportive. Avoid hyperthermia and treat appropriately if it occurs, with rehydration and salt replacement. Use dental prosthetics.

Incontinentia pigmenti

In this rare X-linked dominant disorder girls present in the neonatal period with blistering lesions (cropping circumferentially on the trunk and in a linear distribution on the limbs) that within weeks turn into warty plaques and nodules that resolve to leave streaky hyperpigmentation.

Ultimately, the lesions regress by late childhood to leave atrophic, streaky areas of hypopigmentation (often most noticeable on the back of the calves). This condition is associated with dental, eye, musculoskeletal, and neurological abnormalities. No specific treatment is available.

Dermatitis artefacta

These self-inflicted skin lesions usually affect adolescent girls. Lesions are extremely variable but are usually bizarre and sudden in appearance. The patient is often inappropriately unconcerned.

Occlusive dressing leads to rapid healing. Sympathetic listening is most likely to be helpful. Consider underlying abuse. Psychiatric input may be helpful.

Lichen planus

This disorder is of unknown cause. Itchy, flat-topped violaceous papules develop, usually over flexor aspects of the wrist and trunk. Papules tend to coalesce into hypertrophic plaque. The nails (pits or ridges) and mouth (white lacy network—Wickham's striae) are involved.

Treatment

Apply topical steroids. Lesions may recur for several years.

Mastocytosis

In this developmental, abnormal collection of skin mast cells, single or multiple macular or nodular lesions urticate when rubbed (Darier's sign). Hyperpigmentation develops after several months. There may be systemic involvement.

Treatment

Treat with antihistamines. Lesions and pigmentation will resolve.

Connective tissue disorders

See p. 904. Skin manifestations of connective tissue disorders include the following.

Systemic lupus erythematosus
- Widespread or "butterfly rash" facial erythema; scalp alopecia; chronic discoid patches; light sensitivity

Dermatomyositis
- Violaceous erythema ± edema of the face (especially eyelids), upper chest, elbows, knees, and knuckles and around the nails. Rash may become scaly.

Morphea
In this idiopathic condition there is localized sclerosis of the skin. Usually a large oval plaque of violaceous hue develops, which then gradually becomes indurated, smooth, and shiny. It usually resolves spontaneously.

Treat severe facial or restrictive linear morphea with pulsed IV methylprednisolone and oral methotrexate.

Systemic sclerosis
This condition consists of Raynaud's phenomenon; fingertip ulceration; skin of the face and hands becoming progressively indurated and "bound down" to underlying tissues; restricted facial movements; beaked nose; mouth puckering; skin atrophy; telangiectasia; pigmentation; and calcinosis.

Cutaneous polyarteritis nodosa
Tender nodules (usually lower legs) are surrounded by livedo reticularis. Nodules may ulcerate or become necrotic.

Lichen sclerosus et atrophicus
In this idiopathic chronic inflammatory skin disorder localized distinct atrophic changes occur with associated pallor usually affecting the genital and perianal regions, almost always in females (the male variety is balanitis xerotica obliterans, which causes phimosis). Pruritus, blistering, or erythema may occur.

Treat with emollients, or potent topical steroids if condition is severe.

Pediatric surgery

Symptoms and signs that should cause concern

Neonates and infants

As a pediatrician you will be involved with the surgical care of newborn babies, infants, and older children. It is important that you recognize important symptoms and signs that indicate surgical emergency.

Neonatal intestinal obstruction (see p. 998)

A prompt diagnosis is essential if the small bowel is to be salvaged.

- *Bile-stained vomiting* is the cardinal sign of an intestinal obstruction.
- *Emergency assessment*: Check vital signs and commence resuscitation.
- *X-ray*: All children with bile-stained vomiting should have an abdominal X-ray taken.

Radiology

- Dilated bowel loops on the abdominal X-ray suggest an intestinal obstruction. Loops larger than lumbar vertebral body width are dilated.
- Look for free air to indicate a perforation. In the supine film this might outline the falciform ligament (umbilical vein).

Clinical assessment

- *Anus*: Make sure the baby has an anus, especially females.
- *Meconium*: Most babies pass meconium within 24 hours of birth. Delayed passage of meconium in a baby with abdominal distension could indicate Hirschsprung's disease.
- *Rectal examination*: Do not perform a rectal examination, insert a suppository, or perform a rectal washout without seeking advice first, because some surgeons use lower GI contrast studies for diagnosis and the signs of Hirschsprung's disease may be obscured.

Esophageal atresia (EA) (see also p. 986)

The combination of polyhydramnios and a baby with increased secretions is suspicious of esophageal atresia.

Intussusception in infants (see also p. 996)

Suspect intussusception in any infant with gastroenteritis who is not getting better, is unusually miserable, vomits bile, or has blood in the stool. The classical presentation is an infant with the following:

- Intermittent colicky, abdominal pain
- Episodic drawing up of the knees
- Passing of "red current jelly" stool (late sign)

Incarcerated inguinal hernia (see also p. 1004)

An irreducible swelling in the groin in a baby who is ill and vomiting is probably an incarcerated inguinal hernia.

Older children

Acute appendicitis (see also p. 1000)
This is accompanied by acute pain, usually in the right iliac fossa. The history may be atypical and the abdominal signs are either difficult to decipher or absent in children taking antibiotics.

Acute scrotal pain (see also p. 1012)
Assume that any boy with acute scrotal pain has a testicular torsion.

Congenital abnormalities: upper airway

Choanal atresia

Congenital obstruction of the posterior choana of the nose may be unilateral or bilateral. Babies are obligate nose breathers; bilateral obstruction presents with asphyxia during feeding and sleep. Unilateral obstruction may pass unnoticed. Choanal atresia may be a presenting feature of the CHARGE association:

- **C**oloboma
- **H**eart defects
- **A**tresia of the choanae,
- **R**etardation of growth and development
- **G**enitourinary abnormalities
- **E**ar abnormalities and hearing loss

Diagnosis

- Nasogastric tube: The diagnosis is excluded by passage of a tube down each nostril.
- CT scan will determine whether the obstruction is membranous or bony.

Treatment

- Emergency treatment comprises an oropharyngeal airway and an orogastric tube for feeding.
- Surgery restores patency of the choanae, which is performed through a transnasal approach.

Laryngeal atresia

Laryngeal atresia is a rare condition, invariably fatal at birth. It is relatively easy to detect using antenatal ultrasound because the fetal lungs appear bright and large. Large airways can also be visualized because they are distended with fetal lung fluid. No treatment is available and termination of pregnancy may be considered.

Cleft lip and palate (see also p. 221)

Approximately 1 baby per 1000 is born with a cleft lip and palate, which may be sporadic or familial. A cleft lip is immediately apparent. An isolated cleft palate may not be noticed immediately but will present with feeding difficulties, particularly nasal regurgitation of milk.

A cleft palate will interfere with breast-feeding as it precludes generation of suction. Bottle-feeding may also be difficult unless a squeezable bottle rather than a rigid bottle is used.

Management

- Lip repair at ~3 months of age
- Palate repair at ~6 months of age
- Follow-up includes long-term therapy for speech, dentistry, and hearing.

Pierre Robin sequence

The Pierre Robin sequence (Fig. 23.1) is characterized by three features:

- Micrognathia
- Glossoptosis
- Cleft palate

Management

- The large tongue has a tendency to obstruct the airway, causing apnea, particularly during sleep.
- Prone positioning may help, allowing the tongue to fall forward, but occasionally tracheostomy is necessary.
- Endotracheal intubation is often difficult.
- Tube feeding may be necessary.
- The palate is generally repaired between 9 and 18 months of age.
- The airway problems invariably improve with growth.

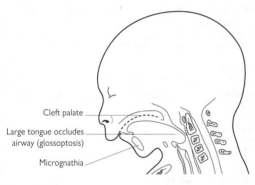

Cleft palate

Large tongue occludes
airway (glossoptosis)

Micrognathia

Figure 23.1 Pierre Robin sequence.

Congenital abnormalities: tracheoesophageal

Tracheoesophageal fistula (TEF)

TEF is usually associated with esophageal atresia (EA). However, an isolated TEF will present with

- Choking or coughing during feeding
- Abdominal distension
- Recurrent lower respiratory tract infection

Although symptoms are present from birth, the diagnosis of isolated TEF (without EA) is frequently not made until later in childhood. The investigations of choice are a tube injection of X-ray contrast into the esophagus and bronchoscopy. Treatment is surgical division of the TEF through a neck incision.

Esophageal atresia and tracheoesophageal fistula (p. 1077)

The incidence of EA and TEF (see Fig. 23.2) is 1:3500 live births.

- >75% babies with EA will have a TEF.
- <5% will have isolated EA, which is usually associated with a long gap or defect.
- <5% have isolated TEF.
- Rare EA with both upper and lower pouch TEFs

Maternal polyhydramnios is common, although antenatal diagnosis is rare. Babies present at birth with

- Excess mucous or oropharyngeal secretions
- Choking and cyanosis on feeding
- Associated malformations in 50%, usually the VACTERL association (see Box 23.1)

Box 23.1 VACTERL association

- **V**ertebral anomalies (fused vertebrae, hemivertebrae)
- **A**norectal anomalies (imperforate anus)
- **C**ardiac anomalies (all types)
- **T**racheo-**E**sophageal anomalies
- **R**enal abnormalities (all types)
- **L**imb abnormalities (radial ray anomalies, e.g., hypoplastic thumbs)

Diagnosis

Diagnosis is confirmed or excluded by

- Passage of a 10F nasogastric or orogastric tube
- Chest X-ray: The tube stops in the upper thorax. Air in the stomach indicates a fistula between the trachea and the distal esophagus (TEF).

Acute management

- The baby should be kept warm, and disturbed as little as possible.
- The upper esophageal pouch should be aspirated regularly by oropharyngeal suction or a Replogle tube.

- Standard intravenous fluids should be started.
- Preoperative antibiotics are only required if there is evidence of aspiration pneumonia.
- Babies who require mechanical ventilation must be repaired urgently because gas may produce progressive gastric distension, which impairs ventilation further and ultimately leads to gastric perforation.
- Echocardiogram and renal ultrasound

Surgery

- Disconnection of the TEF and anastomosis of upper and lower esophagus through a right thoracotomy
- Long-gap EA may require a feeding gastrostomy and a cervical esophagostomy in the neonatal period, followed by esophageal replacement during infancy.
- High-risk babies may have a staged procedure: the TEF is ligated and then the EA repaired a few days or weeks later.
- Complications include anastomotic leak, anastomotic stricture, gastro-esophageal reflux (GER) and recurrent fistula.

Follow-up

- Respiratory morbidity in the early years after EA/TEF repair is relatively high, particularly in the winter months.
- Obstruction of the esophagus by food boluses is common in toddlers and young children after EA repair. Usually it is caused by meat or firm vegetables not being chewed properly. Refer patient for urgent esophagoscopy.

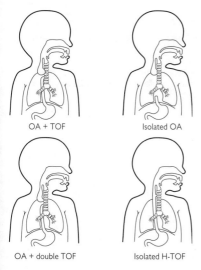

OA + TOF   Isolated OA

OA + double TOF   Isolated H-TOF

Figure 23.2 Types of esophageal atresia (OA) and tracheoesophageal fistula (TOF).

Congenital abnormalities: esophagus

Esophageal stricture

Esophageal strictures in children may be congenital (5%) or acquired (95%). Strictures may be acquired as a result of reflux esophagitis or caustic ingestion or following repair of EA. Congenital esophageal strictures most commonly affect the middle and distal third of the esophagus and rarely cause symptoms in the neonatal period. It may be due to

- Membranous diaphragm
- Segmental submucosal fibrosis
- Presence of ectopic tracheobronchial rests

Presentation
Strictures present with

- Regurgitation of undigested food
- Bolus obstruction
- Failure to thrive

Diagnosis

- Barium swallow
- Esophagoscopy

Treatment

- Peptic strictures are an absolute indication for antireflux surgery.
- Congenital strictures may respond to dilatation but resection or esophageal replacement is often necessary.

Box 23.2 Caustic ingestion

- *Acute phase*: Resuscitate and support with intravenous fluids and antibiotics.
- *Endoscopy*: To confirm the severity of the burn
- *Feeding gastrostomy*: In severe strictures
- *Chronic phase*: Serial esophageal dilatation. Many children require esophageal replacement.

Congenital abnormalities: lung

Congenital cystic adenomatoid malformation (CCAM)

CCAM is a congenital malformation of the lung bud lesion characterized by dysplasia of respiratory epithelium. Most cases of CCAM are now diagnosed prenatally by ultrasound, and high-risk cases will be associated with hydrops. Symptomatic CCAMs should be resected.

- Large CCAMs present at birth with respiratory distress.
- Small CCAMs will be asymptomatic at birth but may present in early childhood with pulmonary sepsis.

Sequestration

Pulmonary sequestrations are segments of lung parenchyma, often with an anomalous blood supply from the aorta. There may be an abnormal bronchial connection with the foregut or tracheobronchial tree. The majority are detected prenatally and management is with resection.

- Large sequestrations will present at birth with respiratory distress or with heart failure from high flow through the feeding vessel.
- Sequestrations may present in infancy or childhood with pulmonary sepsis.

Congenital lobar emphysema (CLE)

CLE is an unusual lung bud anomaly characterized by massive air trapping in the emphysematous lobe. This compresses the surrounding normal lung and may result in mediastinal shift.

- CLE presenting with progressive respiratory distress within the first few weeks or months of life nearly always requires lobectomy. In the acute phase, positive-pressure ventilation may produce rapid worsening of the emphysema.
- Lobar emphysema identified on chest X-ray in the absence of symptoms will need close follow-up and surgery may be avoided.

Congenital abnormalities: chest

Congenital diaphragmatic hernia (CDH)

The incidence of CDH is 1:2400. The main problem is not the diaphragmatic hernia but rather the associated pulmonary hypoplasia that is often severe and determines prognosis. The most common type of diaphragmatic defect is posterolateral (Bochdalek) and left sided, occurring in 90% (see Fig. 23.3 and Fig. 23.4).

Antenatal screening

Most CDHs are identified on antenatal ultrasound; other associated anomalies may be detected as well.

Birth

Clinical findings may include respiratory distress, scaphoid abdomen, and apparent dextrocardia. The prognosis for survival is >80% in specialized centers.

Coincidental

Approximately 10% of CDHs are discovered during early childhood, including most anterior (Morgagni) defects. The prognosis is excellent.

Neonatal management (at a referral center)

- Initial management consists of sedation, endotracheal intubation and mechanical ventilation, and maximizing of cardiac function. Permissive hypercarpnea or "gentle ventilation" should be attempted to avoid barotrauma.
- Place nasogastric tube and avoid bag-mask-valve ventilation.
- If oxygenation is good and pulmonary hypoplasia is not severe, repair of the diaphragmatic defect is undertaken after a few days by either primary suture or insertion of a prosthetic patch.

Hiatus hernia (HH)

Hiatus hernia refers to herniation of the stomach into the chest through the esophageal hiatus in the diaphragm. The lower esophageal sphincter also moves and becomes incompetent. Most children with HH present with GER. Two types of HH are recognized (see Fig. 23.5).
- Sliding (common)
- Rolling or paraesophageal (rare)

Management

- *Diagnosis* is made radiologically by barium meal.
- *Treatment* comprises management of the GER, initially medically.
- *Surgery* is reserved for children who fail to respond to medication or have complicated reflux (i.e., peptic strictures) or paraesophageal hernias (because of the risk of incarceration and infarction of the herniated stomach). Surgery involves repair of the HH and a fundoplication to prevent GER.

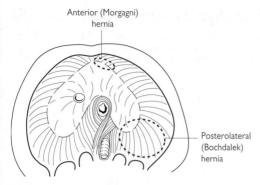

Figure 23.3 Types of diaphragmatic hernia.

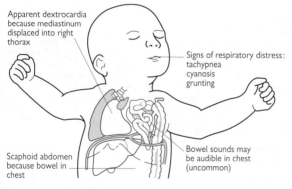

Figure 23.4 Clinical features of congenital diaphragmatic hernia.

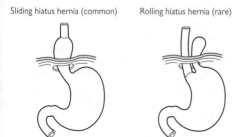

Figure 23.5 Types of hiatus hernia.

Idiopathic hypertrophic pyloric stenosis

The incidence of hypertrophic pyloric stenosis (HPS) is ~3/1000 live births. Boys are affected more frequently than girls. The pylorus enlarges as a result of hypertrophy of the circular muscle to produce the typical "olive." The cause remains unknown. Familial occurrence is well documented.

Clinical features (see Fig. 23.6)

- *Vomiting* is usually, but not always, projectile, starting in the third or fourth week of life. The vomitus is usually nonbilious but it may contain altered ("coffee ground") or fresh blood from esophagitis. Vomiting occurs within an hour of feeding and the baby is immediately hungry. Babies who present early (first or second week) are often misdiagnosed as having GER.
- *Constipation* is common from reduced fluid intake.
- Dehydration, malnutrition, and jaundice are late signs.
- HPS is rare beyond 12 weeks of age.

Diagnosis

Test feed

The baby is allowed to feed from the breast or bottle while the examiner palpates the baby's abdomen. The test feed is best conducted with the baby resting on the mother's lap, cradled on her left arm. The examiner sits opposite the mother, on the baby's left. Visible waves of gastric peristalsis may be seen passing across the upper abdomen. The pyloric olive is usually easiest to feel either early in the feed or after the baby has vomited. Some 60%–90% of olives are palpable. The thickened pylorus is palpable as a firm, "olive-shaped" mass, just above and to the right of the umbilicus during a test feed.

Ultrasound

Ultrasound will confirm or exclude the diagnosis.

Biochemistry

The biochemical abnormality of HPS is a hypochloremic, hypokalemic metabolic alkalosis. Assess the degree of alkalosis at presentation and monitor correction prior to surgery.

Preoperative management

- *Rehydrate* and correct alkalosis before surgery.
- *Intravenous fluids* should be started: 0.45% saline with 5% dextrose and 20 mmol/L potassium chloride at >120 mL/kg/day
- *Feeds*: Withhold—the stomach should be emptied with a nasogastric tube.
- *Electrolytes* should be checked until they return to normal. Correction may require >24 hours if the alkalosis is severe.
- *Blood glucose* should be monitored.

Surgery

Ramstedt's pyloromyotomy

This is the treatment of choice (see Fig. 23.7). It involves splitting the thickened pyloric muscle. Complications include perforation of the mucosa (rarely serious if recognized and repaired) and wound infection.

Oral feeds are usually withheld for <4 hours. Transient postoperative vomiting is common but invariably settles within 36 hours. There are no long-term sequelae.

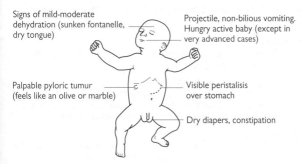

Signs of mild-moderate dehydration (sunken fontanelle, dry tongue)

Projectile, non-bilious vomiting. Hungry active baby (except in very advanced cases)

Palpable pyloric tumor (feels like an olive or marble)

Visible peristalisis over stomach

Dry diapers, constipation

Figure 23.6 Clinical signs of pyloric stenosis.

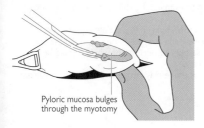

Pyloric mucosa bulges through the myotomy

Figure 23.7 Ramstedt's operation.

Ingested foreign bodies

Swallowed foreign bodies are fairly common in young children (see also p. 294). The incident may have been witnessed. Alternatively, the child may present with

- Drooling
- Regurgitation
- Occasionally cough and stridor

Diagnosis

- Chest X-ray: Most ingested foreign bodies are radio-opaque (coins).

Management

Esophageal

If the foreign body is in the esophagus it should be removed within 24 hours, usually by esophagoscopy.

Button (e.g., watch or calculator) batteries

If these are in the esophagus they must be retrieved within a few hours of ingestion. Electrolytic ulceration of the esophagus occurs rapidly and may lead to perforation or fistulation into the trachea or aorta.

Below the diaphragm

If the foreign body is below the diaphragm it will invariably pass spontaneously per rectum and all that it required is reassurance. Serial radiographs are unnecessary. The only proviso is a child who has had previous abdominal surgery, in which case adhesions may impede passage of the object.

- Parents should be asked to examine the child's stools for the foreign body.
- Colicky abdominal pain and vomiting (i.e., possible signs of intestinal obstruction) warrant review and a repeat X-ray. Provided the child remains asymptomatic, surgery to retrieve the object should be deferred for several months.
- Multiple magnets in the intestine may attract and lead to ischemia and perforation.

Bezoars

Bezoars are foreign-body concretions composed of hair (trichobezoar) or vegetable matter (phytobezoar). The bezoar forms in the stomach and may extend into the small bowel. Bezoars are most commonly seen in young girls who present with
- Weight loss
- Vomiting
- Abdominal pain
- Anemia

Diagnosis
- An abdominal mass may be palpable.
- Barium meal or endoscopy will confirm the abnormality.

Surgical treatment
- *Large bezoars*: Open surgical removal is necessary.
- *Smaller bezoars*: Endoscopic removal

Midgut malrotation and volvulus

During the first trimester of intrauterine development the fetal midgut transiently herniates into the umbilical cord. As it reduces, the mesentery normally rotates to bring the cecum to lie in the right iliac fossa and ligament of Treitz (LOT) to lie to the left of the midline. The midgut mesentery extends diagonally across the back of the abdominal cavity and provides a broad, stable pedicle for the superior mesenteric artery (SMA) to supply the bowel. Malrotation is a failure of this normal rotation that leaves the cecum high in the right upper quadrant and the LOT mobile in midline (see p. 356). The result is a narrow base for the midgut mesentery and a narrow mobile pedicle through which the SMA runs (see Fig. 23.8). Malrotation is usually asymptomatic and only detected by upper GI with small bowel follow-through contrast study.

Midgut malrotation
- Midgut malrotation predisposes to midgut volvulus.
- To prevent this complication, surgical correction of a malrotation is advised, using Ladd's procedure.
- An incidental appendectomy is usually performed.

Midgut volvulus
- It is a catastrophic event that occurs without warning.
- The immediate effect is high intestinal obstruction at the duodenal level that is rapidly followed by infarction of the entire midgut.

Symptoms
- Bile-stained vomiting
- Circulatory collapse
- Tender abdomen

Diagnosis
- An abdominal X-ray may appear similar to one of duodenal atresia with a "double bubble" and paucity of gas elsewhere in the abdomen, or may appear nearly normal (see Fig. 23.9).
- The diagnosis is confirmed by an urgent upper GI contrast study. Time is of the essence.

Surgical treatment
- Immediate laparotomy to untwist the volvulus
- If the bowel is healthy a Ladd's procedure is performed.
- If bowel viability is doubtful, a second-look laparotomy may be necessary after 24 hours. Frequently there is massive intestinal necrosis and the child is left with a very short gut, in which case long-term intravenous feeding is required.

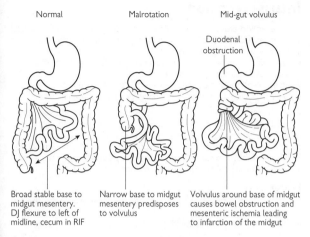

Figure 23.8 ntestinal rotation and volvulus, RIF, right iliac fossa; DJF, duodenojejeunal flexure.

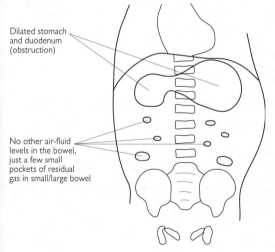

Figure 23.9 Features of volvulus on abdominal X-ray.

Intussusception

Intussusception typically affects infants between 6 and 18 months of age. The incidence is 1:500 children. The majority of intussusceptions occur in association with viral gastroenteritis.

- Enlarged Peyer's patch in the ileum acts as the *lead point* that then invaginates into the distal bowel.
- Intussusceptions in older children and adults are more likely to be due to a *pathological lead point*, e.g., a polyp or Meckel's diverticulum.

Intussusception causes a small-bowel obstruction. The intussuscepted bowel becomes engorged, which causes rectal bleeding and, eventually, gangrenous. Following this, perforation and peritonitis will occur. The most common site for an intussusception is ileocolic (see Fig. 23.10). Small-bowel intussusception may occur as a postoperative complication in infants, typically following resection of retroperitoneal tumors.

Presentation

The typical presentation of an intussusception is an infant with the following symptoms:

- Spasms of colic associated with pallor, screaming, and drawing-up of the legs
- The child falls asleep or becomes unusually lethargic between episodes.
- Later, as the intestinal obstruction progresses, bile-stained vomiting develops and rectal bleeding (i.e., "red current jelly stools") occurs.
- The child will appear ill, listless, and dehydrated.
- In late cases circulatory shock or peritonitis will be present.

Assessment

- In 30% of cases the intussusception will be palpable as a sausage-shaped abdominal mass.
- Blood may be noted on rectal examination.
- Abdominal X-ray shows small-bowel obstruction; occasionally a soft-tissue mass will be visible.
- Ultrasound confirms the diagnosis by showing a characteristic "target sign."

Management

- *Resuscitation*: Often large volumes of intravenous fluid are required to restore perfusion.
- Antibiotics should be deferred until the diagnosis is verified.
- Analgesia
- Pass a nasogastric tube if the infant is vomiting.

Radiological reduction
Provided that there is no evidence of peritonitis, the treatment of choice is for a pediatric radiologist to reduce the intussusception pneumatically by rectal insufflation of air under fluoroscopic control. Risks are incomplete reduction and perforation. The latter is more likely in infants <6 months old and can be particularly dangerous, as a tension pneumoperitoneum develops very rapidly.

Laparotomy or laparoscopy
if pneumatic reduction fails or is contraindicated because of concern about a gangrenous intussusception, laparotomy or laparoscopy is necessary. The distal bowel is gently compressed to reduce the intussusception. If this is not successful the intussusception is resected. There is a recurrence rate of ~10%, regardless of whether the intussusception is treated radiologically or by surgery. Further recurrence should raise the question of a pathological lead point.

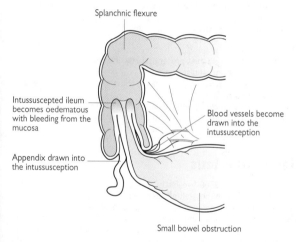

Splanchnic flexure

Intussuscepted ileum becomes oedematous with bleeding from the mucosa

Blood vessels become drawn into the intussusception

Appendix drawn into the intussusception

Small bowel obstruction

Figure 23.10 Ileocolic intussusception.

Duodenal atresia (DA)

The incidence of DA is 1:5000 live births.
- One-third of babies with DA have trisomy 21.
- Babies with DA present at birth with bile-stained vomiting.
- Abdominal X-ray shows "double bubble" sign of gas in the stomach and proximal duodenum (see Fig. 23.11).
- Surgical treatment consists of duodenoduodenostomy. The prognosis is excellent.

Small bowel atresias

The incidence of small bowel atresia is 1:3000 live births. The etiology is thought to be vascular. The pathology of small bowel atresias varies (depending on how deep in the mesentery the vascular accident occurs), from an atresia in continuity with a mucosal membrane to a widely separated atresia with a V-shaped mesenteric defect and loss of gut. Approximately 10% of atresias are multiple.

Clinical aspects
- *Bile-stained vomiting*: Babies present shortly after birth with bile-stained vomiting and abdominal distension.
- *Contrast enema* confirms patency of the colon and distal small bowel prior to laparotomy.
- *Abdominal X-ray* shows multiple fluid levels (see Fig. 23.12).
- *Laparotomy*: End-to-end anastomosis. The prognosis depends on the length of the remaining small bowel.

Meconium ileus

The incidence is ~1:2500 live births. Meconium ileus is associated with cystic fibrosis (CF). Almost all affected infants have CF; 15% of children with CF present with meconium ileus. Lack of pancreatic enzymes results in meconium that is thick and viscous, causing an intraluminal obstruction in the terminal ileum. Occasionally the distended obstructed bowel will perforate or result in volvulus in utero, or meconium peritonitis. Babies present at birth with intestinal obstruction.

Management
Treatment involves relieving of the intestinal obstruction.
- *Contrast enema*: Provided that there is no evidence of intrauterine perforation, the obstruction may be relieved by the contrast, which draws fluid into the bowel lumen, which loosens inspissated meconium.
- *Laparotomy*: For unsuccessful enema or complicated meconium ileus
- Genetic testing for CF in all cases.

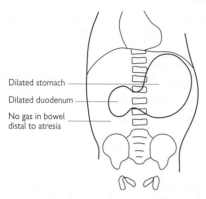

Dilated stomach

Dilated duodenum

No gas in bowel
distal to atresia

Figure 23.11 Features of duodenal atresia on abdominal X-ray.

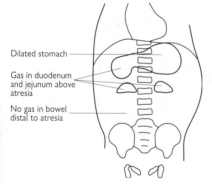

Dilated stomach

Gas in duodenum
and jejunum above
atresia

No gas in bowel
distal to atresia

Figure 23.12 Features of jejunal atresia on abdominal X-ray.

Acute appendicitis

Acute appendicitis is the most common abdominal emergency in children, affecting approximately one-sixth of the population. Acute appendicitis begins with obstruction of the lumen of the appendix, often by a fecalith, causing vague, central abdominal pain.

After 6–12 hours, an inflammatory process involves the full thickness of the wall of the appendix. After a further 24–36 hours the appendix will become gangrenous and perforate. Irritation of the peritoneum results in a more severe abdominal pain localized to the right iliac fossa.

- Pain is aggravated by movement.
- The child may prefer to lie still with knees flexed.
- Mild fever is usual.
- Peritoneal irritation results in involuntary spasm in the muscles of the abdominal wall—"guarding"

Diagnosis

The mortality from appendicitis is very low. However, substantial morbidity is incurred by delayed diagnosis. The diagnosis of appendicitis is clinical and laboratory investigations are minimally helpful.

- The "classic" symptoms and signs of acute appendicitis are seen in about 60% cases.
- Of all children admitted to a hospital with abdominal pain, only ~30% will have acute appendicitis. Only 50%–70% of these cases are obvious at the initial assessment.
- Urinalysis is abnormal in about one-third of children with acute appendicitis: pyuria and even bacteruria may be present.
- The white blood cell count is normal in 10%–20% of children with appendicitis.
- Ultrasound: When in doubt, ultrasound is the investigation of choice. The accuracy of ultrasound in the diagnosis of acute appendicitis is ~90%.
- CT scan is rarely needed, although quite accurate.

Mesenteric adenitis (MA)

MA is a condition that mimics acute appendicitis. It is usually the result of an intercurrent viral infection. Children with MA typically present with

- Fever
- Malaise
- Central abdominal pain

Diagnosis

- Usually a period of observation is necessary, when the symptoms remain static or improve, unlike appendicitis.
- MA accounts for the majority of children who undergo a normal appendectomy.

Meckel's diverticulum (MD)

MD is a persistence of the embryonic vitelline or omphala-mesenteric duct that normally involutes during late fetal development. It is present in 2% of the population and most cases are asymptomatic. MD is a cause of gastrointestinal bleeding, obstruction, inflammation, and umbilical discharge.

Management

- Rectal bleeding from a MD is painless, fresh, and sufficient to cause a drop in hemoglobin. Often a ^{99m}Tc-pertechnetate isotope scan will identify an MD.
- Persistent or recurrent bleeding requires a laparotomy or laparoscopy even if the scan is negative. Diverticulitis or perforation of an MD is clinically indistinguishable from appendicitis.
- Symptomatic MD should be resected.

Gastroschisis

The incidence of gastroschisis is 1:3000 live births, but it is increasing. Most fetuses with gastroschisis are identified on prenatal ultrasound and delivery should be arranged in a regional referral center.

The abnormality is immediately apparent at birth as a defect in the abdominal wall to the right of the umbilicus (see Fig. 23.13). The bowel is eviscerated, not covered by a sac, and thickened and matted. Associated malformations are uncommon, except intestinal atresias (10%).

Management
- *Immediate*: Cover the exposed bowel with a nonadherent dressing and a waterproof barrier such as plastic.
- Keep the baby warm and hydrated.
- *Surgery*: The defect requires surgical closure as rapidly as possible. Often this has to be staged using a silo because the abdomen is too small to accommodate the intestine. The silo is reduced serially, ideally in <7 days, then secondary closure of the defect is performed.
- *Nutrition*: Total parenteral nutrition may be required for many weeks. The long-term outcome is excellent.

Omphalocele

The incidence of omphalocele is 1:3000 live births. It is usually identified on prenatal ultrasound (see Fig. 23.13). It is characterized by the following:
- Hernia into the base of the umbilical cord—the herniated bowel is covered by a sac (amnion).
- Giant omphalocele: Defect >5 cm in diameter

Associated malformations are found in 50% of cases:
- Chromosomal defects: Trisomies 18, 13, and 21 and Turner's syndrome
- Cardiac defects
- Beckwith–Wiederman syndrome
- Pulmonary hypoplasia, particularly with giant omphalocele

Surgical treatment
- Closure of the defect in one or more stages
- The prognosis depends on associated malformations.
- *Giant omphalocele*: Escharotic dressing with delayed surgical closure may be safer because of the pulmonary hypoplasia.

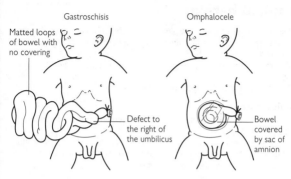

Figure 23.13 Anterior abdominal wall defects.

Inguinal hernias

Groin hernias in children are almost invariably indirect inguinal hernias. Femoral hernias are rare in children. Inguinal hernias
- Are more common in boys
- Are more common on the right side due to later descent of the right testis
- May be associated with pain or fussiness

Clinical care
- A reducible swelling in the groin, often extending into the scrotum (see Fig. 23.14)
- Surgical herniorrhaphy: Infants should be repaired within a few weeks of diagnosis because the risk of incarceration is high. The risk of incarceration lessens after the age of 1 year.

Incarcerated hernia
- Incarceration results in an intestinal obstruction.
- There is a 30% risk of testicular infarction from pressure on the gonadal vessels.
- Treatment of an irreducible inguinal hernia comprises resuscitation of the child then reduction of the hernia by taxis (i.e., gentle but sustained pressure is applied to the sac to reduce the contents).
- Most hernias can be reduced safely, although it may be necessary to give the baby morphine first. If the hernia cannot be reduced, emergency surgical exploration is necessary.
- After reduction a herniorrhaphy should be performed after 24–48 hours to allow for any edema to settle.

Hydroceles

Infantile hydroceles are common.
- They are caused by failure of the processus vaginalis to obliterate after testicular descent through the inguinal canal.
- The clinical signs are a soft swelling around the testis, which transilluminates and above which the examiner can palpate a normal spermatic cord (see Fig. 23.14).
- Most cases resolve by the second year and those that do not should be treated surgically through a short groin incision.
- Check for inguinal hernia.

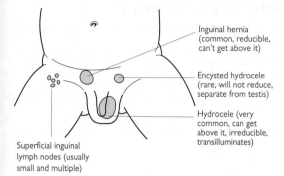

Figure 23.14 Groin swellings.

Inguinal hernia (common, reducible, can't get above it)

Encysted hydrocele (rare, will not reduce, separate from testis)

Hydrocele (very common, can get above it, irreducible, transilluminates)

Superficial inguinal lymph nodes (usually small and multiple)

Hirschsprung's disease (HD)

The incidence of HD is 1:5000 live births. It may be familial (10%) and associated with trisomy 21 (10%).

- It is caused by a failure of ganglion cells to migrate into the hindgut.
- This defect leads to an absence of coordinated bowel peristalsis, and functional intestinal obstruction at the junction ("transition zone") between normal bowel and the distal aganglionic bowel.
- In 80% of cases the transition zone is in the rectum or sigmoid—short-segment disease.
- In 10% of cases the entire colon is involved—long-segment disease.
- Occasionally, children with short-segment disease present in childhood with chronic constipation.

Diagnosis

- HD usually presents within the first few days of life with low intestinal obstruction, i.e., failure to pass meconium, abdominal distension, and bile-stained vomiting. 99% of normal newborns pass the meconium within 24 hours of delivery.
- Abdominal X-ray shows distal intestinal obstruction.
- Contrast enema shows small-caliber rectum with dilated colon proximally (transition zone).
- Rectal biopsy has no ganglion cells in the submucosa.

Surgical treatment

Many surgeons now perform a single-stage pull-through in the neonatal period, managing initial intestinal obstruction with rectal washouts. But traditionally a two-stage procedure is used:

- Defunctioning colostomy, with multiple biopsies to confirm the site of the transition zone
- Pull-through procedure to bring ganglionic bowel down to the anus

Outcome

- Approximately 75% children acquire normal bowel control; 15%–20% have partial control; and 5% never gain control and may end up with a permanent stoma.
- The most important complication of Hirschsprung's disease is entero-colitis, a dramatic gastroenteritic illness characterized by abdominal distension, bloody, watery diarrhea, circulatory collapse, and sepsis. The condition is often associated with *Clostridium difficile* toxin in the stools. Mortality can be as high as 10%.

Rectal prolapse

Rectal prolapse refers to a mucosal or full-thickness herniation of rectum through the anal canal.

- It is most commonly seen in constipated toddlers squatting and straining.
- It is rarely associated with diarrhea, cystic fibrosis, and celiac disease.

Management

- Often the prolapse reduces spontaneously after defecation. Otherwise, gentle digital reduction should be performed.
- Constipation should be treated.
- Recurrent prolapse may be managed with submucosal injection of sclerosing agents such as hypertonic glucose.
- Surgical procedures are sometimes necessary.

Anorectal malformations

The incidence of anorectal malformation is 1:5000 live births. Anorectal malformations comprise part of the VACTERL association (see p. 1066). The abnormality should be identified at birth. The baby presents with

- Failure to pass meconium
- Abdominal distension
- Bile-stained vomiting

Anatomy

The precise anatomy varies, but the malformation can be subdivided into high and low/intermediate anomalies in males and females.

Low/intermediate anomalies

- The rectum is present and passes through a normal sphincter complex.
- In boys (see Fig. 23.15) there is a tiny, fistulous track to the surface of the perineum, often anteriorly onto the scrotum.
- In girls (see Fig. 23.16) the rectum may open into the back of the introitus as a rectovestibular fistula. Normal continence is expected, reconstruction involves division of a common wall between the rectum and vagina. Treatment involves a multistage procedure with defunctioning colostomy, anorectal reconstruction, and then closure of the stoma.
- Vesicoureteric reflux is common.

High anomalies

- These anomalies are common in boys and rare in girls.
- The sphincter complex is poorly developed and the prospects for continence are mediocre.
- In boys the rectum makes a fistulous connection with the urethra. Treatment involves a defunctioning colostomy within the first 48 hours of birth, reconstruction at a few months of age (most commonly involving a posterior sagittal anorectoplasty [PSARP] performed through a midline perineal incision), and then closure of the colostomy.

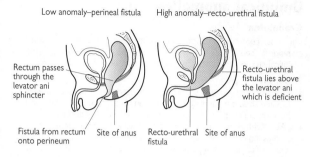

Figure 23.15 Male anorectal malformations.

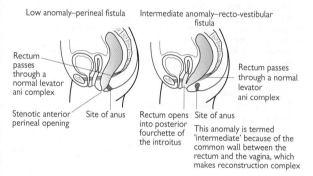

Figure 23.16 Female anorectal malformations.

Umbilical anomalies

Granuloma

The most common umbilical abnormality seen in infants is an umbilical granuloma (see Fig. 23.17). This is a harmless reaction to the resolving umbilical stump and usually disappears by the second to third week.

Treatment

- A persistent granuloma should be cauterized with a silver nitrate stick. Vaseline should be applied round the umbilicus to prevent damage to the surrounding skin. Multiple applications may be necessary.
- CAUTION: A persistent "granuloma" discharging small-bowel contents signifies a patent omphalomesenteric duct (see Fig. 23.17). Treatment involves surgical exploration of the umbilicus and excision of the duct with a small segment of ileum. The diagnosis is clinical.

Urachal remnants

These are uncommon anomalies that present in infancy or early child-hood. The urachus is an embryonic tubular connection between the bladder and the allantois that normally obliterates before birth.

- *Main symptom:* Persistent discharge of urine from the umbilicus
- *Bladder outlet obstruction* (posterior urethral valves) should be excluded by voiding cystourethrography (VCUG). Treatment is surgical closure.

Umbilical hernias (see Fig. 23.17)

- These are common, particularly in African-American children.
- Most will close spontaneously during the first few years of life, regardless of size.
- Complications are rare.
- If the hernia fails to close, surgical repair can be performed at ~5 years of age.

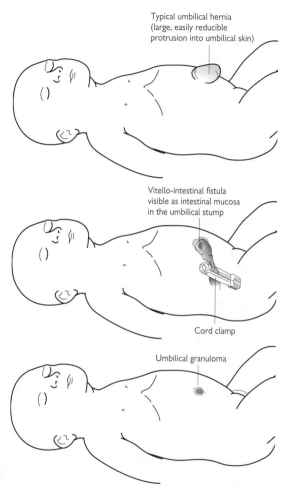

Figure 23.17 Disorders of the umbilicus.

Testicular torsion

Testicular torsion must be excluded in a child with acute scrotal pain (see Box 23.3). Peak incidence is at ~12 years, but it can occur at any age.

Congenital testicular torsion

This is a rare perinatal event. The newborn infant has a hard, painless scrotal mass. The testis has invariably infarcted and exploration is not necessary, nor is fixation of the opposite testis, because the pathology is torsion of the spermatic cord outside the tunica vaginalis.

Torsion outside the perinatal period

This is the result of an abnormally mobile mesentery of the testis inside the tunica vaginalis. This anomaly is bilateral and allows the gonad to twist on its vascular pedicle.

Presentation

Testicular torsion presents with
- Sudden-onset, severe scrotal pain, often with nausea and vomiting
- Tender testis
- Overlying scrotal skin may be reddened and edematous.

Treatment
- Immediate scrotal exploration is mandatory to salvage the testis, which should then be fixed to prevent recurrence.
- The contralateral testis should also be fixed.

Box 23.3 Differential diagnosis of acute scrotal pain
(see also p. 1004)

Testicular torsion
- Sudden-onset pain, swelling, and nausea
- Testis is very tender, and may lie transversely in scrotum
- Scrotal skin may be red

Torsed hydatid
- Gradual onset of less severe pain; no nausea
- Focal tenderness at upper pole of testis
- Torsed hydatid may be visible through scrotal skin as a pea-sized blue/black swelling

Epididymo-orchitis
- Insidious onset of dysuria and fever
- Usually associated with a urinary tract infection
- Red, tender scrotum

Testicular trauma
- History is obvious and there are signs of trauma or hematocele

Idiopathic scrotal edema
- Child is well
- Scrotal skin is cellulitic but the testes are not tender.
- The condition settles spontaneously within a few days.

Orchitis and epididymitis

Orchitis
- Orchitis is an uncommon condition in boys, which presents with fever and testicular pain.
- Approximately 20% of prepubertal patients with mumps develop orchitis.
- Diagnosis is based on a history of recent mumps or parotitis; mumps orchitis is unilateral in 70% of cases.
- In 30% of cases, contralateral testicular involvement follows a few days later.
- This condition is rare in postpubertal boys.
- Bacterial orchitis is usually associated with an epididymitis.

Epididymitis
- Epididymitis is usually associated with concomitant orchitis.
- In children, epididymo-orchitis is usually associated with a urinary tract infection: infected urine refluxes down the vas.
- Structural abnormality in the renal tract should be excluded.
- Epididymo-orchitis presents with fever, urinary symptoms, and scrotal pain.
- In sexually active adolescents, epididymo-orchitis may be caused by gonorrhea or chlamydia.
- Epididymo-orchitis should be managed with antibiotics once urine has been sent for culture. Adolescents should be screened for sexually transmitted infection.

Testicular trauma

A direct blow to the scrotum may rupture a testis. The scrotum is too painful to examine clinically and a gentle ultrasound examination should be performed. If the testis is disrupted, surgical exploration and repair is necessary to prevent atrophy. If the blow is severe, a urethral injury should be suspected and, if necessary, excluded by urethrography.

Undescended testes (cryptorchidism)

The testes descend through the inguinal canal into the scrotum during the first trimester. Cryptorchidism (see Fig. 23.18) is seen in 3% of full-term newborn boys and 1% of boys at 1 year. Spontaneous descent may occur in the first 6 months, but it is unlikely after this. Cryptorchidism is more common in premature infants.

Clinical aspects

Undescended testes are subdivided into palpable and impalpable forms.

Palpable undescended testes (80%)

These are usually at the external inguinal ring. The testes can be brought down into the scrotum with an orchidopexy performed through an inguinal incision.

Impalpable testes (20%)

These cases are intra-abdominal, inside the inguinal canal, or absent. There is risk of malignant degeneration in an intra-abdominal testis (1:70, compared to 1:5000 for normal testis). Laparoscopy is the investigation of choice for an impalpable testis. Ultrasound, CT, and MRI are not helpful. If the vas and vessels enter the deep inguinal ring (30%) then an inguinal orchidopexy is indicated. If the vas and vessels end blindly at the deep ring (30%), the testis has torsed in utero and has resorbed. No further action is necessary. If a testis is seen inside the abdomen it must be removed or brought down with a two-stage orchidopexy.

> *When should boys be referred to a surgeon?*
> - If an undescended testis is noted on routine postnatal check this should be documented in the medical records.
> - Initial follow-up should be with the pediatrician because most of these testes will descend during the first 6 months of life.
> - If still undescended at 6 months, refer patient to a pediatric surgeon or urologist.

Retractile testes

The cremasteric muscle is overactive and the testes retract into the groin. The scrotum is well developed and the parents may notice that the testes are in place when the child is in a warm bath. Examine the child in a warm environment. The testes can be manipulated into the scrotum and will remain there until the cremasteric reflex is stimulated. Surgery is not necessary.

Hypospadias

Hypospadias affects ~1 in 350 male births. It is characterized by an abnormal position of the external urethral meatus and classified according to the location of the meatus (penis down to the scrotum; see Fig. 23.19).

Severe forms of hypospadias may be associated with chordee—a ventral curvature of the penis. The most common consequences of hypospadias are difficulty urinating while standing and a cosmetic appearance of the penis that differs from that of other boys. Sexual function is not affected unless chordee is present, which may cause painful erections.

> *Hypospadius advice*
> - Make sure you document the diagnosis in the notes.
> - Tell the parents NOT to circumcise the child.
> - Give the parents a letter stating this advice.
> - Refer the child to a pediatric surgeon or urologist.

Surgery

Surgical correction involves straightening of any chordee and reconstruction of the urethra to the glans. This may involve tubularizing skin from the prepuce so circumcision is contraindicated. The correction can be completed in one or more operations during early childhood.

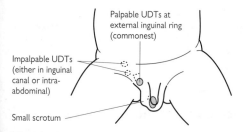

Figure 23.18 Undescended testes (UDTs).

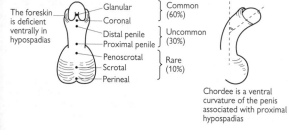

Figure 23.19 Classification of hypospadias.

Phimosis and paraphimosis

The foreskin develops in utero as a protuberance of the penile epidermis, which grows forward over the glans and adheres to it. The prepuce is normally nonretractable during early childhood. During this period it is very common for parents to notice that the child's prepuce balloons during micturition. It is also very common for boys to complain of intermittent redness and discomfort from the prepuce.

This is rarely the result of bacterial or candidal infection but simply a chemical irritation from urine under the foreskin. These symptoms are self-limiting and resolve during childhood without intervention (i.e., circumcision).

Circumcision

The medical indications for circumcision in boys are controversial. Genuine indications for circumcision are given below.

Phimosis

This is almost exclusively caused by balanitis xerotica obliterans (BXO, or lichen sclerosis), which is an uncommon scarring dermatitis characterized by a thickened, indurated, whitish appearance of the tip of the prepuce. BXO affects 2% boys by the age of 17 and is very rare under 5 years of age.

Paraphimosis

The prepuce retracts as the boy gets an erection and becomes stuck behind the glans. The glans becomes swollen and edematous. The paraphimosis should be reduced under general anesthesia and circumcision scheduled a few weeks later to prevent recurrence.

Recurrent balanitis

This is rare.

Balanitis/balanoposthitis

Balanoposthitis is acute inflammation of the glans and foreskin associated with a purulent discharge from the preputial orifice. This condition affects 4% boys, mostly between 2 and 5 years. Recurrent episodes are rare.

- *Urinary tract infection*: *Staphylococcus aureus* is the most common cause.
- *Treatment*: 5-day course of oral trimethoprim or amoxicillin. Topical antibacterials or antifungals are of no value.

Priapism

Priapism is a persistent painful erection. The most common cause in boys is trauma, usually a fall-astride injury to the perineum. Occasionally priapism is a presenting symptom of acute leukemia or sickle cell disease. Treatment is usually conservative.

Penile trauma

The most common penile trauma is from circumcision. Bleeding post-circumcision usually needs exploration under anesthesia. Clotting should be checked to exclude hemophilia in infants. Entrapment of the foreskin in trouser zippers is occasionally seen.

- If the prepuce is caught between the teeth of the zipper, release can be achieved by cutting across the zipper and separating the edges.
- This can usually be managed without surgery or anesthesia. Entrapment between the zip slide and the teeth is more complicated because the slider has to be pried off with bone cutters. This is best performed under anesthesia.

Imperforate hymen

An imperforate hymen usually presents within a few days of life with a lower abdominal mass, sometimes associated with urinary retention. Intrauterine stimulation of the infant's cervical mucous glands by maternal estrogens causes accumulation of secretions (mucocolpos).

The imperforate hymen can be seen bulging through the introitus and treatment consists of incising the hymen. Occasionally, an imperforate hymen presents at puberty with primary amenorrhea or a painful lower abdominal mass from a hematocolpos. Treatment comprises incision of the hymen under general anesthesia.

Labial adhesions in infants

Labial adhesions are common in female toddlers. A rash and exposure to urine causes a chronic irritation of the fragile labia, which adhere. There is invariably a small opening anteriorly through which urine escapes. Labial adhesions cause no symptoms but they are a major source of anxiety to parents.

Treatment is best deferred until the child is out of diapers. Topical application of estrogen cream for 2 weeks will result in separation of most adhesions but occasionally gentle separation under anesthetic may be necessary.

Miscellaneous conditions

Tongue- tie

Tongue-tie is common and rarely causes symptoms. Tongue-tie does not cause lisp, and is not responsible for eating problems in an older child. Division of a tongue-tie does not alter the natural history of either condition. Tongue-tie does affect the ability of newborns to breast-feed, and division of the lingual frenulum within the first week of life will correct this problem. Bottle-feeding is not affected (p. 124).

Dermoid cysts

Dermoid cysts are common in children. Dermoids are non-tender, mobile, subcutaneous cysts filled with keratin, hair follicles, and sebaceous glands. They enlarge slowly and should be treated by excision.

Dermoid cysts occur most frequently along lines of embryological fusion, such as the lateral corner of the eyebrows (external angular dermoid), midline of the neck, over the bridge of the nose, and suprasternal notch.

Thyroglossal duct cyst (TDC)

TDC presents with midline swelling in the neck, just below the hyoid bone. The swelling rises with tongue protrusion and swallowing. TDCs develop from epithelial remnants left after descent of the developing thyroid from the foramen cecum at the base of the tongue.

TDCs gradually enlarge and eventually become infected, which makes excision more difficult. Treatment is surgical removal of the central portion of the hyoid bone along with the cyst and track.

Branchial remnants

Branchial remnants persist from the branchial clefts during embryogenesis of the head and neck. Anomalies of the second branchial cleft are by far the most common. They can be a cyst, a sinus tract, or, rarely, a fistula.

Branchial sinuses

These present as small cutaneous openings along the anterior lower third border of the sternocleidomastoid muscle which discharge mucous (see Fig. 23.20). They can communicate with the tonsillar fossa (branchial fistula). Management is excision to prevent infection.

Branchial cysts

These cysts are uncommon neck swellings along the anterior border of the sternomastoid. The differential diagnosis includes cystic hygroma, which is more common; treatment is surgery.

Cystic hygroma (CH)

CH is a congenital malformation of the lymphatic system, also termed lymphangioma. They present in early childhood as soft, multilocular, cystic swellings that often appear after an intercurrent viral infection. CHs are more often found in the neck and axillae, although they can occur anywhere, including inside the abdomen or thorax.

Large cervical cystic hygromas may present at birth with airway obstruction. Small CHs require no treatment. Large lesions infiltrate the surrounding tissues, making complete surgical excision impossible. Intralesional injection of sclerosants is an alternative to surgery in some cases.

Congenital torticollis (see also p. 861)

Within the first weeks of birth a small swelling in the baby's neck is noticed. A sternocleidomastoid tumor is a palpable area of fibrosis in the lower sternocleidomastoid muscle (SCM) and is a transient phenomenon that will resolve after a few months. Sometimes there is a history of dystocia.

Shortening of the SCM results in torticollis with rotation and tilting of the head to the opposite side. Management is nonoperative in most cases, with passive exercises to achieve full neck movements.

Hemifacial atrophy and strabismus may develop unless full movement is restored. Occasionally it is necessary to divide the SCM, but this is no substitute for physical therapy.

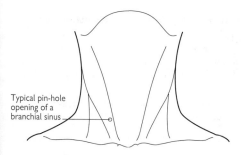

Typical pin-hole opening of a branchial sinus

Figure 23.20 Branchial sinus.

Perioperative care

Preparation of children for elective surgery

- The presenting complaint should be documented and confirmed.
- Previous medical history, medications, and allergies must be recorded.
- A clinical examination should be performed. In the case of undescended testes, hydroceles, and inguinal hernias, a mark (either "yes"
  or the physician's initials) should be made on the child's thigh to
  document the side for operation (away from the surgical field to
  prevent tattooing of the wound).
- If the child is unwell with an intercurrent illness, discuss this with the
  anesthesiologist, who may decide that the child is unfit for anesthesia.

Blood tests

These should be kept to a minimum. Children undergoing major surgery
should have the following elements tested:

- Hematocrit checked and blood cross-matched, according to the nature
  of the operation (usually one unit of blood is sufficient)
- BUN and electrolytes should be checked preoperatively in children
  taking diuretics and in children in renal failure.
- Children at risk of sickle cell disease or thalassemia should be screened
  as outpatients before admission.

Fasting prior to elective surgery

This is essential for safe induction of anesthesia. Recommendations are in
Box 23.4.

> **Box 23.4 Minimum fasting times prior to elective surgery**
>
> - Solid food: 6 hours
> - Formula milk: 6 hours
> - Breast milk: 4 hours
> - Clear fluids (dextrose solution, water): 2 hours

Anesthesiologist

The anesthesiologist will visit preoperatively and discuss anesthesia and
postoperative analgesia with the child and parents. In some instances
premedication may be appropriate.

- Intravenous access will be obtained during induction of anesthesia.

Newborns

Preoperative resuscitation and preparation are essential if the outcome
of surgery is to be successful. Newborns with congenital malformations
will be admitted to a neonatal intensive care unit.

Routine preparation

This should include
- Intramuscular vitamin K
- Full blood count, to determine the hematocrit
- Cross-matching blood. Many laboratories require a sample of maternal blood for typing, and this should accompany the baby if the mother is unable or unfit to travel

Echocardiography

Babies with EA, duodenal atresia, Down syndrome, or anorectal malformations should undergo echocardiography before surgery because of the possible associated cardiac defects.

Renal imaging

Provided the baby passes urine (indicative of functioning nephrons), renal imaging can be arranged electively. Anuria necessitates a renal ultrasound scan to exclude renal agenesis.

Intestinal obstruction

Babies will require the following:
- *Intravenous fluid*: Normal maintenance is required. Babies with gastroschisis lose fluid and heat rapidly from the exposed bowel. The baby's abdomen should be covered in plastic wrap, or the infant's trunk and lower extremities can be placed in a plastic bag. Regular bolus infusions of albumin solution should be considered before closure of the defect.
- *Nasogastric (NG) or orogastric (OG) decompression.* A wide-bore NG or OG tube is necessary to empty the stomach (8 or 10 French gauge). The tube should be aspirated every hour and left on free drainage. Gastric aspirates should be replaced milliliter for milliliter with 0.9% saline with 20 mmol KCl per liter, in addition to maintenance fluids.
- *Biochemistry and acid–base balance* is necessary in babies with prolonged vomiting (e.g., pyloric stenosis).

Box 23.5 Consent for surgery: clinical practice
(see p. 1174, Chapter 31)

The best person to obtain consent is the surgeon performing the operation.

Preparing children
- Whenever possible, the procedure should be explained to the child in language that they can understand.
- Young children are not generally interested in alternative treatments and risk.
- Children are interested to know how long the operation will take, how they will feel afterwards, and how long they will get off school.

Parents
Informed consent must be sought from the parents. This must include
- An explanation of the diagnosis and the proposed operation, along with alternative treatments, risks, and benefits and the likely outcomes
- It is prudent to discuss potential complications and provide an estimate of risk. The risk of adverse reactions to general anesthesia in fit, healthy children is between 1:10,000 and 1:100,000, which is comparable to the risk of injury crossing a road.

Emergency
- In an emergency it is justifiable to treat without parental consent.
- It must, however, be documented clearly that the child's life is in danger and that attempts have been made to contact the parents.
- Ensure that entries in the records are signed, timed, and dated.
- Verbal consent from the parents is acceptable in an emergency and should be recorded on the consent form.

Postoperative care: fluids

Day-case children

Children admitted for day surgery will return to the recovery area once they are alert, able to maintain their airway, hemodynamically stable, and comfortable. The presence of a parent in the recovery room is usually beneficial.

Oral fluids can be offered in most cases on return to the recovery area, if tolerated without nausea, followed by food. Within a few hours most children can be discharged home.

Major surgery

Following major surgery children will return to the ward or intensive care unit. Postoperative orders should include specific instructions regarding antibiotics, catheters, intravenous fluids, etc.

Postoperative intravenous fluids

These will depend on the nature of the surgery. For postoperative fluid, 0.45% sodium chloride with 5% dextrose is most often used. The rate of infusion should be adjusted according to the weight of the child. Potassium chloride 20 mmol/L should be added to fluids after the first day.

Nasogastric aspirates

These should be replaced milliliter for milliliter with 0.9% sodium chloride with 20 mmol KCl/L. It is easy to underestimate "third space losses" (i.e., fluid translocating into the peritoneum, bowel, or chest) after major surgery, and this volume of fluid should be added to the maintenance requirements and fluid given to replace continuing losses (e.g., nasogastric aspirates).

If the child has cool extremities and a prolonged capillary refill time the situation will almost always improve after infusion of 20 mL/kg of additional fluid (lactated Ringer's solution, 0.9% saline, 4.5% albumin, and plasma substitutes are all possibilities, based on the situation).

Hematocrit

Check the hematocrit on the first postoperative day. Blood transfusion is to be avoided whenever possible and, with the exception of oxygen-dependent children, a moderate postoperative anemia is well tolerated.

If transfusion is necessary, every effort should be made to ensure that the child is only exposed to blood from one donor, even if this means that the volume of blood transfused is less than that originally calculated. Routine co-administration of diuretics is not necessary in the surgical patient.

Biochemistry

Children with high urinary or high stoma losses receiving intravenous fluids should have blood urea and electrolytes measured daily. Frequent adjustments to the electrolyte content and rate of infusion may be necessary.

Oral fluids

Following abdominal surgery, most children will have a paralytic ileus for 36–48 hours. After this period, oral intake will resume and IV fluids can be gradually discontinued. If more prolonged IV fluid therapy is necessary, consideration should be given to parenteral nutrition.

Nasogastric tubes

Nasogastric (NG) or orogastric (OG) tubes are usually inserted to keep the stomach empty. In the preoperative period this is useful in a child with an intestinal obstruction. An OG tube may be preferable in newborns who are obligate nasal breathers.

A bile-stained aspirate signifies an intestinal obstruction and emptying the stomach will prevent the child from vomiting. Unless otherwise instructed, the NG tube should be aspirated every hour and the aspirate replaced intravenously milliliter for milliliter with 0.9% saline containing KCl 20 mmol/L.

- It is common practice to insert an NG tube in the OR in a child undergoing abdominal surgery with high risk for paralytic ileus.
- Postoperative management is the same as preoperative. As the ileus resolves after 24–36 hours the volume of the NG or OG tube aspirate will decrease and it will become clear. At this stage, the tube can usually be removed and oral fluids resumed.

Transanastomotic tubes

Following repair of EA in the newborn some surgeons will place a "transanastomotic tube" (TAT). The purpose of the TAT is to allow early resumption of enteral nutrition.

- Do not attempt to repass a TAT that has been removed inadvertently without seeking advice from the surgeon.

Newborns and infants

Newborns and former premature infants <50 weeks post-conception should be transferred to a neonatal or special care unit postoperatively.

The risk of postoperative apnea after general anaesthesia is relatively high. Monitoring for a minimum of 24 hours post-anesthetic should include routine nursing observations of

- Temperature
- Pulse
- Respiration
- Pulse oximetry
- Apnea monitoring

Postoperative care: analgesia

See also p. 1154.

Analgesia for day cases

Operations are painful and analgesia is essential.

- In many cases local anesthetic blocks or wound infiltration will provide complete analgesia for several hours.
- After this, simple analgesics such as acetaminophen or ibuprofen are usually all that is required.
- For older children codeine may be necessary. A prescription for 2–3 days should be given prior to discharge.

Analgesia for major surgery

After major surgery stronger analgesia is required for a longer period. This applies to neonates as well as older children.

Continuous epidural infusions of local anesthetics

There are many advantages to local or regional analgesia, and continuous epidural infusions of local anesthetics (e.g., bupivacaine) work particularly well after major abdominal or thoracic surgery.

- Epidural infusions are not without risk. It is essential that close nursing supervision be maintained (i.e., vital signs and level of the epidural block).
- In many hospitals there is a "pediatric pain team" who supervise the epidural. If this is not available, close liaison should be maintained with the anesthetist responsible.
- If the level of anesthesia seems to be rising to the upper thoracic dermatomes, the infusion should be stopped pending advice.
- If the analgesia is inadequate, advice should be sought before either removing the epidural catheter or starting opiates.

Continuous intravenous infusion of morphine

Infusion of morphine or other opiates is another very effective method of postoperative analgesia. For older children this may be in the form of a patient-controlled analgesia pump with a button the child can press to obtain an increment of analgesic.

- Many hospitals will have a pain management team and/or guidelines on the use of analgesics for children.
- Pain must be treated. Administering strong analgesics will not mask clinical signs. Peritonitis can be detected reliably in a child who has received morphine.

Postoperative care: drains and wounds

Chest drain removal

An adult can be asked to suspend respiration in full inspiration before removal of a chest drain. Children will not cooperate with this.

- The best strategy is to remove the drain quickly. Then cover the site with an airtight transparent dressing (i.e., Tegaderm).
- The dressing should remain undisturbed for 48 hours, after which time the wound can be left open.
- Purse-string sutures are painful and not necessary.
- A chest radiograph should be taken after the drain has been removed to check for a pneumothorax.

Wound care

Routine closure of skin wounds in children is by subcuticular suture. The suture runs along below the surface of the wound and provides a neat and watertight closure. Invariably an absorbable suture is used.

- Dressings are a matter for individual preference. If dressings are used it is wise to keep the wound dry until the dressing is removed.
- If no dressing is used, then keep the wound dry for 24 to 48 hours.
- The appearance of clean surgical wounds should improve progressively each day after surgery.
- Parents should be asked to report increasing redness or tenderness so that the wound can be reviewed.

Advice on care after discharge from the hospital

Before the child is discharged from the hospital parents should be given clear, simple advice regarding analgesia, wound care, and postoperative follow-up. Ideally, written information should also be provided.

- *Following a minor day case*: Children will generally be back to normal within 24 hours. The return to school should be governed by their pain control. They should be excused from sports activities for >7 days.
- *Convalescence following major surgery*: Advice relating to return to school and resumption of sporting activity depends on the operation.

Postoperative care: drains and wound

Chest drain removal

- [text illegible]
- [text illegible]
- [text illegible]
- [text illegible]

Wound care

- [text illegible]
- [text illegible]
- [text illegible]
- [text illegible]
- [text illegible]

Advice on care after discharge from the hospital

- [text illegible]
- [text illegible]

Special senses

Common presentations

The red eye

Careful evaluation is needed when presentation is acute and there is pain, swelling, constant lacrimation, or blurred vision (see Box 24.1).

Box 24.1 Causes and differential diagnosis of red eye

Causes
- Upper respiratory infection
- Viral conjunctivitis
- Irritant conjunctivitis, e.g., chlorinated swimming pool
- Bacterial conjunctivitis
- Allergic conjunctivitis
- Stye (infection of eyelash root)
- Chalazion (meibomian or tarsal cyst)
- Trauma
- Other: Corneal abrasion, ulcer, keratitis; foreign body; preseptal cellulitis; uveitis

Differential diagnosis
Redness of entire eyelid or swollen eyelid
- Preseptal cellulitis
- Orbital cellulits
- Acute ethmoiditis

Associated eye pain or constant eye tearing, blinking
- Corneal ulcer
- Herpes simplex virus keratitis
- Eye foreign body

Blurred vision
- Uveitis

Infant under age 1 month
- Gonorrhea

Ear—pain and discharge

Ear discharge (otorrhea) may be due to drainage of blood, pus, or fluid from the ear. Discharge may also be caused by local ear canal irritation or infection:
- Otitis externa
- Eczema and other skin irritations
- Foreign-object impaction
- Otitis media with perforation of eardrum
- Head injury—CSF leakage

Earache (otalgia) can be a symptom of the conditions noted above. However, it may be the result of pain referred from pathology at another location:
- Teeth and jaw: Impaction molars, dental caries, malocclusion
- Acute tonsillitis
- Temporomandibular joint pain in rheumatologic disease
- Sinusitis
- Parotitis

Hearing assessment

A fetus will respond to sound in the latter part of pregnancy (from third trimester on). At birth, the baby will react to noise with a marked preference for voices. Significant bilateral hearing loss occurs in 0.1%–0.3% of newborn infants and in 2%–4% of the neonatal intensive care population.

Hearing tests

The early detection of hearing loss is important. Deafness impairs speech and language development, cognitive development, and socialization. Some evidence indicates that early detection of hearing loss with initiation of services improves developmental outcome.

Children should be referred for formal audiologic evaluation in any of the following scenarios:

- Any parental concern that the child has hearing loss
- Evidence of speech or language delay, cognitive delay, learning disability, or school failure
- Congenital anomaly of the ear or midface
- Family history of hearing loss
- Medical risk factors for hearing loss: Prematurity, ototoxic drugs, hyperbilirubinemia, hypoxemic–ischemic encephalopathy

Audiologists will conduct pure tone audiometry at a range of frequencies. Hearing threshold is defined by the sound intensity at which the child can hear the stimulus 50% of the time.

0–20 dB	Normal hearing
20–40 dB	Mild hearing loss
40–60 dB	Moderate hearing loss
60–80 dB	Severe hearing loss
>80 dB	Profound hearing loss

Hearing loss of up to 20 dB tends not to affect development but a loss of >40 dB will affect speech and language development.

Universal newborn hearing screening

The American Academy of Pediatrics (AAP) recommends universal hearing screening for all newborns before hospital discharge, with a goal of detecting hearing loss in infants before 3 months of age, and appropriate intervention no later than 6 months of age.

Most screening programs are conducted in nurseries and employ an electrophysiologic technique suitable for infants.

Auditory brainstem response (ABR)

ABR measures action potentials generated by the eighth cranial nerve in response to a click stimulus. Infants must typically be asleep for testing. Approximately 4% of tests result in referral for formal testing.

Otoacoustic emissions (OAE)

OAE testing measures the otoacoustic emissions generated by the normal-functioning cochlea in response to specific stimuli. Infants can be tested while awake, feeding, or using a pacifier. This testing modality is falsely positive when ear canals are occluded by vernix. From 5% to 20% of tests result in audiologic referral.

As with any screening program, failed tests are NOT diagnostic of hearing loss. It is important to reassure parents that a failed test simply means that a more formal audiologic investigation is indicated. For every 1 case of significant hearing loss diagnosed, screening programs typically result in 40 referrals for formal audiologic testing.

Childhood deafness

Hearing loss or deafness may be congenital or acquired and can be divided into sensorineural (SN) or conductive causes.

Sensorineural
Inherited, genetic
- Treacher–Collins syndrome (see Table 24.1)
- Wardenburg syndrome (see Table 24.1)

Antenatal, perinatal
- Congenital infection (e.g., rubella, CMV; syphilis)

Preterm
- Birth asphyxia
- Hyperbilirubinemia

Postnatal, childhood
- Drugs (e.g., aminoglycosides)
- Meningitis
- Head injury

Conductive
- Otitis media with effusion

Eustachian tube dysfunction
- Down syndrome
- Cleft palate
- Micrognathia (e.g., Pierre Robin sequence)
- Midfacial hypoplasia

Table 24.1 Syndromes associated with childhood deafness

Syndrome	Characteristics
Wardenburg syndrome	SN deafness + pigmentation anomalies (white forelock)
Klippel–Feil sequence	Deafness (SN or conductive) + short neck with low hairline
Treacher–Collins syndrome	Conductive deafness + midface hypoplasia
Pierre Robin sequence	Conductive deafness + mandibular hypoplasia and cleft soft palate
Alport syndrome	SN deafness, pyelonephritis, hematuria, and renal failure
Pendred syndrome	SN deafness + hypothyroidism
Usher syndrome	SN deafness + retinitis pigmentosa
Jewel–Lang–Nielson	SN deafness + long QT interval

Disorders of the ear

Acute otitis media (AOM) (see p. 812, Chapter 19)

Infection of the middle ear is associated with pain, fever, and irritability. Examination reveals a red and bulging tympanic membrane with loss of normal light reflection and mobility. Occasionally there is acute perforation.

Causal organisms include the following:

- Viruses (including RSV)
- *Pneumococcus*
- *H. influenzae*
- *Moraxella catarrhalis*
- Group A β-hemolytic streptococcus

Treatment always includes education and analgesia. Because 85% of episodes will resolve without antibiotic therapy, a period of watchful waiting or a plan for delayed prescription of antibiotics can be considered.

If antibiotic therapy is considered, amoxicillin is the typical first-line agent. Children at risk for penicillin-resistant *Pneumococcus* infection (those <2 years old, in child care, or with antibiotic treatment in the preceding 3 months) should be given a high-dose prescription (80–90 mg/kg/day). Erythromycin or TMP-SMX are alternatives for amoxicillin-allergic children.

For most children there is no need for a routine follow-up exam. Young children 12–36 months of age may be returned to the clinic 12 weeks after treatment to verify resolution of associated effusions.

Otitis media with effusion (OME)

This is a middle ear effusion without the inflammatory symptoms and signs of acute otitis media. OME is the result of acute otitis media complicated by residual eustachian tube dysfunction.

Most children are asymptomatic and treatment is not indicated.

Effusions that last more than 12 weeks are less likely to spontaneously resolve. An empiric trial of amoxicillin/clavulanic acid may promote resolution in this subset of patients. Children with chronic effusions should be referred for audiologic screening and may be candidates for insertion of pressure-equalization tubes (PET) through the tympanic membrane to bypass the dysfunctional eustachian tube.

Otitis externa (OE)

Itching or pain of the external ear canal is common in swimmers and after minor trauma. There may be discharge.

Examination reveals an inflamed ear canal that may be edematous. Traction on the ear lobe intensifies or reproduces pain. Often, the tympanic membrane is obscured, but otitis media is rare in the typical clinical circumstances of OE.

Treatment is with a combined antibiotic and steroid preparation applied as eardrops.

holesteatoma

This is an erosive condition affecting the middle ear and mastoid. It may lead to life-threatening intracranial infection. Signs include offensive discharge, conductive hearing loss, vertigo, and facial nerve palsy. Urgent referral to the ENT team is required for surgery and antibiotics.

Acute mastoiditis

This is uncommon but may follow an episode of acute otitis media. In the early stage, symptoms are indistinguishable from acute otitis media but may evolve to include intense pain, swelling, or tenderness over the mastoid process. The latter is due to acute mastoid osteitis and occurs when infection and destruction of the mastoid bony trabeculae have occurred.

Clinical examination may also reveal outward and downward displacement of the pinna, and swelling of the posterior-superior wall of the external ear canal. Purulent discharge may also be present.

Diagnosis is largely clinical, although CT scan is helpful. Admission for intravenous antibiotic treatment and drainage is indicated. Mastoidectomy is sometimes required.

Foreign-body impaction

Parents may observe a child putting an object in the ear canal, which otherwise may take several days to come to notice. On examination with an otoscope, objects that are easily visible (and with a cooperative child) may be extracted using a hook. Some nonorganic objects can also be flushed from the canal with an irrigation syringe and warm water.

Use of forceps should be avoided, as they tend to push the object further down the ear canal and may damage the tympanic membrane. Refer patient to the ENT team.

Common disorders of the nose

Epistaxis

A nosebleed or epistaxis is common in childhood. There is usually no obvious precipitating cause, but may be associated with minor nasal trauma (including nose-picking). Rarely, an underlying coagulation disorder may be present. Purulent, bloody nasal discharge should raise suspicions of foreign-body impaction.

Almost all nosebleeds originate in the vascular beds of the anterior cartilaginous septum. Initial management should include firm pressure applied to the cartilaginous part of the nose with finger and thumb for 10–15 minutes. Lubricant jelly can be applied to the anterior septum to reduce friability and recurrent epistaxis.

If simple measures fail to stop bleeding, refer patient to ENT for nasal packing or cauterization under direct visualization. A blood sample for full blood count, clotting screen, and blood-group testing is warranted in this situation.

Nasal -foreign body

Children may present with a unilateral offensive discharge from the nose. Removal may be attempted if the patient is able to cooperate, by having them trying to blow their nose. Alternatively, removal may be attempted directly by dislodging it with a suitable instrument.

An alligator-type forceps should be used to remove cloth, cotton, or paper foreign bodies. Pebbles, beans, and other hard foreign bodies are more easily grasped using bayonet forceps, or they may be rolled out by getting behind it with an ear curette, single skin hook, or right-angle ear hook.

If these measures are unsuccessful refer patient to the ENT department.

Nasal polyps

Nasal polyps are infrequent in childhood. They are associated with allergic rhinitis or cystic fibrosis. Signs include clear, watery rhinnorrhea, postnasal drip, and nasal obstruction. Increased snoring intensity may also be a feature. Treatment with nasal topical corticosteroids (e.g., beclomethasone) is required.

Nasal malformations

Abnormalities in nasal development may be associated with a number of congenital or inherited conditions.

Low or depressed nasal bridge

- Achodrogenesis syndromes
- Trisomy 21
  - Fetal valproate syndrome
  - Mucopolysaccharoidosis

Broad or wide nasal bridge

- Ehlers–Danlos syndrome (p. 973)
- Fragile X syndrome (p. 1069)
- Waardenberg syndrome

Small nose

- Cornelia de Lange syndrome (p. 1074)
- Fetal alcohol syndrome
- Osteogenesis imperfecta type 2 (p. 882)
- Williams syndrome (p. 1067)

Hypoplastic nares

- Ectodermal dysplasia
- Cleft lip sequence

Prominent nose

- Coffin–Lowry syndrome
- Rubenstein–Taybi syndrome
- Smith–Lemli–Opitz syndrome

Choanae atresia

- CHARGE association (p. 1076)

Disorders of mouth and tongue

Gingivostomatitis

Gingivostomatitis refers to inflammation of the oral mucosa and is characterized by the presence of gum edema and mouth ulcers. The condition is common, particularly among preschool-aged children, and is usually secondary to a viral infection, particularly those that cause common childhood illness such as the following:

- Herpes simplex virus (HSV) causes disease that is predominantly anterior in the mouth (cold sores, perioral vesicles, gingivitis).
- Coxsackie viruses more commonly cause disease posteriorly in the mouth (vesicles on tonsils or soft palate; hand, foot, and mouth disease).

Vesicular lesions may erupt on the lips, gums, tongue, and hard palate. There is a wide spectrum of clinical features ranging from mild to severe, often characterized by the following:

- Pain on eating and drinking
- High fever
- Bleeding from gums
- Extensive ulceration of the tongue, palate, and buccal mucosa
- Cervical lymphadenopathy
- Dehydration due to refusal to eat or drink may occur.

Investigation

Usually no specific tests are required for the diagnosis.

Treatment

- Symptomatic (analgesia) and supportive (fluids). Consider acetaminophen with codeine or similar analgesics.
- Good oral hygiene should be maintained with saline mouth washes as tolerated.
- Young children with high fever and a predominance of anterior oral lesions (lips, face, gums) are more likely to have an initial HSV infection. These children will benefit from oral acyclovir if initiated early in the course of illness.
- Severe infection may require hospital admission for rehydration with IV fluids.

Macroglossia

Macroglossia is tongue enlargement that leads to functional and cosmetic problems. Although this is a relatively uncommon disorder, it may cause significant morbidity. Macroglossia may be congenital or acquired in origin.

Congenital

- Down syndrome (p. 1059)
- Beckwith–Wiedemann syndrome (p. 1075)
- Mucopolysaccharidosis syndromes (p. 1100)

Acquired

- Congenital hypothyroidism (see p. 502)

In infants it poses early difficulty with feeding. In the longer term children may need assistance through speech and language therapy.

Vision assessment

Early visual development

At birth, most babies can fix their gaze and follow objects horizontally. Initially the eyes move independently; this unsteady alignment resolves in most children by 2–4 months.

Visual acuity is about 20/200. Infants see best about 12 inches from their eyes, approximately the location of the mother's face during breast-feeding.

The retina is well developed but the fovea is immature. The development of visual acuity is dependent on the production of well-formed images on the retina. Any obstacle that impedes images from reaching the retina will therefore affect normal development of the optic pathway and visual cortex. Examples include congenital cataract, persistent strabismus, marked discrepancies in visual acuity, and external obstructions (e.g., periorbital hemangioma).

Lack of normal development leads to amblyopia.
- 6 weeks: Both eyes move together and will follow a light source.
- 4 months: A baby should watch their hands and notice toys.
- 6 months: A baby reaches for toys.

Vision screening

Assessment for visual problems should be performed on all children at routine well-child visits, starting at birth.

Box 24.2 Vision screening from birth to 5 years

- *Birth* Verify presence of red reflex. Dark spots in the red reflex can be due to cataracts, corneal abnormalities, or opacities in the vitreous. The red reflex may be absent with a dense cataract. A white reflex is present with cataracts, retinoblastoma, or retinopathy of prematurity.
- *4 months* Gaze should be conjugate most of the time.
- *15 months* Cover–uncover test to detect latent strabismus
- *2 years* Identification of pictures
- *4–5 years* Identification of letters on the Snellen chart

The following problems should raise suspicions if they occur at the age of 6 months:
- Lack of eye contact or visual inattention
- Random eye movements
- Persistent nystagmus or squint

Visual impairment

Severe visual impairment is evident in 1 in 1000 births. Approximately 50% of severe visual impairment is genetic in origin. Early recognition is important to
- Identify those causes amenable to treatment (e.g., congenital cataracts)
- Put in place additional nonvisual stimulation (e.g., touch speech) to aid development
- Provide a safe environment

Legal definitions of blindness vary. One common criterion is vision of 20/200 or less in the better eye with best correction possible.

Causes of visual impairment

Inherited, genetic (50%)
- Trisomy 21
- CHARGE association

Congenital
- Cataract
- Albinism
- Retinal dystrophy
- Retinoblastoma
- Congenital infection e.g., CMV, rubella

Antenatal, perinatal (30%)
- Retinopathy of prematurity
- Hypoxic ischemic encephalopathy
- Cerebral damage
- Optic nerve hypoplasia

Postnatal (20%)
- Trauma
- Infection
  - Ophthalmic herpes simplex
- Juvenile idiopathic arthritis
  - Iritis

The early involvement of specialist preschool teachers for the visually impaired is essential for nonvisual stimulation and development.

Strabismus

Strabismus is an anomaly of ocular alignment. It is common in childhood, affecting 2%–4% of children. Uncorrected strabismus causes diplopia and can lead to suppression of visual input from one eye. This has a significant impact on visual development and can cause amblyopia.

The causes of strabismus may be
- Idiopathic
- Refractive error
- Visual loss
- Ophthalmoplegia (central or peripheral)

Describing strabismus
- Strabismus is described according to the direction of the eye deviation and the conditions under which deviation can be detected.
- Nasal deviation is described with the prefix eso- and temporal deviation with the prefix exo-.
- Strabismus that is present only when the visual axis is interrupted is "latent" and is described as a *phoria* (e.g., esophoria, exophoria).
- Strabismus that is always present is "manifest" and described as a *tropia* (e.g., esotropia, exotropia)
- Pseudostrabismus describes the appearance of strabismus in, typically, young infants with broad nasal bridges and epicathal folds. True strabismus is excluded by observation of a symmetrically placed corneal reflex.

Testing for strabismus
Parental report is often the best clue to latent strabismus.

Some clinicians now use a photoscreener to detect strabismus and anisometropia (significant variation in visual acuity between eyes). This device photographs a light reflex from the child's eyes. Variations in the reflex indicate certain ophthalmologic concerns. The test does not depend on patient cooperation, thus making it an appealing technology for use with infants, toddlers, and developmentally delayed older children.

The Cover–Uncover test is useful for detecting latent strabismus in toddlers and young children (see Fig. 24.1).

Management
The aim of treatment is to get the "weaker" eye "trained up" to prevent amblyopia. Treatments are usually under the supervision of ophthalmologists:
- Correct refractive error—wear glasses
- Wear an eye patch on the good eye to train weaker eye
- Eye muscle exercises
- Eye (muscle) surgery if the above measures fail

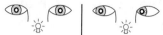

PSEUDOSQUINT Wide epicanthic folds give the appearance of squint
in the eye looking towards the nose. That the eyes are correctly aligned
is confirmed by the corneal reflection.

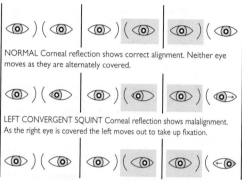

NORMAL Corneal reflection shows correct alignment. Neither eye
moves as they are alternately covered.

LEFT CONVERGENT SQUINT Corneal reflection shows malalignment.
As the right eye is covered the left moves out to take up fixation.

LEFT DIVERGENT SQUINT Corneal reflection shows malalignment.
As the right eye is covered the left moves out to take up fixation.

Figure 24.1 Testing for squints. Reprinted from Collier J, Longmore M, Brinsden
M (eds.) (2006). *Oxford Handbook of Clinical Specialties*, 7th ed., by permission of
Oxford University Press.

Disorders of the eye: infection and inflammatory

Eye infections are common in childhood and largely due to bacterial or viral infections affecting the conjunctiva.

Neonatal conjunctivitis

- Chemical conjunctivitis can occur 2–3 days after birth in response to the ocular chemoprophylaxis applied in most nurseries. This is usually mild and self-limited.
- Gonococcal conjunctivitis should be suspected if purulent discharge with swelling of the eyelids occurs within the first 48 hours of life. Intravenous antibiotic is required. The mother should be referred for care.
- Chlamydial conjunctivitis usually presents at the end of the first week of life. Diagnosis is established by specific monoclonal antibody test performed on conjunctival secretions. A 2-week course of oral erythromycin is required. The mother should be referred for care.

Childhood conjunctivitis

This may be due to bacteria (e.g., gram-positive cocci or *H. influenzae*), virus (e.g., adenovirus), or allergy.

Although most eye infections begin with viral pathogens, secondary bacterial infection is common. Most practitioners will treat infection with antibiotics. Specific antibiotic eye drops or ointment for 5 days is required.

Allergic conjunctivitis is more typically associated with itching, clear discharge, and bilateral presentation. Rhinitis may also be present. Ocular or systemic antihistamines may be prescribed.

Preseptal cellulitis

This is infection of the periorbital skin, usually due to infection by either *Staph. auerus or H. influenzae*. It may occur secondary to paranasal or dental abscess in older children.

Children are often systemically unwell with fever, erythema, and tenderness over the affected area. This requires prompt treatment with antibiotics.

Preseptal cellulitis must be differentiated from orbital cellulitis, an ophthalmologic emergency. Clues to orbital cellulitis include proptosis, limited ocular movement, and decreased visual acuity. A CT scan should be considered to exclude these complications if suspected.

Iritis (see Chapter 20, p. 891)

Also known as anterior uveitis, iritis refers to inflammation of the uveal tract structures (i.e., iris, ciliary body, and choroids). It is characterized by symptoms of

- Ocular pain
- Photophobia
- Excessive lacrimation
- Blurred vision

Signs include

- Redness
- Miosis
- Keratic precipitates on slit-lamp examination
- Long-term disease may be complicated with the development of cataract, glaucoma, and macular eye degeneration.

Causes of iritis

- Local infection, e.g., herpes simplex or zoster virus
- Trauma or surgery: Think about this diagnosis when eye pain and redness worsen in the days after blunt trauma to the eye.
- Systemic disease
- Seronegative arthritides: HLA B27 positive, ankylosing spondylitis, Reiter syndrome, psoriatic arthritis
- Inflammatory bowel disease
- Juvenile idiopathic arthritis
- Sarcoidosis
- Bechet's disease

Referral to an ophthalmologist and treatment with topical steroid drops or ointment and mydriatic agents are required.

Disorders of the eye: retinal disease

Retinopathy of prematurity (ROP)

This is a fibrovascular proliferative retinal disorder occurring in preterm and low birth weight infants (see also Chapter 6, p. 184). Its development has been associated with high concentrations of inspired oxygen during the neonatal period.

Normal retinal vascularization is not complete until full term. In preterm infants this process is interrupted and on restarting may proceed abnormally with aberrant and proliferative new vessel formation.

ROP screening

Infants born <31 weeks gestation or who are <1500 g are screened from 6 weeks of age until the retina has vascularized.

Treatment

Indirect laser therapy is used in severe cases.

Other medical conditions causing retinopathy

Sickle cell disease

The deformed red blood cells in sickle cell disease may cause retinal vascular occlusion or ischemia. A proliferative retinopathy with new vessel formation, or a nonproliferative retinopathy with scarring and fibrosis may develop. Screening is required with laser photocoagulation for new vessel formation.

Diabetes mellitus

Diabetic retinopathy is rarely seen in children with type 1 diabetes and not usually before onset of puberty and teenage years.

Retinitis pigmentosa (RP)

This progressive, degenerative disorder of the retina is characterized by typical pigmented retinal appearances. It is an important cause of night blindness, reduced central and peripheral vision, and cataracts. It may occur as an isolated finding or may be part of a systemic disorder (see Table 24.2).

Table 24.2 Syndromes associated with retinitis pigmentosa (RP)

Usher syndrome	RP + congenital deafness
Bassen–Kornweig syndrome	RP + abetalipoproteinemia, ataxia and malabsorption
Refsum's disease	RP + polyneuropathy, deafness and cerebellar dysfunction
Kearns–Sayre syndrome	RP + ophthalmoplegia, cardiac conduction defect

Eye foreign body

Small foreign bodies are usually cleared by tear film. Occasionally they may lodge underneath the upper eyelid or become embedded in the cornea, causing intense irritation and excessive lacrimation. Examination of the eye to locate and remove the foreign body should be carried out:

- Instill topical anesthetic drops.
- Perform a visual acuity check (where appropriate) and fundoscopy. Examine the anterior chamber and tear film with a bright light and examine the conjunctival sacs.
- Fluorescein examination to rule out corneal abrasion
- A loose foreign body usually adheres to a swab lightly touched to the surface of the conjunctiva, or will be washed out by copious irrigation with saline.

Cataract

Cataract refers to an opacification of the lens. It may be congenital or acquired.

Causes of cataract

- Inherited, genetic
  - Myotonic dystrophy
  - Walker–Warburg syndrome
- Congenital maternal infection, e.g., rubella, toxoplasmosis
- Trauma
- Radiotherapy
- Inflammation, e.g., chronic iritis
- Infection
- Metabolic syndromes
  - Galactosemia
  - Wilson disease
  - Lowe syndrome
  - Fabry disease
- Other syndromes, e.g., trisomy 21
- Drugs, e.g., long-term steroid therapy

Absence of the normal bilateral red reflex or the presence of a white reflex on ophthalmoscopic examination should raise suspicion of an underlying cataract. Referral to an ophthalmologist is required.

Glaucoma

This condition is associated with raised intraocular pressure, disc cupping, and visual-field loss. Primary open-angle glaucoma and secondary closed-angle glaucoma are rare in childhood.

Congenital glaucoma is also rare and may be due to the abnormal development of the anterior chamber angle.

Later-onset glaucoma may result from syndromes that effect eye development. The infant eye, unlike the adult eye, can enlarge enormously with high intraocular pressures (buphtalamous "ox-eye"), developing a hazy cornea and excess lacrimation. The treatment is surgical, but is often unsuccessful.

Visual prognosis is poor and often results in blindness.

Nystagmus

This is a series of involuntary, rhythmic oscillations of one or both eyes in either the horizontal or vertical plane (see Table 24.3). It occurs when there is impairment of the mechanisms controlling conjugate eye movement.

Table 24.3 Types of nystagamus

Type	Characteristics
Pendular	Ocular oscillations equal in speed and amplitude
Jerking	Movement in one direction is faster than in the other. The "direction" of nystagmus is taken from the direction of fastest phase of movement.
Gaze	Jerking nystagmus on lateral gaze. Usually due to a lesion in the brain stem. Also caused by drugs and labyrinthine dysfunction
Fixation	A pendular nystagmus resulting from damage to central vision. Congenital visual defects may produce this type of nystagmus.
Vestibular	Horizontal jerk movements. Secondary to severe middle-ear infection affecting the labyrinth structures, or due to damage to the vestibular nerve (e.g., acoustic neuroma)
Cerebellar	Gaze-paretic nystagmus with jerk movements of eyes to maintain eccentric gaze. Secondary to cerebellar damage

Nystagmus may also occur if there is muscle paralysis or weakness (e.g., secondary to myasthenia gravis).

Genetics

Useful resources

The human genome contains ~30,000 genes, so the few common genetic disorders in this section are a very tiny sample from an enormous range of genetic disorders. Other useful resources for genetic disorders are listed below.

Books

- Cassidy SB, Allanson JE (eds.) (2004). *Management of Genetic Syndromes*, 2nd ed. New York: Wiley.
- Firth HV, Hurst JA, Hall JG (2005). *Oxford Desk Reference Clinical Genetics*. New York: Oxford University Press.
- Harper PS (2004). *Practical Genetic Counselling*, 6th ed., revised reprint. London: Arnold.
- Jones KL (2006). *Smith's Recognizable Patterns of Human Malformation*, 6th ed. Philadelphia: W.B. Saunders.
- Nussbaum RL, McInnes RR, Willard HF, Boerkel CF III. *Thompson and Thompson Genetics in Medicine*, 6th ed. revised. Philadelphia: W.B. Saunders.

Web-based resources

- Online Mendelian Inheritance in Man (OMIM)
  www.ncbi.nlm.nih.gov
- Directory of Clinical Genetics Services in the United States
  www.genetests.org
- GeneReviews
  www.genereviews.org
- National Organization for Rare Disorders (U.S.)
  www.raredisease.org
- Orphanet database on rare diseases and orphan drugs
  www.orpha.net
- March of Dimes
  www.marchofdimes.com

Clinical genetics and genetic counseling

Definition of genetic counseling

In the 1998 edition of *Practical Genetic Counselling*, P.S. Harper defined genetic counseling as "the process by which individuals or relatives at risk for a disorder that may be hereditary are advised of the consequences of the disorder, the probability of transmitting it and the ways in which this may be prevented, avoided or ameliorated."

Role of the clinical geneticist

Clinical geneticists are doctors with special expertise in the assessment and diagnosis of children and adults with multiple congenital anomalies and inherited disorders. Departments of clinical genetics are usually based in large teaching hospitals. During their training and practice, clinical geneticists acquire expertise in a wide variety of rare disorders and the genetics of more common multifactorial disorders.

When families come to the genetics clinic, they usually have a number of questions, which can be summarized as follows:
- What is it?
- Why did it happen?
- Will it happen again?
- If so, what can be done to prevent it?
- What management or treatment is recommended?

The main role of the clinical geneticist is to establish an accurate genetic diagnosis, which is essential to
- Gain an understanding of the condition and possible prognosis
- Guide optimal management for the child and identify other systems that need surveillance, e.g., hearing or vision
- Address concerns about events during pregnancy or delivery
- Enable accurate genetic advice for parents and other family members about the risk of recurrence in future pregnancies.

A basic principle of genetic counseling is that advice is *nondirective*.

When to refer to clinical genetics

A majority of underlying chronic disorders in children are either clearly genetic or have a genetic susceptibility. It is increasingly important for pediatricians to be able to recognize genetic disorders and to know when to enlist the help of a clinical geneticist.

Indications for referral to clinical genetics

Congenital anomalies

- Multiple congenital anomalies (birth defects)
- Isolated congenital anomaly in conjunction with dysmorphic features, developmental delays, abnormal growth parameters, or family history

Dysmorphic features is a term used to describe physical features, particularly unusual facial features, which are not usually found in a child of the same age or ethnic background.

Abnormal growth parameters refer to height or weight or OFC >98th centile or <2nd centile.

Developmental delays (infant, preschool child)

- Unexplained severe developmental delays
- Developmental delays in conjunction with dysmorphic features, a congenital anomaly, abnormal growth parameters, or family history

Dysmorphic features

- Especially if in conjunction with developmental delays, learning disability, a congenital anomaly, or abnormal growth parameters

Family history

- Similar problems affecting more than one member of the family

Learning disability or mental retardation (older child, school age)

- Unexplained severe learning disability
- Learning disability in conjunction with dysmorphic features, a congenital anomaly, abnormal growth parameters, or family history

Multiple problems and no diagnosis

- Child with multiple problems and under the care of many specialists with no unifying diagnosis

New diagnosis of a genetic disorder

- Enables explanation of the genetic basis of the condition
- Essential if the diagnosis may have implications for other relatives
- Important if the parents would like advice regarding future pregnancies

Teenager with a genetic disorder

- If a genetic diagnosis was made in infancy or early childhood, refer back to clinical genetics when the child is in their mid-teens so that the young adult understands the genetic basis of their condition and the risks to their own offspring.
- New information for a known condition or new testing options for a known or as yet undiagnosed condition

Taking a family history

This is a very important tool in clinical genetics. One of the key skills in taking a family history is drawing a family tree. The approach described here is intended for routine use in a general pediatric setting. A more detailed approach is indicated when assessing a patient with a known or possible genetic disorder.

Drawing a basic family tree

- Start with your patient. Draw a ▪ symbol for a boy, ○ for a girl.
- Next draw ▪ or • symbols for your patient's parents and siblings. Record basic information only, such as age and whether they are in good health and whether there are any concerns regarding development. If an individual has died, note the age and cause of death and annotate the family tree with a straight line slash through the ▯ or ⊘ symbol(s).
- Ask whether there are any inherited disorders in the family.
- Ask whether your patient's parents are related (consanguinity increases the chance of an autosomal recessive disorder). Consanguinity is indicated by drawing a double line on the family tree between related individuals.
- Ask the key question, "Has anybody else in your family had a similar problem to the patient?" Be aware that some conditions have variable expression, e.g., del 22q11 may present with cleft palate in one member of the family and congenital heart disease in another.
- Ask if there are any family members with birth defects, developmental delays/mental retardation, or growth problems.
- Extend the family tree to include grandparents, aunts, uncles, and cousins. If you have not revealed a familial problem by this stage, do not go any further, as you are unlikely to have missed an important familial disease with onset in childhood. In the case of a suspected X-linked disorder, extend the family tree further on the maternal side.
- Color-shade those people in the family tree affected by the disorder. This will help determine whether there is a genetic problem, and if there is, to suggest the pattern of inheritance.

Genetic testing

Appropriate situations for genetic testing in a child

- Diagnostic testing in a *child who has features of a genetic disorder*, e.g., chromosome analysis in a child with suspected Down syndrome.
- The child is asymptomatic, but is *at risk for a genetic condition for which preventative or other therapeutic measures are available*, e.g., testing to determine if a child of an affected parent with retinoblastoma (with a known mutation) requires screening by frequent periodic examinations under anesthesia. This is predictive testing and should involve a clinical geneticist.
- The child is *at risk for a genetic condition with pediatric onset for which preventive therapeutic measures are not available*, e.g., SMA type 1.
- Involve a clinical geneticist. The decision to undertake a genetic test requires a careful balancing of benefit and harm; each case is assessed on its individual merits. Generally, testing is done at parental discretion after careful discussion. Most genetic tests are not fully sensitive.

Inappropriate situations for genetic testing in a child

- An asymptomatic child is *at risk for a genetic condition that usually has onset in adult life* for which preventive or effective therapeutic measures are not available, e.g., Huntington disease.
- Testing for *carrier status*, e.g., siblings of a child with cystic fibrosis. Practice does vary, but we recommend that testing be deferred until the child is old enough to provide informed consent, or at least to take part in the discussion about testing. Parents sometimes request testing of young children without having necessarily thought through the difficulties this may lead to later on. We suggest referral to clinical genetics if parents request carrier testing.
- Genetic testing of children for the *benefit of another family member* should **not** be performed unless testing is necessary to prevent substantial harm to the family member.

Chromosome tests

Karyotype analysis

A standard chromosome analysis involves a G-banded karyotype viewed by a cytogeneticist using a light microscope. Using this approach, the maximum resolution is ~5–10 Mb (1 Mb = 1 million base pairs). One of the major advantages of a chromosome analysis is that it is a genomic survey, i.e., it looks in outline at the whole genome. The normal male karyotype is 46,XY. The normal female karyotype is 46,XX.

Fluorescence in situ hybridization

Targeted studies are possible at higher resolution using specific fluorescence in situ hybridization (FISH) probes. Using FISH, it is possible to see the submicroscopic deletions responsible for Williams syndrome (7q) and Angelman syndrome (15q), but only if the clinician specifically requests this.

Currently, high-resolution genome-wide techniques such as array CGH (microarray-based comparative genomic hybridization) are being implemented to complement conventional chromosome analysis and may supersede standard karyotyping in the future.

Molecular genetic analysis

The human genome contains ~3,000,000,000 DNA base pairs and ~30,000 genes. In genetic disorders, the pathology may range from a whole extra chromosome (i.e., Down syndrome) to a single base-pair alteration (i.e., achondroplasia). Molecular genetic tests (i.e., gene probes) are highly specific tests that only reveal information about one specific gene, usually selected on clinical grounds.

- If *commonly occurring mutations exist*, analysis is simple and comparatively inexpensive, e.g., cystic fibrosis (standard kit test for the most common mutations in the Caucasian population) and achondroplasia (two common mutations, G1138A and G1138C in the *FGFR3* gene, account for ~98% of mutations in children with achondroplasia).
- If the *mutation in a family is known*, analysis is usually straightforward and takes a few weeks for most tests. Such tests, based on information obtained from other family members, should involve a clinical geneticist.
- If the *mutation is unknown* an entire gene may have to be sequenced. In this situation genetic testing can be labor intensive and expensive (often several thousand dollars), and only a small proportion may be available as diagnostic tests. Reporting times are highly variable. Consult a clinical geneticist on whether genetic testing is appropriate in these circumstances.

Practical issues relating to genetic testing

Counseling the family before testing

Diagnostic testing

Think carefully about the potential impact of the diagnosis you may make with a genetic test. Some genetic conditions are relentlessly progressive and life limiting (i.e., Duchenne muscular dystrophy). Others imply lifelong impairment of a child's ability to learn and communicate (i.e., Angelman syndrome, fragile X syndrome).

If you make a genetic diagnosis, it is likely to remain a permanent aspect of that child's life. There may be some treatable elements to the condition, but it is unlikely to be transient or curable.

On the other hand, a scientifically confirmed biomedical diagnosis allows parents to obtain appropriate medical and educational resources for their child. The diagnosis may have implications for other family members.

Preferably, the family should be counseled by a clinical geneticist or genetic counselor before a genetic test is performed. Ensure that the parents understand what you are testing for and why. Explain how long it may take to obtain a result and make careful arrangements for communicating the result.

Predictive testing

The circumstances in which this may be appropriate can be complex and vary for different disorders. Predictive testing should be arranged through a clinical geneticist.

Common chromosomal disorders

Klinefelter syndrome (47,XXY)

- Affects ~1/600 to 1/800 boys
- Most cases are caused by non-disjunction during maternal oogenesis.
- Boys with Klinefelter syndrome enter puberty normally, but by mid-puberty the testes begin to involute and the boys develop hypergonadotropic hypogonadism with decreased testosterone production. (They are often tall compared to siblings and may develop female habitus.) Testes are small in adult life, and men with Klinefelter syndrome are generally infertile (azoospermia). Gynecomastia develops at puberty in ≥50%. Boys with Klinefelter syndrome typically have an IQ ~15 points lower than that of their siblings.
- Many boys with Klinefelter syndrome remain undiagnosed throughout childhood, with the diagnosis only coming to light during investigation of infertility.
- Diagnosis is by chromosome analysis.

Trisomy 13 (Patau syndrome)

- Incidence is ~1/6000 births
- ~75% of cases are caused by non-disjunction during maternal oogenesis, ~20% have Robertsonian translocation, ~5% result from mosaicism.
- Trisomy 13 may be diagnosed by antenatal ultrasound scan, since the majority of affected babies have multiple congenital anomalies.
- Typical malformations include holoprosencephaly; small for gestational age (SGA); microcephaly; microphthalmia; cleft lip/palate; congenital heart disease, e.g., atrial (ASD) or ventricular septal defect (VSD); renal anomalies, e.g., fused kidneys; postaxial polydactyly; together with severe or profound mental retardation.
- If there is clinical suspicion of trisomy 13, a physician should discuss these concerns with the parents.
- The diagnosis is confirmed by a chromosome analysis (additional chromosome 13). Most cytogenetics laboratories are able to offer a rapid analysis, e.g., interphase FISH to confirm the diagnosis quickly.

Trisomy 18 (Edwards syndrome)

- Incidence is ~1/8000 births
- Most cases are caused by non-disjunction during maternal oogenesis.
- Babies with Trisomy 18 are usually SGA (mean birth weight, 2240 g) with an OFC <3rd centile. Other common features include congenital heart disease, usually VSD ± valve dysplasia; short sternum; overriding fingers; and "rocker-bottom" feet. There is a strong female excess. Median life expectancy is ~4 days, although some affected babies live for several months and even longer.
- If there is clinical suspicion of Trisomy 18, a physician should discuss these concerns with the parents.
- Investigation is as for Trisomy 13, with initial rapid interphase FISH testing followed by formal chromosome analysis (additional chromosome 18).

Turner syndrome (45,X) (see p. 551)

Down syndrome

Incidence
- ~1 in 600–700 live births (incidence increases with advancing maternal age)

Cause
The great majority (~95%) of babies with Down syndrome have trisomy 21, usually due to non-disjunction during maternal oogenesis. Approximately 2% are the result of a Robertsonian translocation; ~2% are mosaic, with a normal cell line as well as the trisomy 21 cell line.

Clinical features
- Usually presents at birth
- Generalized hypotonia and marked head lag
- Facial features include small ears, up-slanting eyes, prominent epicanthal folds, a flat facial profile, and protruding tongue; later, Brushfield spots are apparent in the iris (whitish spots)
- Flat occiput (brachycephaly) and short neck
- Typical limb features include short, broad hands (brachydactyly); short, incurved little fingers (clinodactyly); single transverse palmar crease; and a wide "sandal" gap between the first and second toes.
- Mild short stature
- Intellectual impairment becomes apparent. IQ scores range from 25 to 70.
- Social skills often exceed other intellectual skills.

Associated conditions
- ~40%–50% have congenital heart disease, most commonly atrioventricular canal, ASD, VSD, and tetralogy of Fallot
- GI problems include duodenal atresia, anal atresia, Hirschsprung's disease
- Increased risk of infection
- Developmental hip dysplasia
- Atlantoaxial instability or subluxation of the cervical spine
- Eczema
- Deafness, both sensorineural and conductive
- Cataracts
- Leukemia (1%)
- Acquired hypothyroidism

Diagnosis
If there is clinical suspicion of Down syndrome, a pediatrician should discuss his or her concerns with the parents. The diagnosis is confirmed by chromosome analysis showing an additional chromosome 21. Most cytogenetics laboratories are able to offer a rapid analysis, e.g., interphase FISH, to establish the diagnosis quickly.

Management

- Refer patient for a detailed cardiac assessment and audiology evaluation.
- Genetic counseling by a clinical geneticist should be offered. It is not necessary to undertake parental chromosome analysis if the cause is non-disjunctional trisomy 21 or mosaic trisomy 21, but this is very important if the karyotype shows a translocation.
- Putting the parents in contact with support organizations is often helpful, such as the National Down Syndrome Society, at: www.ndss.org, or National Down Syndrome Congress, at: www.ndsccenter.org.
- Long-term follow-up should ideally be a multidisciplinary team led by the primary-care pediatrician, with expertise provided by appropriate specialists as needed. Physical therapy to improve tone and posture is often required.
- Routinely test thyroid function and hearing annually.
- Almost all children with Down syndrome are now educated in main-stream schools with appropriate educational support.
- Atlantoaxial instability can be evaluated at 3–5 years, especially if the child plans to participate in sports such as in the Special Olympics.
- Refer to the American Academy of Pediatrics (2001). Health supervision for children with Down syndrome. *Pediatrics* **107**(2):442–449.

Prognosis

If deaths from congenital cardiac disease are excluded, life expectancy is well into adult life, although somewhat shortened, as almost all individuals with Down syndrome develop Alzheimer disease by age 40 years. Most adults can live semi-independently with supervision.

Genetic disorders with cardiac features

Many chromosomal disorders and genetic syndromes are characterized by congenital heart disease.

Deletion 22q11 syndrome/velocardiofacial syndrome (VCFS)/Di George syndrome

- Incidence is ~1/4000
- Caused by a microdeletion on chromosome 22q11.2. Most children have a de novo microdeletion, but in ~15% of cases the condition is inherited from an affected parent
- Apart from cardiac defects, usually involving aortic arch, features include subtle dysmorphism (wide, prominent nasal bridge, down-slanting eyes, small mouth), parathyroid aplasia or hypoplasia (hypocalcemia), and thymus aplasia (T-cell deficiency). Short stature is common.
- Consider this condition in all children diagnosed with tetralogy of Fallot or aortic arch abnormalities, e.g., interrupted aortic arch (~20% will have del(22q11)).
- Also consider this condition in any child with congenital heart disease, e.g., VSD, who has hypernasal speech, a cleft palate, including submu-cous cleft palate, hypocalcemia, recurrent infections, or learning difficulties, especially speech and language delays.
- Diagnosis will be missed on a routine chromosome analysis; it requires a FISH study.

Marfan syndrome (MFS)

- Incidence is ~1/5000 births
- This variable autosomal dominant multisystem disorder is caused by mutation in the *FBN1* gene on chromosome 15q. There is a high new mutation rate (~30%)
- Features include tall and slim body build with long limbs; pectus chest deformity; scoliosis; high, narrow palate; long fingers (arachnodactyly); and joint laxity. Most affected children are myopic and some may develop lens dislocation (a major diagnostic feature).
- Cardiac features: Initially, there may be a floppy mitral valve. With time, dilatation of the aortic root (another major diagnostic feature) may occur, leading eventually to ascending aortic aneurysm and dissec-tion. Treatment with β-blockers may slow the progression of aortic dilatation. New therapies such as losartan (an angiotensin II receptor antagonist) are being evaluated.
- If genetic confirmation of the diagnosis is required, this is possible (in conjunction with a clinical geneticist) by mutation analysis of the *FBN1* gene.
- Other causes of aortic dilatation and dissection in childhood include mutations in *TGFBR1* and *TGFBR2*, also known as Loeys–Dietz aortic aneurysm dissection syndrome.

Noonan syndrome (NS)

- Incidence is ~1 in 2500 births
- An autosomal dominant disorder, NS is genetically heterogeneous, with ~50% of cases caused by mutation in the *PTPN11* gene on 12q. Other genes that cause NS or related disorders have been identified.
- Features include short stature, congenital heart disease (especially pulmonary stenosis), a broad neck, chest deformity with pectus carinatum superiorly and pectus excavatum inferiorly, mild developmental delays, undescended testes, and typical facial features (hypertelorism, ptosis, ear abnormalities).
- If genetic confirmation of the diagnosis is required, this may be possible (in conjunction with a clinical geneticist) for some children by mutation analysis of the *PTPN11* or other genes.

Williams syndrome (WS)

- Incidence is 1 in 7500 live births
- WS is caused by a microdeletion on 7q11, which encompasses the elastin gene.
- An associated cardiac defect is supravalvular aortic stenosis, often with peripheral pulmonary branch stenosis.
- Facial features include periorbital fullness; full cheeks; anteverted nares; wide mouth with full lips; and small, widely spaced teeth. Most affected individuals have mild mental retardation with strengths in language but poor visuospatial skills.
- The typical behavioral phenotype is that of overfriendliness, short attention span, and anxiety.
- ~15% of infants have hypercalcemia.
- Diagnosis is by FISH study for the 7q11 microdeletion.
- Further information, including growth charts, is available at: www.williams-syndrome.org/fordoctors

Turner syndrome (45,X) (see p. 551)

Genetic testing in cognitive impairment

Among children with severe mental retardation, a high proportion will have a genetic cause (see also p. 1068). This can be elucidated in ~50% of children, with chromosomal disorders being the largest group. Referral to clinical genetics should be considered for all children with unexplained severe global developmental delays or mental retardation.

The referring pediatrician may choose to undertake some basic diagnostic genetic testing, including the following.

Chromosome analysis

Investigation has a higher yield for children with more severe forms of unexplained developmental delays. Specific FISH tests for submicroscopic microdeletions, e.g., Williams, 22q11 syndrome, can be requested, but molecular cytogenetic approaches such as array comparative genomic hybridization (CGH) are likely to be of greater yield in the near future.

Fragile X analysis

This is the most common cause of inherited learning disability, but remains a rare disorder. As it is often difficult to diagnose on clinical grounds, genetic testing should be offered to all children with developmental delays.

Creatine kinase in boys

Duchenne muscular dystrophy may present with speech delays and delayed motor milestones and/or global delays.

Amino and organic acids

Inborn errors of metabolism are individually rare, but may present with nonspecific features, e.g., developmental delays and/or FTT. Plasma and urine samples should be arranged if there is developmental regression, episodic decompensation, parental consanguinity, a family history, or physical examination findings consistent with a metabolic disorder, e.g., microcephaly, macrocephaly, and hepatosplenomegaly. "Nonspecific" abnormalities are more common than true diagnoses.

Urine glycosaminoglycans (mucopolysaccharidoses)

Consider this test if there is developmental regression, coarse features, macrocephaly, short stature, or signs of dysostosis multiplex.

Ophthalmological consultation

This is important especially if there is concern regarding vision, eye signs (e.g., nystagmus), neurological signs, or microcephaly.

Audiology assessment

Obtain this assessment especially if there is speech delay or concern regarding hearing.

Consider congenital infection

Consider such infection in children with intrauterine growth retardation, microcephaly, and eye and hearing signs. Culture of appropriate body fluids in the infant with serial maternal serologies may be diagnostic. It is useful for children up to ~18 months of age.

Angelman syndrome (AS)

- Incidence ~1/40,000
- AS is caused by impaired or absent function of the maternally imprinted *UBE3A* gene on chromosome 15q11.13.
- AS is a distinctive neurobehavioral condition with severe developmental delays, profound speech impairment, an ataxic wide-based gait, and a specific behavioral phenotype (excitable personality, hand-flapping, and inappropriately happy affect). Seizures are common.
- The genetics of AS are complex. Refer to a clinical geneticist.

Fragile X syndrome (FRAXA)

- Incidence is ~1/5500 males. It is the most common inherited cause of mental retardation.
- FRAXA is caused by a full expansion (>200 repeats) in the $(CGG)_n$ triplet repeat in the FRAXA gene on chromosome Xq27.3
- Boys with fragile X syndrome typically have global developmental delays, often with gaze avoidance, autism, stereotyped repetitive behaviors such as hand-flapping, and resistance to change of routines.
- Up to 50% of girls with a full *FRAXA* expansion will have learning and behavioral difficulties that are similar to but less severe than those seen in affected boys.
- Genetic counseling is very complex and there will be genetic implications for relatives; referral to a clinical geneticist is recommended.

Prader–Willi syndrome (see p. 1075)

Rett syndrome

- Affects ~1/10,000 female births
- Caused by mutation in the *MECP2* gene on Xq28. Girls with Rett syndrome appear normal in the first 6 months of life. A second gene, *CDKL5*, causes a Rett-like syndrome in girls with early-onset, intractable seizures.
- This is a severe neurodevelopmental disorder that almost exclusively affects girls. It presents after age 1 year, usually with developmental regression and loss of purposeful hand movements. The child may develop seizures, scoliosis, erratic breathing with episodes of breath-holding and hyperventilation, and stereotypic hand-wringing. The condition is more variable than initially described.

Smith–Magenis syndrome

- Affects at least 1/25,000 children
- Usually caused by a de novo microdeletion on chromosome 17p11.2
- Typical features include a broad face with midface hypoplasia, brachydactyly, obesity, developmental delays or learning disability with behavioral disturbance, especially of sleep (nighttime waking and daytime somnolence)
- The diagnosis may be missed on a routine chromosome analysis and may require FISH for the 17p11.2 microdeletion.

Williams syndrome (see p. 1067)

Genetic disorders with neuromuscular features

The vast majority of severe neuromuscular disorders affecting infants and children have a genetic basis. In addition to accurate assessment and examination of the child, a detailed family history and examination of parents may sometimes be very helpful in establishing the diagnosis.

Congenital myotonic dystrophy (see also p. 612)

- Caused by a triplet repeat expansion $(CTG)_n$ in the *DM1* gene on 19q. Congenitally affected infants usually have a huge expansion of the triplet repeat with >1000 repeats.
- Occurs in affected babies born to women who also have myotonic dystrophy (an autosomal dominant disorder with onset usually in adult life), even when mild or undiagnosed.
- Typically, there is polyhydramnios, and at delivery the baby is floppy and may require ventilatory support.
- Diagnosis is usually possible by careful examination of the mother (grip myotonia and inability to bury eyelashes) and analysis of a DNA sample from the infant.
- Mortality is ~50%. Survivors have static or slowly progressive muscle weakness. Many have associated moderate intellectual impairment.

Duchenne muscular dystrophy (DMD) (see also p. 612)

- Affects ~1/3500 male births, DMD is the most common and severe form of childhood muscular dystrophy.
- DMD is caused by mutations (deletions, duplications, and point mutations) in the dystrophin gene on Xp21.
- DMD presents with developmental delays, especially late walking and speech delays. In the early phase of the disease, boys have difficulty rising from the floor (using Gowers maneuver—the child climbs up their thighs with their hands to get up off the floor). Later there is early loss of ambulation (mean age ~9 years), and death occurs in the late teens or early 20's. Affected boys develop progressive cardiomyopathy. ~30% of boys with DMD have a mild learning disability that is not progressive.
- Serum creatine kinase (CK) is grossly elevated, usually >10× normal levels. Diagnosis is often possible by genetic testing, avoiding the need for muscle biopsy.
- DMD follows X-linked recessive inheritance, and expert genetic counseling is an essential part of management.
- Death from cardiorespiratory failure or infection usually occurs in the early 20's.

Spinal muscular atrophy (SMA) (see also p. 608)

- An autosomal recessive disorder caused by mutations in the *SMN1* gene on 5q13. ~95% of infants with type 1 SMA are homozygously deleted for exon 7 of the *SMN1* gene.
- Symmetrical proximal muscle weakness is a consequence of degeneration of the anterior horn cells of the spinal cord. Intelligence is
- unaffected.
- There are several types:
  - *Type 1 SMA* (severe): Onset is in first few months of life. The child is never able to sit or walk. Death is from respiratory failure, usually by age 6–12 months.
  - *Type 2 SMA* (intermediate): Onset is before age 18 months. The child is able to sit, but not to walk unaided; survival into adult life is usual.
  - *Type 3 SMA* (mild): Onset of proximal muscle weakness is after age 2 years. The child has the ability to walk independently initially. Survival is into adult life.
- Diagnosis can be made by molecular genetic testing.

Genetic disorders with dermatological features

Sometimes the cutaneous features are the key to diagnosis of a genetic disorder (see also Chapter 22).

Ehlers–Danlos syndrome (EDS) (see p. 973)

- Incidence is ~1 in 5000 births
- There are numerous types of EDS. Classical EDS is autosomal dominant and caused by mutation in the *COL5A1* and *COL5A2* genes.
- All forms of EDS are characterized by skin fragility, excessive bruising and scarring, musculoskeletal pain, and susceptibility to osteoarthritis. The skin is soft and hyperextensible with easy bruising and thin, atrophic, "cigarette paper" scars, joint hypermobility, varicose veins, and a risk of premature delivery in affected fetuses.
- Hypermobile EDS is a common and usually mild autosomal dominant disorder characterized by soft skin with hypermobility of large and small joints.
- Vascular EDS is caused by mutations in the *COL3A1* gene. Affected individuals are prone to rupture of large arteries as well as hollow viscera, such as bowel and pregnant uterus. Joint signs are less prominent and typically the skin is translucent with prominent veins visible.

Neurofibromatosis type 1 (NF1) (see also p. 617)

NF1 has a prevalence of ~1 in 4000. It is an autosomal dominant condition caused by mutation in the *NF1* gene on 17q11.2. For a clinical diagnosis of NF1, the patient should have two or more of the following features:

- Six or more café-au-lait spots (≥0.5 cm in children)
- Two or more neurofibromas of any type (dermal neurofibromas are small lumps in the skin that appear in adolescence) or one or more plexiform neurofibroma
- Freckling in the axilla, neck, or groin
- Optic glioma (tumor in the optic pathway)
- Two or more Lisch nodules (benign iris hamartomas)
- A distinctive bony lesion, e.g., sphenoid wing dysplasia, or dysplasia or thinning of the long bone cortex, e.g., pseudoarthrosis of the tibia
- A first-degree relative with NF1

NF1 is a highly variable disorder with a small risk of serious complications, e.g., scoliosis, pressure effects of tumors or malignant change, e.g., neural crest tumors, and hypertension. Regular surveillance, e.g., annual physical examination, is recommended to try and detect these early.

X-linked hypohidrotic ectodermal dysplasia

- The condition follows X-linked recessive inheritance and is caused by mutation in the *EDA-1* gene.
- Boys have reduced/absent sweating, which may cause dangerous hyperpyrexia in infancy. Oligodontia and dental problems are prominent.
- Carrier females may be mildly affected.

Tuberous sclerosis (TSC) (see also p. 616)

- Affects ~1/10,000 individuals
- This highly variable autosomal dominant multisystem disorder is caused by mutation in the *TSC1* gene on 9q or the *TSC2* gene on 16p.
- It is characterized by hamartomas in the brain, skin, and other organs.
- It commonly presents with infantile spasms. Seizures and mental retardation are often associated.
- Hypomelanotic macules ("ash-leaf" spots) occur in ~95% of affected individuals by the age of 5 years. A Woods light (UV light) may be needed to visualize these. Angiofibromas occur in later childhood in a butterfly distribution over the nose and cheeks. Other cutaneous features include forehead fibrous plaques, shagreen patches, ungual fibromas, and dental pits.
- Half of individuals with TSC have normal intelligence, but children who develop infantile spasms and severe epilepsy in the first year of life often have learning disability.
- Thorough clinical evaluation, e.g., cranial MRI, eye exam, renal ultrasound, is indicated to make the diagnosis prior to genetic testing.
- Renal disease can include angiomyolipomas, cysts, and renal cell cancer, which is especially prevalent in adults. In females, lymphangiomyomatosis may manifest with shortness of breath or spontaneous pneumothorax.
- Expert genetic advice, with careful evaluation of the parents, is important. ~60% of cases arise as a result of new mutations.
- Genetic testing is possible by mutation analysis of *TSC1* and *TSC2*, but it is helpful to establish a clear clinical diagnosis before embarking on genetic testing. Severe polycystic kidney disease may coexist due to contiguous gene involvement of *PKD1* and *TSC2*.

Incontinentia pigmenti

- This rare X-linked dominant disorder is caused by mutation in the *NEMO* gene on Xq28 (~80% carry a common deletion).
- Affected male pregnancies almost invariably die in utero. Girls present in the neonatal period with blistering lesions, cropping circumferentially on the trunk and in a linear distribution on the limbs. Ultimately, lesions regress by late childhood or in adult life to leave atrophic, streaky areas of hyperpigmentation or hypopigmentation (often most noticeable on the backs of the calves). The child remains well and continues to feed. There is often a marked eosinophilia in the blood.
- Roughly 50% of patients have associated abnormalities of dentition, eyes (cataracts), or the CNS (seizures, microcephaly).
- Genetic testing is possible; ~80% of affected individuals carry a large deletion in the *NEMO* gene.
- No specific treatment is available.

Genetic disorders of growth

Assessment of growth plays an important role in deciding whether a child may have an underlying genetic disorder. Measurements <0.4th centile, or >99.6th centile nearly always merit further assessment, unless there is a clear explanation. Measurements between the 0.4th and 2nd centiles or 98th–99.6th need to be interpreted in context and may be clinically significant. If in doubt, discuss with a clinical geneticist.

Intrauterine growth restriction (IUGR)
Russell–Silver syndrome
- Incidence is unclear (1/100,000 births). There is an equal sex ratio.
- ~10% of children have maternal uniparental disomy for chromosome 7 (UPD7). Imprinting defects at 11p15.5 have also been implicated.
- This is a genetically heterogeneous condition characterized by intrauterine and postnatal growth retardation with short stature and FTT. Typically, babies have a disproportionately large head (OFC usually in the 3rd–25th centile), triangular facies, down-turned mouth, and limb asymmetry.

Cornelia de Lange syndrome
- Rare, incidence is ~1/50,000 live births
- Intrauterine and postnatal growth impairment, limb anomalies, microcephaly, hirsutism, and distinctive facial features (arched eyebrows, short, upturned nose, thin lips with down-turned corners of the mouth)
- Approximately half of affected children have mutations in the gene *NIPBL* on chromosome 5p13. A few males have an X-linked form caused by mutations in the *SMC1A* gene.

Short stature
Turner syndrome (see also p. 551)
- Affects ~1/2500 females
- Most girls have a single X chromosome (45,X), usually due to non-disjunction.
- As well as short stature, the typical phenotype includes broad neck; ptosis; wide, carrying angle at elbows (cubitus valgus); widely spaced hypoplastic nipples; low posterior hairline; and excessive pigmented nevi. Puffiness of the hands and feet is a common neonatal finding.
- Associated abnormalities include congenital heart disease (15%–50%), especially coarctation of the aorta and VSD; structural renal anomalies (~30%), e.g., horseshoe kidney or unilateral renal agenesis; and hypoplastic "streak" ovaries (primary amenorrhea and infertility).
- Girls with this condition often have specific visuospatial difficulties.
- The phenotype can be very subtle and is easily missed; thus, chromosome analysis should be considered for all girls with unexplained short stature.

Tall stature
Marfan syndrome (see p. 559)

Obesity

Bardet–Biedl syndrome (BBS)

- Rare condition, incidence in the U.S. population is <1/100,000
- Genetically heterogeneous with at least 12 genes identified to date. In the majority of families, inheritance is autosomal recessive.
- Features include pigmentary retinopathy, postaxial polydactyly, obesity from infancy, cognitive impairment, renal defects, and hypogonadism.

Prader–Willi syndrome (PWS)

- Affects ~1/10,000 individuals
- Caused by defects in paternally derived imprinted domain on 15q11-13
- Babies are floppy with feeding difficulties and may fail to thrive in infancy.
- There is rapid weight gain between the ages of 1 and 6 years.
- Older children have truncal obesity, mild to moderate learning difficulties, and short stature. Typically, children have an insatiable appetite with food-foraging and other behavioral problems.
- Diagnosis is by molecular genetic analysis (*SNRPN* methylation assay).

Overgrowth

Beckwith–Wiedemann syndrome (BWS)

- Incidence is ~1/14,000
- The genetic basis is complex; it is caused by defects in the imprinted region on chromosome 11p15.
- BWS usually presents in the perinatal period with macrosomia. Birth weight is usually >97th centile and length is usually over +2 SD. Polyhydramnios or preterm delivery commonly occurs.
- There may be associated congenital anomalies: omphalocele/umbilical hernia; dysmorphic features, e.g., earlobe creases, nevus flammeus, macroglossia (large tongue); visceromegaly; hemihypertrophy
- Neonates are at risk for severe hypoglycemia and should be monitored closely.
- Macrosomia continues through early childhood and then becomes less dramatic with increasing age.
- Some children with BWS are at increased risk for Wilms and other abdominal tumors, requiring screening throughout childhood.
- The genetics of BWS are complex. Refer to a clinical geneticist if clinical confirmation is required.

Sotos syndrome

- Incidence is ~1/15,000 children
- Due to mutation or deletion in the *NSD1* gene on chromosome 5q35. Most are isolated de novo mutations but familial cases do occur.

Sotos syndrome is characterized by prenatal overgrowth (birth weight ~4200 g in males, ~4000 g in females), which persists in childhood, especially through the preschool years. Final adult height is often in the upper normal range. The OFC is also increased and bone age is advanced. Affected children typically have a tall skull with a prominent broad forehead and pointed chin. Developmental delays are almost always present, but vary from mild to severe. Some children have seizures.

Miscellaneous genetic conditions

See Table 25.1.

Table 25.1 Miscellaneous genetic conditions

Syndrome	Features	Inheritance	Chromosome	Gene
Achondroplasia	Short limbs, large head, 'trident' hand, flat midface, lumbar lordosis	AD	4p16	FGFR3
Apert	Craniostenosis, beaked nose, cleft palate, severe syndactyly ('mitten hand'). ↓ IQ	AD	10q26	FGFR2
CHARGE (see p828)	**C**oloboma, congenital **H**eart disease, choanal **A**tresia, **R**etarded growth (short stature), hypo**G**enitalism, external **E**ar abnormality and deafness	AD (usually de novo)	8q12	CHD7
5p- (Cri du chat)	Hypoplastic larynx (cat-like cry), small stature, microcephaly, micrognathia, low-set ears, hypertelorism, ↓ IQ	Sporadic	5p deletion (5p-)	
Crouzon	Craniostenosis, brachycephaly, prominent forehead, proptosis, beaked nose	AD	10q26	FGFR2
Holt–Oram	Hypoplastic thumbs ± radius, ASD, VSD	AD	12q	TBX5
Primary AR microcephaly	Sloping forehead, OFC << 0.4th centile (< 4SD), moderate mental retardation	AR	Various	MCPH1-7
Smith–Lemli–Opitz (SLO)	Ptosis, anteverted nostrils, narrow frontal region, hypospadias, toe syndactyly, ↓ IQ	AR	11q12–13	DHCR7
Thanatophoric dysplasia	Large head, small thorax, short limbs, lethal	Sporadic	4p16	FGFR3
Treacher–Collins	Malar hypoplasia, micrognathia, down-slanting eyes, ear malformations, deafness, lower eyelid coloboma	AD	5q32	TCOF1
Zellweger	Prominent forehead, large fontanelles, flat facies, hypotonia, stippled epiphyses, nystagmus, hepatomegaly	AR	Various	PEX1-14

Miscellaneous congenital malformations

See Table 25.2.

Table 25.2 Miscellaneous congenital malformations

Condition	Features	Cause
Amniotic bands	Congenital facial clefts, limb constrictions, amputations, syndactyly or talipes	Annular amniotic bands
Diabetic embryopathy	Macrosomia, organomegaly (particularly heart and liver), polycythaemia, caudal regression syndrome (sacral and femoral agenesis or hypoplasia), transient hypertrophic cardiomyopathy, neural tube defects	Maternal diabetes mellitus
Fetal compression syndrome	Joint contractions/dislocation, talipes, micrognathia, cleft palate, skull deformity	In utero compression, eg. maternal pelvic abnormality
Fetal alcohol syndrome	IUGR, hirsutism, microcephaly, mid-face hypoplasia, short palpebral fissures, long smooth philtrum, ↓ IQ, low weight for height.	Excessive maternal alcohol ingestion in pregnancy
Fetal anticonvulsant syndrome	2–3× increase in major malformations, growth retardation, midface hypoplasia, ↓ IQ. Maternal valproate causes a 10× increased incidence of neural tube defects	Maternal anticonvulsant therapy in pregnancy
Goldenhar syndrome	Asymmetric facial hypoplasia, eye coloboma/dermoid, ear hypoplasia, preauricular skin tags, vertebral defects, cardiac defects (Fallot's tetralogy, VSD)	Unknown. Usually sporadic
Klippel–Feil syndrome	Cervical vertebral fusion, low hair line, webbed neck, torticollis, kyphoscoliosis, deafness	Usually sporadic
Moebius syndrome	Immobile face, strabismus, limb defects, syndactyly	Unknown, usually sporadic
Pierre–Robin sequence (see p829)	Micrognathia, glossoptosis, cleft palate	Unknown (need to exclude del22q11). Usually sporadic
Potter's sequence	Depressed nasal bridge, crumpled low set ears, talipes equinovarus, joint contractures, lung hypoplasia and respiratory failure. Lethal	Severe oligohydramnios due to renal or urethral abnormalities
VATER association (see p830)	Vertebral defects, Anal atresia, Tracheo-oEsophageal fistula, Renal defects. (VACTERL = additional cardiac and radial limb defects)	Unknown. Usually sporadic

Inherited metabolic disorders

General principles

Inherited metabolic disease (IMD) may present at any age, and the signs and symptoms may result from the following:
- Accumulation of substrate, which leads to a toxic effect
- Accumulation of a minor metabolite, which in excess is toxic
- Deficiency of a product of a specific reaction
- Deficiency of energy production
- Secondary metabolic phenomena

The most common error in managing infants and children with IMD is a delay in diagnosis, resulting in further hindrance of initiating treatment. Failure to recognize an IMD occurs because its clinical features may be confused by the following:
- Genetic heterogeneity
- A presenting intercurrent illness
- Similarity with other common, acquired conditions in which the differential diagnosis has not been fully explored

Acute metabolic decompensation includes hypoglycemia, lactic acidosis or ketoacidosis, hyperammonemia, intractable seizures, cardiomyopathy, rhabdomyolysis acute encephalopathy or coma, and acute liver failure.

A useful approach is to consider certain "syndromes" and use this as a framework for investigation (see Clarke JTR (2006), *A Clinical Guide to Inherited Metabolic Diseases*, Cambridge University Press). This approach is widely used and should serve the purpose (see Table 26.1).

Table 26.1 Differential diagnosis of inherited metabolic syndromes

IMD syndrome	Nonmetabolic differential
Neurology (p. 582) Encephalopathy	Infections: Enterovirus, herpes
	Drug reaction: CNS depressants, antihistamines, anticonvulsants
Metabolic acidosis (p. 1084) Lactic acidosis	Drug reaction: Alcohol, methanol, ethylene glycol, salicylates (see p. 96)
	Deficiency: Thiamine
Hypoglycemia (p. 148)	Hormonal disturbances: Hyperinsulinism, hypopituitarism
Storage or dysmorphism (p. 1080)	Infections: Congenital CMV, congenital toxoplasmosis
	Hematological disorders: See p. 705
Hepatic (p. 412)	Infections: Hepatitis, enterovirus, infectious mononucleosis
	Drug reaction
	Hematological disorders: See p. 705
Cardiac (p. 289)	Infections: Enterovirus
	Drug reaction

Laboratory evaluations for every suspected metabolic patient with an acute illness should include the following:

- Basic workup
  - *Blood*: Gases, electrolytes, glucose, lactate and pyruvate, ammonia, CBC, liver function tests, CK, uric acid, creatinine, coagulation studies
  - *Urine*: Ketones, reducing substances
- Special investigations
  - *Blood*: Amino acid analysis, acylcarnitines analysis
  - *Urine*: Organic acid analysis
  - *CSF*: Glucose, lactate, amino acids, neurotransmitters

Metabolic syndromes: neurological

Acute encephalopathy

Deterioration in the level of consciousness resulting from IMD
- May occur in a previously healthy child
- Usually shows no focal features, but ataxia may be present
- May start with unusual behavior
- Progresses rapidly even to the stage of coma

The likely causes are hyperammonemia (urea cycle) (p. 1092), amino acidopathy (p. 1094), organic aciduria (p. 1096), fatty-acid oxidation defect (p. 1103), mitochondrial defect (p. 1104), and hypoglycemia (p. 148).

Epileptic encephalopathy

Disorders of cerebral gray matter frequently accompany the seizures. Neuronal ceroid-lipofuscinosis, peroxisomal disorders, mitochondrial disorders, and lysosomal storage disorders should be considered.

Laboratory investigation should include urine purine pyrimidine analysis, creatine metabolites, serum transferring isoelectric focusing (IEF) for congenital disorders of glycosylation (CDG), biotinidase, and CSF amino acid and neurotransmitters.

Stroke

The IMDs associated with stroke or stroke-like episodes are as follows:
- Homocystinuria
- Fabry disease
- Organic acidopathy: Methylmalonic acidemia, propionic acidemia, isovaleric acidemia, glutaric aciduria I and II
- Ornithine transcarbamylase deficiency
- MELAS
- Congenital disorder of glycosylation type 1A (CDG-1A)
- Familial hemiplegic migraine

Chronic encephalopathy

Gray matter: developmental delay, psychomotor retardation

Developmental delay is a common problem (see p. 530), but the features that warrant investigation for IMD include the following:
- Global delay affecting all areas of development
- Progressive course with loss of developmental milestones
- Objective evidence of neurological dysfunction (e.g., special senses, pyramidal tract, extrapyramidal, cranial nerves)
- Severe behaviors including irritability, impulsiveness, aggressiveness, and hyperactivity
- Seizures (complex partial or myoclonic) originating early in life that are resistant to usual therapy

Causes

Causes include vitamin B_6 dependency, biotinidase deficiency, neuronal ceroid–lipofuscinosis, GM2 gangliosidosis, cherry-red spot myoclonus syndrome (sialidosis type I), Leigh disease, Alpers disease, and MELAS—**M**itochondrial **E**ncephalopathy–**L**actic **A**cidosis and **S**troke-like episode syndrome.

White matter: gross motor delay, weakness and incordination
- *Central involvement only*: Canavan disease, Alexander disease, GM2 gangliosidosis, GM1 gangliosidosis, X-linked adrenoleukodystrophy (ALD), amino acidurias, organic acidurias
- *Central and peripheral involvement*: Metachromatic leukodystrophy (MLD), Krabbe leukodystrophy, peroxisomal disorders

Chronic encephalopathy with abnormalities outside the CNS
- *Muscle*: Mitochondrial myopathy
- *Hepatosplenomegaly ± bone*: Gaucher disease, Niemann–Pick disease, mucopolysaccharidosis (MPS) I–IV (Hurler disease, Hunter disease, Sanfilippo disease, Sly disease), GM1 gangliosidosis, sialidosis II, Zellweger syndrome
- *Skin ± connective tissue*: Homocystinuria, Menkes disease, fucosidosis, multiple sulfatase deficiency, galactosialidosis, prolidase deficiency

Movement disorders

- *Ataxia*: Maple-syrup urine disease, pyruvate dehydrogenase deficiency, Friedreich ataxia, abetalipoproteinemia
- *Choreoathetosis and dystonia*: Glutaric aciduria I, Lesch–Nyhan disease, triose-phosphate isomerase deficiency
- *Parkinsonism*: Wilson disease, tyrosine hydroxylase deficiency

Myopathy

- *Acute intermittent muscle weakness*: Hyperkalemic periodic paralysis, paramyotonia congenita, hypokalemic periodic paralysis
- *Progressive muscle weakness*: Glycogen storage disease II (GSD, Pompe disease), GSD III
- *Exercise intolerance with cramps and myoglobinuria*: Myophosphorylase deficiency, carnitine palmitoyltransferase II
- *Myopathy as a manifestation of multisystem disease*: Mitochondrial myopathies

Autonomic dysfunction

The causes include dopamine β-hydroxylase deficiency, neurovisceral porphyrias, Fabry disease, MPS I–III, occipital horn syndrome, and mitochondrial neurogastrointestinal encephalomyopathy.

Psychiatric problems

The causes include the following:
- *Child:* MPS II, MPS III, X-linked ALD, Lesch–Nyhan syndrome
- *Adolescent:* Late-onset MLD, late-onset GM2 gangliosidosis, porphyria, Wilson disease, Wolfram syndrome, cerebrotendinous xanthomatosis, urea cycle disorder, homocystinuria, adult-onset neuronal ceroid lipofuscinosis

Metabolic syndromes: metabolic acidosis

The emergency care of acid–base problems is discussed on p. 102. Metabolic acidosis may occur as a result of
- Abnormal loss of bicarbonate.
- Abnormal accumulation of hydrogen ions in association with a non-volatile organic anion.

These two states can be differentiated by calculating the anion gap (i.e., the difference between plasma $[Na^+]$ and the sum of plasma $[Cl^-]$ and $[HCO_3^-]$). The normal anion gap is 10–15 mmol/L.

Abnormal bicarbonate loss

When metabolic acidosis is due to bicarbonate loss from either the gut or kidney:
- The anion gap is normal.
- Hyperchloremia is usually present.
- History of diarrhea will distinguish between hyperchloremia due to gastrointestinal losses and renal tubular losses.

IMDs associated with renal tubular acidosis (RTA) include galactosemia, hereditary fructose intolerance, hepatorenal tyrosinemia, cystinosis, GSD I, Fanconi–Bickel syndrome, congenital lactic acidosis, Wilson disease, vitamin D dependency, osteopetrosis with RTA, and Lowe syndrome.

Accumulation of organic anion

When metabolic acidosis is due to accumulated organic anion:
- It is associated with failure to thrive (p. 362).
- Tachypnea may be present.
- Secondary hypoglycemia leads to a neurologic syndrome (p. 148).
- Organic anion may lead to a distinct smell of sweat or urine.

Odor	Substance	Disorder
Mouse urine	Phenylacetate	PKU
Maple syrup	Sotolone	MSUD
Sweaty feet	Isovaleric acid	IVA
Cabbage	2-OH butyric acid	Tyrosinemia I

- The anion gap is raised.

The causes include the following:

- *Lactic acidosis*: Pyruvate accumulation (e.g., pyruvate dehydrogenase deficiency, pyruvate carboxylase deficiency, multiple carboxylase deficiency); NADH accumulation (e.g., defect of mitochondrial electron chain).
- *Ketoacidosis*: Secondary to IMD (e.g., maple syrup urine disease, organic acidopathies, GSD, disorders of gluconeogenesis); rare primary disorders of ketone utilization (e.g., β-ketothiolase deficiency, succinyl-CoA:3-ketoacid transferase deficiency).
- *Organic aciduria*: A large spectrum of disorders (see p. 1096).

Metabolic syndromes: dysmorphism

Box 26.1 IMDs associated with significant dysmorphic features

Lysosomal disorders (p. 1099)
- Mucopolysaccharidoses
- Glycoproteinoses
- Sphingolipidoses

Peroxisomal disorders (p. 1076)
- Zellweger syndrome
- Rhizomelic chondrodysplasia punctata

Mitochondrial disorders (p. 1104)
- Glutaric aciduria type II
- Pyruvate dehydrogenase deficiency

Disorders of sterol synthesis
- Smith–Lemli–Opitz syndrome

Other
- Menkes disease (p. 1112)
- Homocystinuria (page 1094)

Lysosomal disorder

The characteristic features of the storage dysmorphic syndrome are
- Coarse faces
- Bone changes (dysostosis multiplex)
- Short stature
- Organomegaly (hepatosplenomegaly)

Peroxisomal disorder

The characteristic features of the Zellweger phenotype are
- Psychomotor retardation
- Hypotonia and weakness
- Seizures
- Hepatocellular dysfunction
- Impaired special senses

Investigations

The initial investigation should include the following:
- *Urine*: Mucopolysaccharide and oligosaccharide screen, organic acids
- *Plasma*: Lactate, pyruvate, very long-chain fatty acids, phytanic acid, amino acids, isoelectric focusing of transferrin

Metabolic syndromes: hepatic syndromes

There are four possible ways in which IMD may present with hepatic involvement.

Jaundice (see p. 368)

Severe neonatal jaundice can occur in peroxisomal disorders, α_1-antitrypsin deficiency, Niemann–Pick type C, galactosemia, bile acid synthesis defects, progressive familial intrahepatic cholestasis, and Alagille syndrome.

Hepatomegaly (see p. 398)

The liver enlargement associated with IMD is usually persistent and not tender. The causes include the following:
- GSD type I presents in infancy with hypoglycemia.
- GSD type III presents in early infancy with failure to thrive, hyperlipidemia, ketosis during fasting, and deranged liver function.
- GSD type VI: hepatic phosphorylase deficiency
- Hereditary tyrosinemia type I
- Lysosomal storage disease
- Disorders of gluconeogenesis
- Congenital disorders of glycosylation

Hypoglycemia (see p. 148)

Common IMD causes
- Disorders of fatty acid oxidation
- Organic acidemia
- GSD type III and type 0
- Gluconeogenesis defects
- Mitochondrial disorder
- Fructose intolerance

Hepatocellular dysfunction (see also p. 398)

IMD with characteristic, severe liver involvement may present at different ages.
- *Infancy*: Failure to thrive, mild to severe hyperbilirubinemia, hypoglycemia, hyperammonemia, deranged liver function tests, bleeding, edema, and ascites
- *Children*: Presentation with chronic active hepatitis (fatigue, anorexia, hyperbilirubinemia, tender hepatomegaly), cirrhosis (edema, gynecomastia, ascites, clubbing, spider nevi), or neuropsychiatric disease

Some causes with distinguishing features in <u>infancy</u> include the following:
- Galactosemia: Hyperbilirubinemia, hemolytic anemia, coagulopathy, E. coli sepsis (see p. 1098)
- Hepatorenal tyrosinemia: Coagulopathy
- α_1-antitrypsin deficiency: Jaundice, failure to thrive, intracranial and other hemorrhages

- Congenital disorders of glycosylation: failure to thrive, chronic vomiting and diarrhea, seizures, developmental delay
- Mitochondrial hepatopathy due to mtDNA depletion

Some causes with distinguishing features in childhood include:
- GSD type III: skeletal myopathy (see p. 1098)
- Gaucher disease type III: Massive hepatosplenomegaly, failure to thrive, abdominal protuberance, anemia, ascites, bleeding diathesis, myoclonic seizures (see p. 589)
- Niemann–Pick disease, type C: Neurodegeneration, hepatosplenomegaly
- Wilson disease: Chronic hepatitis, hemolysis, neuropsychiatric disturbance (see p. 1112)

Box 26.2 Investigation of liver function

Tests of cholestasis
- Bilirubin (conjugated and unconjugated)
- Alkaline phosphatase
- γ-glutamyltranspeptidase
- Bile acids (urine)

Blood tests of active liver disease
- Aspartate aminotransferase
- Alanine aminotransferase

Tests of synthetic function
- Albumin
- Prothrombin (PT) and partial thromboplastin time (PTT)
- Clotting factor levels VII, V
- Ammonia

Specific tests for IMD
- Copper and ceruloplasmin (Wilson disease)
- α-fetoprotein (tyrosinemia)
- α₁-antitrypsin (PI phenotype, ZZ for deficiency)
- Plasma/urine amino acids
- Plasma acylcarnitines
- Urine organic acids
- Red cell galactose-1-phosphate uridyltransferase (galactosemia)
- Lysosomal enzymes
- Liver biopsy
- Carbohydrate-deficient transferrin

Metabolic syndromes: cardiac syndromes

Cardiomyopathy

This may be the dominant or only clinical problem in a variety of IMDs.

Glycogen metabolism (hypertrophic cardiomyopathy)

- *Pompe disease* (GSD II) presents in early infancy with marked skeletal myopathy and massive cardiomegaly (large QRS, left axis deviation, shortened PR, T-wave inversion).

Fatty acid metabolism (dilated cardiomyopathy)

- *Systemic carnitine deficiency* presents with skeletal myopathy, hypotonia encephalopathy, and hepatic syndrome (hepatomegaly, hypoglycemia, hepatocellular dysfunction).
- *Long-chain 3-hydroxyacyl-CoA dehydrogenase deficiency* or very long-chain acyl-CoA dehydrogenase deficiency presents with myopathy, exercise intolerance with myoglobinuria, hypotonia, encephalopathy, and hepatic syndrome ± hyperammonemia.

Organic acidopathy (dilated cardiomyopathy)

- *Propionic academia* features intermittent metabolic acidosis, ketosis, hyperammonemia, and neutropenia.

Mitochondrial cardiomyopathy (hypertrophic or dilated)

- *Barth syndrome* (3-methylglutaconic aciduria type II)

Sphingolipidoses (hypertrophic cardiomyopathy)

- *Fabry disease* presents with chronic neuritis pain in the hands and feet, angiokeratomata, corneal opacities, progressive renal failure, cardiac arrhythmias (intermittent SVT), and cerebrovascular disease.

Mucopolysaccharidosis (hypertrophic cardiomyopathy)

Congenital disorders of glycosylation

Box 26.3 Investigation of cardiomyopathy

Initial studies
- *Plasma*: Lactate, carnitine (free and total), acylcarnitine profile, ammonia, liver function tests, urea, creatinine, and electrolytes
- *Urine*: Organic acids, ketones

Suspected fatty acid oxidation defect
- Fibroblast cultures, enzyme studies, or DNA sequencing

Suspected mitochondrial electron transport defect
- *Plasma*: Lactate–pyruvate ratio
- *CSF*: Lactate
- *Imaging*: MRI, MRS
- *Electrophysiology*: Evoked potentials
- *Tissue*: Muscle and skin biopsy studies

Suspected lysosomal storage disease
- *Urine*: Mucopolysaccharide and oligosaccharide screen, glycolipids
- *Imaging*: Skeletal radiology
- *Blood, skin fibroblasts*: Lysosomal enzyme studies, α-glucosidase

Arrhythmias

IMD-related cardiomyopathy may be complicated by arrhythmias, including:
- *Heart block*: Mitochondrial cytopathy, Fabry disease, carnitine-acylcarnitine translocase (CACT) deficiency, propionic acidemia
- Tachyarrhythmia: fatty acid oxidation defects, CAC

Coronary artery disease (CAD)

CAD occurs in Fabry disease, familial hyperlipidemias, and familial hypercholesterolemia (FH). FH affects 1 in 500 individuals:
- *Homozygotes*: Severe cholesterolemia, ischemic heart disease in infancy or childhood, cholesterol accumulation in the skin (tuberous xanthomas, subcutaneous nodules), and arcus senilis
- *Heterozygotes*: Fatal myocardial infarction in the third decade

Familial hyperlipidemias causing premature CAD
- *Type IV*: Hyperlipidemia (increased very low-density lipoproteins)
- *Type IIa, familial hypercholesterolemia*: Hypercholesterolemia (increased low-density lipoproteins) with tuberous xantomas, tendinous xanthomas, and arcus senilis
- *Type IIb*: Combined hyperlipidemia (increased low- and very low-density lipoproteins)
- *Type III, familial dysbetalipoproteinemia* Very low-density lipoproteins with eruptive tuberous xanthoma, planar xanthomas, and peripheral vascular disease

Specific metabolic disorders: urea cycle disorders

The urea cycle disorders (UCDs) are a group of conditions resulting from enzyme deficiencies in protein degradation and waste nitrogen excretion through the conversion of ammonia into urea for excretion in urine. Enzyme deficiencies result in nitrogen accumulation and hyperammonemia, which may cause vomiting, seizure, encephalopathy, coma, brain damage, and death. Together they are estimated to occur in 1 in 10,000 births.

Presentation

Infants may present in the newborn period often with progressive signs of poor feeding, lethargy, vomiting, and irritability and are often confused with septic shock. Older children and adults may have recurrent hyperammonemia, often triggered by illness, fever, dehydration, or malnutrition, manifesting as the following:

- Protein intolerance
- Recurrent nausea and vomiting
- Failure to thrive
- Headache
- Psychomotor retardation
- Increased somnolence
- Decreased mental clarity
- Cerebellar ataxia

Diagnosis

Plasma concentrations of ammonia are elevated. There is no hypoglycemia or metabolic acidosis, but respiratory acidosis is frequently seen from hyperventilation. Specific disorders are differentiated by quantitative plasma and urine amino acids, including elevations in glutamine and alanine (the major nitrogen-carrying amino acids) and elevations of orotic acid on urine organic acids (see Table 26.2).

Table 26.2 The urea cycle disorders

Disorder	Amino acid profile	Inheritance
N-acetylglutamate synthetase deficiency (NAGS)	Low citrulline, arginine	AR
Carbamoyl phosphate synthetase deficiency (CPS)	Low citrulline, arginine	AR
Ornithine transcarbamylase deficiency (OTC)	Low citrulline, arginine High orotic acid	X-linked
Argininosuccinic acid synthetase (citrullinemia) deficiency (AS)	High citrulline Low arginine	AR
Argininosuccinase acid lyase deficiency (argininosuccinic aciduria) (AL/ASA)	High argininosuccinic acid	AR
Arginase deficiency (argininemia) (ARG)	High arginine	AR

Treatment

It is essential to closely monitor the blood ammonia in any patient with unexplained neurological symptoms. Acute hyperammonemia can be treated through restriction of protein intake, sodium benzoate, sodium phenylbutyrate, and sodium phenylacetate for alternative nitrogen removal, supplementation with L-arginine or L-citrulline, and glucose with insulin to provide adequate caloric intake to promote anabolism. Long-term management targets restriction of protein intake while providing essential amino acids to achieve normal growth and development. Hemodialysis must be promptly started if ammonia is >500 uM/L.

Disorders of amino acid metabolism

Amino acid disorders are due to defects in the synthesis, breakdown, or cellular transport of amino acids. Elevations of specific amino acids or their derivatives, or absence of the products lead to symptoms of disease. Diagnosis is established by detecting abnormal plasma and urinary amino acid profiles.

Phenylketonuria (PKU)

One of the first inherited metabolic diseases identified for which an effective treatment was found, PKU was the original target of newborn screening; it occurs in 1 in 12,000 newborns. Classic untreated hyperphenylalanemia due to a deficiency in phenylalanine hydroxylase will lead to impaired brain development, progressive mental retardation, and seizures. Children often have fair hair and blue eyes, and a mouse-like odor may be noted.

- *Treatment*: Lifelong adherence to a diet low in phenylalanine and high in tyrosine will prevent neurological problems.
- *Maternal PKU*: Children of women with elevated phenylalanine levels during pregnancy have a significantly increased risk of mental retardation, microcephaly, and other congenital birth defects. Strict control of phenylalanine levels in women who may become pregnant is essential.

Homocystinuria (HCY)

Classic HCY results from a deficiency in cystathionine β-synthase. Individuals with this disorder have increased plasma and urine homocysteine and methionine levels. Clinical manifestations resemble Marfan syndrome (see p. 1066), in addition to a high risk of thromboembolism often presenting as myopia or stroke in children and adults. Alternative forms may be due to disorders of vitamin B_{12} metabolism.

- *Treatment*: High-dose pyridoxine and low-methionine diet, supplemented with cysteine. Some patients may respond to hydroxycobalamin or betaine.

Maple syrup urine disease

This is a disorder of leucine, isoleucine, and valine metabolism. Deficiency of branched-chain α-ketoacid dehydrogenase produces alloisoleucine, a specific finding. Severely affected infants present in the first week of life with poor feeding, lethargy, and coma. Mildly affected children will have mental retardation and episodic vomiting and a sweet, sugary smell to their urine.

- *Treatment*: Acute implementation of glucose and insulin to suppress catabolism, and hemodialysis. Dietary restriction of branched-chain amino acids.

Tyrosinemia

This disorder is due to deficiency in fumarylacetoacetate hydrolase. Elevated tyrosine and methionine levels are detected and succinylacetone is diagnostic on urine organic acids. Untreated children will have severe liver disease, hypoglycemia, and renal Fanconi syndrome. Chronic manifestations include hepatocellular carcinoma, rickets, neurological crisis, and renal failure. The urine may have a cabbage-like smell.

- *Treatment*: Dietary restriction of phenylalanine and tyrosine. NTBC will prevent accumulation of metabolites.

Disorders of organic acid metabolism

This large group of disorders is characterized by a broad range of clinical symptoms and signs varying in seriousness from trivial to lethal, including developmental delay, poor growth, and episodic illnesses with vomiting and metabolic acidosis. Some of these disorders may be precipitated by prolonged fasting or minor viral infection. They may be associated with hypoglycemia and ketosis or hyperammonemia.

- They are characterized by urinary excretion of abnormal types and amounts of organic acids.
- Diagnosis is by urinary organic acid profile.
- *Treatment:* Avoid prolonged fasting. During acute illness extra carbohydrate and temporary restriction of protein is necessary with correction of acute acidosis, dehydration, and hyperammonemia. .

Methylmalonic acidemia (MMA)

MMA is caused by methylmalonyl-CoA mutase deficiency. It commonly presents in the newborn period with the following features:

- Severe metabolic acidosis
- Acute encephalopathy
- Hyperammonemia
- Neutropenia and thrombocytopenia

Differential diagnosis with cobalamin metabolism defect is required. It requires either skin fibroblast study or DNA sequencing.

Propionic acidemia (PA)

- Caused by propionyl-CoA carboxylase deficiency.
- Severe metabolic acidosis, acute encephalopathy, and hyperammonemia are common in the newborn period.
- Complication includes pancreatitis and cardiomyopathy.

Isovaleric acidemia (IVA)

IVA is caused by isovaleryl-CoA dehydrogenase deficiency. A mild form detected early by newborn screening with early intervention has favorable prognosis.

Glutaric aciduria (GA)

GA type 1 is caused by deficiency of mitochondrial glutaryl-CoA dehydrogenase. The condition presents in infancy with episodes of hypotonia, dystonia, opisthotonus, grimacing, fisting, tongue thrusting, and seizures. GA type II is caused by deficiency of mitochondrial electron transport flavoprotein or dehydrogenase. It may present as the following:

- *Neonatal disease:* With or without dysmorphism (abnormal facies, muscular defects of the abdominal wall, hypospadias in boys, cystic kidneys), hypotonia, hepatomegaly, hypoketotic hypoglycemia, metabolic acidosis, hyperammonemia.
- *Later-onset disease:* Episodic metabolic acidosis, failure to thrive, hypoglycemia, hyperammonemia, and encephalopathy.

3-hydroxy-3-methyl-CoA (HMG-CoA) lyase deficiency

This disorder may present in the newborn period with severe metabolic acidosis, poor feeding and vomiting, lethargy, altered level of consciousness, hypoglycemia, and hyperammonemia.

Disorders of carbohydrate metabolism

Disorders of galactose and fructose metabolism

Classical galactosemia

This is due to complete or near-complete deficiency of galactose-1-phosphate uridyltransferase enzyme. Partial deficiency is usually benign. The disorder is characterized by failure to thrive; cataracts, hepatomegaly, jaundice, vomiting, diarrhea, and mental retardation (if untreated). Treatment is with a galactose-free diet.

Nonclassical galactosemia

Uridine diphosphate galactose 4-epimerase (GALE) with profound deficiency resembles classic galactosemia. Galactokinase deficiency results in cataract formation without symptoms of intolerance.

Hereditary fructose intolerance

Fructose-1-phsophate aldolase deficiency results in failure to thrive; hypoglycemia, metabolic or lactic acidosis, vomiting; and GI bleeding.

Glycogen storage diseases (GSD types 0 to X)

(see Table 26.3)

- Specific enzyme defects prevent mobilization of glucose from glycogen, resulting in abnormal storage in the liver and/or muscle.
- GSD often presents with one or more of the following: episodic hypoglycemia, lactic acidosis, poor growth, and hypotonia; mental retardation or developmental delay, and vomiting; cramps, myoglobinuria, and muscle weakness.
- Major liver forms of GSD include types I, III, IV, VI, IX, and 0. Major muscle forms of GSD include types V, VII, and IX and phosphoglycerate kinase deficiency.

Table 26.3 Glycogen storage disease (GSD) types I–V

GSD type	Enzyme defect	Tissue	Key clinical features
Type I Von Gierke	Glucose-6-phosphatase	Liver +++	Poor growth Hypoglycemia Hepatomegaly
Type II Pompe	Lysosomal α-glucosidase	Liver ++ Muscle +++	Cardiac failure Hypotonia
Type III Corri	Glycogen debrancher (amylo-1,6–glucosidase)	Liver ++ Muscle +	Poor growth Muscle weakness Hypoglycemia
Type IV Andersen	Glycogen branching (amylo-1,4 -1,6 transglucosidase)	Liver +++ Muscle +	Failure to thrive Liver failure Muscle weakness
Type V McArdle	Myophosphorylase	Muscle ++	Muscle weakness Cramps

Disorders of lipoprotein metabolism

This is a heterogeneous group of disorders resulting in abnormalities of the blood lipid profile. They may predispose to cardiovascular disease (see p. 1090).

Lysosomal storage diseases

This is a large group of disorders due to defects in lysosomal function.

Mucopolysaccharidoses (MPS)

This is a group of IMDs caused by deficiency in lysosomal enzymes needed to break down glycosaminoglycans (long-chain carbohydrate molecules formerly called mucopolysaccharides). They affect bone, cartilage, tendons, eyes, skin, and connective tissue, leading to accumulation of glycosaminoglycans and progressive cellular and tissue damage (see Table 26.4). They are typically autosomal recessive in inheritance.

Clinical features are not apparent at birth but progress with time as storage of glycosaminoglycans impacts tissues and organs. Typical features include the following:

- *Skeletal disease:* Coarse facies, bone dysostosis multiplex, contractures.
- *Organ disease:* Hepatosplenomegaly, valvular heart disease.
- *Neurological disease:* Learning disability, behavioral problems, progressive mental retardation; hearing loss (conductive or sensory), hydrocephalus; corneal clouding, glaucoma, or retinal degeneration.

Table 26.4 Mucopolysaccharidosis (MPS) types I–VI

MPS type	Enzyme defect	Tissue	Key features
Type I Hurler	α-L-iduronidase	Skeletal Organ Neurologic	Mild form known as Scheie ERT
Type II Hunter	Iduronate-2-sulphatase	Skeletal Organ Neurologic	X-linked recessive inheritance No corneal clouding ERT
Type III Sanfilippo	4 subtypes each with enzymes in heparan sulphate metabolism	Neurologic	Often with no or mild skeletal or organ disease
Type IV Morquio	2 subtypes with enzymes in keratan sulphate metabolism	Skeletal	Severe Normal intelligence
Type VI Maroteaux–Lamy	N-acteylgalactos-amine-4-sulphatase (arylsulfatase B)	Skeletal Organ	ERT

Enzyme replacement therapy (ERT)
- Improvements are seen in liver and spleen size.
- Bone changes, stabilization
- Does not cross blood–brain barrier

Sphingolipidoses

Clinically the sphingolipidoses show variable severity. They cause progressive peripheral and CNS disease (psychomotor retardation, myoclonus, weakness, and spasticity). Variants of Gaucher and Niemann–Pick disease that do not affect the nervous system are termed non-neuronopathic.

GM2-gangliosidoses (Tay–Sachs disease)

This disease is autosomal recessive and is due to a deficiency of hexosaminidase A; deficiency of hexosaminidase B is known as Sandhoff disease. Accumulation of GM2-ganglioside results in macrocephaly and neurological regression. Affected infants may have a cherry-red spot on retinal exam and a typical startle response. There is a common mutation in the Ashkenazi Jewish population.
- *Treatment*: Supportive; seizures are typically responsive to therapy.

Fabry disease

This disease is X-linked recessive and due to a deficiency of $\alpha\alpha$-galactosidase A, resulting in the accumulation of globotriaosylceramide within blood vessels and other tissues. Clinical features become evident in early childhood and increase in severity with age: anhidrosis, fatigue, skin lesions (angiokeratomas: tiny, painless papules), and burning pain of the extremities. Renal failure, heart disease, and stroke increase with age. Other symptoms include tinnitus, vertigo, nausea, and diarrhea.
- *Treatment*: ERT is highly effective.

Gaucher disease

This is the most common lysosomal storage disorder; it is autosomal recessive. It is due to deficiency in $\beta\beta$-glucocerebrosidase and leads to intracellular accumulation of glucosylceramide (glucosylcerebroside) within cells of mononuclear phagocyte origin (producing characteristic Gaucher cells).

Type I

This is the most common type of Gaucher disease. There is no primary CNS involvement. It affects infants to adults and has a wide spectrum of severity including hepatosplenomegaly, bone marrow infiltration with anemia, and thrombocytopenia. Severe orthopedic complications occur, including vertebral compression, avascular necrosis of the femoral head, and pathologic fractures of long bones. There is a common mutation in the Ashkenazi Jewish population.
- *Treatment*: ERT helps with pancytopenia and bone disease.

Type II (acute neuronopathic)

Type II presents in infancy with rapid progression of hepatosplenomegaly, developmental regression, spasticity, ophthalmoplegia, and growth arrest within a few months of age. Death is often by 2 years of age.

Type III (subacute neuronopathic)
This is similar to type II, and may have hepatosplenomegaly, seizures, and dementia with a later age of onset and slower progression.

GM1-gangliosidosis
This autosomal recessive disorder results from a deficiency of β-galactosidase. Neonates are hypotonic and may have peripheral edema, skeletal changes, neurological regression, and dysmorphic features. Later-onset types have ataxia or dystonia without skeletal involvement.
- *Treatment*: Supportive.

> **Other types of sphingolipidoses**
> - Krabbe disease (globoid cell leukodystrophy)
> - Metachromatic leukodystrophy
> - Niemann–Pick disease types A and B

Other lysosomal disorders
Neuronal ceroid lipofuscinosis
In this autosomal recessive disorder, progressive blindness from retinal degeneration is common to nearly all types. It may present with behavioral changes, seizures, and neurological regression in infants to adults.
- *Treatment*: Symptomatic. Some antiepileptics may worsen seizure activity.

Cystinosis
Cystinosis is autosomal recessive and due to a defect in lysosomal transport of cystine. The nephropathic infantile form often presents as failure to thrive, generalized aminoaciduria (renal Fanconi disease), and metabolic acidosis. Corneal crystals are common. Long-term survival is associated with multi-organ disease. Juvenile and adult forms exist and may be progressive.
- *Treatment*: Supportive; cysteamine will decrease cystine accumulation.

Glycoproteinosis
This is a heterogeneous group of disorders of glycoprotein storage. A spectrum of phenotypes includes neurological deterioration, growth retardation, visceromegaly, and seizures. Coarse facial features, angiokeratoma corporis diffusum, spasticity, and delayed development also occur.
- Mucolipidosis II (I—cell disease)
- Mucolipidosis III (pseudo-Hurler polydystrophy)
- Defects in glycoprotein degradation: Aspartylglucosaminuria, fucosidosis, mannosidosis, sialidosis (mucolipidosis I)

Disorders of fatty acid oxidation

Disorders of fatty acid metabolism may be due to deficiency in the acyl–CoA dehydrogenase enzyme complex and β-oxidation, deficiency in carnitine, or carnitine transport. All disorders together may be present in 1 in 10,000 newborns.

Clinical presentation

These disorders are characterized by hypoketotic hypoglycemia resulting in acute encephalopathy, recurrent vomiting, lethargy, drowsiness, and seizures. Hepatomegaly and hyperammonemia may be present. Presentation is usually in the first 2 years of life during a period of prolonged fasting or by intercurrent illness associated with poor feeding.

Diagnosis

Diagnosis is by demonstration of characteristic abnormalities in plasma acylcarnitine profiles and urine organic acid and acylglycine analysis. Abnormalities may not be present when the child is well. Molecular genetic testing is also available. Infants can now be identified on expanded newborn screening before presenting with clinical illness.

Treatment

These disorders are successfully managed by avoidance of prolonged fasting, IV glucose, a bedtime snack, a high-carbohydrate diet, and carnitine (50–100 mg/kg/day) supplementation. During intercurrent illness, administration of carbohydrates (either IV or PO) is essential.

Medium chain acyl-CoA dehydrogenase deficiency (MCAD)

This is the most common fatty acid oxidation disorder (1 in 10,000 births). Historically this presented with fulminant hepatic failure (Reye-like illness) or as sudden infant death. Now, with newborn screening, this is a highly manageable disease, with asymptomatic individuals now being identified. Individuals have elevations of C8 and C10-acylcarnitine species.

Very-long chain acyl-CoA dehydrogenase deficiency (VLCAD)

Originally thought to be a disorder of LCAD (long-chain acyl-CoA dehydrogenase), VLCAD has three clinical presentations: severe neonatal-onset cardiomyopathy and mortality, an intermediate childhood form with episodic fasting hypoketotic hypoglycemia, and an adult-onset skeletal myopathy and rhabdomyolysis. Individuals have elevations of C14, C16, and C18-acylcarnitine species.

Long chain 3-hydroxy-acyl-CoA dehydrogenase deficiency (LCHAD)/ mitochondrial trifunctional protein deficiency

Clinical presentation of these disorders ranges from cardiomyopathy, hypotonia, liver disease, neuropathy, to retinopathy. Mothers of affected fetuses may develop AFLP or HELLP syndrome. Individuals have elevations of C16-hydroxy and C18-hydroxy acylcarnitine species.

Mitochondrial disorders

Mitochondrial diseases are a clinically heterogeneous group involved in generation of ATP, especially in organs with high energy requirements such as brain, muscle, heart, kidney, or eyes. Dysfunction of mitochondrial respiratory chain could be due to mutations in either nuclear genes or mitochondrial DNA. Therefore, the inheritance may be autosomal dominant, autosomal recessive, X- linked, or mitochondrial (i.e., maternal).

Disorders of mitochondrial function result in a wide spectrum of clinical problems (see Box 26.4).

Box 26.4 Disorders of mitochondrial function: clinical problems

Common clinical features
- Lactic acidosis
- Muscle weakness, hypotonia
- Poor growth or short stature
- Neurodevelopmental delay
- Seizures

Other recognized features
- Eyes: Ophthalmoplegia; retinal degeneration
- Ears: Sensorineural deafness
- Cardiovascular: Cardiomyopathy; arrhythmias
- Respiratory: Periodic breathing
- Diabetes mellitus
- Stroke
- Renal tubular dysfunction
- Anemia and thrombocytopenia

Investigations
- Lactate and pyruvate, organic acids, amino acids, CSF study
- MRI, MRS
- *Muscle biopsy*: Immunohistochemical studies, electron microscopy, enzyme studies. Presence of "ragged-red" fibers in skeletal muscle biopsy is characteristic but not common in childhood.
- *Molecular studies* for a specific syndrome (for examples, mtDNA depletion, Pearson, MELAS, MERRF)

Leigh's syndrome
- Relapsing subacute encephalomyelopathy; lactic acidosis; hypotonia; seizures; ± cardiomyopathy; ± hepatic or renal tubular dysfunction
- *Genetic defects*: mtDNA mutations and various nuclear genes, particularly complex I deficiency and PDHC deficiency

Pearson's syndrome
- Failure to thrive; lactic acidosis; sideroblastic anemia/pancytopenia; hypoparathyroidism; diabetes mellitus
- *Genetic defects*: Large deletions of mtDNA

Barth syndrome
- Cardiomyopathy, neutropenia, myopathy, 3-methylglutaconic aciduria in organic acid analysis
- *Genetic defects*: mutations in Taffazin (X-linked)

MELAS
- Encephalomyopathy, lactic acidosis, stroke-like episodes
- *Genetic defects*: mtDNA mutations

MERRF
- Myoclonic epilepsy with ragged red fibers
- *Genetic defects*: mtDNA mutations

MNGIE
- Myoneurogastrointestinal encephalopathy, frequent episode of intestinal pseudo-obstruction
- *Genetic defects*: mtDNA depletions, thymidine phosphorylase deficiency

Peroxisomal disorders

Peroxisomes are ubiquitous cellular organelles that function to rid the cell of toxic material. Their oxidative enzymes have an important role in the metabolism of fatty acid molecules. Diagnosis through characteristic biochemical abnormalities (particularly very long chain fatty acids [C22 to C26 carbon chain lengths], phytanic acid, and bile salt metabolites) is confirmed by enzyme assay on skin fibroblasts, liver biopsy, and electromicroscopy morphologic studies.

Box 26.5 Classification of peroxisomal disorders

Disorders of peroxisome development
- Zellweger syndrome
- Neonatal adrenoleukodystrophy
- Infantile Refsum disease

Defects in peroxisome function
- Rhizomelic chondrodyslpasia punctata (RCDP)
- DHAP acyltransferase deficiency
- Acyl-CoA oxidase deficiency
- D-bifunactional protein deficiency
- Classical Refsum disease
- *X-linked adrenoleukodystrophy
- *Primary hyperoxaluria type 1
- *Acatalasemia

Note: Those marked with * may not present with the severe peroxisome phenotype.

Most peroxisomal disorders are associated with severe peroxisome phenotype and share many common features:

- Severe neurodevelopmental delay
- Neurological regression
- Hypotonia, weakness
- Seizure, encephalopathy
- Hepatitis, hepatomegaly
- Retinopathy, cataract
- Impaired hearing and deafness
- Sudanophilic leukodystrophy

Neonatal and early-childhood presentation

Infants may demonstrate profound hypotonia and may die within a few months of birth. Infants may have dysmorphic features with Zellweger syndrome, calcific epiphyseal stippling with RCDP, neonatal adrenoleukodystrophy, or D-bifunctional protein deficiency. Infantile Refsum disease is the least severe of this group and children may survive to adulthood.
- *Treatment*: Supportive.

Late-childhood to adult presentation

Children may develop failure to thrive, hearing loss, vision loss, and neurological regression. Those with classical Refsum disease will have retinal degeneration and an increased plasma phytanic acid.

- *Treatment*: A phytanic acid–restricted diet may slow progression of retinopathy and polyneuropathy and reduce cardiac arrhythmias.

X-linked adrenoleukodystrophy

This X-linked recessive disorder is the most common peroxisomal disorder (1 in 20,000). It presents with behavioral changes and neurological regression, with or without adrenal dysfunction or Addison's disease. X-linked adrenomyeloneuropathy presents in adult men and women with spastic paresis and cerebral demyelination.

- *Treatment:* Supportive. Lorenzo's oil has not been found to be effective. Bone marrow transplant may have a limited role early in the disease progression.

Disorders of nucleotide metabolism

This group of disorders is characterized by abnormalities in enzymes responsible for metabolism and removal of the purine and pyrimidine components of proteins and amino acids.

Box 26.6 Classification of disorders of nucleotide metabolism

Disorders of purine metabolism
- Lesch–Nyhan syndrome
- Renal lithiasis (adenine phosphoribosyltransferase [APRT] deficiency)
- Xanthinuria (xanthine oxidase deficiency)
- Adenosine deaminase deficiency

Disorders of pyrimidine metabolism
- Hereditary orotic aciduria
- Dihydropyrimidine dehydrogenase (DPD) deficiency
- Dihydropyriminidase deficiency

Common clinical features
- *Renal*: Nephrolithiasis, renal failure
- *Neurological*: Seizures, spasticity, dystonia, self-mutilation
- Muscle cramps and wasting
- Anemia, immunodeficiency with recurrent infections

Investigations
- Uric acid in serum and urine
- Purine and pyrimidine metabolites in urine

Lesch–Nyhan syndrome
This X-linked recessive syndrome is due to a deficiency in hypoxanthine-guanine phosphoribosyltransferase (HGPRT) leading to the formation of excessive uric acid. A partial HGPRT deficiency may present with gouty arthritis and a normal neurological exam (although some patients do have spasticity, dysarthria, and spinocerebellar syndrome).

Children are normal at birth and symptoms and signs develop in the first few months. Classic clinical features include the following:
- Severe neurodevelopmental impairment
- Behavioral problems including self-mutilative biting of fingers and lips
- Spastic cerebral palsy
- Choreoathetosis
- Uric acid urinary or renal stone development
- Megaloblastic anemia
- Short stature
- Vomiting

Biochemical analysis demonstrates increased plasma and urinary uric acid levels. Detection of HGPRT enzyme activity in red blood cells or molecular genetic testing for mutations in HGPRT gene is available.

Adenosine deaminase deficiency

Most patients present with a profound impairment of humoral and cellular immunity within the first weeks or months after birth. Diarrhea, failure to thrive, and progressive neurological symptoms including spasticity are common.

- *Diagnosis:* Increased adenosine, hypogammaglobulinemia, lymphopenia
- *Treatment:* Bone marrow transplantation, enzyme replacement

Disorders of porphyrin metabolism

The *porphyrins* are the main precursors of heme and are essential constituents of hemoglobin, myoglobin, the respiratory and P450 liver cytochromes, and other enzymes (catalases and peroxidases). Deficiency in porphyrin pathway leads to accumulation of precursors, which are toxic to tissues in high concentration. The chemical properties of these precursors determine the site of tissue accumulation and whether they induce photosensitivity.

The porphyrias may be inherited or acquired. They are broadly classified as hepatic or erythropoietic, based on the site of the overproduction and main accumulation of the porphyrins. They manifest with either skin problems or neurological complications (or occasionally both) and present either acutely or nonacutely (see Table 26.5).

Table 26.5 Types of porphyria

Porphyria type	Inheritance/ site	Enzyme	Acute/ non- actute	System in volved
Acute	AR/Hep	ALA dehydratase	A	Neurovisceral
Acute/ intermittent (AIP)	AD/Hep	Porphobilinogen deaminase	A	Neurovisceral
Hereditary coproporphyria	AD/Hep	Coproporphy-rinogen oxidase	A	Neurovisceral + cutaneous
Variegate porphyria	AD/Hep	Protoporphyrinogen oxidase	A	Neurovisceral + cutaneous
Congenital erythropoietic porphyria	AR/Erthyro	Uroporphyrinogen III cosynthase	N-A	Cutaneous
Porphyria cutanea tarda	AD/Erthyro	Uroporphyrinogen decarboxylase	N-A	Cutaneous
Hepatoery-thropoietic porphyria	AR/Erthyro	Uroporphyrinogen decarboxylase	N-A	Cutaneous
Erythropoietic protoporphyria	AD/Erthyro	Ferrochetalase	N-A	Cutaneous

AR = autosomal recessive; AD = autosomal dominant; Hep = hepatic; Erythro = erythropoietic.

Erythropoietic porphyrias

These include congenital erythropoietic porphyria, hereditary coproporphyria, and erythropoietic protoporphyria. Presentations range from a severe, mutilating form (CEP) in infancy with photosensitivity including light-sensitive blistering rash and increased hair growth to milder solar urticaria or eczema.

- *Treatment*: The skin rash occuring in erythropoietic porphyrias generally requires use of sunscreens and avoidance of bright sunlight. Chloroquine may be used to increase porphyrin secretion.

Acute hepatic porphyrias

These include acute, intermittent porphyria, variegate porphyria, hereditary coproporphyria, and 5-ALA dehydratase deficiency. They may present with acute neurological episodes that can become life threatening, manifesting as hyperthermia, hypertension, seizures, neuropathy, behavior problems, psychosis or hallucinations. Muscle (back) pain, vomiting, and abdominal pain are also common. Acute episodes may be triggered by exposure to certain drugs (e.g., alcohol, oral contraceptive agents, menstruation, certain antibiotics) and by other chemicals and certain foods. Fasting can also trigger attacks.

- *Treatment*: High-carbohydrate diet and avoidance of precipitating factors. Heme arginate (early in acute episode). Symptomatic treatment.

Diagnosis

Spectroscopic and biochemical analysis for abnormalities in porphyrin metabolite profile in urine and stools is required for diagnosis. In nearly all cases of acute porphyria syndromes, urinary porphobilinogen is markedly elevated (except in ALA dehydratase deficiency) and can be collected on a random sample. Collection of urine or feces during symptoms is preferable. Initial screening ideally consists of 24-hour quantitative urine porphyrins and urine aminolevulinic acid along with urine organic acids and heavy metals for acquired porphyrias.

Disorders of metal metabolism and transport

Wilson disease

This autosomal recessive (1 in 30,000 births) disease is due to mutation in the *ATP7B* gene that encodes for a cell membrane ATP-sensitive copper pump. The condition results in a buildup of intracellular hepatic copper with subsequent hepatic dysfunction, neurological abnormalities, and hemolytic anemia.

Symptoms and signs

Symptoms usually develop after the age of 10 years (rare <5 years). Half of patients first present with chronic active hepatitis (which may lead to cirrhosis), and half with neurological symptoms including mood disorder, psychosis, and features consistent with Parkinson disease. Hemolysis is usually present in severe hepatic failure cases. Other features seen include renal tubular acidosis, renal stones, and cardiomyopathy.

Diagnosis

- Low plasma concentrations of copper and ceruloplasmin (in 80% of patients). Elevated 24 -hour urinary copper excretion.
- Slit-lamp examination to detect Kayser–Fleischer rings (although its absence does not rule out Wilson disease).
- DNA sequencing and/or liver biopsy

Treatment

- Lifelong chelating agents (e.g., trientine, penicillamine) or zinc
- Liver transplantation may be needed in severe disease.

Menkes disease

This X-linked recessive disease is caused by mutation in the gene encoding Cu(2+)-transporting ATPase (*ATP7A*). The disease is characterized by the following:

- Early-onset growth retardation
- Hypotonia, seizures, microcephaly, and osteoporosis
- Peculiar hair development (sparse, steely, or kinky hair)
- Focal cerebral and cerebellar degeneration
- Predisposition to intracranial hemorrhage is also recognized
- A milder form, occipital horn syndrome, may be seen in up to 15% of patients.

Diagnosis

- Biochemical analysis reveals low plasma levels of ceruloplasmin and copper
- Catecholamine metabolites in CSF, plasma
- DNA sequencing

Hemochromatosis

At least four inherited iron-overload disorders have been identified:

- *Classic hemochromatosis (HFE 1)*: Autosomal recessive, affecting 1 in 200 to 1 in 400 populations. Common mutations are C282Y and H63D in the *HFE* gene (on 6p21.3) or hemojuvelin gene (*HJV*) (1q21).
- *Juvenile hemochromatosis (HFE 2)*: Common mutation is G320V in the *HFE2* gene. Autosomal recessive.
- *Hemochromatosis type 3 (HFE 3)*: Transferrin receptor protein 2 gene. Autosomal recessive.
- *Hemochromatosis type 4 (HFE4)*: Ferroportin gene. Autosomal dominant.

The clinical features of hemochromatosis are wide ranging and include the following:

- Hepatomegaly
- Splenomegaly
- Cirrhosis of the liver
- Hypermelanotic pigmentation of the skin
- Heart failure (cardiomyopathy)
- Joint stiffness and arthritis
- Involvement of the endocrine glands can lead to diabetes mellitus, adrenal insufficiency, gonadal failure, and hypopituitarism.
- Increased susceptibility to certain infections is recognized (e.g., *Salmonella*; *Klebsiella*).

Primary hepatocellular carcinoma complicating cirrhosis is responsible for about one-third of deaths in affected homozygotes.

Diagnosis

- Increased serum iron and ferritin levels. Liver biopsy

Treatment

- Repeated therapeutic phlebotomy; deferoxamine
- Restriction of dietary iron, iron supplements, excess vitamin C, or uncooked seafood.

Community and child health

The health of a child is inextricably intertwined with the health of his or her family, neighborhood, and community. Community pediatrics acknowledges that the major determinants of well-being for most children are not found in the clinic, nor do they arise from the individual interactions between clinicians and their patients.

Robert J. Haggerty, MD, has noted that community pediatrics provides a "realistic and complete clinical picture by taking responsibility for all children in a community, providing preventive and curative services, and understanding the determinants and consequences of child health and illness, as well as the effectiveness of services provided."[1]

Thus, the unique feature of community pediatrics is its concern for all of the population—those who remain well but need preventive services, those who have symptoms but do not receive effective care, and those who seek medical care in either a physician's office or a hospital.

More succinctly, the National Public Health Performance Standards Program describes community health as "a perspective on public health that assumes community to be an essential determinant of health and the indispensable ingredient for effective public health practice. It takes into account the tangible and intangible characteristics of the community—its formal and informal networks and support systems, its norms and cultural nuances, and its institutions, politics, and belief systems."[2]

1 Haggerty RJ (1994). Community pediatrics: past and present. *Pediatr Ann* **23**:657.
2 http://www.cdc.gov/od/ocphp/nphpsp/

Trends in child health

Over the last 100 years, dramatic advances in medical care and technology have decreased child mortality and morbidity from infectious disease and injury, and improved survival following premature birth. However, a growing number of children are struggling with the "new morbidities" of obesity, asthma, depression, behavioral issues, school failure, and the consequences of risk taking, interpersonal stress, or social inequities.

Important trends in child health include the following:

- Concentration of *poverty* in childhood. Following the enactment of Medicare, which decoupled ill health from poverty in the elderly, children became—and remain—the poorest group in U.S. society.
- Growing *inequalities in income and wealth*. Between 1982 and 1998, the top 1% of U.S. households saw wealth increase by 42%. Over the same period, the poorest 40% of households lost 76% of their wealth. Income inequality in a society is associated with poor child-health outcomes, independent of absolute income levels.
- *Infant mortality* has improved for all groups over the last 20 years, mainly due to innovations in the care for preterm infants. The rate of preterm birth has not declined, however, and, in fact, rates of very low weight births are increasing.
- The prevalence of *chronic medical conditions* in children has increased over the last 30 years, with 15% of U.S. children now affected. While some of this increase results from more inclusive diagnostic criteria, conditions such as chronic asthma, obesity, and developmental disabilities are increasingly common.
- Despite reduction in *child injury mortality* of 45% or more over the last 30 years, unintentional and inflicted injuries remain the most common causes of death in childhood after infancy.

Indicators of child health

Understanding the health of a population requires access to reliable data with trends observed over time. The Federal Interagency Forum on Child and Family Statistics publishes an annual compilation of measures of child well-being in the United States. Highlights from 2005–06 are provided below.[1]

Demographics

- In 2006, there were 73.7 million children ages 0–17 in the United States, comprising 25% of the population, down from a peak of 36% at the end of the "baby boom" (1964).

Family and social environment

- 67% of children ages 0–17 lived with two married parents, down from 77% in 1980.
- 20% of school-age children spoke a language other than English at home and 5% of school-age children had difficulty speaking English.

Economics

- 18% of all children ages 0–17 lived in poverty; among children living in families, the poverty rate was 17%.

Health care

- 89% of children had health insurance coverage at some point during the year, down from 90% in 2004.
- 48% of children ages 2–4 had a dental visit in the past year, compared with 84% of children ages 5–11 and 82% of children ages 12–17.

Physical environment and safety

- 60% of children lived in counties in which concentrations of one or more air pollutants rose above allowable levels.
- Injury remains the leading cause of death for all children outside of infancy. In 2004, the injury death rate for children ages 1–4 was 13 deaths per 100,000 children.

Behavior

- The percentages of 8th-, 10th-, and 12th-grade students reporting illicit drug use in the past 30 days remained stable from 2005 to 2006. However, past-month use among all three grades has declined significantly since 1997.
- 47% of high school students reported ever having had sexual intercourse. This was statistically the same rate as in 2003 and a decline from 54% in 1991.

Education

- The percentage of children ages 3–5 not yet in kindergarten who were read to on a daily basis by a family member was higher in 2005 than in 1993 (60% vs. 53%).
- In 2005, 69% of high school completers enrolled immediately in a 2- or 4-year college.

Health

- The percentage of infants with low birth weight was 8.2% in 2005, up from 7.9% in 2003 and 8.1% in 2004 and has increased steadily since 1984 (6.7%).
- 5% of children ages 4–17 were reported by a parent to have serious (definite or severe) emotional or behavioral difficulties.
- The proportion of children ages 6–17 who were overweight grew from 6% in 1976–1980 to 11% in 1988–1994 to 18% in 2003–2004.

About 9% of children ages 0–17 currently have asthma, and about 5% of children had one or more asthma attacks in the previous year. The prevalence of asthma in children is particularly high among African-American non-Hispanic, and Puerto Rican children (13% and 20%, respectively).

Data sources

For more information, or to find data customized to specific states, cities, or population groups, visit the following resources online:

- *Childstats* (http://www.childstats.gov/). Published by the Federal Interagency Forum on Child and Family Statistics
- *Childtrends* (http://www.childtrends.org/). Indicator data and reports that interpret and synthesize data trends for policy makers and advocates.
- *Healthy People 2010* (http://www.healthypeople.gov/). Tracks 10 leading health indicators for the United States.
- *Healthy Youth* (www.cdc.gov/healthyyouth/). CDC site with data from the Youth Risk Behavior Surveillance Survey
- *Kidscount* (www.kidscount.org) A project of the Annie E. Casey Foundation. Includes indicator data from the 50 largest U.S. cities.
- *WISQARS* (www.cdc.gov/ncipc/wisqars/). CDC site with easily accessible data on fatal and nonfatal injury.

---

1 From Eunice Kennedy Shriver National Institute of Child Health and Human Development, NIH, DHHS (2007). *America's Children: Key National Indicators of Well-Being 2007*. Washington, DC: Government Printing Office.

Disparities in health

The Institute of Medicine (IOM) report *Unequal Treatment* defined health disparities as "racial or ethnic differences in the quality of health care that are not due to access-related factors or clinical needs, preferences and appropriateness of intervention."

Racial and ethnic minorities account for almost 40% of all children in the United States. Disparities in health and health care have been documented in many aspects of child health.

- *Mortality*: African-American and American Indian/Alaska Native children have death rates 1.5 to 2 times higher than those of White children.
- *Infant mortality*: Black infants are more than twice as likely as White infants to die during their first year, due primarily to higher rates of preterm birth and a higher incidence of sudden infant death syndrome (SIDS).
- *Access to health-care services*: Racial and ethic minority children are likely to have a higher burden of unmet health-care needs, and these are not completely determined by economic status.
- *Quality of health-care services*
  - Immunizations, receipt of anticipatory guidance, controller medications for asthma and medical treatment of diagnosed ADHD varies by race and ethnicity.
  - Language and communication barriers are common and may lead to misunderstanding, poor compliance, or medical errors.

Steps to elimination of disparities include the following:
- Reframing disparity as a social-justice issue reaching beyond health care
- Incorporation of health disparities indicators into individual and institutional quality measures
- Legislative measures (S-CHIP) to improve access to care for children living in families with limited financial resources
- Improved communication across language and cultural barriers, with special emphasis on low health-literacy populations
- Diversification of the health-care workforce

- Ethnomed (http://ethnomed.org/) provides information about cultural beliefs and medical issues pertinent to the health care of recent immigrants.
- Health Literacy—Ask Me 3 Campaign (http://www.npsf.org/askme3/)
- National Healthcare Disparities Report (http://www.ahrq.gov/qual/measurix.htm)

---

1 Institute of Medicine (2002). *Unequal Treatment: Confronting Racial and Ethnic Disparities in Health Care.* New York: IOM.

Access to health care

Access to health care has been defined by the IOM as the "timely use of personal health services to achieve the best possible health outcomes." Barriers to obtaining needed services include inadequate insurance coverage, geographic distance to a health-care provider, and linguistically or culturally inaccessible services.

Health insurance is a major determinant of access to care. Children who are uninsured are more likely to have unmet health-care needs and less likely to have received preventive services. Uncovered health-care costs are a leading cause of bankruptcy.

- Access is related to health outcomes when services provided are effective in correcting or preventing morbidity. This connection was easier to demonstrate when the major causes of ill health were acute infections; pediatric health-care providers are now challenged to address the new morbidities of asthma, obesity, mental health, and risk-taking behaviors.
- Access is also related to disparities if services are effective. Inequalities in access to effective services will worsen health disparities, while unequal access to ineffective services may not impact health outcomes.

In 2007:
- 11.7% of children—or 8.7 million—were uninsured. Of these, 5 million uninsured children were eligible for Medicaid/SCHIP but not enrolled.
- 22.1 million children (30%) were covered by a public source of health insurance.

Box 27.1 Public sources of health-care coverage

- *Medicaid*: A federal–state program for certain low-income people that covers health and long-term care services for 51 million Americans, including children, the aged, blind, disabled, and people who are eligible to receive federally assisted income maintenance payments.
- *State Children's Health Insurance Program (SCHIP)*: A federal–state program enrolling children from families that earn too much to qualify for Medicaid but not enough to afford private health insurance.
- *Federally qualified health centers*: Community-based and consumer-run organizations that serve populations with limited access to health care.

For more information on this issue, see Cover the Uninsured, at: http://covertheuninsured.org

Public health systems

The public health system in the United States is a complex amalgam of federal agencies; state, tribal, and territorial health authorities; local health departments; health-care providers; and voluntary organizations.

Federal leadership for public health is based at the Centers for Disease Control and Prevention (CDC) (http://www.cdc.gov).

Most public health authority, such as mandatory disease reporting, licensing of health-care providers and facilities, and quarantine authority, is based with states as an extension of their police powers.

Children may encounter the public health system in various ways:
- Immunization requirements for school entry
- Reporting and tracking of certain diseases
- Licensing of child-care facilities
- Outreach and education campaigns to promote health or prevent disease
- In some areas, health departments provide "safety net" health-care services to families otherwise unable to access care.

Public health surveillance

Surveillance, a core function of the public health system, is the systematic collection, analysis, and interpretation of health-related data essential to planning, implementation, and evaluation of public health practice. Surveillance systems can be used to detect outbreaks, evaluate control measures, allocate resources, and facilitate planning.

You should familiarize yourself with local disease-reporting requirements. A comprehensive list is available from the Nationally Notifiable Diseases Surveillance System, at: http://www.cdc.gov/ncphi/disss/nndss/nndsshis.htm

Disaster preparedness

Many disaster plans fail to adequately consider the unique needs of children in disasters or mass-casualty incidents. Pediatric providers may be called upon to provide care or information in these situations.

Creation of a "family disaster plan" (Box 27.2) can be encouraged at well-child visits. Online materials are available through the AAP.

Box 27.2 Creating a "family disaster plan"

1. Talk with children about the danger of disasters that are common in your area and how to prepare for each of them. Make sure they know where to go in the home and school to stay safe during an earthquake, tornado, hurricane, or other disaster.

2. Teach children to recognize alarms. Let them know what smoke detectors, fire alarms, and community warning systems (horns and sirens) sound like and what to do when they hear them.

3. Explain to children how and when to call for help. Keep emergency phone numbers where family members can find them.

4. Pick an out-of-state family contact person who family members can check in with if separated during an emergency.

5. Agree on a meeting place away from your home (a neighbor or relative's house or even a street corner) where you would get together if you were separated in an emergency.

6. Put together a disaster supplies kit for the family.

7. Children with special health-care needs and children dependent on technology are especially vulnerable in community disruptions. Parents should work with providers to develop and record individual health-care plans for these children.

8. Practice the family disaster plan every 6 months, so everyone will remember what to do in an emergency.

In mass-casualty incidents, children may be *separated from parents*. The National Center for Missing and Exploited Children (1-800-843-5678) and the Red Cross (1-866-GET-INFO) have hotlines to help family members find each other.

Pediatricians should also consider the *feeding needs of infants* during complex emergencies. Breast-feeding can be supported whenever possible as the cleanest, safest, and most reliable food source for infants.

The following online sources provide details on pediatric-specific management of chemical, biological, and radiological exposures as well as the psychological needs of children and families caught up in humanitarian emergencies:

- American Academy of Pediatrics (AAP):
  http://www.aap.org/terrorism/
- U.S. Department of Health and Human Services (DHHS):
  http://www.hhs.gov/disasters/
- National Child Traumatic Stress Network: http://www.nctsnet.org
- Agency for Healthcare Research and Quality (AHRQ):
  http://www.ahrq.gov/prep

Schools and health

Local schools are an important context for child health and well-being. While the primary aim of public schools is clearly education, there is ample evidence that health conditions can affect readiness to learn and that school-based services can address unmet health-care needs, promote healthful behaviors, and improve the health of school populations.

The coordinated school health model[1] envisions schools as a venue for coordination of eight services:

1. Health education: K–12 curriculum that addresses the physical, mental, emotional, and social dimensions of health. The curriculum is designed to motivate and assist students to maintain and improve their health, prevent disease, and reduce health-related risk behaviors.

2. Physical education: K–12 curriculum that provides cognitive content and learning experiences in a variety of areas, promoting activities that all students enjoy and can pursue throughout their lives. Qualified, trained teachers teach physical activity.

3. Health services: Services designed to ensure access or referral to primary health-care services, control communicable disease, and provide emergency care for illness or injury

4. Nutrition services: Access to a variety of nutritious and appealing meals that accommodate the health and nutritional needs of all students

5. Counseling and psychological services: Services provided to improve students' mental, emotional, and social health. These services include individual and group assessments, interventions, and referrals.

6. Healthy school environment: The physical surroundings and the psychosocial climate and culture of the school

7. Health promotion for staff: Opportunities for school staff to improve their health status through activities such as health assessments, health education, and health-related fitness activities. Health promotion activities have improved productivity, decreased absenteeism, and reduced health insurance costs.

8. Family and community involvement: An integrated school, parent, and community approach for enhancing the health and well-being of students

Poverty

The official poverty measure in the United States focuses narrowly on income and is based on patterns of food expenditure from the 1950s. It is an incomplete measure of economic well-being. On average, families need an income 200% of the federal poverty level to make ends meet. Those making less than 200% of the poverty level are "low income."

In 2007, the federal poverty level for a family of four was $20,650. See http://aspe.hhs.gov/poverty for current definitions.

Children are the poorest group in American society. In 2007, 17% of children lived in poverty; 39% were low income. There is significant racial and ethnic variation in child poverty (see Fig. 27.1).

Federally funded public-assistance programs intended to mitigate the effects of poverty on low-income children[1]:

- *Medicaid* provides health insurance coverage for low-income children. http://www.cms.hhs.gov/home/medicaid.asp
- *Head Start* targets families below the poverty level to provide child development preschool programs for 3- and 4-year-old children. http://www.acf.hhs.gov/programs/hsb/
- *Food Stamp Program*: Benefits are provided on an electronic card that is accepted at most grocery stores. http://www.fns.usda.gov/fsp/
- *WIC* (Supplemental Food Program for Women, Infants, and Children) Provides food, nutritional counseling, and screening/referral for low-income women and children up to age 5. http://www.fns.usda.gov/wic/
- *National School Lunch Program* (and School Breakfast Program) provides low-cost or free lunches to children each school day. http://www.fns.usda.gov/cnd/Lunch/
- *Housing assistance* is provided to low-income families as project-based housing or as vouchers to subsidize rent in qualified Section 8 units. http://www.hud.gov/renting/
- *Child-care subsidies.* Tax credits are provided to offset the cost of child care. http://www.childcareaware.org/

---

1 National Center for Children in Poverty, at: http://www.nccp.org/

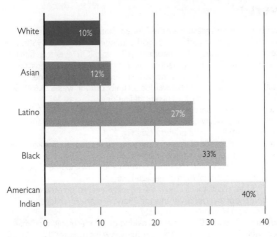

Figure 27.1 Reprinted with permission from NCCP, National Center for Children in Poverty.

Child care

The quality and availability of child care is a growing concern:
- Over 60% of women with young children are employed.
- About 25% of children live in households headed by single women.

High-quality child care has the following features:
- Appropriate supervision and discipline
- Nurturing care
- Low staff-to-child ratio and group size (see Table 27.1)
- Written immunization requirements
- Hand washing and diapering sanitation
- Director qualifications
- Developmentally appropriate toys and activities
- Staff teacher qualifications
- Staff training
- Plans for medical administration
- Emergency plan and contact
- Fire drills
- Appropriate outdoor playground
- Safe storing of toxic substances

High-quality care keeps children safe and healthy, promotes development, and enhances school readiness.

Table 27.1 Recommended adult-to-child ratios by age

Age	Child:staff ratio	Maximum group size
0–24 months	3:1	6
25–30 months	4:1	8
31–35 months	5:1	10
3 years old	7:1	14
4–5 years old	8:1	16

Child care also includes before- and after-school programs. After-school programs can reduce high-risk behaviors such as substance abuse, juvenile delinquency, and teen pregnancies.

- Healthy Child Care America (AAP): http://www.healthychildcare.org/
- Federal Child Care Bureau: http://www.acf.hhs.gov/programs/ccb
- National Institute on Out-of-School Time: http://www.niost.org/

Foster care

- Over 500,000 U.S. children reside in some form of foster care.
- Children are placed into foster care for many reasons:
  - Abuse or neglect
  - Parental illness, incapacity, or death
  - Severe behavior problems of the child
- One-third of children in foster care have significant mental health issues.
- There is a higher proportion of children of color in the foster-care system than in the general U.S. population. However, child abuse and neglect occur at about the same rate in all racial and ethnic groups.
- On average, children spend 28 months in foster care.
- About 20,000 youth "age out" of the foster-care system every year. These 18-year-olds tend to be disconnected from societal networks and lack family support. This group is at high risk for homelessness and poor health outcomes.
- Reimbursement rates for foster parents are lower in most states than the true costs of providing routine care for the child.

Important challenges for foster parents:
- Limits to their emotional attachment to the child
- Mixed feelings toward the child's biological parents
- Difficulties letting the child return to birth parents
- Dealing with the complex emotional and physical needs of children in their care
- Working with social service agencies and caseworkers
- Finding support services in the community
- Dealing with the child's emotions and behavior following visits with the biological parents

Children in foster care have often had many transitions in living situation and health-care provider. Extra effort is required to gather relevant past medical information and records.

Some states provide "medical passports," or brief, portable records of important health information.

For more information on foster care in the United States, contact:
- Child Welfare League: http://www.cwla.org/
- National Foster Care Coalition http://www.nationalfostercare.org/

Juvenile justice

- Each year in the United States about 2.3 million juveniles under age 18 are arrested and encounter the juvenile justice system.
- Residential placement occurs when youth are detained (pending adjudication, for example) or committed (after a hearing).
- Approximately 97,000 U.S. youth are in custody on any given day (see Box 27.3). About 15% of this population is female.

Box 27.3 Custody rates per 100,000 vary by race and ethnicity, 2006

White	190
Black	754
Hispanic	348
American Indian/Alaska Native	496
Asian	113

Custody rates per 100,000 vary by state, from 96 (Vermont) to 632 (South Dakota)

From the Office of Juvenile Justice and Delinquency Prevention (OJJDP) Statistical Briefing Book. 2006.

Youth in custody are a high-risk population:
- Risk behaviors begin before youth are 11 years old.
- 60% have sexual intercourse by age 12.
- 30% have sexually transmitted infections.
- 25% have experienced fight-related injuries within the past year.
- Up to 75% have mental health concerns.
- 22% report suicidal ideation.
- 60% have substance abuse problems.

Access to health services in many detention centers is limited. However, incarceration may be the only time for contact with a health-care provider outside of an emergency setting.

Youth leaving custody should be directed to a medical home for aftercare. However, many low-income youth have been removed from Medicaid benefits during custody and experience financial barriers to health-care access.

Advocacy

Advocacy is not a pediatric subspecialty: it is an integral part of pediatric practice. Clinicians "advocate" on behalf of children in many ways, some private, some very public:

1. At the level of the **individual child and family**, pediatricians advocate to help their patients gain access to needed resources, social supports, or community benefits.
2. At the level of the practice or health-care organization, pediatricians advocate for systems and services to promote child health and safety and to meet the unique developmental and medical needs of their patients.
3. In the local community, pediatricians can work with schools, charitable organizations, and other institutions to promote the well-being of children.
4. Some pediatricians engage in legislative or policy advocacy to change laws, allocate resources, modify environments, or improve systems that impact the health and well-being of children on a local, state, or national scale.

Tips for successful advocacy

- Be familiar with local resources to which parents and patients can be referred for help in the community. Look for help in solving problems that happen outside the medical sphere (consider, for example, the Medical-Legal Partnership for Children: http://www.mlpforchildren.org/)
- Follow your passion. Successful advocacy at any level is driven by your commitment and interest.
- Coordinate your efforts with others interested in working on similar issues. Consider joining local and state chapters of your professional medical organization. See, for example, AAP and Resident Section Advocacy (http://www.aap.org/sections/ypn/r/advocacy/)
- Know your elected representatives and keep in contact with their offices. A phone call is better than e-mail (refer to http://www.usa.gov/Contact/Elected).

Child protection

Definitions

Child protection

This is the decisive action taken to safeguard children from harm.

Child abuse

Child abuse is defined as either
- deliberate or unreasonably reckless infliction of harm to a child, or
- knowingly not preventing harm to a child.

Children may be abused in the family home, in an institutional setting or, rarely, by a stranger. Most young people who are abused know their abuser. It is estimated that several children die each week from abuse.

Child abuse may be categorized as
- Neglect
- Physical
- Sexual
- Emotional

Neglect

Neglect is defined as the persistent failure to meet a child's basic physical or psychological needs, which is likely to result in serious impairment of the child's health and development. It may involve the following:
- Failing to provide adequate food
- Failing to protect the child from physical harm or danger
- Failure to access appropriate health care or treatment

Presentation
- Failure to thrive
- Consistently unkempt and dirty appearance
- Repeated failure by caretakers to prevent accidental injury
- Lack of social responsiveness and/or developmental delay when there are other concerns about the environment at home
- Failure to follow through on unmet medical, dental, educational, nutritional, or mental health needs

Physical abuse

Physical abuse involves any activity that causes physical harm to a child (e.g., hitting, shaking, burning, suffocating; see Box 28.1). Fabricated illness is also usually included in this category (see p. 1138).

Box 28.1 Presentation of physical abuse

Typical presentations of physical abuse include the following:

Bruises
- Symmetrical bruised eyes, without nasal or brow injury
- Bruising of soft tissues of the face, especially in small babies. Pre-mobile babies should not get bruises or other injuries.
- Bruising of mouth or ears
- Finger marks on the face, legs, arms, or chest (the latter occasionally has associated rib fractures)
- Unexplained bruising of different ages
- Linear bruising on buttocks or back
- Distinct patterns of bruising (i.e., handprint marks, implements, kicks)
- Uncommon sites for accidents (i.e., stomach, chest, genitalia, neck)

Burns or scalds
- Contact burns with clear outlines, on usually protected body surfaces; multiple burns; or small, clearly imprinted round burns (e.g., cigarette burns)
- Limb or buttock immersion scalds

Fractures
It is rare for a child <1 year of age with normal bones to sustain an accidental fracture. Bone disorders (i.e., osteogenesis imperfecta [see p. 882] or rickets) are rare but should be clinically evaluated. Consider:
- Fracture type should be evaluated to see if it is consistent with the mechanics of the injury history.
- Long bones (arms, legs) in pre-mobile infants
- Rib fractures, particularly posterior.
- Multiple fractures of various bones and ages are usually from abuse.
- Metaphyseal avulsion injuries
- Fractures of unusual bones or unusual fracture types of normally injured bones

Bite marks
- Adult bites are differentiated from child bites by forensic dentistry.
- Blood group and DNA evidence should be collected in serious cases.

Scars
- Especially if patterned or in unusual locations

Poisoning
- This may accidental as a consequence of neglect, or deliberate (as in fabricated illness or attempts to quiet a fussy child).
- Abusive intoxications should be considered when severe, recurrent symptoms or signs such as coma, seizures, or severe gastrointestinal upset (vomiting or diarrhea) remain medically unexplained.

Investigations
Skeletal survey and other imaging
Infants localize pain poorly, hence skeletal injuries may be missed. X-rays must be carefully planned with the radiology team and the correct views carried out. X-rays may need repeating if they are inconclusive; alternatively, consider a radioisotope bone scan.

- *X-rays*: Full skeletal survey for children <2–3 years old with evidence of physical trauma, and X-rays of individual sites of symptoms for older children.
- *Bone scan*: If X-rays are inconclusive and immediate information is needed. A bone scan is useful for assessing rib fractures, but less so for metaphyseal or skull fractures.
- *CT or MRI scan of brain*: In infants and young children who present with seizures, apnea, irritability, or coma. Obtain CT or MRI for children who are asymptomatic from head injury, and for children <6 months old with other physical-abuse findings, even if they are without CNS signs.

Clotting screen
Perform tests if there is extensive or unusual bruising, or unexplained cerebral hemorrhage.

- This test is more necessary when only bruising or bleeding is present than when burns or fractures are also found.
- It is not mandated for patterned injuries resulting from slaps or recognizable blows from implements.

Ophthalmology examination
In cases of suspected inflicted head injury, examination by an experienced ophthalmologist is needed to look for evidence of retinal hemorrhages.

Sexual abuse

Sexual abuse involves the forcing or enticing of a child or young person to take part in sexual activities, regardless of whether the child is aware of what is happening. This may include physical contact or penetrative or nonpenetrative acts. It may also involve non-contact activities such as looking at or being involved in the participation of pornographic or other sexual activities.

Presentation

Children who have been victims of sexual abuse may present in a number of ways:

- Sexually transmitted infections: Gonorrhea, *Chlamydia*, *Trichomonas vaginalis*
- Pregnancy
- Vaginal bleeding in prepubertal children
- Behavioral changes
  - Self-harm
  - Withdrawal
  - Aggression
  - Sexualized behavior
  - Unexplained deteriorating school performance
- Disclosure by the child
- Secondary wetting and/or fecal soiling

Signs

Few physical signs are diagnostic, and most victims, even of penetrating vaginal injury, lack abnormal physical findings.

Acute signs

- *Girls*: Acute tears in the hymen, vaginal bleeding, bruising around the genital area and "hand" grip marks
- *Boys*: Bruising to the genital area, urethral injury, torn frenulum of the penis
- *Anal signs*: Anal fissure, gaping anus, swelling of the anal margin (all are very nonspecific for abuse)
- *Note*: Signs of sexual abuse may disappear or heal rapidly.

Chronic

- These signs are more difficult to interpret and may be suggestive of previous, penetrative trauma:
  - Scar in posterior fourchette
  - Old tear/cleft or scar of the hymen
  - Attenuation of hymen (very hard to measure and nonspecific)

Emotional abuse

Emotional abuse is persistent, emotional ill treatment of a child that results in severe impairment of emotional development.

This may involve the following:
- Conveying to children that they are worthless or unloved
- Imposing age- or developmentally inappropriate expectations
- Causing children to frequently feel frightened and threatened
- Failure to seek care for emotional problems

This form of abuse often coexists with other forms of ill treatment.

Presentation

This is almost always gradual and difficult to diagnose. Symptoms are largely behavioral and may include the following:
- Excessively clingy
- Attention-seeking behavior
- Excess aggression
- Excess anxiety
- Over-serious
- Anxious to please

Parental behaviors are a clue to the diagnosis. Any of these must be persistent and severe and have a major impact on the child to reach the threshold for emotional abuse:
- Persistently negative view of the child
- Inconsistent and unpredictable responses
- Behavioral expectations that are very inappropriate
- Induction of a child into bizarre parental beliefs

Fabricated or induced illness by caretakers

This is an unusual form of child abuse. It has also been referred to as Munchausen syndrome by proxy (MSbP). The salient feature is that the child is harmed by being presented for medical attention with symptoms or signs that have been falsified by the caretaker.

- The child is the victim of the abuse and the perpetrator is the person who fabricates the illness.
- Existing mental health difficulties in the perpetrator (the child's natural mother in 90% of cases) have been described, but are usually personality or mood disorders and are not essential for the diagnosis.

Presentation

There is a wide spectrum of severity of harm:

- False medical history
- Fabrication of symptoms and signs (e.g., warming a thermometer under hot water, blood placed on clothing, diaper or sugar added to a urine specimen)

The *most serious* presentations include fabrication of illness by directly induced events, such as poisoning or suffocation.

Symptoms

Children may present with a range of symptoms:

- Seizures, collapse, coma
- Apnea
- Vomiting and diarrhea
- Failure to thrive
- Polyuria and polydipsia
- Purpura
- Recurrent fever
- Multiple and unusual allergies and treatment sensitivities
- Virtually all natural illnesses have been the subject of falsification.
- Failure of normal illnesses to respond to normal treatments
- Hematuria

Diagnosis

- It is important to realize that the medical profession may add to the harm of these children by unnecessary investigations and treatments.
- The diagnosis can be established by resolution of the problems when the child is separated from the perpetrator and should be considered when investigations for other usual illnesses are persistently normal.
- Very careful attention should be paid to the medical history, particularly as to who witnessed the events and when they occurred.
- The caretaker's own history and their family's history are often floridly abnormal.

Seek an opinion from an experienced colleague who should arrange a strategy meeting between health-care professionals to decide on what further action is necessary.

Medical involvement in child protection

All health professionals have a role ensuring that children and families receive the care, support, and services they need to promote child health and development. Health professionals are often the first to have contact with children or families in difficulty. Participation in child protection encompasses a range of activities:

- Recognizing children in need of support or protection and parents who may need extra help in raising their children
- Reporting victims to proper authorities for further investigation
- Contributing to enquiries about a child or family
- Assessing the needs of children and the capacity of parents to meet their children's needs
- Planning and providing support for vulnerable children and families
- Participating in child protection conferences
- Planning support for children at risk of significant harm
- Providing therapeutic help to abused or neglected children and parents under stress
- Contributing to case reviews
- Providing testimony in legal proceedings

Initial concerns

When there are concerns about a child, and when there is reasonable belief that a child is at serious risk of immediate harm, doctors should act immediately to protect the interests of the child. This will almost always involve contacting one or both of the statutory bodies with responsibilities in this child protection:

- State social services or protective services
- Police

A full report of concerns will be required. The precise action taken is governed by the procedures set out by the individual state's child protection laws.

Referral to other agencies

An experienced or senior member of the medical team should be involved when there are child protection concerns.

Agencies

- *Social services or protective services* are the lead agency for investigation of child abuse.
- *Police* are frequently involved in the initial joint investigation or when criminal prosecution is likely.

Referral procedure

- Parents should normally be informed that protective-services referrals are being made, unless that information would increase the risk to the child or impair the investigation (e.g., in MSbP, where the caretaker is at risk to actively make the child ill to "prove" the reality of the child's illness, or with sexual abuse, where the child's history might by suppressed by the caretaker before the authorities investigate).
- In cases of serious abuse, immediate reporting to not only protective services but also the police is most likely to aid in identifying the perpetrator.
- Referral does not need parental permission and is legally mandated.
- Specific concerns should be clearly stated.
- Telephone referrals must be confirmed in writing in some states.
- Referrals should be followed up if no acknowledgement or action is taken.

The child's safety is of equal importance to their medical treatment.

If hospitalization for medical treatment is not indicated, the child should not be discharged without a clear plan and decision about place of safety and future follow-up. This will be a joint decision and the responsibility of the multidisciplinary agencies (social services and police), advised by the medical assessment. The police should be immediately informed if the parents or caretakers attempt to remove the child from the hospital before these decisions are made.

Medical assessment

The purpose of the medical assessment is to
- Assess whether the child has been injured and/or whether there are any other medical or developmental concerns
- Provide appropriate investigations and treatment for the child
- Provide an opinion about possible cause

When assessing a child who may have been the victim of child abuse, it is important to inform and involve your senior colleagues at an early stage. The assessment should be carried out (along with an experienced or senior colleague, if possible) in an environment that provides a sufficient degree of comfort for the child and their parents or caretakers, as well as sufficient access and lighting for examination. It is good practice to have a nurse or other health professional present at the time of history taking and examination.

History

- A thorough history is required. Stick to your medical history; confrontational interviewing is the job of the police.
- The presenting problem should be documented chronologically, outlining the sequence of events and circumstances leading up to presentation and referral.
- The family history, past medical history (i.e., clotting defects, bone disorders, psychiatric), birth and developmental history, and social history should be detailed.
- Medical or social-work history should include who was taking care of the child at given time points and any social risk factors, such as past abuse of the parent as a child, domestic violence, or substance abuse.

Examination

This should include a general examination of all the systems.
- Weight, head circumference, and height should be plotted on a growth chart.
- Neurodevelopmental assessment is appropriate in infants and toddlers.
- External injuries should be recorded in detail, including a description of their location, size, tenderness, induration, and appearance.
- Photographs should be taken (see next page).
- Examination of children with suspected sexual abuse, beyond that required for management of acute issues, such as serious genital bleeding, should be undertaken by specially trained sexual-abuse examiners.

Child protection register

When there are concerns about a child, inquiries should be made to the local child protection registry, which is a confidential list of names of children who have been reported or substantiated as abuse victims. The register is maintained within the state social-services department or protective-services agency. Its specific registrants, access, and information vary by state.

Consent

This is an important consideration that needs to be taken into account before proceeding with the medical assessment of any child. If the child is deemed to have sufficient understanding to make an informed decision, consent should be obtained from them. Children of sufficient understanding cannot be medically examined without their consent even when an emergency protection order has been made.

Record keeping

Clear, detailed notes are required.
- *Written or dictated notes:* Full and contemporaneous notes should be kept, including statements made by the parents and the child. All notes must be signed and dated with the name of the doctor printed underneath an entry.
- *Diagrams:* Particularly body maps to illustrate location of injuries
- *Photographs* should be obtained for children with visible injuries. They should be dated, include the child's identity, and include a ruler or other size standard for patterned injuries. Both distant photos to locate injuries on the child's body and detailed close-ups should be obtained.

Assessment by social services

Social services and the police will undertake an assessment and will collect the relevant information from all professionals involved. Referrals may result in

- No further action being taken
- Provision of support and help for the child and their family through a voluntary agreement
- Fuller assessment of the needs and circumstances of the child
- Legal dependency for the child with either supervised, in-home care by the child's family or placement outside the home

Reporting to child protection services

Those members of the medical team directly involved in the initial assessment and/or subsequent management of the child should write a medical report. Parents and their attorneys have the right to see reports before legal proceedings. Important points in writing these reports include the following:

- Distinguish facts from opinions and allegations.
- Relevant information should be used from current and past records.
- Explain medical terms for the benefit of laypersons.
- Include observations and relevant statements from the child and caretaker.
- Attribute these statements to their source.
- State clearly the degree of medical certainty as to whether the injury is the result of normal childhood events or of abuse.
- State your medical opinion, not legal opinion.

Confidentiality and disclosure of medical information

The Health Insurance Portability and Accountability Act's (HIPAA) confidentiality previsions are specifically superseded in the act, by the individual state's reporting requirements for cases of suspected child abuse. All states mandate reporting of child abuse, but the specific reporting thresholds and pathways of whom to report to and in what time frame vary by state.

In general, reporting is required for reasonable suspicion of abuse, not certainty, and the reporter is immune from civil liability for filing good-faith reports. Most states attach criminal liability for failure to report, and civil liability would also be risked. Because of the variable requirements, review of one's own state's law is advised.

- Information can be disclosed to protective services and the police without consent in cases of a serious crime (including child abuse).
- In the absence of consent, confidential medical information about parents or third parties only should be shared when relevant and necessary to protect the safety and welfare of the child. The more sensitive this information is, the greater the child's needs must be to justify disclosure.
- Normally, permission from parents should be obtained to disclose parental health information unless it is reasonable to conclude that this would hinder inquiries or place the child at greater risk.

Prevention strategies

Most children referred to social services will be those in need, rather than those requiring protection. Children in need are those whose vulnerability is such that they are unlikely to reach or maintain a satisfactory level of health or development without the provision of support services.

The role of social services in prevention is to undertake an initial assessment and implement a plan to maximize the child's health and development, including

- Referral to support services (i.e., health visitors, parenting groups, school nurses, nursery placement, home support)
- Referral to specialist services (i.e., mental health [adult or child], substance abuse treatment, pediatric care)

Pharmacology and therapeutics

Prescribing for children

Licensing

Many medicines prescribed are not licensed for use in children because pharmaceutical companies have not sought licenses from the regulatory authorities for uses in children. Hence, many medicines used in children are used *off label*—i.e., the drugs are used at doses, routes, ages, or indications that are different from those specified within the product licenses.

Benefit versus risk should be determined before prescribing any medication for children, particularly for off label use.

Disease states

Certain diseases (i.e., cystic fibrosis) or clinical conditions (i.e., shock) may affect drug metabolism. Both liver and renal failure can delay drug elimination and may require dosage reduction.

Breast-feeding

Most medicines taken by a breast-feeding mother are safe for her infant. Mothers should not be discouraged from breast-feeding because of uncertainty about possible toxic effects. Refer to the AAP policy (*Pediatrics* 2001; 108:776–789).

Medication errors

Medication errors are a significant problem in children. **Most health professionals will commit a medication error during their careers!** Types of medication errors include the following.

Incorrect dose

This is the most common error, and the type most likely to be associated with a fatality. Knowledge of the child's actual weight and checking of dose calculation is vital, especially on the neonatal unit and with parenteral medicines. Avoid 10-fold errors caused by decimal misplacement.

Incorrect drug

This is the second most common type of error and is associated with significant fatalities.

Incorrect route

This is a particular problem with intrathecal drugs, a procedure for specialists.

Other errors

Other errors include incorrect rate of administration, duplicate dosing, and administration of the drug to the *incorrect patient.*

Adverse drug reactions

Over 9% of children in the hospital and 1.5% of outpatients will experience an adverse drug reaction (ADR), and ~1 in 8 of these will be severe. ADRs are responsible for 2% of children admitted to the hospital. Differences in drug metabolism make some ADRs greater problems in children than in adults (i.e., valproate hepatotoxicity), or less of a problem (i.e., paracetamol hepatotoxicity following an overdose).

The mechanisms of ADRs specifically affecting children are illustrated with examples below.

Mechanisms of ADRs

Impaired drug metabolism

When first used in neonates, chloramphenicol led to development of the gray-baby syndrome (vomiting, cyanosis, cardiovascular collapse, and, in some cases, death). Newborn infants metabolize chloramphenicol more slowly thando adults and require a lower dose of this antibiotic. Reduction in the dosage prevents gray-baby syndrome.

Children, particularly neonates, are more likely to have lower capacities to metabolize drugs than do adults. Therefore, lower doses are usually required.

Altered drug metabolism

Children may have lower activities of major hepatic enzymes associated with drug metabolism than of the corresponding activities in adults. To compensate for this, children may use other enzyme pathways. This is thought to be one of the factors contributing to the increased hepatotoxicity from sodium valproate in children under the age of 3 years. This risk is increased by the concurrent use of other anticonvulsants.

Sodium valproate should not be used as a first-line anticonvulsant in children under the age of 3 years.

Protein-displacing effect on bilirubin

The use of the sulfonamide sulfisoxazole in ill neonates in the 1950s was associated with the development of fatal kernicterus (see p. 144). This condition is due to drug displacement of protein-bound bilirubin in the blood, because of the higher binding affinity of albumin for sulfisoxazole.

The protein-displacing effect of medicines should be considered, particularly in sick preterm neonates.

Percutaneous absorption

Percutaneous toxicity can be a significant problem in the neonatal period, due to the higher surface area-to-weight ratios in neonates than in older children and adults. An example of this is the use of antiseptic agents, such as hexachlorophene, that have been associated with neurotoxicity.

Drug interactions

Skin reactions to the anticonvulsant lamotrigine are more likely to occur in children than in infants. The incidence is significantly increased by co-medication with sodium valproate along with the lamotrigine. The mechanism of this drug interaction is unknown.

Drug interactions may increase the risk of an ADR.

Unknown

We do not understand the mechanisms responsible for some ADRs. Salicylates given during a viral illness increase the risk of development of Reye's syndrome in children of all ages. Since the use of salicylates has been avoided in children, the incidence of Reye's syndrome has decreased dramatically.

Propofol has minimal toxicity when used to induce general anesthesia. Used as a sedative in critically ill children, however, propofol has been associated with death in children. The propofol infusion syndrome is thought to be related to the total dose of propofol infused, i.e., high-dose or prolonged duration is more likely to cause problems.

Propofol should not be used as a sedative in critically ill children.

Suspect ADRs

One should always consider the possibility of an ADR being responsible for a child's symptoms. Some of the serious ADRs associated with widely used medicine are listed in Table 29.1.

Table 29.1 Serious ADRs associated with medicines

Drug	ADR
Corticosteroids	Adrenal insufficiency or sepsis
Cytotoxics	Neutropenia
Carbamazepine	Stevens–Johnson syndrome
NSAIDs (including ibuprofen)	Gastrointestinal hemorrhage
Opiates	Respiratory depression
Sodium valproate	Hepatotoxicity

Preventing ADRs

Recognition of patients at greater risk for ADRs can help reduce the overall incidence. Health professionals should follow guidelines.

Reporting ADRs

Suspected ADRs should be reported to the FDA.

Pharmacokinetics

Pharmacokinetics defines the relationship between the dose of a drug and its concentration in different parts of the body (usually plasma) in relation to time. This relationship is measured and defined numerically. Knowledge of several key terms is needed to understand pharmacokinetic principles.

Absorption
If a drug is given intravenously, 100% of the dose enters the blood stream. If a drug is given orally, usually only a fraction is absorbed. The term *bioavailability* is used to describe the percentage of the drug administered that reaches the systemic circulation. Absorption is often reduced following oral administration in the neonatal period.

Volume of distribution (V_D)
This is an apparent volume into which the drug would have to distribute to achieve the measured concentration. Water-soluble drugs, such as gentamicin, have V_Ds that are similar to the extracellular fluid volumes. Drugs that are highly bound to plasma proteins have lower V_Ds.

Lipophilic (fat-soluble) drugs can exhibit V_Ds that are much larger than the total mass of the patient, especially in patients with large amounts of body fat. Children differ from adults in their body compositions (neonates and young children have a higher proportion of body water) and lower plasma protein concentrations.

Clearance
Clearance describes the removal of a drug from the body and is defined as the volume (usually of plasma) that is completely cleared of drug in a given time. In adults, clearance is described in relation to volume/time (mL/min).

In children, clearance is also described in relation to body weight (mL/min/kg). Clearance rates are usually lower in neonates but may be higher in infants and young children than in adults.

Elimination half-life
This is the time taken for the concentration of a drug (usually in plasma) to fall to half of the original value. Elimination half-lives are inversely related to rates of clearance. Fifty percent of the dose will be eliminated in one half-life, and 97% of a drug will be eliminated after 5 half-lives; this is also the time required for steady state to be achieved following initial administration of the drug.

Mathematical formulas are available in standard texts that describe the interrelationships among clearance, volume of distribution, and elimination half-life.

Drug metabolism

The major pathways involved in drug metabolism are divided into phase I (oxidation, reduction, hydrolysis, and hydration) and phase II (glucuronidation, sulfation, methylation, and acetylation) reactions. As a general rule, rates of clearance of drugs in neonates are lower than those in adults. For many drugs, adult clearance values are reached by the age of 2 years.

Phase I pathways

The major pathway is oxidation, which involves the cytochrome P450 (CYP) enzymes. The major CYP enzymes are CYP3A4 and CYP1A2.
- *CYP3A4* is responsible for the metabolism of many drugs (i.e., midazolam, cyclosporin, fentanyl, nifedipine). CYP3A4 activities are lower in neonates and newborn infants than in adults. Enzyme activities between individuals vary considerably, which can lead to a large range of plasma concentrations after the same dose of a drug.
- *CYP1A2* accounts for 13% of total CYP enzyme activity in the liver. Caffeine and theophylline are metabolized via the CYP1A2 pathway. Enzyme activities are low in the neonatal period but increase rapidly, such that by the age of 6 months, activities approach those in older children and adults.

Phase II pathways

Glucuronidation and sulfation are the two major phase II pathways. Glucuronidation rates are lower in neonates than in adults, but sulfation rates are higher.

The development of glucuronidation varies for different drugs. For example, children who are 2 years old have rates of glucuronidation of morphine that are similar to those in adults, whereas adult rates of glucuronidation of acetaminophen are not reached until puberty.

Pain management

See also p. 926.

Assessment

It is important to always assess the presence of pain in all pediatric patients. Accurate assessment requires an age-appropriate, validated pain assessment scale. Self-reporting is the ideal, but the child needs to be ≥3 years old to be able to do this. Do not use pain scales validated for acute pain to assess chronic pain.

Self-report scales

Implementation of these scales usually involves the child pointing to a photograph of a child in pain (the Oucher) or a diagram of a child in pain (Bieri Faces Pain Scale or Wong–Baker Faces Pain Scale). The Oucher has been validated in children as young as 3 years of age, whereas the Bieri Faces Pain Scale has only been validated in children aged ≥6 years.

The Wong–Baker Faces Pain Scale is more reliable in children aged 8–12 years than in the 3- to 7-year age group. The Adolescent Pediatric Pain Tool is for children between the ages of 8 and 17 years.

Behavioral pain scales

Rely on assessment of the child's behavior. These scales are validated for children aged 1–5 years. Examples include the Toddler–Preschooler Postoperative Pain Scale (TPPPS) and the Children's Hospital Eastern Ontario Pain Scale (CHEOPS). The FLACC has been validated for children aged 2 months to 7 years.

Neonatal pain scales

Examples include the Children's Revised Impact of Events Scale (CRIES), Neonatal Facial Coding System (NFCS), Neonatal/Infant Pain Scale (NIPS), and Premature Infant Pain Profile (PIPP). These rely on behavioral observation and, in some, measurements of pulse, blood pressure, and O_2 saturation.

It is important to use a pain scale that has been validated for the gestational age of the infant, i.e., is it valid only in full-term neonates?

Management

It is best to consider pain as being mild, moderate, or severe.

Mild pain

Acetaminophen is the safest analgesic available and is the first-line drug to be used for mild pain in all ages.

Moderate pain

Children who are unresponsive (or unlikely to respond) to acetaminophen should receive either a nonsteroidal anti-inflammatory drug (NSAID), such as ibuprofen, or diclofenac.

Alternatively, codeine or dihydrocodeine can be administered orally, but codeine is not metabolized to morphine and therefore will not be effective, in ~7% of Caucasians.

Severe pain
Morphine is the drug of choice. It can be given IV (including as patient-controlled analgesia [PCA]), intranasally, or orally.

Procedural pain
For certain painful procedures (i.e., dressing change in burn patients) it may be better to use inhaled entonox. This is an effective and safe analgesic with a short duration of action, which the child can control.

Sedation

Sedation is required most often during procedures and while receiving pediatric intensive care. Sedation is not analgesia, and painful procedures or conditions require analgesia.

Procedural sedation

All sedative agents can have significant toxicities. The choice of sedative agent depends on the requirement for rapidity of onset and duration of action.

If a child is expected to be difficult to sedate, consider whether a short-acting general anesthetic, administered by a pediatric anesthetist, is more appropriate for the patient. Similarly, a pediatric anesthetist should be consulted, if loss of airway secondary to sedation is a concern.

Prolonged sedation (critical care)

The purpose of sedation in the pediatric intensive care unit (PICU) is to help the child during a time of invasive tests and procedures. Midazolam administered IV is the drug of choice on admission. Subsequently, when nasogastric feeds are tolerated, chloral hydrate and promethazine have been shown to be more effective than midazolam.

Although the first-line drug in many situations requiring long-term sedation, propofol use is accompanied by risk of a fatal ADR, and use should be considered carefully and monitored closely.

Fever

Fever is a sign of an underlying illness. It is more important to treat the underlying illness than the fever itself. Fever is reduced to make the child more comfortable. The two most used antipyretics (acetaminophen and ibuprofen) are also analgesics (see p. 706).

Management

Acetaminophen is the drug of choice. It is less likely to be associated with a significant ADR than is ibuprofen. Ibuprofen is appropriate to use as an antipyretic agent if acetaminophen has failed.

Although the safest of all NSAIDs, acetaminophen should not be used in children with gastroenteritis or other gastrointestinal symptoms. Acetaminophen should be used with caution in children with asthma or viral-induced wheeze. NSAIDs should be avoided in children with kidney disease.

International health and travel

Global health: childhood illness

Ninety percent of children under 5 years old live in the developing world. Over 10 million children under 5 die each year, most from preventable or treatable causes.

Child mortality rates vary among world regions, and these differences are large and increasing (see Fig. 30.1).

Worldwide, half of the deaths in children under the age of 5 years are due to
- Pneumonia
- Diarrhea
- Malaria
- Measles (see Fig. 30.2)

Undernutrition is a major factor contributing to these deaths. Two-thirds of them could be prevented by interventions already available and feasible today for implementation in low-income countries.

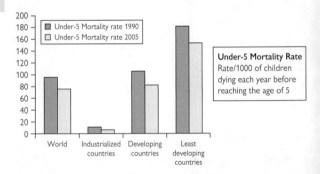

Under-5 Mortality Rate
Rate/1000 of children dying each year before reaching the age of 5

Figure 30.1 Reprinted from Rosenberg, M. Global child health: Burden of disease, achievements, and future challenges. *Current Problems in Pediatric and Adolescent Health Care*, October 2007 (Vol. 37, Issue 9, pages 338–362, DOI: 10.1016/j.cppeds.2007.07.003), with permission from Elsevier.

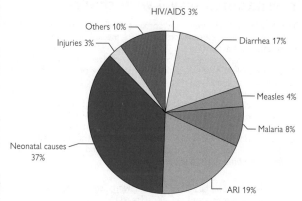

Figure 30.2 Major causes of mortality, children <5 years old. ARI, acute respiratory infections. From WHO *World Health Statistics, 2007*.

International travel with children

Over 2 million U.S. children travel abroad annually. Health risks for these children vary by age, risk behaviors, underlying medical conditions, location, and duration of travel.

Not all children seek medical advice before travel and fewer still have access to established "travel clinics." You should be prepared to screen these children for modifiable risks and offer appropriate preventive services and counseling.

The most common reported health problems among children traveling abroad are diarrheal illnesses, malaria, and motor vehicle- and water-related injuries. Children who are visiting family or relatives living in developing countries are at high risk for a variety of travel-related health problems, including malaria, intestinal parasites, and tuberculosis. Risk increases with time spent in endemic areas.

> For up-to-date travel health advice along with disease risk assessments for specific countries, visit the CDC's Travel Health page: http://wwwn.cdc.gov/travel/

Immunizations

Children should be up to date with routine immunizations before travel. In addition, some routine vaccines can be given on an accelerated schedule to provide optimal protection before travel.

- *DTaP* immunization may be started as soon as the infant is 6 weeks of age, with the second and third doses given 4 weeks after each preceding dose.
- Children12 months of age and older should receive two doses of *MMR* separated by at least 28 days. Children age 6–11 months can receive MMR before departure, but this should not be counted in the routine immunization schedule.
- *Hemophilus influenzae type b* is endemic worldwide and can cause meningitis, epiglottitis, and other fatal illnesses in susceptible children. If previously unvaccinated, infants younger than 15 months of age should receive at least two vaccine doses before travel. An interval as short as 4 weeks between these two doses is acceptable.
- *Meningococcal meningitis* is epidemic in Sub-Saharan Africa. Meningococcal conjugate vaccine is indicated for persons 11 years or older Children 2–10 years of age can receive meningococcal polysaccharide vaccine. Antibody response to the polysaccharide is seen in some children as young as 3 months. Immunization of infants traveling to high-risk areas should be considered.

- *Hepatitis A* vaccine is recommended for all children at 12–23 months. The first dose should be administered 4 weeks before travel to allow time for an adequate immune response to develop. Children less than 1 year of age who are traveling to high-risk areas should receive immune globulin (IG). This may also be given to children older than 1 year who will be traveling less than 4 weeks after receipt of the first dose of hepatitis A vaccine. The vaccine and IG can be administered at the same time. IG can interfere with the response to live injected vaccines. Administration of MMR should be delayed for 3 months after IG, and IG should not be administered for 2 weeks after MMR.
- *Yellow fever* is transmitted by mosquitoes in certain areas of Africa and South America. Proof of yellow fever vaccination is required for entry into some countries. Infants and children older than 9 months of age should be vaccinated if they travel to countries with endemic yellow fever. Infants are at high risk for developing encephalitis from yellow fever vaccine; it should never be given to infants younger than 6 months of age
- *Typhoid fever* is a febrile illness caused by the bacterium *Salmonella enterica Typhi*. Two typhoid vaccines are available: a Vi capsular polysaccharide vaccine (ViCPS) administered intramuscularly, and an oral, live, attenuated vaccine (Ty21a). The ViCPS vaccine can be administered to children who are at least 2 years of age. The Ty21a vaccine is a series of four capsules ingested every other day and can be administered to children 6 years of age and older. All the capsules should be taken at least 1 week before potential exposure.
- *Rabies* occurs throughout the world and is endemic in most countries. Decisions regarding vaccination should include planned activities, likely exposures, and availability of antirabies biologics at the destination. Rabies vaccine may be administered to infants and children and are given as a series of injections on days 0, 7, and 21 or 28.

Diarrhea and dehydration

Diarrhea is the most common travel-related problem affecting children. Infants and children with diarrhea can become dehydrated more quickly than adults.

For young infants, breast-feeding is the best way to reduce the risk of food-borne and waterborne illness. Travelers should use only purified water for drinking, preparing ice cubes, brushing teeth, and mixing infant formula and foods.

Parents should be counseled on the use of oral rehydration solution (ORS). Immediate medical attention is required for an infant or young child with diarrhea who has signs of moderate to severe bloody diarrhea, fever higher than 38.5°C (101.5°F), or persistent vomiting. ORS should be provided to the infant by bottle or spoon while medical attention is being obtained.

The greatest risk to the infant with diarrhea and vomiting is dehydration. Dehydration is best prevented and treated by use of ORS, in addition to the infant's usual food. ORS packets are available at stores or pharmacies in almost all developing countries.

ORS is prepared by adding one packet to the correct volume of boiled or treated water. An infant or child who vomits the ORS will usually keep it down if it is offered by spoon in frequent small sips. Oral syringes available for oral medications can be useful for the administration of ORS.

Children weighing less than 10 kg who have mild to moderate dehydration should be administered 60–120 mL ORS for each diarrheal stool or vomiting episode. Children who weigh 10 kg or more should receive 120–240 mL ORS for each diarrheal stool or vomiting episode.

Breast-fed infants should continue nursing on demand. Formula-fed infants should continue their usual formula during rehydration.

The use of antimotility agents in children younger than 2 years of age is not recommended. Ondansetron orally disintegrating tablets may be useful in reducing nausea and emesis. Probiotics, such as lactobaccillus GG, may reduce duration of diarrhea.

Few data are available regarding empiric administration of antibiotics for diarrhea in children. In some studies, azithromycin has been found to be as effective as fluoroquinolones in treating traveler's diarrhea in adults. Azithromycin may be considered for empiric treatment. The suspension does not require refrigeration; however, it should be used within 10 days of mixing.

Malaria

Malaria is one of the most serious travel-related illnesses in children. Pediatric patients are at increased risk for severe complications of malaria, including shock, seizures, coma, and death.

Protection from mosquito bites is an important strategy for malaria prevention. Measures include the following:
- Staying in well-screened areas between dusk and dawn
- Using insecticide-treated bed netting
- Covering most of the body with clothing
- Using insect repellant with DEET (concentrations up to 50% are acceptable for infants older than 2 months)

Chemoprophylaxis

All children traveling to malaria-risk areas should take an antimalarial drug. In the United States, antimalarial drugs are available only in tablet form and taste quite bitter.

Overdose of antimalarial drugs can be **fatal**. Medication should be stored in childproof containers out of the reach of children.

- Chloroquine is the drug of choice for children traveling to areas without chloroquine-resistant *P. falciparum*.
- Mefloquine is an option for use in infants and children of all ages and weights who are traveling to areas with chloroquine-resistant *P. falciparum*.
- Doxycycline may be used for children who are at least 8 years of age.
- Atovaquone/proguanil may be used for prophylaxis for infants and children weighing at least 5 kg. Atovaquone/proguanil is available in pediatric tablet form; dosage is based on weight (see Table 30.1).

Table 30.1 Dosages of atovaquone/proguanil by weight

Weight (kg)	Atovaquone /proguanil (mg)	Dosing
5–8	31.25/12.5	1/2 pediatric tablet
8–10	46.88/18.75	3/4 pediatric tablet
10–20	62.5/25	1 pediatric tablet
>20–30	125/50	2 pediatric tablets
>30–40	187.5/75	3 pediatric tablets
>40	250/100	1 adult tablet

Safety
Motor vehicle–related injuries
These injuries are the leading cause of death in children who travel.
- While traveling in automobiles and other vehicles, children should be restrained in age- and weight-appropriate car seats or booster seats.
- These seats should be carried from home, since well-maintained and approved seats may not be available abroad. In general, children are safest traveling in the rear seat; however, many developing countries have cars without rear seatbelts.
- Up to 80% of road traffic injuries in the developing world occur to pedestrians. Children must be supervised at all times in the road traffic environment.

Drowning
This is the second leading cause of death in young travelers; close supervision is essential.
- Personal floatation devices are not likely to be available abroad, so families should consider bringing these from home.

Interpersonal safety

This is a concern in any country. Common sense is indispensable. Infants and children should carry identification and contact information in case they are separated from their caregivers.

- Because of concerns about illegal transport of children across international borders, if only one parent is traveling with the child, he or she may need to carry relevant custody papers or a notarized permission letter from the other parent.

Air travel

- Serious injury or death can occur during air travel when children are unrestrained during turbulence or survivable crashes. Children under 40 pounds should be secured in the aircraft with an approved car safety seat.
- Air travel is safe for healthy newborns and infants; however, children with chronic heart or lung problems may be at risk for hypoxia during flight.
- Ear pain during air travel reflects eustachian tube dysfunction. Pressure equalization can be facilitated by swallowing or chewing; infants should nurse or suck on a bottle. Older children can try chewing gum. Antihistamines and decongestants have not been shown to have benefit.

Illness after international travel

Approximately 3% of people traveling internationally have fever for a short period. Children will require a full assessment of fever, as discussed in Chapter 19.

When a history of recent travel is known, the additional information needed in your assessment should include the following:
• Review of travel itinerary
• Exposure history
• Duration of fever
• Likely incubation period
• Immunization status
• Use or non-use of antimalarial chemoprophylaxis

Incubation period

Determining an approximate incubation period is particularly helpful when you are trying to rule out possible causes of fever. It is also useful to consider causes according to key features. For example, is the fever
• nonspecific?
• associated with hemorrhage?
• associated with central nervous system involvement?
• associated with respiratory symptoms?
• associated with exposure to blood?
• associated with eosinophila

Table 30.2 summarizes the likely causes by incubation period and key features, and can be used to guide your history.

Once the travel exposure and likely duration of symptoms have been identified, additional workup could include the following:
• Thick and thin blood films for malaria
• Full blood count and differential white cell count
• Liver function tests
• Urinalysis
• Culture of blood, stool, and urine
• Chest X-ray
• Specific serology based on the likely incubation period

Specific discussion about some of the infections in Table 30.2 is provided in Chapter 19.

Table 30.2 Likely causes of illness by incubation period

Incubation period <14 days	Region
Nonspecific fever	
• Malaria (*Plasmodium* species)	Tropics, subtropics, temperate
• Dengue (virus serotypes 1–4)	Tropics, subtropics
• Rickettsial spotted fever	Worldwide
• Scrub virus	Asia, Australia
• Leptospirosis	Tropics
• *Campylobacter, Salmonella, Shigella*	Developing countries
• Typhoid fever	Developing countries
• East African trypanosomiasis	Sub-Saharan East Africa
Fever with hemorrhage	
• Meningococcemia, leptospirosis, bacterial infection, malaria	
• Viral hemorrhagic fever	
Fever with CNS involvement	
• Meningococcal meningitis	
• Bacteria and viral meningitis and encephalitis	
• Malaria, typhoid, and typhus	
• Rabies	Africa, Asia, and Latin America
• Arbovirus encephalitis	Worldwide
• Eosinophilic meningitis	
• Poliomyelitis	
• East African trypanosomiasis	
Fever with respiratory findings	
• Influenza	Widespread, seasonal
• Legionellosis	Widespread
• Acute histoplasmosis	Americas
• Acute coccidioidomycosis	Americas
• Q fever	Worldwide
Incubation period 14–55 days	
• Malaria	
• Typhoid fever	
• Hepatitis A	Widespread
• Hepatitis E	Widespread
• Acute schistosomias	
• Amoebic liver abscess	
• Leptospirosis	
• Acute HIV	
• East African trypanosomiasis	
• Viral hemorrhagic fever	
• Q fever	

Table 30.2 (*Contd.*)

Incubation period >55 days
- Malaria
- Tuberculosis   Worldwide
- Hepatitis B and E   Worldwide
- Visceral leishmaniasis   Africa, Asia, South America,
- Lymphatic filariasis   Mediterranean basin
- Schistosomiasis   Tropics
- Amoebic liver abscess

Bioethics

Pediatric bioethics is the systematic analysis of the reasons and justifications for pediatricians' value-based clinical decisions. Legal analysis is related to but distinguished from ethics. Pediatricians must be aware of state and federal laws that relate to ethical practice, but should consult with legal counsel before making decisions based on their own legal analysis.

Ethical practices are also distinguished from our moral intuitions about what is right and wrong. These intuitions are important and provide guidance that must be balanced with ethical analysis.

The complex relationship between the parents, the child, and the pediatrician distinguishes ethical issues in pediatrics. This relationship is not static and changes according to parental decisions and attitudes and the maturity of the child. This chapter illustrates examples of issues that may arise in routine and complex pediatric care.

The principles and approaches described in this chapter can be applied to other issues not covered here, such as parental refusals for immunizations, parental requests for genetic testing of adult-onset diseases, parental reluctance to provide chronic care for serious physical or behavioral issues, and issues related to organ donation. A separate chapter focuses specifically on issues of child abuse and neglect (Chapter 28).

Most health systems and hospitals have ethics committees and ethics consultants to provide specific advice and recommendations.

The doctor–parent–child relationship

Most professionals do not have difficulty with the idea that competent adult patients should be involved in their treatment. In the case of children, parents are the proxy decision makers. In this regard:

- All doctors have a duty to act in the best interests of their patients.
- Parents have the right to make decisions about a procedure on behalf of their child.
- Parents do not have the right to insist on a doctor doing something that the doctor does not consider to be in the child's best interest. Given this responsibility, there will be times when a doctor may decide not to do what parents request.
- As long as the parent's approach does not directly harm the child, the most productive approach is to accommodate the family's views and focus on maintaining a trusting relationship with the family.

Involving children in decision making about their own care is important for both developmental and ethical reasons. It is only through the process of increasing involvement in decisions that children develop the skills and reasoning that we expect of them as adults. As a child develops those capacities, parents and physicians should respect the role of the child in decision making.

One of the challenges facing parents and doctors is when to override children's wishes and preferences for health-care decisions because of concerns that the decision will be harmful to the child. Parents override young children's decisions more frequently. As children become older, a greater threshold of harm is necessary to override children's wishes. This is not only because of the ethical importance of respecting their decision-making authority but also because their cooperation is necessary in continued care and treatment.

Informed consent, parental permission, and child assent

Informed consent is a central doctrine in bioethics that protects the rights of patients with decision-making capacity to have sufficient information for making voluntary health-care decisions. Not only should the appropriate information be disclosed, but also health-care providers have an obligation to ensure that a patient understands the information before making health-care decisions. A patient's decision for or against a particular test or treatment should also be voluntary (free from "controlling influences").

The concept of consent is relevant to older adolescents, who typically have the capacity to make many health-care decisions. When making decisions for young children, parents do not provide consent, but give permission. This distinction explains the justification for overriding parental permission in circumstances where the consent of an adult would be respected (e.g., refusing an amputation in a life-saving situation).

The term *assent* is used to describe the process of involving a child in their health-care decisions. The American Academy of Pediatrics recommends that assent include at least the following elements:

- *Helping the patient achieve a developmentally appropriate awareness* of the nature of his or her condition.
- *Telling the patient what he or she can expect* with tests and treatment.
- *Making a clinical assessment of the patient's understanding* of the situation and the factors influencing how he or she is responding (including whether there is inappropriate pressure to accept testing or therapy).
- *Soliciting an expression of the patient's willingness to accept* the proposed care. No one should solicit a patient's view without intending to weigh them seriously. In situations in which the patient will have to receive medical care despite his or her objection, the patient should be told that fact and should not be deceived.

The American Academy of Pediatrics suggests that clinicians seek the assent of the school-age patient as well as informed permission of the parent for procedures such as

- *Venipuncture* for diagnostic study in a 9-year-old
- *Orthopedic surgery device* for scoliosis in an 11-year-old

The pediatrician should present information in a manner suited to the child's developmental level. Other professionals, such as child psychiatrists and developmental specialists, can provide additional insights into a particular child's developmental level and comprehension of the information presented. The capacity to make decisions is not global but must be assessed according to the particular context:

- Nature and the purpose of the therapy
- Risk and consequences of therapy, and of not having therapy
- Benefits and the probability that therapy will be successful
- Feasible alternatives (see Chapter 21)

Defining whether an adolescent demonstrates this capacity or not may be difficult. Fundamentally, the adolescent must possess the qualities associated with self-determination and self-identity, as well as the appropriate cognitive abilities to rationalize and reason hypothetically. Understanding, intelligence, and experience are also important qualities that may influence capacity.

While clinicians can make an ethical assessment of whether an adolescent has the capacity to provide informed consent, state regulations and case law can provide legal guidance.

Many states have provisions for "mature minors" that permit adolescents to give consent for certain medical interventions (e.g., treatment for sexually transmitted diseases, contraception, and drug use). Most states also have categories of "emancipated minors," who can give consent because of particular circumstances, such as their martial status. In some states, these determinations can only be made after a judicial review.

It is important to seek guidance from the hospital counsel and ethics committee about rules that apply in a particular state.

Confidentiality, truth telling, and disclosure

Health providers have a responsibility to protect the privacy of a patient's health information in the clinical encounter. The obligation to protect the confidential nature of the physician–patient relationship stems from an obligation to respect the autonomy of a patient and from the importance of maintaining a trusting relationship with one's patients.

Confidentiality is especially important in treating adolescents, given the importance of encouraging them to seek treatment when needed. Confidentiality should be protected when adolescents seek advice or treatment for issues such as: contraception, abortion, sexually transmitted infection, substance misuse, mental health issues, or family problems. In this regard:

- The duty of confidentiality owed to adolescents is the same as that owed to any other person.
- Confidentiality is not absolute and may be breached when there is serious risk to the health, safety, or welfare of the adolescent or others.
- Disclosure should only take place after consulting with the adolescent.

Objections to disclosure of information should be respected, although in certain situations disclosure may be required by law for the purposes of protecting the adolescent or others from significant harm (as in the case of reporting abuse or suicidal ideation). Legal guidance should be sought when complex situations arise.

Breach of confidentiality may be acceptable in the following situations:

- History of current or past sexual abuse
- History of current or recent suicidal thoughts or self-harm behavior
- Homicidal intentions

The patient should always be informed that the information will be disclosed and the reason why. Attempts should be made to encourage the patient to agree to disclosure.

Even in circumstances where the pediatrician should honor the confidentiality of the adolescent, it may be appropriate to encourage and facilitate the adolescent to share the information with parents or other supportive adults. For example, when the pediatrician has reason to believe that the parents can provide emotional support for the adolescent, the reluctant adolescent may need the pediatrician's support to involve the parents.

Conversely, some parents may request that pediatricians not disclose information to young children because the parents worry about upsetting the child. Some parents may request nondisclosure of a serious diagnosis, such as cancer or HIV, or nondisclosure of a prognosis. Depending on the age of the child, it may be appropriate to honor a parent's request for nondisclosure.

However, it is important to recognize that parents sometimes underestimate a child's ability to process the information, or awareness of his or her condition. Given the importance of promoting a child's understanding and engagement, the pediatrician should encourage disclosure and offer to facilitate the disclosure.

In circumstances where parents are still reluctant, it is important to explain that the information will likely be learned eventually. The child may ask the pediatrician directly, and obligations and expectations to tell the truth will require honest answers.

Even if not asked, the child may learn the information inadvertently from other health-care providers who are not aware of the desire for secrecy. This is particularly problematic for the child who becomes aware of the diagnosis, and is also aware that the parent does not want to talk with the child, so the child deals with the information in silence.

Withholding or withdrawing life-sustaining treatment in children

There are medical situations in which either death is imminent or the quality of life for a child is such that it is appropriate to withdraw or withhold treatments that would be appropriate in other circumstances. Such treatments might range from ECMO, mechanical ventilation, and dialysis, to antibiotics, nutrition, and hydration.

Ethical framework

Substituted judgment

Respect of persons requires that adults be permitted to refuse medical treatments even if it will result in their death. Adults can provide "advance directives" indicating their preferences in the event that they lose the capacity to express their wishes.

Even if an adult has not explicitly expressed a preference, surrogate decision makers can make a "substituted judgment" based on what they believe the adult would have decided, given their familiarity with the person and his or her values.

Best interest

Because most children will not have expressed such preferences, parents may have to make such decisions on the basis of the child's interests. Such assessments are inherently subjective, but necessary. Parents are given the authority to make life-and-death decisions for their children because it is assumed that 1) they are in the best position to make assessments of the child's interests, and 2) the parent's own interests in self-determination generally extend to decisions about their children.

Respect for children's rights

Although assessments about quality of life are subjective, there may be occasional circumstances when parents request withholding or withdrawing treatments that pediatricians think are in the child's interest.

Two examples for which there is both an ethical and legal consensus for treatment despite parental objections are the use of blood transfusions in infants whose parents are Jehovah's Witnesses, and surgery to correct gastrointestinal atresia in infants with Down syndrome. In either of these circumstances, or others where pediatricians are concerned about parental decisions, it may appropriate to obtain an ethics consult.

Futility

Some parents may request interventions that pediatricians think are not appropriate. Such issues arise routinely in general pediatric practice, such as requests for antibiotics for viral infections, MRIs for ankle sprains, or Ritalin to study for the SATs. There may be a number of reasons for pediatricians to not accommodate such requests, such as lack of efficacy, harm to the child or others, and cost.

One reason to not provide life-sustaining interventions is "futility," although use of this term is debated. Persistent requests related to genuine futility, where the requested intervention will simply not work, are rare.

More typically, futility is invoked to indicate that the clinicians do not think that the child's quality of life would justify further treatment. In such cases, the true issue is not futility but rather might include a range of concerns such as harm and suffering to the child, distress of the caregivers, and resource allocation. By identifying the alternative concern, a solution may be more apparent. These concerns should be directly discussed with the family.

In some cases, the best recourse is to accommodate a parent's request, since they are the ones who will live with the experience of their child's life and death for the rest of their lives. Requests for interventions in seriously ill children are particularly complex, because the consequence of not providing the requested treatment may be perceived by the family as the proximate cause of death of their child.

Pediatricians also have the responsibility of caring for the family, particularly when their child is dying.

Withholding and withdrawing interventions

While some argue that it is acceptable to withhold life-sustaining treatment but not to withdraw the same treatment, ethically there is little difference. Both will result in death of the child. Psychologically, it may feel that withdrawing treatment is more directly causing the child to die.

However, there are pragmatic advantages of withdrawal over withholding.

First, withdrawal of treatment can offer more time to make a decision or to wait for the arrival of family members.

Second, it allows more information to be gathered prior to making further decisions.

Third, appreciating that decisions to treat are not "irreversible," withdrawal of treatment may enable the parents to be willing to begin therapies when the outcome is not yet clear.

Nutrition and hydration

When a family and pediatrician agree that a child's death is an appropriate outcome, withdrawal of a ventilator and withdrawal of feeding are ethically equivalent. While withdrawal of nutrition and hydration is common in adult medical practice, it poses a special problem for providers who may consider feeding the "essence" of pediatric care. Withdrawal of nutrition and hydration is a less familiar experience for pediatric health-care professionals, which can add to staff discomfort.

Death following withdrawal of a ventilator will typically occur in a range of minutes to hours, whereas death following withdrawal of fluids and hydration will typically occur in days to weeks.

Families may choose to be at home with palliative care and hospice support. When withdrawal of fluids and hydration is considered in an inpatient setting, it is important to engage the staff about the ethical and psychological issues, and ethics consultation is advisable.

One ethical advantage of withdrawal of nutrition and hydration over withdrawal of a ventilator is that parents may want to use nutrition for a period of time (weeks to years) before they are ready to make a decision that death is an appropriate outcome. Many children are only on the ventilator transiently, which may not be enough time for the parents to make a decision. Permitting the later withdrawal of nutrition and hydration may encourage more families to initially provide treatment in the face of uncertainty.

Children with profound developmental disabilities

Decisions about providing or withdrawing tracheostomies and feeding tubes in children with profound developmental disabilities are particularly complicated because of the broad range of views about the quality of life for children. Parents are typically given discretion regarding the use or non-use of technological assistive devices such as feeding tubes and tracheostomies.

However, because of the broad range of social views, it is common for a health-care professional to raise concerns that are contrary to the parents' decision. Pediatricians should give parents broad latitude in making decisions that are consistent with the family's values. These issues become even more difficult when the decisions for care involve intensive home-care resources, which may be scarce or beyond the family's financial means.

The ultimate resource scarcity relates to organs. While organ transplants are more commonly provided to children with moderate developmental disabilities, as the profoundness of the disabilities increases, the decision to offer organ transplant may be deemed unreasonable.

Approach to decision making

Making a decision about withholding or withdrawing life-sustaining treatment requires time. The whole team must be involved, and all must wait until enough information and evidence about the child's condition are available. The decision to withhold or withdraw life-sustaining therapy should always be associated with consideration of the child's overall palliative or terminal-care needs.

One approach is to ask the family how they envision the death of their child. Do they want their child to die at home on in the ICU? Do they envision their child having CPR in the last moments of life, or holding their child in their arms? Such questions can help the pediatrician make recommendations about hospice, palliative care, "do not attempt resuscitation (DNR) orders," etc.

Following are a few practical suggestions:

• *Don't ask if the parents want everything done.* Most parents would do anything for their child to continue living a good-quality life, so this question can be difficult to say no to. Instead, be specific about the medically appropriate options.

- *Don't ask, "What do you want us to do?"* Most parents have not faced such decisions before. While the intent of the question is to respect the parent's wishes, making a specific recommendation based on the child's condition and knowledge of the parents' values may be more appropriate. You can also let them know that they do not have to follow the recommendation if they are not comfortable.
- *Don't offer options that you are hoping they will refuse,* because you think the option is not ethically appropriate. This becomes problematic if they give the "wrong" answer and request that option. Instead, simply mention the option and explain why it is not being offered on medical and ethical grounds.
- *If you are concerned that a parent's decision is not ethically appropriate, share your concern directly with the family.* Explain that the decision is difficult for you, rather than saying that their decision is wrong.

Index